T0402080

W. Konrad Karcz

Oliver Thomusch (Eds.)

Principles of Metabolic Surgery

W. Konrad Karcz
Oliver Thomusch (Eds.)

Principles of Metabolic Surgery

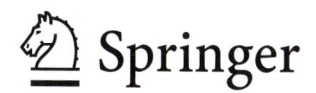
Springer

Dr. W. Konrad Karcz
Prof. Dr. Oliver Thomusch
Universitätsklinikum Freiburg
Abt. Allgemein- und Viszeralchirurgie
Hugstetter Str. 55
79106 Freiburg

ISBN 978-3-642-02410-8 Springer-Verlag Berlin Heidelberg New York

Bibliographic information Deutsche Bibliothek
The Deutsche Bibliothek lists this publication in Deutsche Nationalbibliographie;
detailed bibliographic data is available in the internet at <http://dnb.ddb.de>.

Springer Medizin
Springer-Verlag GmbH
Ein Unternehmen von Springer Science+Business Media

springer.de
© Springer- Verlag Berlin Heidelberg 2012
Printed in Germany

Editor: Diana Kraplow, Heidelberg
Project Manager: Ulrike Dächert, Heidelberg
Copyediting: Mary Schäfer, Buchen-Hettingen
Drawings: Alexandra Szypowska
Typesetting: TypoStudio Tobias Schaedla, Heidelberg
Cover Design and Layout: deblik Berlin
SPIN: 12700264

Printed on acid free paper: 5 4 3 2 1 0

Dedication

To medical professionals dealing with obesity-related metabolic disorders, at all levels, in the quest for knowledge

Preface

Metabolic surgery is an area of increasing specialization that aims at opening new perspectives in the treatment of morbid obesity and its associated diseases. The knowledge and expertise accruing in this interdisciplinary field are currently driving this specialization rapidly forward. However, because so many experts and disciplines are involved in promoting metabolic surgery, it is difficult to efficiently communicate novel ideas, models, and skills. Metabolic surgery is thriving in large centers, where the newest standards can be met and where patients may expect the highest competence.

The objective of this book is to provide a comprehensive insight into the latest developments in metabolic surgery, thus serving the purpose of all those who are invested in treating and managing patients suffering from morbid obesity. All medical doctors should possess the knowledge and clinical skills to provide sufficient treatment in this multidisciplinary field.

The editors succeeded in recruiting international experts, each of whom helps individually to shed light on the diversity of current treatment options. Each chapter provides the foundation for rational decision-making at a given stage of therapy. Additionally, the book elucidates proper perioperative management and adequate substitution strategies, as well as conservative therapeutic approaches.

Contents

II Preoperative Evaluation and Indications for Surgery

III Surgical Procedures

IV Accessory Medical Problems after Metabolic Surgery

V Secondary and Redo Operations

I Introduction

History of Obesity and Metabolic Surgery

Oliver Thomusch, MD

Obesity has become an epidemic worldwide condition, especially in the Western world. For example, the percentage of adults in the United States who are obese (defined as having a BMI of 30 kg/m^2 or more) increased from 15.3% in 1995 to 23.9% in 2005 [1]. Approximately 4.8% are considered to be extremely or morbidly obese (having a BMI of 40 kg/m^2 or more) [2]. An equivalent trend is observed in Europe. Nowadays, it is estimated that worldwide more than 300 million people are obese [3]. Due to the wide range of severe co-morbidities related to obesity and especially to morbid obesity, health-care systems are increasingly burdened in times of sparse resources. In 2000, obesity was estimated to contribute to approximately 400 000 deaths in the United States [4] and it may be assumed that the increasing rate of obesity will lead to a decline in overall life expectancy in the United States [5] in the 21st century and very likely all over the world.

The pathophysiology of obesity is complex and still poorly understood, but it includes a multifactorial genesis including genetic, behavioral, psychological, and other causes. Family studies strongly suggest that heredity may explain 67% of the population variance in BMI [6]. However, genetic factors are unlikely to account fully for the rapid increase in the prevalence of obesity. Declining rates of physical activity [7] coupled with a steady increase in the consumption of energy-dense foods may play a crucial rule [8].

To date, non-surgical treatments have not been very effective in treating obesity, regardless of the approach used, with rates of recurrence up to 90% [9, 10]. There are currently no effective pharmacological agents to treat obesity. Due to a lack of effective alternative treatments, surgery is currently accepted as the only treatment approach, with the greatest and longest-lasting success in achieving weight loss. Bariatric surgery has gained popularity in the past two decades as an alternative to weight-loss diets.

The history of bariatric surgery can be traced back to the 1950s; it is an extraordinary example of how new therapeutic ideas and new surgical techniques influence the development of a surgical field. As always, history and progress can be followed and demonstrated by the work of pioneers in the field. Many innovations and improvements have since been made to make the bariatric procedures safer and more effective. Weight-loss operations can be divided into restrictive procedures and malabsorptive procedures. Malabsorptive procedures reduce the absorption of calories, proteins, and other nutrients. In contrast, restrictive bariatric procedures decrease food intake and promote a feeling of fullness (satiety) following meals. Some operations are a combination of both.

1.1   Surgical Procedures

The first pioneers of bariatric surgery were J.H. Linner (❏ Fig. 1.1) and A.J. Kremen [11]. Linner and Kremen performed the first bariatric procedure in 1954. The idea was to decrease the amount of food processed in the intestine by reducing digestive and absorptive sections of the small intestine so that the body absorbs fewer calories. They bypassed most of the intestine while keeping the stomach intact. A similar procedure was developed by Henriksson, a Swedish physician [12], at about the same time. In his procedure the redundant portion of the small intestine was removed. Although the weight loss with jejunoileal bypass (JIB; ❏ Fig. 1.2) was good, too many patients developed complications such as diarrhea, night blindness (from vitamin-A deficiency), osteoporosis (from vitamin-D deficiency), protein-calorie malnutrition, and kidney stones. Later the jejunocolic shunt was introduced by Payne and DeWind [13] in 1963, which connected the upper small intestine to the colon. Patients also experienced uncontrollable diarrhea, and the procedure was converted to end-to-end anastomosis to allevi-

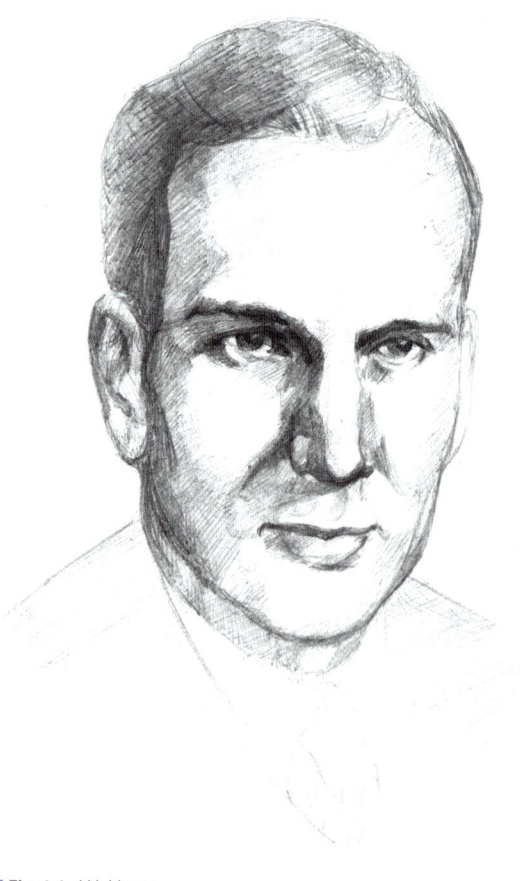

❏ **Fig. 1.1.** J.H. Linner

ate symptoms. In 1970, Scott et al. [14] tried to bypass smaller lengths of small intestine. With respect to the malabsorptive approach of the described procedures, the most worrisome complications of extensive small intestine bypasses were associated with the toxic overgrowth of bacteria in the bypassed intestine. These bacteria caused liver failure, severe arthritis, skin problems, and flu-like symptoms. Overall, after an initial excellent weight reduction, these bariatric procedures demonstrated severe complications in the long-term follow-up. Intestinal modification was therefore abandoned, and modifications in the upper gastrointestinal tract were introduced, based on the principle of restricting the amount of food [15].

Scopinaro et al. [16] (◘ Fig. 1.3) first performed the biliopancreatic diversion (BPD; ◘ Fig. 1.4) which was designed to be a safer malabsorptive alternative to JIB. The portion of the upper stomach that remains (nearly 70% of the stomach is removed) is far larger than the small pouch created for the Roux-en-Y gastric bypass (RYGBP). This allows patients to eat larger volumes before feeling satiety. After entering the upper stomach, food passes through an anastomosis into the small intestine (alimentary limb). This alimentary limb is connected to the so-called biliopancreatic channel 50–100 cm before the colon (common channel, where digestion and absorption of food is possible). This anatomy is very similar to the RYGBP, except that the length of the intestine from the stomach to the colon is much shorter, creating enhanced malabsorption. Long-term studies have demonstrated 72% of excess weight loss maintained over an 18-year observation period.

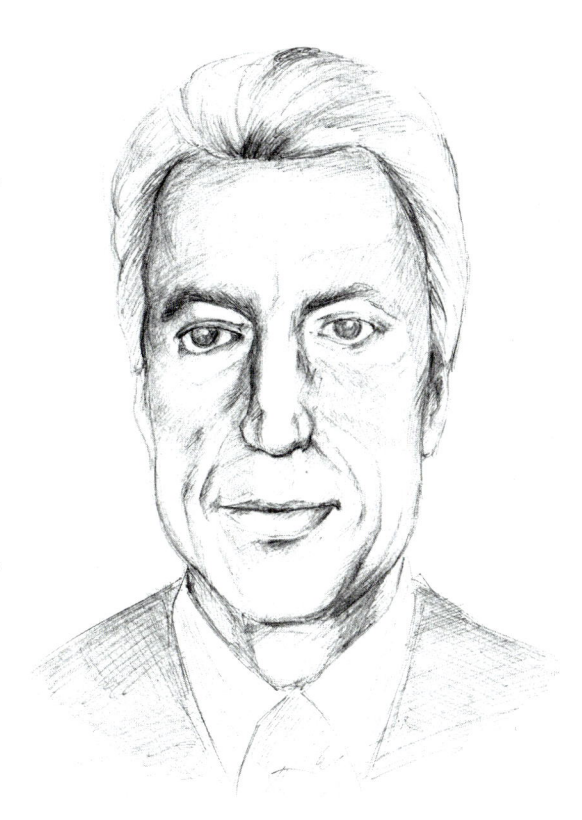

◘ **Fig. 1.3.** N. Scopinoro

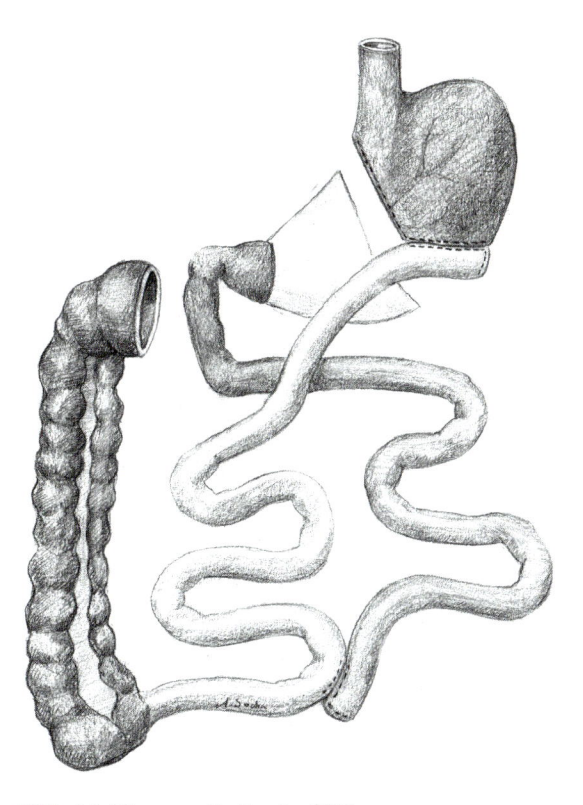

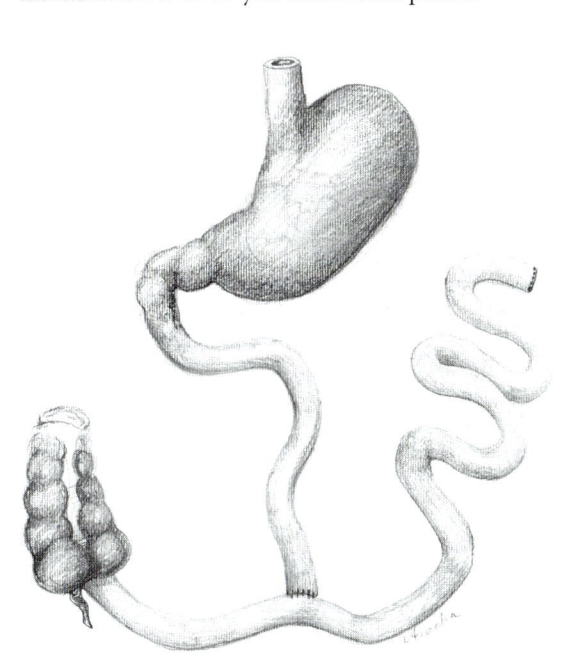

◘ **Fig. 1.2.** Jejunal-intestinal bypass (JIB)

◘ **Fig. 1.4.** Biliopancreatic diversion (BPD)

1

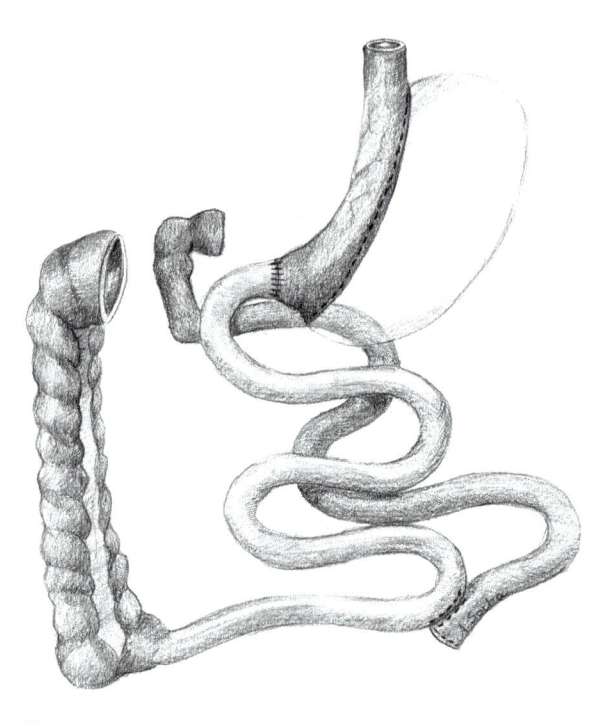

The duodenal switch (DS; ▪ Fig. 1.5) is a modification of the BPD and was first performed by Hess in 1988 [17] (▪ Fig. 1.6). The DS was designed by Hess to prevent gastric ulcers, to increase the amount of gastric restriction, and to minimize the incidence of dumping syndrome. The DS works through an element of gastric restriction as well as malabsorption. The stomach is shaped into a small tube, preserving the pylorus, transecting the duodenum, and connecting the intestine to the duodenum above the point where digestive juices enter the intestine. Anatomically, the main difference between the DS and the BPD is the shape of the stomach. Instead of cutting the stomach horizontally and removing the lower half, the DS cuts the stomach vertically and leaves a tube that empties into a very short (2–4 cm) segment of duodenum.

Both the BPD [18] and the DS [19] can be performed laparoscopically. Long-term follow-up and daily vitamin supplements are crucial to the success of both operations, with life-long monitoring to prevent nutritional and mineral deficiencies.

The modern era of gastric procedures for weight loss began with the observation that some patients who

▪ **Fig. 1.5.** Duodenal switch

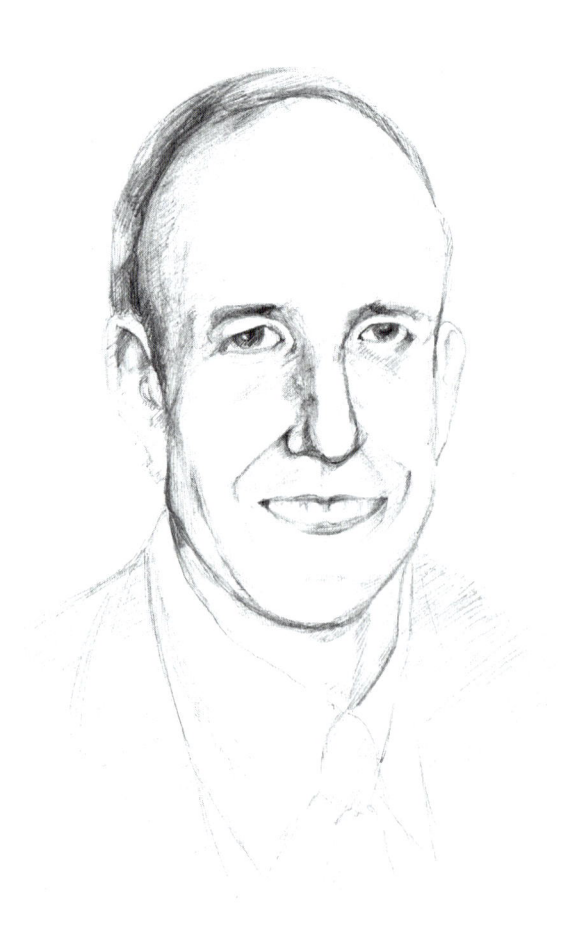

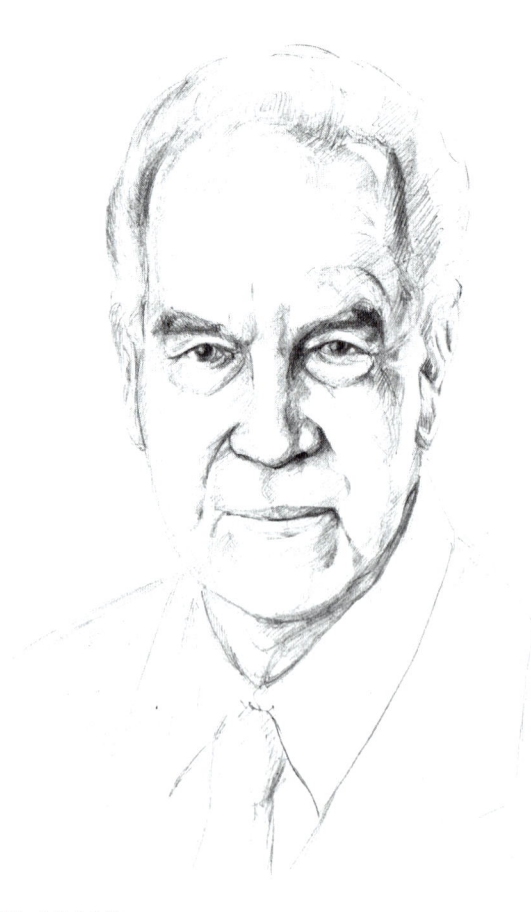

▪ **Fig. 1.6.** D. Hess

▪ **Fig. 1.7.** E.E. Mason

underwent stomach ulcer surgery lost weight afterwards. The horizontal gastroplasty was designed in the early 1970s by Edward E. Mason [20] (■ Fig. 1.7) to be a safer alternative to the RYGBP and the JIB. Gastroplasty was the first purely restrictive bariatric procedure. The original (horizontal) gastroplasty involved stapling the stomach into a small partition and leaving only a small opening for food to pass from the upper stomach pouch into the lower one. Unfortunately, due to dilation of the food pathway, this form of gastroplasty resulted in very poor long-term weight loss and, following several attempted modifications, was abandoned. In 1982, Mason [21] introduced the vertical banded gastroplasty (VBG; ■ Fig. 1.8), with a pouch based on the lesser curvature of the stomach and a polypropylene mesh or Silastic ring around the outlet of the pouch.

Though there were complications in the initial procedure, further refinements were made by reducing the pouch size to increase the restrictive component and thus improve postoperative overweight reduction. While this method proves effective initially, the band and the pouch tend to stretch after a few years, accompanied by renewed weight gain.

A later innovation in the field of bariatric surgery was the development of the gastric bypass (■ Fig. 1.9) and the Roux-en-Y-gastric bypass (■ Fig. 1.10), introduced by Mason and Ito [22], which combined the principles of gastric restriction and the dumping syndrome. Here, the surgeon creates a pouch by stapling the upper stomach and attaching it to the small intestine. The small pouch causes reduced intake and less digestion of food. This procedure proved to be technically difficult but led to long-term sustained weight loss, no protein-calorie malabsorption, and minimal vitamin or mineral deficiency. Initially, this operation was performed as a loop bypass with a much larger stomach. Because of bile reflux that occurred with the loop configuration, the operation is now performed as a Roux-en-Y with a limb of intestine connected to a very small (20 ml) stomach pouch. The remaining stomach and first segment of the small intestine are bypassed. In the standard RYGBP, the amount of intestine bypassed is not enough to create malabsorption of protein or other macronutrients. In bypassing the duodenum and the very first jejunum, the absorption of calcium and iron is decreased, so that lifelong follow-up with mineral supplementation is mandatory. Other clinically important deficiencies that may also occur include vitamin B_1 (thiamine) and vitamin B_{12}.

Although the open RYGBP can be performed with relatively low morbidity and mortality, morbidly obese patients are probably the best candidates for minimal invasive surgery. In 1994, Wittgrove (■ Fig. 1.11) and Clark

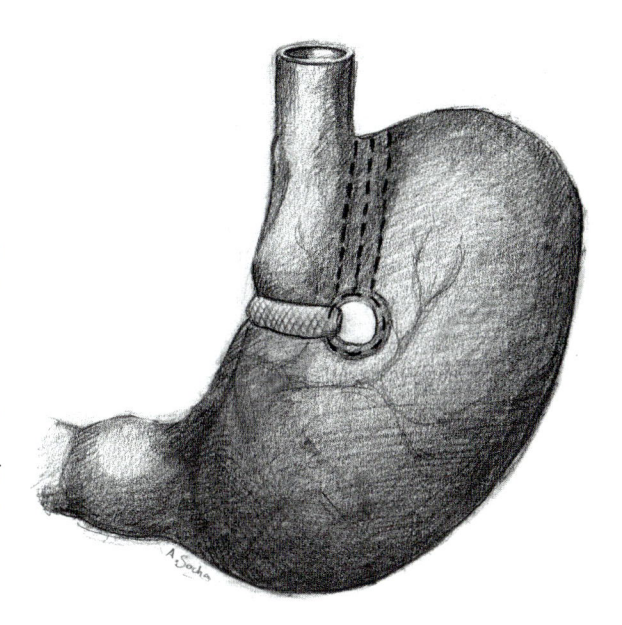

■ **Fig. 1.8.** Vertical banded gastroplasty

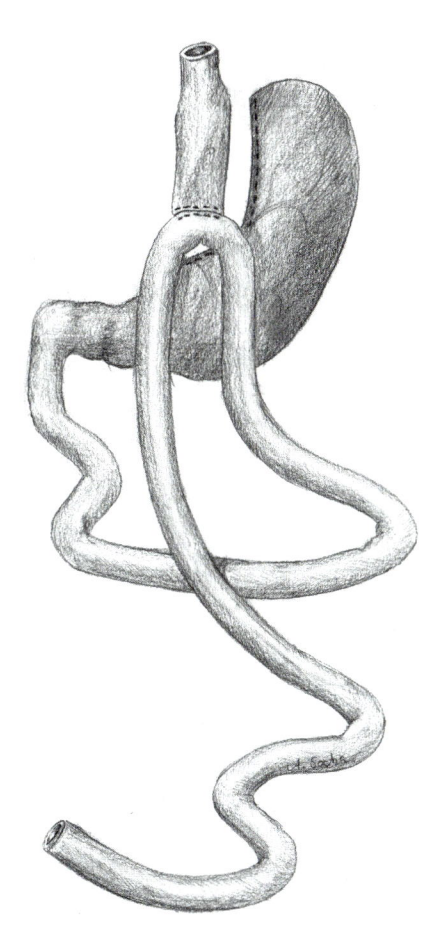

■ **Fig. 1.9.** Loop gastric bypass

1

[23] reported the first case series of laparoscopic RYGBP. Prospective randomized studies demonstrated that long-term weight loss following laparoscopic and open RYGBP did not differ, but that the laparoscopic technique was superior with respect to less intraoperative blood loss, shorter hospitalization, reduced postoperative pain, fewer pulmonary complications, faster recovery, better cosmesis, and fewer wound complications (incisional hernias and infections).

The RYGBP has been proven in numerous studies to result in long-term weight loss and improvement in overweight-related diseases. Half of the weight loss often occurs during the first postoperative year, with a weight-loss peak after 18–24 months postoperatively. Later, due to adaptation of the intestinal tract with dilatation of the small stomach pouch and the jejunum just behind the gastroenterostomy, a small weight gain will occur. To avoid this late postoperative relapse of weight gain, Fobi [24] (◘ Fig. 1.12) introduced the Silastic ring gastric bypass in 1998 (◘ Fig. 1.13).

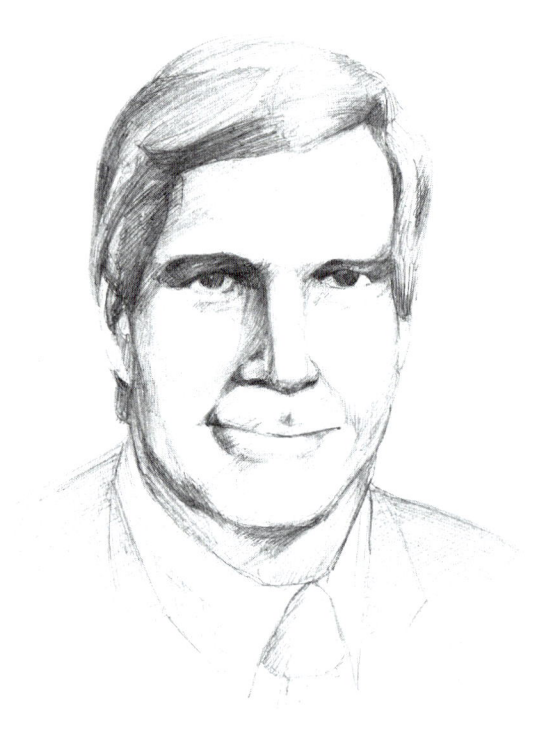

◘ **Fig. 1.11.** A.C. Wittgrove

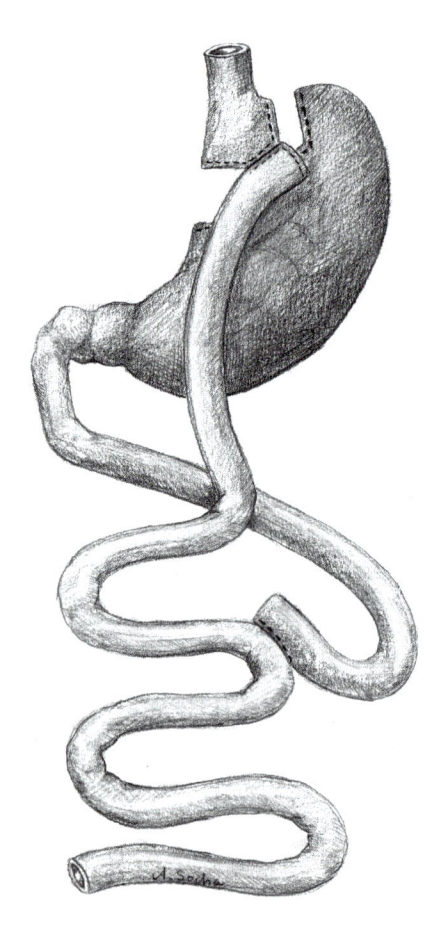

◘ **Fig. 1.10.** Roux-en-Y gastric bypass

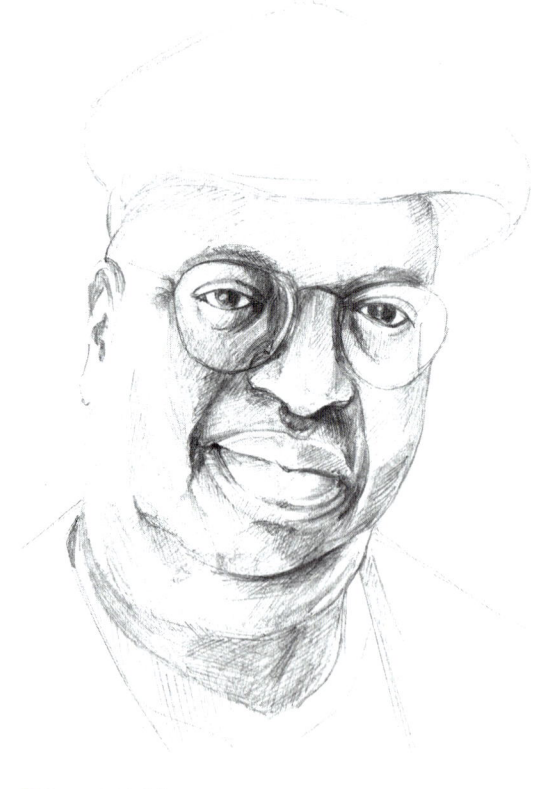

◘ **Fig. 1.12.** M. Fobi

A Silastic ring is placed around the vertically constructed gastric pouch above the anastomosis between the pouch and the intestinal Roux limb. This modification protects the gastric pouch and the upper jejunum against dilation and saves the restrictive component of the gastric bypass. This leads to an enhanced early postoperative and improved long-term weight loss in comparison to the conventional RYGBP. Although the RYGBP is nowadays the gold standard of bariatric surgery, some surgeons modify the RYGBP to incorporate an element of malabsorption to augment weight loss. This modification is called the "distal RYGBP", which may result in more severe nutritional complications than the "conventional (proximal) RYGBP". Whether long-term weight loss is superior or whether the malabsorptive complications are worth the possible improvements in weight loss are questions still under discussion.

Another example of a purely restrictive procedure is the nonadjustable gastric banding. It was first performed in 1976 by Wilkinson [25], who applied a 2-cm Marlex mesh around the upper part of the stomach, creating a stoma to restrict food intake and to achieve a feeling of satiety. Later, in 1980, Molina described the gastric segmentation procedure, in which a Dacron vascular graft was placed around the stomach. The gastric pouch was smaller than Wilkinson's procedure. Because of severe adherence, the Dacron graft was replaced by one made of PTFE (Gore-Tex®). In 1983, Kuzmak [26, 27] (◘ Fig. 1.14) began using a 1-cm silicone band to create a small 30- to 50-ml upper stomach pouch.

The adjustable gastric band (◘ Fig. 1.15) was also developed by Kuzmak, who designed a silicone band with an inflatable balloon in 1986. This small balloon is connected to a small port reservoir under the skin so that the diameter of the stoma is adjustable. The first laparoscopic procedure with the adjustable gastric band was performed by Belachew [28] in 1994.

Another non-invasive approach to creating a sense of earlier satiety is the endoscopic implantation of the intragastric balloon [29] (◘ Fig. 1.16). It was developed to offer a nonsurgical and reversible approach to obesity control. However, the intragastric balloon was removed from the

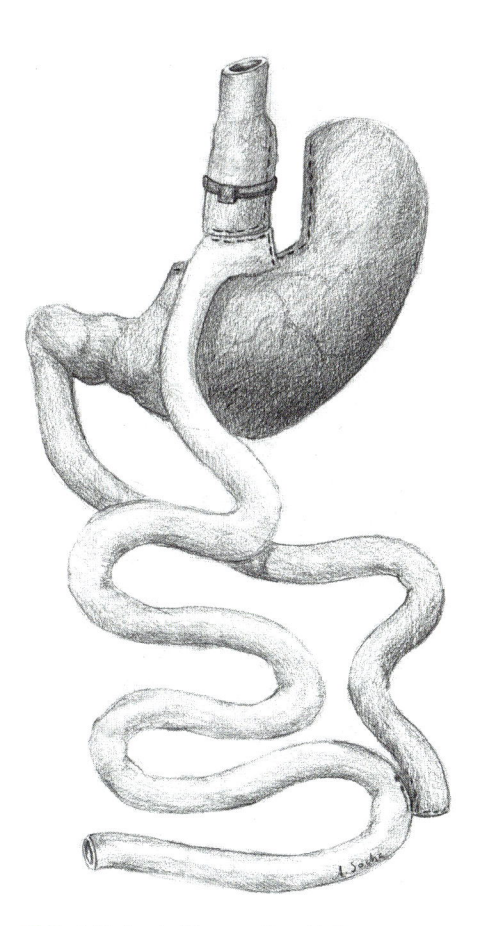

◘ **Fig. 1.13.** Banded Roux-en-Y gastric bypass

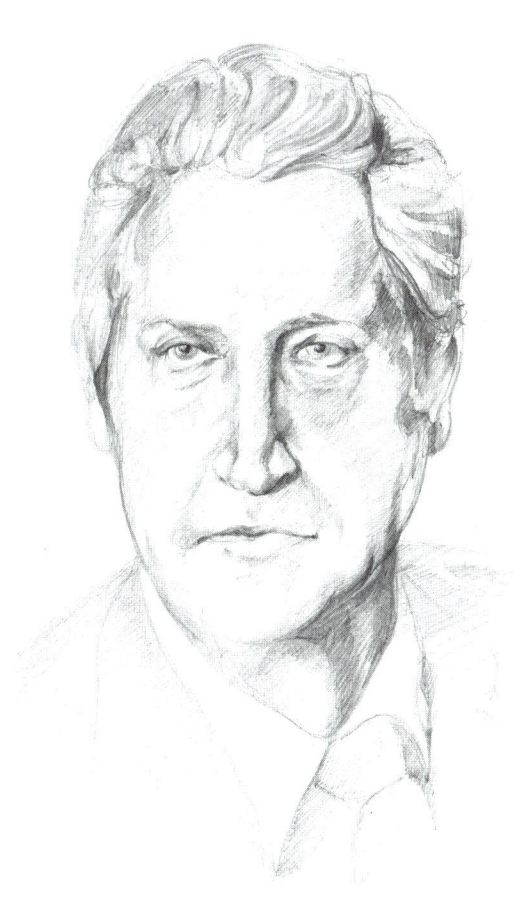

◘ **Fig. 1.14.** L. Kuzmak

1

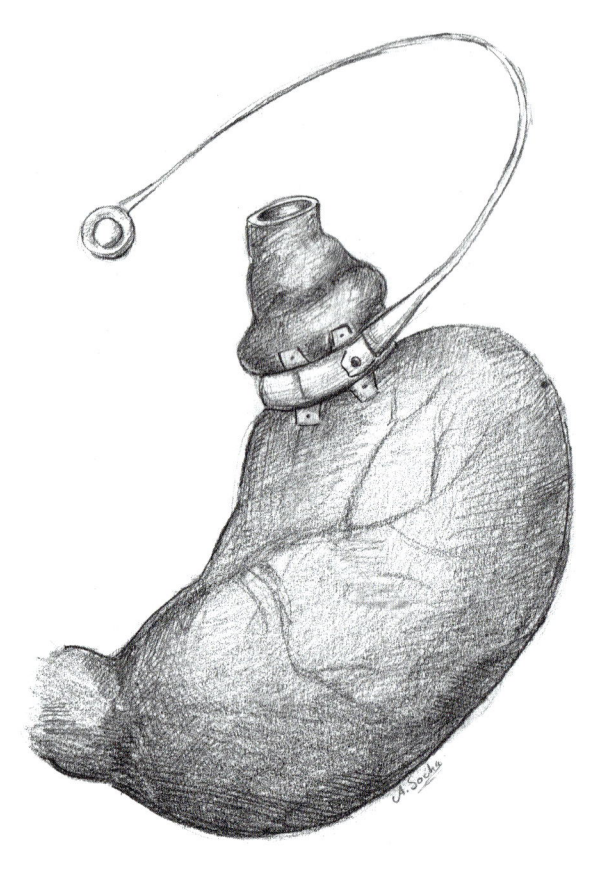

■ **Fig. 1.15.** Laparoscopic adjustable gastric banding (LAGB)

US market after several publicized deaths resulted from obstruction secondary to the passage of partially digested intragastric balloon. In Europe and elsewhere in the world, the intragastric balloon is still used temporarily, for periods of up to 6 months, as a "bridge" to bring severely obese patients down to a weight where they can undergo a permanent bariatric operation with less perioperative risk.

The vertical sleeve gastrectomy (■ Fig. 1.17) was first performed as a distinct operation in 2001 [30] with the intent to remove approximately 90% of the stomach, leaving a narrow tube or "sleeve" which greatly reduces the stomach volume and creates satiety. The procedure minimizes the complications of dumping by preserving the pylorus. The rule of vertical sleeve gastrectomy as a single and definitive bariatric procedure is unclear to date, because long-term results are still lacking. Usually, the restrictive component of the vertical sleeve gastrectomy is used as an initial multiple-step approach in super obese patients. After the initial weight loss that follows vertical sleeve gastrectomy, this procedure can be changed in a more effective malabsorptive operation such as the biliopancreatic diversion with duodenal switch [31, 32]. Similar to that for other forms of gastroplasty, the perioperative risk for sleeve gastrectomy appears to be relatively low, even in high-risk patients. Published complication rates range from 0 to 24%, with an overall reported mortality of 0.39%.

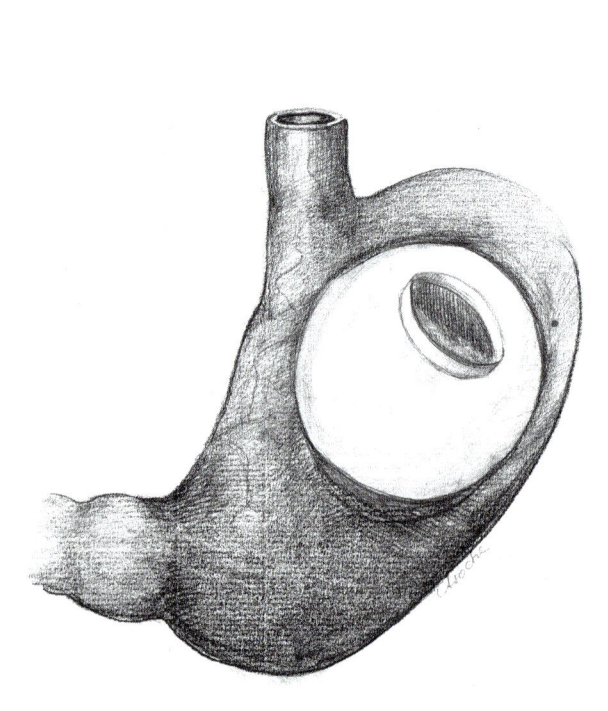

■ **Fig. 1.16.** Gastric balloon

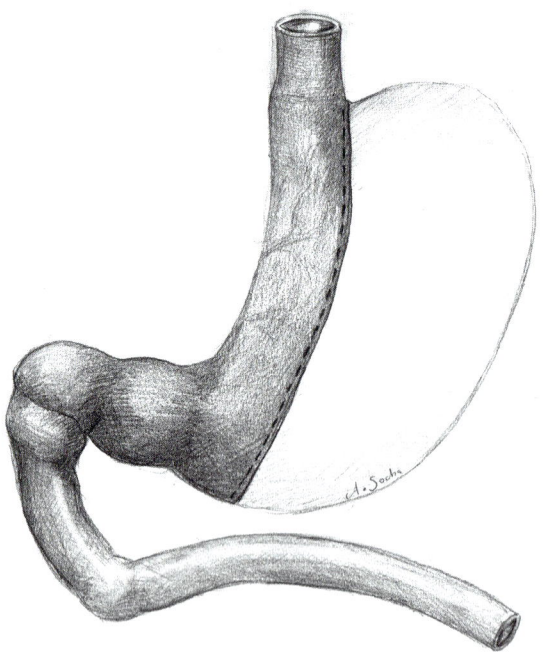

■ **Fig. 1.17.** Sleeve gastrectomy

1.2   Conclusion

The history of bariatric and metabolic surgery shows a changing popularity of specific bariatric surgical procedures over time, suggesting that the ideal procedure has not yet been definitely established. The future will show whether treatment strategies in bariatric surgery will be individualized for each patient with respect to the underlying eating behavior, the spectrum of co-morbidities, and the genetic background.

On the horizon for clinical application are devices for neuromodulation of the vagal nerve [33], which is involved in the control of digestion, intestinal motility, and the feeling of fullness. The intent of this approach is to slow the rate of stomach emptying in order to promote a sense of satiety. Preliminary results showed an inferior weight loss in comparison to established bariatric operations. Long-term results are still lacking and the costs and replacement of the battery unit for this device are probably a significant limitation [34]. Other less invasive endoluminal approaches are also being investigated, which utilize endoscopes to introduce devices through the mouth (natural orifice transgastric endoscopic surgery = NOTES) to achieve weight loss. Active areas of research involve approaches that include:

- Stapling from within the stomach to restrict the volume of the stomach
- Lining the intestinal tract with a sheath to prevent contact between food and digestive enzymes and thereby reduce absorption of food
- Ribbons, gels, or polymers which can fill the stomach to restrict volume
- Endoscopically implanted neuromodulation devices

Besides the technical and clinical progress in bariatric and metabolic surgery, several questions are still under discussion and awaiting a solution in the near future. To date the potential benefit of bariatric surgery for patients with mild obesity (BMI of 30–35 kg/m^2) remains unclear. Also uncertain are whether severely obese patients are appropriate candidates for bariatric surgery and what role bariatric procedures may have in patients outside the commonly defined age range (18–60 years) [35].

References

1.   (2006) State-specific prevalence of obesity among adults – United States, 2005. MMWR Morb Mortal Wkly Rep 55:985–988
2.   Ogden CL, Carroll MD, Curtin LR, McDowell MA, Tabak CJ, Flegal KM (2006) Prevalence of overweight and obesity in the United States, 1999–2004. JAMA 295:1549–1555
3.   Haslam DW, James WPT (2005) Obesity. Lancet 366:1197–1209
4.   Li Z, Bowerman S, Heber D (2005) Health ramifications of the obesity epidemic. Surg Clin North Am 85: 681–701
5.   Mokdad AH, Marks JS, Stroup DF, Gerberding JL (2004) Actual causes of death in the United States, 2000. JAMA 291:1238–1245
6.   Maes HHM, Neale MC, Eaves LJ (1997) Genetic and environmental factors in the relative body weight and human adiposity. Behav Genet 27:325–351
7.   Brownson RC, Boehmer TK, Luke DA (2005) Declining rates of physical activity in the United States: what are the contributors? Annu Rev Public Health 26:421–443
8.   Ledikwe JH, Blanck HM, Khan LK, et al (2006) Dietary energy density is associated with energy intake and weight status in US adults. Am J Clin Nutr 83:1362–1368
9.   National Institutes of Health (2000) The practical guide: identification, evaluation, and treatment of overweight and obesity in adults. NIH publication No. 00-4084
10.   Colquitt J, Clegg A, Loveman E, Royle P, Sidhu MK (2005) Surgery for morbid obesity. Cochrane Database Syst Rev 4: CD003641
11.   Kremen AJ, Linner JH, Nelson CH (1954) An experimental evaluation of the nutrional importance of proximal and distal small intestine. Ann Surg 140:439–448
12.   Henriksson V (1952) Is small bowel resection justified as treatment for obesity? Nordisk Med 47:744
13.   Payne JH, DeWind LT (1969) Surgical treatment of obesity. Am J Surg 118:141–147
14.   Scott HW, Law DH, Sandstead HH, Lanier VC, Younger RK (1970) Jejuno-ileal shunt in surgical treatment of morbid obesity. Ann Surg 171:770–782
15.   Griffen Jr WO, Bivins BA, et al (1983) The decline and fall of jejunoileal bypass. Surg Gynecol Obstet 157:301–308
16.   Scopinaro N, Gianetta E, Civalleri D, Bonalumi U, Bachi V (1979) Bilio-pancreatic bypass for obesity. II. Initial experience in man. Br J Surg 66: 619–620
17.   Hess DS, Hess DW (1998) Biliopancreatic diversion with a duodenal switch. Obes Surg 8:267–282
18.   Ren CJ, Patterson E, Gagner M (2000) Early results of laparoscopic biliopancreatic diversion with duodenal switch. A case series of 40 consecutive patients. Obes Surg 10:514–523
19.   De Csepel J, Burpee S, Jossart G, Andrei V, Murakami Y, Benavides S, Gagner M (2001) Laparoscopic biliopancreatic diversion with a duodenal switch for morbid obesity: a feasibility study in pigs. J Laparoendosc Adv Surg Tech A 11:79–83
20.   Printen KJ, Mason EE (1973) Gastric surgery for relief of morbid obesity. Arch Surg 106:428–431
21.   Mason EE (1982) Vertical banded gastroplasty for obesity. Arch Surg 117:701–706
22.   Mason E, Ito C (1967) Gastric bypass in obesity. Surg Clin North Am 47:1345–1351
23.   Wittgrove AC, Clark GW, Tremblay LJ (1994) Laparoscopic gastric bypass, Roux-en-Y: preliminary report of five cases. Obes Surg 4:353–357
24.   Fobi M, Lee H, Holness R, Cabinda D (1998) Gastric bypass operation for obesity. World J Surg 22:925–935
25.   Wilkinson LH, Peloso OA (1981) Gastric (reservoir) reduction for morbid obesity. Arch Surg 116:602–605
26.   Kuzmak LI (1991) A review of seven years' experience with silicone gastric banding. Obes Surg 1:403–408
27.   Kuzmak LI (1986) Silicone gastric banding: a simple and effective operation for morbid obesity. Contemp Surg 28:13–18
28.   Belachew M, Legrand M, Jaquet N (1993) Laparoscopic placement of adjustable silicone gastric banding in the treatment of

morbid obesity: an animal model experimental study. Obes Surg 3:140

29. Durrans D, Taylor TV, Holt S (1991) Intragastric device for weight loss. Effect on energy intake in dogs. Dig Dis Sci 36:893–896

30. Marceau P, Biron S, Bourque RA et al (1993) Biliopancreatic diversion with a new type of gastrectomy. Obes Surg 3:29–35

31. Lee CM, Cirangle PT, Jossart GH (2007) Vertical gastrectomy for morbid obesity in 216 patients: report of two-year results. Surg Endosc 21:1810–1816

32. Cottam D, Qureshi FG, Mattar SG, et al (2006) Laparoscopic sleeve gastrectomy as an initial weight-loss procedure for high-risk patients with morbid obesity. Surg Endosc 20:859–863

33. Laskiewicz J, Krolczyk G, Zurowski G, Sobocki J, Matyja A, Thor PJ (2003) Effects of vagal neuromodulation and vagotomy on control of food intake and body weight in rats. J Physiol Pharmacol 54:603–610

34. Bohdjalian A, et al (2006) One-year experience with TANTALUS. Obes Surg 16:627–634

35. DeMaria EJ (2007) Bariatric surgery for morbid obesity. N Eng J Med 356:2176–2183

Conservative Treatment of Overweight and Obesity

Hartmut Bertz MD, Andrea Engelhardt MD

2

Conservative therapy of overweight and obesity is difficult, time-consuming and dependent on many different factors:

- The patient, who has to agree to participate in a program of many months to reduce his weight and afterwards to keep that weight level
- The doctor; only a few colleagues are trained in the therapy of overweight and they all have to learn that weight reduction takes time and backlashes are common. During their medical education and career, doctors receive little or no education on this problem. Further, they do not have enough time to concentrate on physical and psychosocial problems of the obese patient.
- In many countries insurance companies do not appropriately reimburse the high costs of treating morbidly obese patients. To achieve a long-lasting positive result, a team is necessary to monitor the weight reduction program for these patients, consisting of:
    - A physician trained in nutritional therapy
    - A dietician
    - A psychologically trained person (doctor or psychologist)
    - A physiotherapist

2.1   When to Start

Depending on the age of the patient, the body mass index (BMI) should be between 22 and 28 kg/m². According to World Cancer Research Fund Report guidelines [1], the individual weight should be within these borders; an indication for intensive, combined weight-reduction therapy is given if (a) BMI is >30 kg/m² or (b) BMI is 25–30 kg/m² and other internal diseases (e.g. hypertension, diabetes mellitus) or psychosocial problems are present. The modern Cardiodiabetology focused the attention also on the WHR (Waist to Hip Ratio) waist 94 cm (m) / 88 cm (f) as a risk factor. There are individuals with overweight and without further signs of morbidity, who will benefit from keeping weight stable [2]. In most cases patients are interested in reducing their weight by the time they have physical (cannot walk, sweating), psychological (appearance), and social (mobbing, exclusion) problems. There is no indication for intensive weight reduction during adolescence, pregnancy, for patients with hyperuricemia, heart failure, older than 60y with low muscle mass or risk for osteoporosis, (eating disorder) or preexisting consuming disease.

2.2   Nutrition

For weight reduction the energy intake must be less than the energy expenditure [3]. This requires a reduction of the daily calorie intake. The diet can consist of fewer than 800 kcal/day (very low calorie diet) or between 800 and 1500 kcal/day (low calorie diet), or it can be 500–800 kcal fewer than the typical daily calorie intake (moderate diet; depending on the daily intake). The first, a very low calorie diet, cannot be recommended in general and should be followed only if a very quick weight loss is necessary and good medical monitoring is available. Otherwise vitamin and protein deficiencies may occur. The last, a moderate diet, is recommended to achieve a weight reduction of 5–10% of body weight or 0.5–1 kg/ week [4]. Many additional efforts may help to achieve the desired goal, such as change in eating-rhythm during the day, meal replacement therapy, or adding fiber [5]. On the other hand, it is possible to decrease energy intake by designing a healthy meal plan without compromising palatability [6].

Low-Carb Diet. A low-carbohydrate diet consists of fewer than 60 g carbohydrates daily. The Atkins diet starts with less than 20 g and subsequently increases the amount slowly. When low-fat diets were compared with low-carb diets the latter effected a significantly higher weight loss in the first 6 months [7, 8]. Additionally, low-carb diets lead to lower glucose and triglyceride levels and to higher HDL cholesterol but also higher LDL cholesterol levels.

Low-Fat Diet. Low-fat diets are a subject of controversy [9]. In a standard diet, fat is restricted to less than 30% of calories. A low-fat diet consists of 15% fat, 15% protein, and 70% carbohydrates. Some studies demonstrated a weight loss of more than 10 kg/year with a diet of less than 10% fat [8].

Low-Glycemic-Index Diet. A low-glycemic-index diet consists of foods which do not considerably increase the blood glucose level at 2 h after consumption. Compared with standard diets, no improvement in weight loss was observed with these diets in randomized trials [10]. However, diets with a low gylcemic index lead to a reduction of overweight-associated risk factors [11].

Very-Low-Calorie Diet. The daily calorie intake is between 800 and 1200 kcal/day, or between 200 and 400 kcal/day with meal replacement/formula diets. Fat should amount to less than 30% and proteins should be calculated at 25–50% to achieve satiation. It is possible to lose

10–30 kg in 3 months. Meal replacement with formula diets is feasible [12] but should not be performed for longer than 12 weeks, because metabolic changes such as ketonemia may occur.

High-Protein Diet. In high-protein diets carbohydrates are replaced by protein and fat. They may lead to higher satiety, thermogenesis, and decreased energy efficiency. In a meta-regression more weight loss was observed with calorie-restricted diets where carbohydrates were reduced to 35–41% energy intake and differences in body composition were seen, especially when protein was > 1.05g/kg and studies were conducted for >12 weeks. [13]. However, when a high-carb diet (64% of energy) was compared recently with a high-protein diet (34% of energy), small diffenrence in weight loss, but no differences in reducing cardiovascular risk factors between the two were demonstrated [14].

Fasting Zero Diet. Total fasting is drinking only energyfree liquids to maintain a urine production of 2000 ml/ day. It has the highest success regarding weight reduction (250–400 g body wt/day), but it is associated with many side effects; therefore, if at all, total fasting should be done for only a short time and with intensive medical surveillance. Micronutrients and electrolytes will be reduced, acidosis may occur, and catabolism will change body composition. The patient becomes weak, complains of dizziness and epigastric pain, and loses muscle protein. No nutritional society recommends total fasting.

Commercial Diets. Many commercial diets or diet plans are available for people who want to lose weight. They are generally named after the person who introduced the diet and consist of the three nutritional components (carbohydrates, fat, and protein) in differing composition. Further programs substituting normal food with industrially produced nutrition drinks are available, which result in more satiety compared with natural food (meal replacement, formula diet). They consist mainly of soya or milk powder and contain the recommended doses of fat, carbohydrates, and vitamins. They do not always include the necessary daily amount of micronutrients. Minimal energy consumption is 700 kcal/ day with an expected weight loss of 1.5–3.0 kg/ week. Important with every diet is the adherence to a minimum daily ingestion of 2.5–3 l liquid. Meal replacement therapy should not be utilized for longer than 3 months. In Europe and the USA, randomized trials were performed comparing commercial diet plans: Ornish (fat restriction), Atkins (carbohydrate restriction) Zone (40% carb, 30% fat and 30% protein), Weight Watchers (calorie restriction), or Slim-Fast plan (meal replacement) [15–17]. All approaches led to the desired reduction of weight and fat mass. One trial compared all four diets and showed no difference in weight loss after 1 year. Another trial compared the Atkins and the Zone diet; the Atkins diet resulted in more weight loss. Overall, all diets reduced blood pressure, blood glucose, insulin, and total cholesterol. In general, no one commercial diet or diet plan has an extraordinary advantage over another. The often higher costs of a commercial diet should be taken into account when one participates in such a plan or program. Often, the ingredients of a diet are cheaper elsewhere and must not be purchased at great expense; a brand name tends to elevate the price. The problem of all diets to reduce weight is the high long term relapse; after five years 80-90% of the individuals regains their initial weight or even go higher [18].

2.3 Guidelines of the German Obesity Society

The German Obesity Society recommends every diet that leads to an energy deficiency, starting at the lowest level [19].

Level 1:
- calorie reduction 500kcal /day, by fat reduction
- with a maximum of 60 g fat/day
- goal: weight reduction of 4 kg in 1 year

Level 2:
- balanced calorie reduced diet, recommended as standard
- energy deficiency of 500–800 kcal/day
- goal: weight reduction of 5 kg in 1 year

Level 3
- formula diet
- energy: 500–1000 kcal/day
- goal: reduction of 0.5–1.5 kg/week in 3 months

2.4 Sports and Physiotherapy

Increasing physical activity is part of the lifestyle program for weight reduction in the recommendations of the WCRF [1] and of national organizations such as the German Obesity Society (DGA) or the Canadian guidelines [19, 20], but only in combination with calorie restriction can physical activity lead to more than modest weight reduction [21]. However, it is possible by increasing physical activity to reduce adipose abdominal tissue and improve insulin resistance [22]. Furthermore, the combination of physical activity and dietetic restriction reduces not only weight but also triglyceride levels and blood pressure [23] and increases HDL cholesterol levels [24].

Mechanism. Regular physical activity has a positive influence on the energy balance. It increases energy expenditure, muscle mass and resting energy expenditure. After additional pharmacotherapy is discontinued, continued physical activity can maintain the weight reduction [25]. It is not an approved method for reducing weight very fast, however [26].

Consequences for the Vascular System. Besides the weight loss, physical activity also has substantial positive consequences for the vascular system:
- Reduction of fat mass
- Increased reduction of visceral (abdominal) fat
- Improved performance
- Reduction of blood pressure
- Reduction of heart rate
- Improvement of dyslipidemia
- Reduction of hyperinsulinemia
- Improvement of insulin action
- Improvement of strength and coordination
- Improved self-confidence
- Less depression

Predictors. The patient should start physical activity under the observation of a physiotherapist or a sports scientist trained in contact with overweight/obese patients. Physical activity can continue or include the sports activities the patient has performed earlier, because physical activity should be pleasurable for the patient and not torture. In the beginning, a simple program should be conducted according to the patient's level of fitness and co-morbidities, and later the intensity can be increased slowly. The program should be integrated into the patient's weekly routine, and training with friends or in a group shows the best results and higher adherence over a long time compared with training by oneself. Protocols and results should be monitored at regular intervals to motivate the patient and to set objectives, but overall, flexible management is better than rigid. Due to their overweight/obesity, most of the patients have problems with their joints, especially their knees. Physical activity should therefore concentrate on training that spares the knees, and it should be something that works out many muscle groups of the body dynamically, such as:

- Ergometer Training, Gerätetraining like rowing
- Gymnastics
- Cycling
- Swimming or aqua fitness
- Dancing, Walking, Walking on an incline, Nordic walking, Running: for well trained, or lower weight subjects.

At the beginning of physical activity, many obese patients cannot participate in outdoor exercises; they have to start very slowly with chair gymnastics or a cycle ergometer for 4–12 weeks, learning again to experience their body and training their sense of balance. This slow start is necessary to avoid injuring muscles, joints of the lower extremities, ligaments, or tendons. If possible, training in a group should be preferred. Endurance training has a lot of impact on obesity [27], plasma leptin levels, insulin resistance, and lipoprotein-subfractions [28]. Alone or in addition to an exercise program, physical activity during daily life can be intensified by doing house and garden work, using the stairs and not the elevator and by walking instead of going by car [29].

Intensity of Physical Activity. The intensity of the physical activity should be adapted individually. To increase the energy expenditure it is better to perform an extensive, long-lasting exercise without exhaustion of the patient than a short, intensive, exhausting program [22]. By adhering to this, an up to fivefold increase in energy consumption is possible. In untrained patients (mainly all overweight persons) the intensity should not exceed 45% of their maximal effort or 60% of the maximum heart rate increase. The training should be performed three times a week for a minimum of 30 min and can be increased to 60 min to achieve a better therapeutic effect [1, 30]. Overall, physical activity is an essential part of the lifestylechange program for overweight persons.

2.5 Psychotherapy

The third pillar of conservative therapy is behavioral therapy to change the patient's lifestyle [31, 32].

Psychosocial Predictors of Weight Control. Many studies have looked for psychosocial pre-treatment predictors of short- and long-term weight loss in overweight and obese patients. The following have been recognized as positive predictors [33]
- Few previous attempts at weight loss
- An autonomous, self-motivated cognitive style
- Higher initial body mass index (BMI)

Behavioral Therapy. The goals of life style modification are
- To reduce food intake and change eating habits
- To increase physical activity
- To cope with overweight-associated psychosocial stress

The intervention should include long-term therapy, fixed in a contract between the therapist and the patient. The basics of the therapy include self-control, self-assessment, and self-monitoring. The patient should write a protocol and the therapy should be performed in an individual or small-group setting [34]. At the beginning a weekly session of about 60–90 min is necessary; after half a year it results in weight loss of up to 10% [35] and the frequency can be extended. If necessary, individual therapy or therapy in a smaller group, or personal discussions can be interposed.

Self-control. Overweight patients have unrealistic goals for reducing their weight. Because they cannot reach them, they will be frustrated and will stop the intervention early. Therefore, the patient first has to accept his disease, and then he can start the intervention. The intervention includes [36]:
- Weekly or daily weight protocol
- A nutrition protocol under guidance of a dietician
- A daily eating protocol with notes about the patient's well-being
- A protocol about physical activity, including kind, expenditure and intensity

During the intervention period the patient needs intensive social support from the family, other relatives, colleagues, and friends. The behavioral therapy includes such different approaches as:
- Overcoming stress
- Controlling impulses
- Continuous motivation with realistic goals of weight reduction
- Flexible control of eating [37]
- Self-management
- Achieving social competence
- Techniques for reinforcement by the group, friends, or the therapist
- Avoiding relapse (weight regain) [38]: learning to cope with situations where the patient will be misled to eat

Predictors of Success. Predictors of success are a good initial weight reduction in the first 1, 3, or 6 months; this leads to good self-esteem and persisting motivation. The main problem is to avoid the yo-yo effect. Patients starting with a high BMI who follow the usual reduction diet will lose more weight and be more motivated than patients with a lower basic BMI. Adherence to group meetings is a positive predictor for successful long-term weight reduction, as is completing the above-mentioned protocols for nutrition, physical activity, and eating habits.

2.6 Psychoactive Drugs

In addition to behavioral therapy, pharmacotherapy can be added for support. This includes the drugs mentioned in the chapter on antidepressive medications, first among them the newer serotonin-specific reuptake inhibitors (SSRIs).

2.7 Psychodynamic Therapy

Many overweight patients have had psychological problems leading to nutrition malpractice during their youth or adolescence. Some women in particular may use their obesity to avoid contact with men (to be unattractive), and some have been sexually abused. Therefore, in addition to behavioral therapy, some patients need psychoanalytical / or in-depth psychological therapy.

It is important to address the high psychological exposure patients with obesity are confronted, as mobbing, loss of work, as well as social isolation.

2.8 Pharmacological Therapy

Pharmacological therapy to support weight reduction until now is disapointing; during the last years several substances were used, but they all showed toxic side effects and little benefit and were taken from the market. Orlistat is the only medicament still available, but only recommended for limited time. In addition some antidiabetic medicaments may help to control weight, whereas insulin may induce weight gain.

Orlistat
Mechanism of Action. By covalent binding, Orlistat selectively inhibits all lipases of the gastrointestinal tract (stomach and pancreas) which are responsible for fat absorption. It is a synthetic derivative of lipstatin (Tetrahydrolipstatin). Inhibition of the hydrolysis of triglycerides reduced the resorption of monoglycerides and free fatty acids in up to 39% of subjects [39].

Side Effects. Gastrointestinal side effects are chiefly seen, such as:

- Fatty and soft stool
- Oily spotting
- Flatus with discharge
- Increased defecation
- Stool incontinence
- Bowel pain

Due to the mechanism of Orlistat, a reduced absorption of lipid-soluble vitamins (A, D, E, and K) may be possible but was not observed in long-term follow-up. Furthermore, no electrolyte imbalances were seen.

Efficacy and Studies. Weight reduction is dose dependent. A daily dose of 3 x 120 mg with the main meals in combination with a fat-reduced diet led to a reduction of up to 10.3 kg body wt in 1 year [40, 41]. Further, reduction of blood triglycerides (up to 7.5%) and increase of HDL-cholesterol (plus 13%) were seen as well [41]. In a study with type-2 diabetes patients [42], plasma insulin levels were significantly reduced and insulin sensitivity increased, leading to weight loss and reduction of visceral fat mass. The licensed and recommended duration of medication is 2 years.

Exenatide

Glucagon-like-peptide-1 (GLP-1) stimulates insulin secretion, stops glucagon production, and slows stomach emptying [43]. Extenatide is a homologue to GLP-1 with an extended half-life. It is licensed for diabetes type 2 in Germany and reduces blood glucose and stomach emptying [44]. Besides controlling blood glucose, Exenatide has been shown to cause weight reduction of more than 2 kg in a few weeks [45]. Nausea and vomiting are rare side effects and are due to the slow stomach emptying. Further, it is necessary to inject the drug subcutaneously.

Biguanide /Metformin

Besides controlling diabetes type 2, metformin led to weight loss of 2.1 kg in 2 years compared with only 0.1 kg in the placebo group in a diabetes intervention program [46].

Drugs not Recommended or not Licensed

Drugs such as amphetamines, diuretics, and several antidepressives or anticonvulsives [47] cannot be recommended for weight reduction, mainly because of their side effects. Rimonabant, an endocanabinoid, is blocking the canabinoid-receptor CB1. It was licensed from 2006-2008 for weight reduction in Europe, never in the US due to the rise of psychiatric diseases as depression and suicides. Since October 2008 the licensure in Europe is suspended. For Sibutramin license is suspended in europe since january 2010 because of low weight reduction and even increase in cardiovascular risc factors.

Others

Owing to the increasing incidence of overweight and obesity, many substances are under investigation (leptin, olestra, medium-chain triglycerides, sumatriptan, PYY3-36). Others have been used and their use has been discontinued because of their side effects, e.g., thyroxine, diuretics, teas, beta2- and 3- agonists, cellulose, ephedrine and caffeine [48].

2.9   Conclusion

Weight reduction in overweight or obese patients is possible if the patients adhere to a conservative program that aims to achieve long-term change in eating behaviour and physical activity. Malnutrition of micronutrients and vitamins may occur after diets and fasting. Patients should be alerted to watch for malnutrion associated changes and then recommended to supplement micronutrients (e.g.vitamin D). Because of limited longterm success further efforts have to be done, to better understanding of the complex metabolic mechanisms of obesity and how to find pathways of prophylaxis, to reduce morbidity associated to obesitiy.

References

1. World Cancer Research Fund / American Institute for Cancer Research (2007) Food nutrition, physical activity and the prevention of cancer: a global perspective. AICR, Washington, DC
2. Sorensen Th.I.A. et.al. Intention to lose weight weight changes and 18-y mortalitiy in overweight individuals without comorbidities 2005, journal.pmed.0020171
3. Ledikwe JH, Rolls BJ, Smiciklas-Wright H, et al (2007) Reductions in dietary energy density are associated with weight loss in overweight and obese participants in the PREMIER trial. Am J Clin Nutr 85:1212–1221
4. McDonald SD (2007) Management and prevention of obesity in adults and children. CMAJ 176:1109–1110
5. Eckel RH (2008) Clinical practice. Nonsurgical management of obesity in adults. N Engl J Med 358:1941–1950
6. Poortvliet PC, Bérubé-Parent S, Drapeau V, Lamarche B, Blundell JE, Tremblay A (2007) Effects of a healthy meal course on

spontaneous energy intake, satiety and palatability. Br J Nutr 97:584–590

7. Foster GD, Wyatt HR, Hill JO, McGuckin BG, et al (2003) A randomized trial of a low-carbohydrate diet for obesity. N Engl J Med 348:2082–2090

8. Stern L, Iqbal N, Seshadri P, et al (2004) The effects of low-carbohydrate versus conventional weight loss diets in severely obese adults: one-year follow-up of a randomized trial. Ann Intern Med 140:778–785

9. Willett WC (2002) Dietary fat plays a major role in obesity: no. Obes Rev 3:59–68

10. Sloth B, Krog-Mikkelsen I, Flint A, et al (2004) No difference in body weight decrease between a low-glycemic-index and a high-glycemic-index diet but reduced LDL cholesterol after 10-wk ad libitum intake of the low-glycemic-index diet. Am J Clin Nutr 80:337–347

11. Halton TL, Willett WC, Liu S, et al (2006) Low-carbohydrate-diet score and the risk of coronary heart disease in women. N Engl J Med 355:1991–2002

12. Heymsfield SB, van Mierlo CA, van der Knaap HC, Heo M, Frier HI (2003) Weight management using a meal replacement strategy: meta and pooling analysis from six studies. Int J Obes Relat Metab Disord 27:537–549

13. Krieger JW, Sitren HS, Daniels MJ, Langkamp-Henken B (2006) Effects of variation in protein and carbohydrate intake on body mass and composition during energy restriction: a meta-regression. Am J Clin Nutr 83:260–274

14. Clifton PM, Keogh JB, Noakes M (2008) Long-term effects of a high-protein weight-loss diet. Am J Clin Nutr 87:23–29

15. Gardner CD, Kiazand A, Alhassan S, et al (2007) Comparison of the Atkins, Zone, Ornish, and LEARN diets for change in weight and related risk factors among over-weight premenopausal women: the A TO Z Weight Loss Study: a randomized trial. JAMA 297:969–977

16. Dansinger ML, Gleason JA, Griffith JL, Selker HP, Schaefer EJ (2005) Comparison of the Atkins, Ornish, Weight Watchers, and Zone diets for weight loss and heart disease risk reduction: a randomized trial. JAMA 293:43–53

17. Truby H, Baic S, deLooy A, et al (2006) Randomised controlled trial of four commercial weight loss programmes in the UK: initial findings from the BBC "diet trials". BMJ 332:1309–1314

18. Hauner H, Buchholz G, Hamann A, et al (2007) Prevention and therapy of adipositas; guidelines of the German Adipositas Society. Adipositas Spektrum 5: 20–25

19. Warburton DE, Katzmarzyk PT, Rhodes RE, Shephard RJ (2007) Evidence-informed physical activity guidelines for Canadian adults. Can J Public Health 98 [Suppl 2]:S16–68

20. Sjöström L, Lindroos AK, Peltonen M et al. (2004) Lifestyle, diabetes, and cardiovascular risk factors 10 years after bariatric surgery N Engl J Med 351(26):2683–93

21. Slentz CA, Duscha BD, Johnson JL, et al (2004) Effects of the amount of exercise on body weight, body composition, and measures of central obesity: STRRIDE – a randomized controlled study. Arch Intern Med 164:31–39

22. Wilmore JH, Després JP, Stanforth PR, et al (1999) Alterations in body weight and composition consequent to 20 wk of endurance training: the HERITAGE Family Study. Am J Clin Nutr 70:346–352

23. Villareal DT, Miller BV 3rd, Banks M, Fontana L, Sinacore DR, Klein S (2006) Effect of life-style intervention on metabolic coronary heart disease risk factors in obese older adults. Am J Clin Nutr 84:1317–1323

24. Wood PD (1994) Physical activity, diet, and health: independent and interactive effects. Med Sci Sports Exerc 26:838–843

25. Stiegler P, Cunliffe A (2006) The role of diet and exercise for the maintenance of fat-free mass and resting metabolic rate during weight loss. Sports Med 36:239–262

26. Wirth A, Kern E, Vogel I, Nikolaus T, Schlierf G (1986) Combination therapy of obesity with a reducing diet and physical training. Cardiovascular and metabolic effects. Dtsch Med Wochenschr 111: 972–977

27. Venables MC, Jeukendrup AE (2008) Endurance training and obesity: effect on substrate metabolism and insulin sensitivity. Med Sci Sports Exerc 40:495–502

28. Sari R, Balci MK, Balci N, Karayalcin U (2007) Acute effect of exercise on plasma leptin level and insulin resistance in obese women with stable caloric intake. Endocr Res 32:9–17

29. Jakicic JM, Marcus BH, Gallagher KI, Napolitano M, Lang W (2003) Effect of exercise duration and intensity on weight loss in overweight, sedentary women: a randomized trial. JAMA 290:1323–1330

30. Jakicic JM, Clark K, Coleman E, et al (2001) American College of Sports Medicine position stand. Appropriate intervention strategies for weight loss and prevention of weight regain for adults. Med Sci Sports Exerc 33:2145–2156

31. Wadden TA, Berkowitz RI, Womble LG, et al (2005) Randomized trial of lifestyle modification and pharmacotherapy for obesity. N Engl J Med 353:2111–2120

32. Wing RR, Gorin AA (2003) Behavioral techniques for treating the obese patient. Prim Care 30:375–391

33. Teixeira PJ, Going SB, Sardinha LB, Lohman TG (2005) A review of psychosocial pre-treatment predictors of weight control. Obes Rev 6:43-65

34. Wadden TA, Anderson DA, Foster GD, Bennett A, Steinberg C, Sarwer DB (2000) Obese women's perceptions of their physicians' weight management attitudes and practices. Arch Fam Med 9:854–860

35. Foster GD, Makris AP, Bailer BA (2005) Behavioral treatment of obesity. Am J Clin Nutr 82 [Suppl]:230S–235S

36. Butryn ML, Phelan S, Hill JO, Wing RR (2007) Consistent self-monitoring of weight: a key component of successful weight loss maintenance. Obesity (Silver Spring) 15:3091–3096

37. Westenhoefer J, Stunkard AJ, Pudel V (1999) Validation of the flexible and rigid control dimensions of dietary restraint. Int J Eat Disord 26:53–64

38. Poston WS, Hyder ML, O'Byrne KK, Foreyt JP (2000) Where do diets, exercise, and behavior modification fit in the treatment of obesity? Endocrine 13:187–192

39. Markham A (1999) Orlistat: a review of its use in the management of obesity. Drugs 58:743–760

40. Van Gaal LF, Wauters MA, Peiffer FW, De Leeuw IH (1998) Sibutramine and fat distribution: is there a role for pharmacotherapy in abdominal/visceral fat reduction? Int J Obes Relat Metab Disord 22 [Suppl 1]:S38–S40

41. Sjöström L, Rissanen A, Andersen T, et al (1998) Randomised placebo-controlled trial of orlistat for weight loss and prevention of weight regain in obese patients. European Multicentre Orlistat Study Group. Lancet 352:167–172

42. Hollander PA, Elbein SC, Hirsch IB, et al (1998) Role of orlistat in the treatment of obese patients with type 2 diabetes. A 1-year randomized double-blind study. Diabetes Care 21:1288–1294

43. Patriti A, Facchiano E, Sanna A, Gullà N, Donini A (2004) The enteroinsular axis and the recovery from type 2 diabetes after bariatric surgery. Obes Surg 14:840–848

44. Edwards CM, Stanley SA, Davis R, et al (2001) Exendin-4 reduces fasting and postprandial glucose and decreases energy intake in healthy volunteers. Am J Physiol Endocrinol Metab 281:E155–161

45. Heine RJ, Van Gaal LF, Johns D, Mihm MJ, Widel MH, Brodows RG, GWAA Study Group (2005) Exenatide versus insulin glargine in patients with suboptimally con-trolled type 2 diabetes: a rand-omized trial. Ann Intern Med 143:559–569
46. Knowler WC, Barrett-Connor E, Fowler SE, et al (2002) Diabetes Prevention Program Research Group. Reduction in the incidence of type 2 diabetes with lifestyle intervention or metformin. N Engl J Med 346:393–403
47. Toplak H, Hamann A, Moore R, Masson E, et al (2007) Efficacy and safety of topi-ramate in combination with metformin in the treatment of obese subjects with type 2 diabetes: a randomized, double-blind, placebo-controlled study. Int J Obes (Lond) 31:138–146
48. Batterham RL, Cohen MA, Ellis SM, et al (2003) Inhibition of food intake in obese subjects by peptide YY3-36. N Engl J Med 349:941–948

Obesity in Children – a Therapeutic Challenge

Ulrike Korsten-Reck, MD

Obesity in children is a chronic disease with a genetic and environmental etiology. In treating obese children, priority ought to be given to primary and secondary prevention, identification of risk groups, and early disease management. In light of the growing prevalence of overweight and obesity in children and the decrease in overall physical activity during childhood and adolescence, the training of competent therapists and the establishment of centers qualified for the early management of risk groups are imperative. Studies illustrate that patients who are affected do not recognize obesity as a chronic disease, despite a growing awareness of this syndrome in society. Intervention programs ought to focus on sports and on counseling of daily activities. Furthermore, statements of commitment from parents and teachers should be obtained early on in therapy. If this strategy is further promoted by insurance companies, programs such as the Freiburg Intervention Trial for Obese Children (FITOC) may be successful in battling this weighty epidemic.

3.1   Introduction

The etiological factors leading to obesity in the young have not all been delineated. Nonetheless, altered environmental and living conditions may be said to have a decisive influence. Leisure activities, eating habits, and current family structures strongly promote the development of overweight [1–5]. On the other hand, while we do not know how strongly a genetic predisposition contributes to this disease, it seems safe to say that children with a predisposition react more sensitively to the above-mentioned changes in lifestyle than do children without [5]. Obesity in the young is associated with numerous severe and impeding co-morbidities as well as with a greater risk of developing obesity in adulthood. In light of these circumstances, it appears crucial to offer early preventive measures and to develop well-planned, nationwide intervention programs in order to identify and adequately treat risk groups.

3.2   Epidemiology

Childhood obesity is a chronic disease with reduced quality of life and increased morbidity and mortality. In fact, the World Health Organization (WHO) assumes it to be a global epidemic and has declared it to be one of today's most significant health-political challenges. In the USA, extensive data have been collected on the physical development of school children and adolescents between 6 and 17 years of age. These studies illustrate a massive increase in the prevalence of obesity since the 1980s. Importantly, these data also indicate an association with diseases such as hypertension and metabolic disorders. In Europe, on the other hand, weight trends over such a long period have not been documented. Thus, international comparison is difficult. A uniform definition of overweight and obesity in children and adolescents was first worked out in 2000 by the *Arbeitsgemeinschaft Adipositas im Kindes- und Jugendalter* (AGA) [6] on the basis of BMI percentile curves. In Germany, the 90th percentile is used to define overweight and the 97th to define obesity. By contrast, the 85th and 90th percentile, respectively, are referred to internationally, thus yielding very different prevalence data.

3.3   Pathophysiology

The causes and pathogenesis of obesity are complex and involve increased caloric intake, genetic disposition, lack of exercise, and changes in dietary behavior [7]. Basically, obesity is the consequence of a positive energy balance. Studies show that a mere imbalance of 2%, i.e., roughly 125 kJ/day, leads to obesity in the long term [8]. Energy balance depends on caloric intake and energy expenditure. Total energy expenditure entails basic expenditure, thermogenesis, and physical activity. Basic expenditure denotes the sum of metabolic activity in the resting body and may individually account for up to 60% of total metabolism. Thermogenesis denotes the energy required for uptake, digestion, and storage of nutrients and accounts for roughly 10% of total energy expenditure. Thus, physical activity accounts for only about 30%. A positive energy balance means that more energy is consumed than expended. This balance may additionally be affected by the autonomic nervous system and by numerous metabolic and biochemical factors in an individual way [9, 10].

3.4   Genetic Factors

We know that there is a genetic disposition for obesity in adulthood [11]. It is assumed that there is a genetically determined "set point" which regulates individual weight. This central system regulates body fat via leptin, a hormone that is produced in lipocytes and influences feelings of hunger and satiation when values lie below or above the individual set point. Furthermore, genetic factors influence basic energy expenditure, body tissue composition, appetite regulation, insulin sensitivity, and even physical activity.

Results of twin, adoption, and family research indicate an impact of genetic factors of between 60% and 80% [12]. This finding is corroborated by the fact that up to 80% of school children between 11 and 14 years of age, one or both of whose parents are obese, will themselves become obese. The human genetic equipment is designed for the storage of fat. This is vital for survival during times when nourishment is scarce. In light of these "thrifty genes", we are not suited for our affluent society, which is characterized not only by an abundance of food but also by a lack of exercise [13].

3.5 Diagnostics

Adequate somatic and laboratory diagnostics as well as a thorough medical history ought to differentiate between symptomatic and alimentary forms of obesity. Additionally, early examination should identify obesity-related health problems. The gravity of obesity in childhood and adolescence arises from the limitations in everyday living and from the many consequences, which often do not become manifest until adulthood. Some of the somatic consequences are hypertension, type 2 diabetes, hyperandrogenemia in girls, hyperuricemia, steatosis, and cholecystolithiasis, as well as orthopedic problems [11, 14]. Other clinical findings might include acceleration of growth and skeletal maturity, striae distensae in girls, and pseudogynecomasty and pseudohypogenitalism in boys (often associated with great psychological suffering).

3.6 Pediatric Obesity and Lipid Metabolic Changes

Much research has been dedicated to the pathogenesis of pediatric and adolescent atherosclerosis over the past decades [15–20]. Early atherosclerotic lesions were found in adolescents with high total LDL and high total cholesterol values [21]. High-fat overeating and a lack of physical exercise appear to contribute significantly to these early changes [22–24]. Furthermore, the metabolic syndrome, which is frequently associated with obesity, is the main risk factor for atherosclerotic coronary heart disease (CHD). Due to these correlations, one of the objectives of the FITOC is to normalize the lipid profile. Data from the Bogalusa Heart Study show that the incidence of cardiovascular events increases with body weight in both sexes [15, 17, 19]. However, the cardiovascular risk depends not only on the extent of obesity, but also on the distribution of fat. As in adults,

children with a greater proportion of visceral fat develop a metabolic syndrome more often than those whose fat accumulation is more peripheral [25]. Furthermore, overweight children more frequently develop insulin resistance and dyslipoproteinemia, both of which lead to accelerated atherosclerosis in adolescence and early adulthood [15].

3.7 Physical Activity

Insufficient physical activity is now considered the "central health problem of the third millennium". Its causes are manifold and entail changes in leisure activities, increased media use, and attendant indoor passivity. Especially in large cities, children live in experience-poor environments with limited space for exercise. There is a close connection between physical inactivity and the development of overweight [26]. Studies show that overweight children spend considerably less time in moderate (e.g. playing outdoors) to strenuous everyday activity (e.g. catching games). The most overweight children are those who show the greatest media use coupled with the consumption of high-calorie snacks and the least exercise [7, 26, 27]. Interestingly, involvement in non-organized sports appears to play a greater role in the prevention of overweight than do athletic activities in clubs or groups [28]. This underlines the importance of exercise-rich everyday life in the prevention and therapy of overweight and obesity.

3.7.1 Epidemiology

The importance of physical activity in prevention and rehabilitation is well-documented for adults [29]. A stunning 45% of German adults nonetheless fail to engage in any sport, 30% are hardly active, and only 13% exercise enough to achieve a preventive effect. Physical activity is understood to mean any activity that leads to energy conversion. An equivalent of 2000–3000 kcal in weekend leisure activities alone can significantly reduce cardiovascular risks. The maximum preventive effect through physical activity is cited at 30 min or more daily, or three to four training units per week with intensive physical stress of more than 6 MET [29].

3.7.2 Physical Activity during Childhood

Exercise and playing are the foundation for developing sensorimotor skills and for healthy cognitive, social, and personal development [30, 31]. A one-sided focus on educational content at the expense of exercise is not justified, and studies effectively illustrate that development of emotional and physical skills are connected. It therefore comes as no surprise that good and poor students differ not only with respect to their grades, but also in their physical coordination. In general, there appears to be a deterioration of physical condition and coordination. This is observed by sports teachers and confirmed by the Federal Youth Games. On the basis of 54 studies, Hebebrand and Bos conclude that the motor performance capacity has decreased by 10% over the past 25 years. According to exercise diaries, an average elementary school child these days engages in the following activities: lying down 9 h, sitting 9 h, standing 5 h, and moving only 1 h [3]. It is easy to categorize "sedentary behavior" as a risk for the onset of obesity because inactivity is relatively easy to measure. Physical activity, on the other hand, is a complex, multidimensional behavior that is difficult to quantify. The methodical difficulties in recording physical activity apply especially in children under 10 years of age because their everyday life often consists of spontaneous, unstructured activities. Small children are not able to keep records of their everyday activities or to assign activities to certain time periods. Data based on questionnaires can thus hardly be interpreted. It is therefore not surprising that there are only few studies for this age-group that address the relationship between physical activity and body fat. For this reason, studies increasingly implement physical procedures to measure activity (e.g. accelerometry). This way, time spent in activity or inactivity can be reproducibly measured [32–36]. Moreover, some measuring devices are capable of differentiating between various intensities of activity. Unlike questionnaires, these measurements enable direct comparisons between populations. Sex and age differences in physical activity among children have been documented by studies using accelerometric data. They show a marked decrease in moderate physical activity of children before puberty and throughout adolescence. Overall, girls spend significantly less time in moderately strenuous physical activity than boys, even at an early age. This difference increases later on [37]. There are few data available on the development of physical activity during childhood during the past decades. However, the low number of children who walk or ride a bike to school is taken as an indicator of the decreasing activity level [38]. The National Travel Survey of 2001 showed that the average distance travelled without motorization has drastically decreased [39]. The importance of sports in school is frequently emphasized [35]. Basic motor principles can be acquired through physical education.

Interestingly, a study of 9-year-old children showed that despite great differences in the number of hours of physical education at various schools, the total activity level of the children as recorded through accelerometers was the same. Children who have fewer hours of physical education in school usually compensate for this by being more active outside of school. Studies to date conclusively illustrate the difficulty of formulating general guidelines concerning interventions in everyday activity. Current guidelines from England and the USA recommend at least 60 min of moderate to strenuous activity per day for normal weight development [32, 40].

3.7.3 Physical Activity and the Onset of Overweight

Studies using objective methods of measuring activity levels are usually designed as cross-sectional studies and compare the activity levels of normal-weight and overweight children. The few prospective studies performed to date report on pre-pubescent children and yield inconsistent results concerning the relationship between physical activity and the onset of overweight. In 2004, Marshall performed a meta-analysis with the keywords "physical activity", "sedentary behavior", "inactivity", "TV", and "computer" [7, 26, 27]. No significant correlations were found. However, the methods of documentation differed widely among the studies (definition of obesity, self-report of physical activity versus objective test procedures, etc.) In our opinion, the conclusion to be drawn from this meta-analysis is that, in addition to watching television and inactivity, other disruptive factors such as eating high-calorie snacks must be present for obesity to develop. Furthermore, there is no doubt that television is the dominant leisure activity of today's children and adolescents. A child in the USA watches an average of 2.5 h of television per day. This is ten times the amount of time spent in intensive exercise per day.

3.8 Therapeutic Principles and Objectives

Therapy of obesity in the young is a long-term endeavor. Short-term, realistic goals have to be set to motivate the patient and his family. A psychosocial, basic diagnostic interview often yields important background information and ought to be carried out regularly during the therapy. The most important therapeutic objectives are [14]:
- Long-term weight loss or stabilization
- Improvement of eating and exercise behavior

- Improvement of obesity-associated co-morbidity
- Prevention of adverse therapy effects, e.g. eating disorders
- Promotion of normal physical, emotional and social development and performance capacity

These goals can be achieved only by means of holistic therapy with an interdisciplinary team, consisting of a physician, a dietary specialist, sports instructors, and psychologists. For this reason, the FITOC was designed as an interdisciplinary intervention program for the outpatient therapy of obesity in children and adolescents. It consists of a combination of organized sports, dietary training, and behavioral therapy [41].

3.9 Integration of Sports into Therapy

Physical activity is particularly important in overcoming obesity, especially in children. Performance capacity should be increased as soon as possible by integrating routine exercise in kindergartens, registering with sports clubs, etc. The age window between 8 and 11 years is especially favorable for therapy due to the motor and cognitive development during this phase [3]. Special efforts ought to be directed at children with inactive parents due to their enormously increased risk of becoming inactive themselves [42]. Psychologically, obese children usually suffer most due to their psychosocial isolation, far more indeed than due to the medical consequences of their disease. Frequently, they are teased by their peers, derided and discriminated against. This leads to insecurity and social withdrawal, thus creating a vicious cycle of inactivity and inactivityrelated overweight. Intervention must therefore end this inappropriate behavior and motivate patients to participate in sports with other overweight children and adolescents [43]. Self-motivation and restructuring can be achieved only by breaking down fears of exercise, by experiencing success, by appropriate demands in the sports program, and by offering new and known exercise situations at a realistic level of success. The exercise program should motivate the patient in a differentiated way without being too performance-oriented. Its goals ought to be:

- To convey joy and fun in exercise
- To rediscover and develop body awareness
- To increase self-worth and self-confidence
- To improve performance
- To induce the patient to participate in "lifetime sport"
- To support weight loss and constancy

3.9.1 Complications and Contraindications

An orthopedic examination is absolutely mandatory at the beginning of therapy in order to point out obesity related weak spots such as genu varu, hyperlordosis, malpositioning of the foot, or similar problems. The additional stress on joints due to existing overweight ought to be minimized by exercising in water, walking instead of jogging, training with a Thera-Band in a sitting position, and other analogous techniques. From an internal medicine point of view, there is no contraindication with the exception of certain cardiological diseases. A healthy cardiovascular status should be ascertained by taking the patient's history and performing an ECG prior to beginning therapy.

3.9.2 Results

Results from the FITOC illustrate that obese children can redevelop motor skills and a natural urge to exercise. The program includes three scheduled sports sessions per week – swimming is included in one of them. Coordination, flexibility, endurance, strength, and speed improve through therapy, thus imparting improved body perception. Sports-motor tests evaluate the individual status at the start and following an intervention in order to monitor success [44]. Increasing the patient's everyday activity and working on individual sports skills enable overweight children to re-establish equality with their peers at school and in everyday life (❏ Fig. 3.1). In addition, activity in the family setting is promoted through activity diaries and "homework". In general, the following aspects ought to be taken into consideration:

- Mobilization of the patient's resources, including his parents
- Age- and gender-specific differences
- Parental involvement in changing dietary and activity behavior
- Non-accusatory instruction of parents, teachers, and children
- Inclusion of all actors in networks of kindergarten, day-care centers, and schools

3.10 Influence of Intervention on Lipid Metabolism Parameters

To date, only few studies have examined the influence of intervention programs on the concentration of lipoproteins of obese children. Our own results suggest a difference between girls and boys: A significant decrease of total and

3

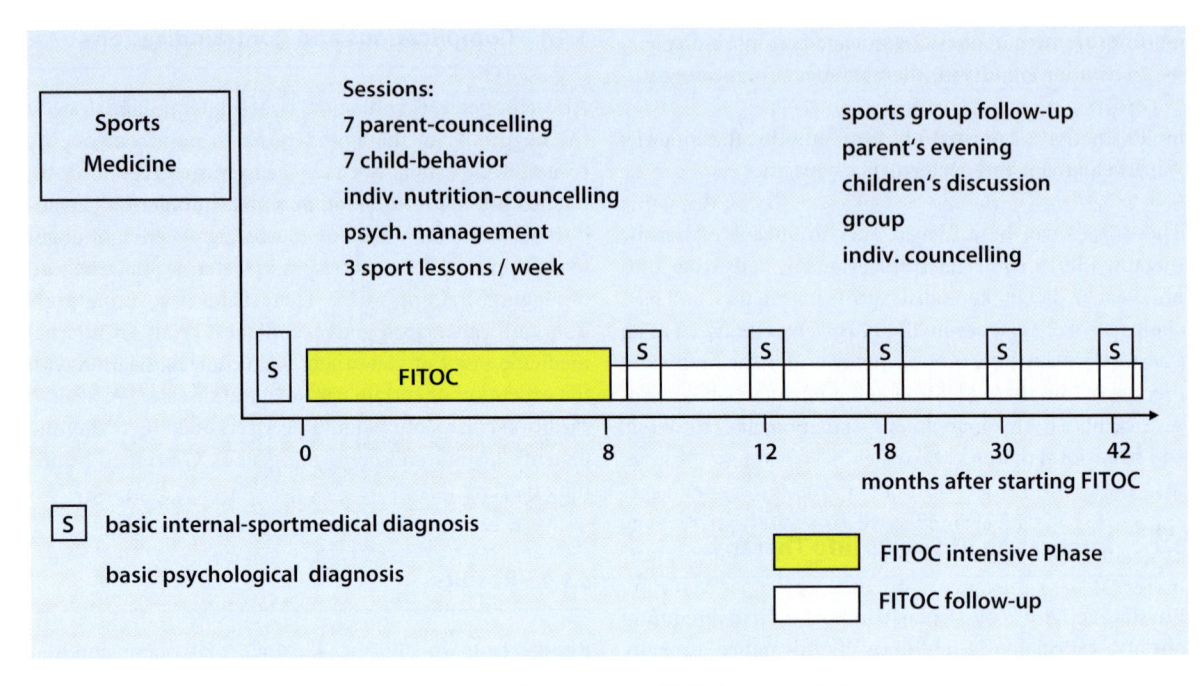

□ **Fig 3.1.** Course of the standardized Intensive Phase and Follow-up-Phase of FITOC (long-term plan)

LDL-C was observed in boys following therapy, while only the LDL-C was significantly reduced in girls. HDL-C appears to be slightly increased in both sexes. Generally, HDL-C has a negative correlation with testosterone and a positive correlation with estrogen [45, 46]. Other metabolic factors, such as elevated apolipoprotein B, an increase in homocysteine, and an increase of CRP, are also considered risk factors for the onset of atherosclerosis-related CHD [47, 48]. A study of children assigned to four groups according to BMI and physical fitness showed that the group of overweight children with the highest level of fitness had the lowest inflammatory parameters [48]. Additionally, obesity in childhood is associated with elevated triglyceride values, even when HDL and LDL-C values are normal. The TG level is co-responsible for the presence of hypo-HDL type in the sense of a metabolic syndrome, as apparent from the BMI-SDS and performance capacity within the four groups. Since atherosclerosis has been proven to begin in childhood, the importance of beginning therapy at an early age is clear.

3.11   Results of Various Intervention Approaches

A significant reduction in the proportion of body fat and an increase in fitness can be achieved in therapy groups with physical training [49–52]. The best results were achieved in therapy programs that involved the patients' parents and combined dietary and physical training [53–65]. These parameters are decisively impacted by the child's parents [66–69]. Parents in higher social classes appear to give their children more adequate support, both cognitively and financially [70, 71]. Flegal illustrated that income and parental educational level play just as important a role in the onset and therapy of obesity as exercise and diet [72]. Children from lower social classes, who are considered to be less-well integrated in schools, are at greater risk for the development of obesity [73–75]. These results have been corroborated by other publications on social status and obesity [71]. In the FITOC, weight stability during growth or weight reduction was achieved in both boys and girls. By contrast, the BMI increased in a control group. The BMISDS was constant. A reduction of LDL-cholesterol was also achieved only in the therapy groups. Importantly, an increase in physical performance capacity was also achieved, while only an age-dependent, non-significant increase was observed in the control group. The increased performance in children under therapy is closely tied to exercise during the therapy program [44, 76]. However, the improvement may also be attributed in part to changes in the children's everyday activity. The sports activities were clearly influenced by the intervention. Although a questionnaire was available as a subjective recording instrument for determining exercise behavior; the result is supported by the objective measurement of performance capacity in watt per kg body weight. Prior to treatment, one third of the boys and one quarter of the girls were athletically inactive. At the end of the intervention, this applied to fewer than 5% of the children. A direct comparison of our intervention results with those of other outpatient therapy programs is difficult due to the differences in program design. For example, the efficacy of sports activity versus inactivity was examined in various studies without additional dietary training. Other studies compare dietary training plus sports with dietary training alone [62, 63, 65, 77, 78]. Reinehr et al. [79] reported a decrease of 0.4 BMI-SDS following an intervention program with comparable therapy components. However, the drop-out rate was 27%, which is considerably higher than our own rate of 7–11%. In summary, training alone appears to be relatively ineffective, since the higher energy expenditure is apparently compensated by higher calorie intake [80]. On the other hand, programs offering dietary training alone are equally ineffective in the long run. In the FITOC, both approaches are combined. Additionally, the patient's parents are intensively involved in dietary training and information. This changes not only their cognition of eating, but also their selection of foods. Our results show that children's knowledge of nutrition can be improved and promoted. In general, behavioral therapy in childhood appears to be helpful. Surgical therapy ought to be very restrictively handled due to a lack of data on the benefits in this young population. We strongly believe that obesity in children is a chronic epidemic disease with a growing prevalence that requires interdisciplinary primary prevention and intensive long-term therapy. In Germany, several political efforts are being made to counteract this worrisome phenomenon. Nonetheless, obesity in children and adolescents will undoubtedly remain one of the greatest social challenges in the future.

References

1. Bouchard C (1995) The genetics of obesity: from genetic epidemiology to molecular markers. Mol Med Today 1:45–50
2. Bray GA (1991) Barriers to the treatment of obesity. Ann Intern Med 115:152–153
3. Hebebrand J, Bös K (2005) Umgebungsfaktoren – Körperliche Aktivität. In: Wabitsch M et al (eds) Adipositas bei Kindern und Jugendlichen. Springer Verlag, Heidelberg
4. Hebebrand J, Friedel S, Schauble N, Geller F, Hinney A (2003) Perspectives: molecular genetic research in human obesity. Obes Rev 4:139–146
5. Plagemann A (2006) Perinatal nutrition and hormone-dependent programming of food intake. Horm Res 65 [Suppl 3]:83–89
6. Kromeyer-Hauschild K, Wabitsch M, Kunze D (2001) Perzentile für den Body-Mass-Index für das Kinder- und Jugendalter unter Heranziehung verschiedener deutscher Stichproben. Monatsschr Kinderheilkd 149:807–818
7. Dietz WH (2004) Overweight in childhood and adolescence. N Engl J Med 350:855–857
8. Goran MI, Carpenter WH, McGloin A, Johnson R, Hardin JM, Weinsier RL (1995) Energy expenditure in children of lean and obese parents. Am J Physiol 268:E917–E924
9. Ravussin E, Swinburn BA (1993) Metabolic predictors of obesity: cross-sectional versus longitudinal data. Int J Obes Relat Metab Disord 17 [Suppl 3]:S28–S31
10. Ravussin E, Smith SR (2002) Increased fat intake, impaired fat oxidation, and failure of fat cell proliferation result in ectopic fat storage, insulin resistance, and type 2 diabetes mellitus. Ann NY Acad Sci 967:363–378
11. Lobstein T, Baur L, Uauy R (2004) Obesity in children and young people: a crisis in public health. Obes Rev 5 [Suppl 1]:4–104
12. Hebebrand J, Wermter A, Hinney A (2004):Genetic aspects. In: Kiess W, Marcus C, Wabitsch M (eds) Obesity in childhood and adolescence. Karger, Basel, pp 80–90
13. Neel JV, Weder AB, Julius S (1998) Type II diabetes, essential hypertension, and obesity as „syndromes of impaired genetic homeostasis": the „thrifty genotype" hypothesis enters the 21st century. Perspect Biol Med 42:44–74
14. Wabitsch M, Kunze D (2002) Leitlinien der Arbeitsgemeinschaft Adipositas im Kindes- und Jugendalter. Ref Type: Report
15. Berenson GS, Srinivasan SR, Bao W, Newman WP III, Tracy RE, Wattigney WA (1998) Association between multiple cardiovascular risk factors and atherosclerosis in children and young adults. The Bogalusa Heart Study. N Engl J Med 338:1650–1656
16. Freedman DS, Srinivasan S, Berenson GS (2002) Risk of cardiovascular complications. In: Burniat W, Cole TJ, Lissau I, Poskitt EM (eds) Child and adolescent obesity. Causes and consequences; prevention and management. Cambridge University, Cambridge, pp 221–239
17. Freedman DS, Khan LK, Serdula MK, Dietz WH, Srinivasan SR, Berenson GS (2004) Inter-relationships among childhood BMI, childhood height, and adult obesity: the Bogalusa Heart Study. Int J Obes Relat Metab Disord 28:10–16
18. Freedman DS, Dietz WH, Tang R, Mensah GA, Bond MG, Urbina EM, et al (2004) The relation of obesity throughout life to carotid intima-media thickness in adulthood: the Bogalusa Heart Study. Int J Obes Relat Metab Disord 28:159–166
19. Frontini MG, Srinivasan SR, Berenson GS (2003) Longitudinal changes in risk variables underlying metabolic syndrome X from childhood to young adulthood in female subjects with a history of early menarche: the Bogalusa Heart Study. Int J Obes Relat Metab Disord 27:1398–1404
20. Srinivasan SR, Bao W, Wattigney WA, Berenson GS (1996) Adolescent overweight is associated with adult overweight and related multiple cardiovascular risk factors: the Bogalusa Heart Study. Metabolism 45:235–240
21. Tracy RE, Newman WP, III, Wattigney WA, Berenson GS (1995) Risk factors and atherosclerosis in youth autopsy findings of the Bogalusa Heart Study. Am J Med Sci 310 [Suppl 1]:S37–S41
22. Steinberger J, Moorehead C, Katch V, Rocchini AP (1995) Relationship between insulin resistance and abnormal lipid profile in obese adolescents. J Pediatr 126:690–695
23. Steinberger J (2003) Diagnosis of the metabolic syndrome in children. Curr Opin Lipidol 14:555–559
24. Steinberger J, Daniels SR (2003) Obesity, insulin resistance, diabetes, and cardiovascular risk in children: an American Heart Association scientific statement from the Atherosclerosis, Hypertension, and Obesity in the Young Committee (Council on Car-

3

diovascular Disease in the Young) and the Diabetes Committee (Council on Nutrition, Physical Activity, and Metabolism). Circulation 107:1448–1453

25. Moreno LA, Pineda I, Rodriguez G, Fleta J, Sarria A, Bueno M (2002) Waist circumference for the screening of the metabolic syndrome in children. Acta Paediatr 91:1307–1312

26. Marshall SJ, Biddle SJ, Gorely T, Cameron N, Murdey I (2004) Relationships between media use, body fatness and physical activity in children and youth: a meta-analysis. Int J Obes Relat Metab Disord 28:1238–1246

27. Gortmaker SL, Must A, Sobol AM, Peterson K, Colditz GA, Dietz WH (1996) Television viewing as a cause of increasing obesity among children in the United States, 1986–1990. Arch Pediatr Adolesc Med 150:356–362

28. Tremblay MS, Willms JD Is the Canadian childhood obesity epidemic related to physical inactivity? Int J Obes Relat Metab Disord 2003 27:1100-1105

29. Löllgen H (2003) Primärprävention kardialer Erkrankungen. Dsch Ärztebl 100: 828-834 15:828–834

30. Ayres AJ (2002)Bausteine der kindlichen Entwicklung, 4th edn. Springer Verlag, Berlin, Heidelberg

31. Bittmann F Pfiffikus durch Bewegungsfluss – ein Projekt der integrativen Motorik- und Kognitionsförderung in der KITA. http://www.mbjs.brandenburg.de/media/lbm1.a.1231.de/Pfiffikus.pdf . 2006, Ref Type: Internet Communication

32. Daniels SR, Arnett DK, Eckel RH, Gidding SS, Hayman LL, Kumanyika S et al (2005) Overweight in children and adolescents: pathophysiology, consequences, prevention, and treatment. Circulation 111:1999–2012

33. Livingstone MB, Robson PJ, Wallace JM, McKinley MC (2003) How active are we? Levels of routine physical activity in children and adults. Proc Nutr Soc 62:681–701

34. Mallam KM, Metcalf BS, Kirkby J, Voss LD, Wilkin TJ (2003) Contribution of timetabled physical education to total physical activity in primary school children: cross-sectional study. BMJ 327:592–593

35. Rennie KL, Livingstone MB, Wells JC, McGloin A, Coward WA, Prentice AM et al (2005) Association of physical activity with body-composition indexes in children aged 6–8 y at varied risk of obesity. Am J Clin Nutr 82:13–20

36. Trost SG, Sirard JR, Dowda M, Pfeiffer KA, Pate RR (2003) Physical activity in overweight and non-overweight preschool children. Int J Obes Relat Metab Disord 27:834–839

37. Riddoch CJ, Bo AL, Wedderkopp N, Harro M, Klasson-Heggebo L, Sardinha LB, et al (2004) Physical activity levels and patterns of 9- and 15-yr-old European children. Med Sci Sports Exerc 36:86–92

38. Korsten-Reck U (2007) Sport zur Prävention und Therapie von Übergewicht bei Kindern. Dtsch Ärztebl 104: A35-9 7 A.D.

39. National Travel Survey Unit (2001) Focus on Personal Travel. Her Majesty's Stationary Office, London, Ref Type: Report

40. Strong WB, Malina RM, Blimkie CJ, Daniels SR, Dishman RK, Gutin B, et al (2005) Evidence-based physical activity for school-age youth. J Pediatr 146:732–737

41. Korsten-Reck U, Kromeyer-Hauschild K, Wolfarth B, Dickhuth HH, Berg A (2005) Freiburg Intervention Trial for Obese Children (FITOC): results of a clinical observation study. Int J Obes Relat Metab Disord 29:356–361

42. Moore LL, Lombardi DA, White MJ, Campbell JL, Oliveria SA, Ellison RC (1991) Influence of parents' physical activity levels on activity levels of young children. J Pediatr 118:215–219

43. Korsten-Reck U, Korsten K, Haeberle K, Kromeyer-Hauschild K, Dickhuth H-H, Schulz E (2009)The psychosocial situation of obese

children: psychological factors and quality of life. Psychol Res Behavior Management 1:23–29

44. Korsten-Reck U., Kasper T, Rücker G, Jotterand S, Bös.K, Berg A (2004) Physical fitness of obese children: Comparison to a reference group and effects of the therapy program FITOC. Isokinetics Exercise Sci 12:87–88

45. Beaglehole R (1988) Oestrogens and cardiovascular disease. BMJ 297:571–572

46. Sorva R, Kuusi T, Dunkel L, Taskinen MR (1988) Effects of endogenous sex steroids on serum lipoproteins and post-heparin plasma lipolytic enzymes. J Clin Endocrinol Metab 66:408–413

47. Halle M, Berg A, Keul J (1999) Overweight as a risk factor for cardiovascular diseases and its possible significance as a promoter of an increased inflammatory reaction [in German]. Dtsch Med Wochenschr 124:905–909

48. Halle M, Korsten-Reck U, Wolfarth B, Berg A (2004) Low-grade systemic inflammation in overweight children: impact of physical fitness. Exerc Immunol Rev 10:66–74

49. Gutin B, Owens S (1999) Role of exercise intervention in improving body fat distribution and risk profile in children. Am J Human Biol 11:237–247

50. Gutin B, Barbeau P, Owens S, Lemmon CR, Bauman M, Allison J, et al (2002) Effects of exercise intensity on cardiovascular fitness, total body composition, and visceral adiposity of obese adolescents. Am J Clin Nutr 75:818–826

51. Owens S, Gutin B, Allison J, Riggs S, Ferguson M, Litaker M, et al (1999) Effect of physical training on total and visceral fat in obese children. Med Sci Sports Exerc 31:143–148

52. Owens S, Gutin B (1999) Exercise testing of the child with obesity. Pediatr Cardiol 20:79–83

53. Davison KK, Birch LL (2001) Child and parent characteristics as predictors of change in girls' body mass index. Int J Obes Relat Metab Disord 25:1834–1842

54. Eliakim A, Kaven G, Berger I, Friedland O, Wolach B, Nemet D (2002) The effect of a combined intervention on body mass index and fitness in obese children and adolescents – a clinical experience. Eur J Pediatr 161:449–454

55. Epstein LH, Valoski A, Wing RR, McCurley J (1990) Ten-year follow-up of behavioral, family-based treatment for obese children. JAMA 264:2519–2523

56. Epstein LH, Myers MD, Raynor HA, Saelens BE (1998) Treatment of pediatric obesity. Pediatrics 101:554–570

57. Epstein LH, Paluch RA, Gordy CC, Saelens BE, Ernst MM (2000) Problem solving in the treatment of childhood obesity. J Consult Clin Psychol 68:717–721

58. Epstein LH, Paluch RA, Raynor HA (2001) Sex differences in obese children and siblings in family-based obesity treatment. Obes Res 9:746–753

59. Epstein LH, Paluch RA, Consalvi A, Riordan K, Scholl T (2002) Effects of manipulating sedentary behavior on physical activity and food intake. J Pediatr 140:334–339

60. Golan M, Weizman A, Apter A, Fainaru M (1998) Parents as the exclusive agents of change in the treatment of childhood obesity. Am J Clin Nutr 67:1130–1135

61. Hills AP, Parker AW (1988) Obesity management via diet and exercise intervention. Child Care Health Dev 14:409–416

62. LeMura LM, Maziekas MT (2002) Factors that alter body fat, body mass, and fat-free mass in pediatric obesity. Med Sci Sports Exerc 34:487–496

63. Reybrouck T, Vinckx J, Van den BG, Vanderschueren-Lodeweyckx M (1990) Exercise therapy and hypocaloric diet in the treatment

of obese children and adolescents. Acta Paediatr Scand 79: 84–89

64. Summerbell CD, Ashton V, Campbell KJ, Edmunds L, Kelly S, Waters E (2003) Interventions for treating obesity in children. Cochrane Database Syst Rev 3:CD001872

65. Summerbell CD, Douthwaite W, Whittaker V, Ells LJ, Hillier F, Smith S et al (2009) The association between diet and physical activity and subsequent excess weight gain and obesity assessed at 5 years of age or older: a systematic review of the epidemiological evidence. Int J Obes (Lond) 33 [Suppl 3]:S1–92

66. Bellisle F, Altenburg de Assis MA, Fieux B, Preziosi P, Galan P, Guy-Grand B, et al (2001) Use of 'light' foods and drinks in French adults: biological, anthropometric and nutritional correlates. J Hum Nutr Diet 14:191–206

67. Bellisle F, Dalix AM, Mennen L, Galan P, Hercberg S, de Castro JM, et al (2003) Contribution of snacks and meals in the diet of French adults: a diet-diary study. Physiol Behav 79:183–189

68. Ebbeling CB, Sinclair KB, Pereira MA, Garcia-Lago E, Feldman HA, Ludwig DS (2004) Compensation for energy intake. from fast food among overweight and lean adolescents. JAMA 291:2828–2833

69. Rolland-Cachera MF, Bellisle F, Deheeger M (2000) Nutritional status and food intake in adolescents living in Western Europe. Eur J Clin Nutr 54 [Suppl 1]:S41–S46

70. Muller MJ, Asbeck I, Mast M, Langnase K, Grund A (2001) Prevention of obesity – more than an intention. Concept and first results of the Kiel Obesity Prevention Study (KOPS). Int J Obes Relat Metab Disord 25 [Suppl 1]:S66–S74

71. Muller MJ, Mast M, Asbeck I, Langnase K, Grund A (2001) Prevention of obesity – is it possible? Obes Rev 2:15–28

72. Flegal KM (1999) The obesity epidemic in children and adults: current evidence and research issues. Med Sci Sports Exerc 31[Suppl 11]:S509–S514

73. Strauss RS, Knight J (1999) Influence of the home environment on the development of obesity in children. Pediatrics 103:e85

74. Strauss RS (2000) Childhood obesity and self-esteem. Pediatrics 105:e15

75. Strauss RS, Pollack HA (2003) Social marginalization of overweight children. Arch Pediatr Adolesc Med 157:746–752

76. Kasper T, Korsten-Reck U, Rucker G, Jotterand S, Bös.K., Berg A (2003) Sportmotorische Fähigkeiten adipöser Kinder: Vergleich mit einem Referenzkollektiv und Erfolge des Therapieprogramms FITOC. Aktuel Ernaehr Med 28:300–307

77. Epstein LH, Coleman KJ, Myers MD (1996) Exercise in treating obesity in children and adolescents. Med Sci Sports Exerc 28:428–435

78. Epstein LH, Roemmich JN (2001) Reducing sedentary behavior: role in modifying physical activity. Exerc Sport Sci Rev 29:103–108

79. Reinehr T, Kersting M, Wollenhaupt A, Alexy U, Kling B, Strobele K, et al (2005) Evaluation of the training program "OBELDICKS" for obese children and adolescents [in German]. Klin Padiatr 217:1–8

80. Parizkova J, Maffeis C, Poskitt EM (2002) Management through activity. In: Burniat W (ed) Child and adolescent obesity. Causes and consequences; prevention and management. Cambridge: Cambridge University Press, pp 307–326

Obesity and Modern Nutrition

Volker Schusdziarra, MD, Johannes Erdmann, MD

During evolution a system of feeding regulation has emerged that is based on permanent and unpredictable energy expenditure in conjunction with varying uncertain periods of food deprivation and starvation and rather limited phases of nutrient abundance. This system is adapted to an energy density of natural foods and has never had to consider liquid calories except for a short postnatal period. Furthermore, within 3–4 decades the exponential agricultural and technical progress has led to a greater availability of food items with an overall higher energy density together with a greater variety and palatability. All these factors are the basis for a substantially greater challenge to the underlying neuroendocrine feeding regulation by cognitive and sensory mechanisms. Thus, an increasing mismatch between feeding conditions and feeding regulation has evolved. The battle of the obesity epidemic requires a multifactorial effort that has to compensate the short-comings of feeding regulation by dietary recommendations requiring great individual acceptance

4.1   Obesity – a Disease

The prevalence of overweight and obesity in most developed countries has been increasing markedly over the past 2–3 decades. The most recent survey in Germany revealed a prevalence of overweight and obesity of 66% among men and 50.6% among women [1]. The health consequences of obesity are many, ranging from an increased risk of premature death to several non-fatal but disabling conditions that impact on the immediate quality of life. Obesity is a major risk factor for cardiovascular diseases, type-2 diabetes, and cancer, where it affects not only morbidity but also mortality [2–4]. In addition, the development of many other conditions, such as gallbladder disease, hypertension, dyslipidemia, osteoarthritis, lower back pain, sleep apnea, fatty liver, steatohepatitis, and psychosocial disorders, is substantially promoted by overweight and obesity [5]. The most important health problem as a consequence of obesity is cardiovascular disease, which comprises coronary heart disease (CHD), stroke, and peripheral vascular disease. CHD and stroke account for a large proportion of deaths among men and women in most industrialized countries. Obesity predisposes to a number of cardiovascular risk factors such as hypertension, raised cholesterol, and impaired glucose tolerance but is also an independent risk factor for CHD-related morbidity and mortality [6, 7]. The association between hypertension and obesity is well-documented and concerns both systolic and diastolic blood pressure increase with BMI [8]. The risk of developing hypertension increases with the duration of obesity. While many large studies have examined the relationship between obesity and CHD, there has not been the same emphasis on stroke, but an important role of obesity in this often fatal and especially disabling disease cannot be denied [9]. A number of studies have found a positive relationship between overweight and the incidence of cancer of the colon, breast, endometrium, kidney, esophagus, gastric cardia, pancreas, gall bladder, and liver [4]. At present, the strongest empirical support for mechanisms to link obesity and cancer risk involves the metabolic and endocrine effects of obesity in the form of insulin resistance and the resulting hyperinsulinemia. The important and central role of insulin resistance as the major pathophysiological factor (◘ Fig. 4.1) becomes most evident for the positive association between obesity and type-2 diabetes mellitus [10]. Insulin resistance, defined as the inability of insulin to adequately promote glucose transport, primarily in skeletal muscle but also in other insulin-dependent organs, begins very early in the course of weight gain. An increase of 6 kg within the normal weight range is sufficient to impair glucose transport [11]. The consequence of insulin resistance is a peripheral hyperinsulinemia, which is initially due to reduced hepatic insulin clearance and switches to augmen- ted pancreatic insulin secretion with greater weight gain [11, 12]. When insulin resistance and hyperinsulinemia are associated with an appropriate genetic background, the degree of insulin resistance reaches a level that makes maintenance

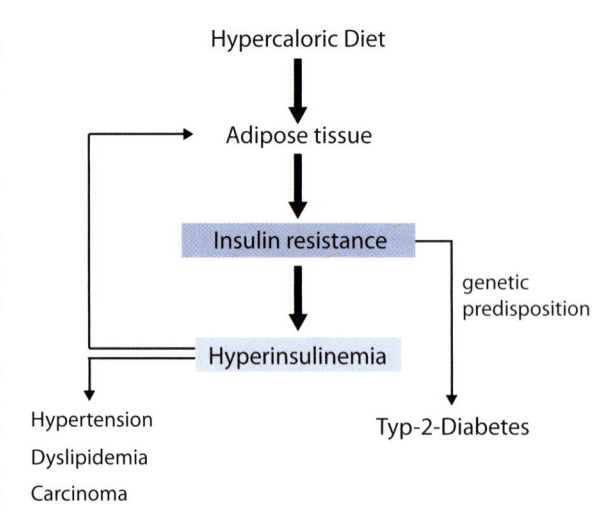

◘ **Fig. 4.1.** Relationship between hypercaloric nutrition in conjunction with the resulting increase of adipose tissue on the development of insulin resistance and hyperinsulinemia. The latter is an important pathophysiological factor for the development of various co-morbidities

4.2 · Obesity-disturbed Regulation or the Nutritional Rape of Evolution?

33   **4**

of normal glucose metabolism impossible, leading to type-2-diabetes. While knowledge about the association between body weight and the development of various disease states is extremely important, the impact of weight loss on the reduction of the aforementioned health problems is of even greater importance and cannot be overemphasized. Thus, the development of type-2 diabetes can already be substantially prevented by moderate reduction of body weight [13–15]. Furthermore, long-term weight loss with surgical treatment modalities has reduced the incidence and prevalence of type-2 diabetes threefold [16]. Moreover, total cardiovascular, diabetes- and cancer-related mortality has been shown to decrease dramatically with weight reduction [17, 18].

4.2 Obesity-disturbed Regulation or the Nutritional Rape of Evolution?

Body weight is the result of the relationship between food-related energy intake and energy expenditure. In the course of human evolution, lifestyle has changed from a struggle for survival to a striving for pleasure and leisure. The consequence of this development is evident: both overweight and obesity have reached epidemic proportions [19]. Energy expenditure by physical activity was necessary in three situations: (a) the search for nutrients, (b) flight and fight in order to avoid becoming a nutrient for other species, and (c) sexual activity to preserve the individual's species. All this was excess energy expenditure on top of the guaranteed daily energy deficit caused by the basal metabolic rate. On the other hand, adequate food intake to compensate for lost energy has never been guaranteed. Considering the obligatory amount of energy expended in the attempt to survive in relation to the uncertainty of food availability, regulation of energy balance must be extremely tight in times of deprivation and starvation. Rapid storage of the available energy surplus must be possible when food is abundant and can be life-saving in periods of starvation. In view of this ancient problem of breaking even with the daily energy balance, it seems to be more reasonable to continue feeding in times of food availability. Nevertheless, virtually all higher species feed not continuously but intermittently. Satiety is normally reached within 30–45 min after the onset of eating (◘ Fig. 4.2). This means that, at best, only 25% of the day is spent on acute food intake, and this behavior persists even after prolonged periods of negative energy balance. Thus, the interruption of acute food intake cannot be meant as a restriction to a positive energy balance. Rather, the interruption of food intake is necessary to assure a maximum of substrate and energy transfer into the organism, since optimal digestion and assimilation of nutrients requires certain time periods that cannot be shortened without any disadvantage. Thus satiety, defined as the interruption of food intake, is an important regulatory component to reach a positive energy balance and to build up fat stores if possible. Therefore, all factors involved in the regulation of feeding behavior have to be coordinated with the capacity of the gastrointestinal digestive system for a proper assimilation of ingested food, to ensure that as little energy and substrate as possible is lost in the feces. It is most reasonable that such a control system originates in the stomach, which is the ideal temporary reservoir to ensure the availability of a certain amount of energy and substrates without the organism having to be afraid of losing it to hungry competitors. Subsequently, the coordinated emptying of the gastric contents into the small intestine, depending on the intragastric reduction of particle size, adaptation of osmolarity, and adequate liquefaction, is a key function. When it is lost, as in patients with distal gastric resection, maldigestion with weight loss is a frequent problem. Once the stomach is empty, the feeding drive can return. Accordingly, the storage capacity of the stomach and the time course of digestion and absorption have to determine the extent of food ingestion and the duration of feeding interruption. In an environment where both sides of the balance, energy expenditure and food intake, were of unpredictable duration and magnitude, an overconsumption of energy followed by an increase of adipose tissue substantially assured survival. However, within an extremely short period of approximately 50 years, energy expenditure and food intake have become predictable as a consequence of an exponential technological development at least in certain parts of

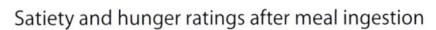

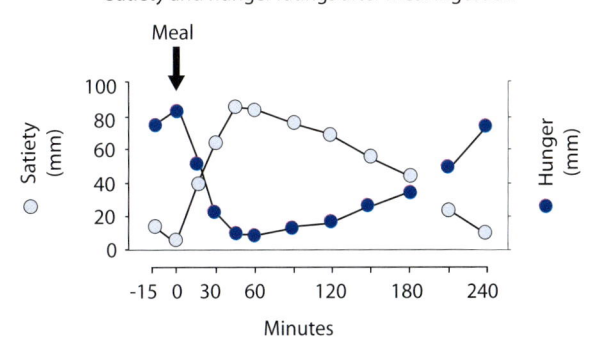

◘ **Fig. 4.2.** Satiety and hunger ratings by means of a visual analogue scale before and after the ingestion of satiating quantities of a mixed meal (mean values of 22 normal-weight subjects)

the world. Under these modern lifestyle conditions a tight limitation of energy intake could be established at no risk for survival due to excess and permanent food availability. However, this would require a modification of neuroendocrine feeding regulation that is able to counterbalance the challenges presented by the modern food supply, such as food items with high energy density that would require registration of ingested calories, regulation of liquid energy, and a great variety of foodstuffs with optimally tuned taste, texture, palatability, etc., requiring more resistance towards cognitive and sensory cues.

4.3   Regulation of Food Intake

For a proper regulation of these perturbations of hunger/satiety sensations that recur several times a day, several key structures are necessary (◘ Fig. 4.3). Satiety signals for termination of food intake originate in the gastrointestinal tract, which also contributes to the recurrence of appetite and hunger. This permits a direct and immediate modification of food intake in relation to (a) the extremely variable quality and quantity of available food items and (b) the digestive capacities required for optimal

assimilation. It is important that all these mechanisms can respond acutely to the phasic changes of feeding. A second regulatory system is required that is the mirror image of the overall nutritional and energetic state of the organism. This should ideally originate in the adipose tissue itself and permit a tonic feedback modulation of the phasic regulatory system. Finally, signals from the phasic and tonic regulatory systems must be integrated into the central nervous system, together with the very important influence of sensory and cognitive information.

4.3.1   Gastrointestinal Mechanisms

Origin of Satiety Signals. Experimental studies in animals and human beings have demonstrated that the stomach plays a major role in terminating food intake [20–25]. Except in monkeys [26], the small intestine does not generate satiety signals during physiological nutrient loads [25, 27]. Intestinal signals were observed only when supraphysiological quantities of food were infused into the small bowel of rats [28, 29] and dogs [30]. Similarly, in man, intrajejunal or intraileal infusions of lipids have been reported to reduce subsequent food intake when fat was administered into the distal small intestine at the extremely high rate

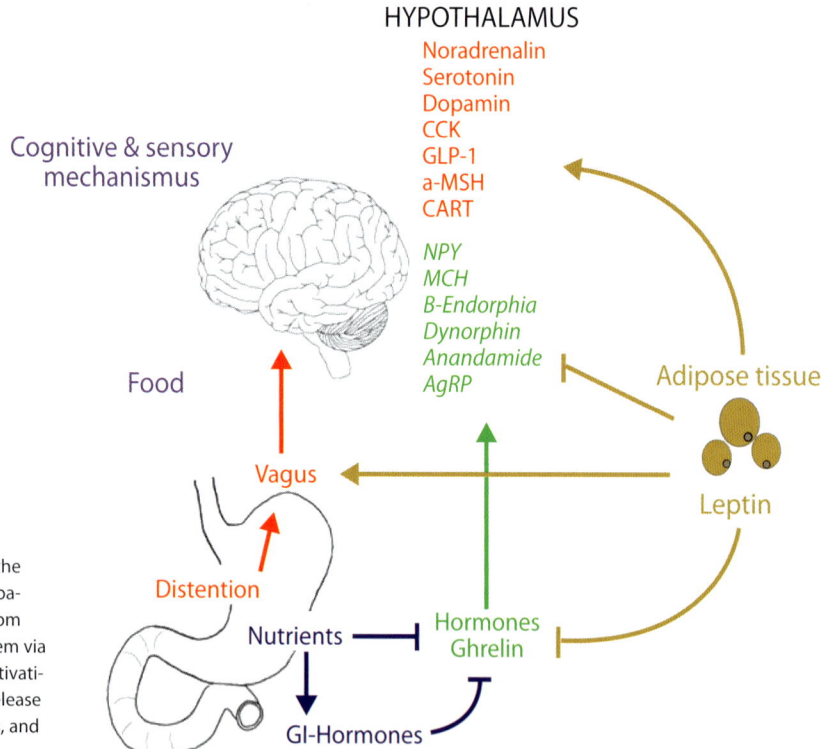

◘ **Fig. 4.3.** Mechanisms contributing to the regulation of hunger and satiety. Major pathways are (1) the signal transduction from the stomach to the central nervous system via vagal afferent fibers with subsequent activation of anorectic neuropeptides, (2) the release of ghrelin and orexigenic neuropeptides, and (3) the feedback exerted by leptin

of 3–5 kcal/min [31–33]. Such an amount of fat never reaches the lower gut under physiological conditions, since the physiological rate at which fat is emptied from the stomach is already much lower and rarely exceeds 1 kcal/min [34, 35]. Moreover, a recent study has shown that an even a high-calorie (3 kcal/min) fat infusion has no effect on food intake when given intraduodenally [36]. The fact that physiological and even supraphysiological duodenal nutrient loads do not alter food intake virtually excludes a major role of neuroendocrine signals originating in the small and large bowel, as well as postabsorptive mechanisms of circulating metabolites. Extremely important in this context is the clinical observation that patients without a stomach following surgical gastrectomy have a total lack of hunger and satiety feelings, indicating that in man, the loss of gastric regulatory systems cannot be compensated by orosensory, intestinal, pancreatic, or postabsorptive metabolic events.

Role of Distension. Distension and filling of the stomach is important for activation of satiety signals in many species. A volume of 400 ml or more is necessary to reduce food intake in man [37–39]. More recently, Rolls et al. came to similar results when administering different volumes of liquid food directly into the stomach or by increasing the volume of more natural food items in various ways [40–42].

Role of Macronutrient Composition. Apart from the role of meal size, the satiating efficacy of the three macronutrients is of great interest for dietary counseling of obese subjects, but this is a matter of debate. Fat, protein, and carbohydrates have been compared with regard to food and energy intake, extent and duration of hunger/ satiety sensations, and subsequent food intake following the respective test meals. Fat and carbohydrates were compared in three longterm studies over 14 days [43–45] in which the amount of food intake was identical. In two experimental settings energy intake was also identical [43, 44], while in one study, due to the higher energy density of the fat-rich meals, energy intake was greater and associated with weight gain [45]. In line with these long-term studies are the results of acute feeding experiments that registered satiety and hunger sensations parallel to ad libitum food intake. In these studies, no differences were observed when carbohydrate-rich pasta was compared with protein-rich meat balls [46] or when bread was compared with protein- or fat-rich meat [47], or a high-protein with a highcarbohydrate breakfast [48]. In obese subjects, ad libitum intake of satiating quantities of bread or protein-rich pork steak gave identical hunger/satiety ratings and comparable amounts of ingested food [49]. A different approach to comparing macronutrient effects is to feed a defined preload and register thereafter hunger/satiety ratings and/or subsequent food intake. Some studies have compared the effects of fat- and carbohydrate- rich preloads on an isocaloric basis. Given the varying energy densities, it is not really surprising that carbohydrate-rich food has a greater effect on satiety than fat, because of substantial differences in meal size [50– 52]. Apart from the effect of such preloads on hunger/ satiety sensations, the alteration of subsequent meal intake can be examined. When energy density is considered and the preload volume is identical, carbohydrates and fat have comparable effects on subsequent food intake when administered directly into the stomach or when ingested orally [51, 53–58]. With regard to protein-rich preloads, some studies have suggested that protein has a greater effect than carbohydrates on satiety [44; 59-62]. It must be mentioned that in three of these studies the protein preload had an effect on satiety and hunger sensations but not on subsequent food intake [44, 59, 62]. These results, however, are not confirmed by other studies that showed identical effects on hunger/satiety ratings and subsequent food intake [45–49, 52, 56, 57, 63]. In summary, the majority of data suggest that the three macronutrients have no nutrientspecific effect on satiety apart from volume or meal size. In this context it is also important to consider the time course of hunger/satiety sensations in relation to the time point of meal ingestion. It has been suggested that as long as satiety and hunger scores are still different after the preload, food intake will be reduced [50, 52] while at a later time point, when satiety is largely back to baseline, subsequent food intake is no longer different [50]. Previous reports showing that a prolonged period of hunger sensations between 30 and 120 min has no effect on subsequent food intake [64–67]. The observation made in these acute experiments can also be demonstrated in "free-living humans". The analysis of dietary protocols of overweight and obese subjects recorded during 10 consecutive days shows clearly that energy intake during dinner was virtually identical on the days with an additional afternoon snack and on those days when the same subjects had no meal between lunch and dinner and accordingly a prolonged period of greater hunger sensations and less satiety [68].

Role of Energy Density. As outlined above, the quantity of ingested food is important for the generation of satiety signals and interruption of feeding. For body weight, however, the control of energy intake would be of greater relevance. The experimental evidence suggests

4

that the energy content of a meal is not registered and accordingly acute energy intake will be tightly related to the energy density (kilocalorie per gram ingestible food) of the respective food items. Long-term studies over 14 days have shown that covertly increased energy densities of food maintaining the macronutrient ratio lead to a greater energy intake [67, 69–71] associated with a rise in body weight [67, 70]. Similarly, epidemiological studies demonstrate a strong relationship between energy intake and energy density of the consumed food [72]. Several acute short-term studies have shown that both single meal intake and total daily calorie intake were much greater with diets of greater energy density. When large portion sizes are required for a person to become satiated, the consumption of high energy-dense food will inevitably lead to a positive energy balance in most subjects [45, 73–79]. While most studies have examined the role of fat as the major contributor to high energy-dense food, several studies found similar effects with carbohydrates. The reduction of energy density by replacing sucrose with aspartame to sweeten various products led to a 25% reduction of energy intake over a period of 2 weeks [80]. Similarly, the exchange of aspartame for high-fructose corn syrup in soft drinks resulted in a reduction of energy intake and body weight over a 3-week period [81]. In this context, it is noteworthy that overconsumption and development of obesity because of protein-rich food items has never been reported. Another important finding is that excess energy intake due to a greater energy density

of meals does not change the time pattern of recurring hunger sensations, so that subsequent meal frequency will not be affected. Moreover, subsequent energy intake is not reduced by any compensatory mechanisms [47, 49, 65, 76, 82–84]. In one study a small caloric compensation was observed, but only in the lean subjects [45]. Thus, the inability to register energy density and finally the caloric content of meals prevents a tight balance of energy intake in relation to expenditure during single meals and also during one day. Accordingly, each individual has great day-to-day perturbations of energy intake which are masked in a group analysis of feeding behavior as illustrated in ◘ Fig. 4.4a. The mean values of these 250 overweight and obese subjects give the impression of tightly regulated energy intake, whereas the energy-intake data for two single subjects are characteristic for individual eating habits. A ranking of the days from those with each individual's lowest energy consumption to the day with the highest caloric intake reveals the true range of day-to-day perturbations in these 250 overweight and obese subjects (◘ Fig. 4.4b).

Role of Liquid Food and Energy-containing Beverages. The satiating effect of liquids is substantially less than that of solid food. Water has virtually no effect when served with a food but not contained in a food [40]. This is not too surprising, considering that 250 ml of water will leave the stomach within 10 min even when co-ingested with solid food [83, 85]. Nutrient-contai-

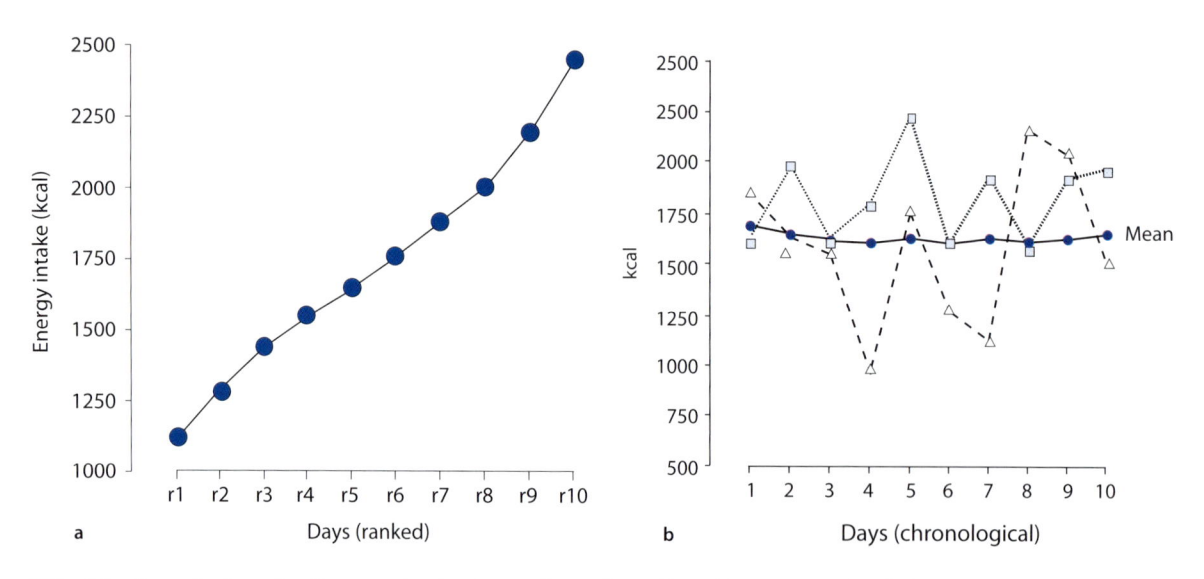

a   Days (ranked)

b   Days (chronological)

◘ **Fig. 4.4. a** Energy intake during 10 consecutive days in two obese subjects (dotted lines) compared with the mean values of a group of 250 overweight and obese subjects. **b** Energy intake of 250 overweight and obese subjects when caloric intake is ranked from the lowest (r1) to the highest value (r2) in each individual

ning (i.e., pri- marily sugar) but also alcohol-containing beverages are emptied much faster than solids. The emptying rate of sugar-containing beverages decreases with increasing osmolarity [86]. Thus, very concentrated sugar solutions will remain in the stomach longer and result in greater and prolonged distention. Studies with energy-containing liquids such as soup, soft drinks, or alcoholic beverages have shown fairly small effects on satiety ratings and food intake [87–98]. Reduction of hunger sensations by soup was approximately 10–25% of that observed after a solid meal, depending on the ingested volume but not the energy density [87]. There was little or no effect on subsequent food intake. Similarly, carbohydrate- or ethanol-containing drinks had either no or even a stimulating effect on solid food ingestion [88, 98]. A reduction of subsequent food intake of 15% was observed only after a glucose-containing liquid preload of extremely high osmolarity (75 g in 200 ml water), while other sugars or polysaccharides had no effect [89]. On the other hand, when the sugar content of beverages and also desserts is replaced with aspartame, substantial reductions of energy intake can be observed [81]. All these data demonstrate that liquid calories have no or only minor satiating effects because they bypass the regulatory effect of gastric filling and distention. Since liquid calories do not displace calories ingested in solid form, they favor high intake of excess energy and the development of obesity [97–100].

4.3.2 Signal Transduction from GI Tract to CNS

Neural Pathways. Gonzalez and Deutsch have shown that distention-induced satiety can be abolished by vagotomy while reduction of food intake as a result of the gastric nutrient content remains unaffected [101]. Furthermore, physiological stimulation of gastric functions leads to an activation of the gastric-vagal-hypothalamic axis [102]. The intragastric instillation of a meal stimulates the release of anorectic neuropeptides, as demonstrated for cholecystokinin (CCK) from neurons of the lateral hypothalamus in cats and monkeys [103, 104]. This increase is due to meal-induced gastric distention, since an identical volume of water without nutrients elicits virtually the same response [105]. On the other hand, bilateral afferent vagotomy did not change the feeding pattern and weight gain in rats studied for a period of 10 weeks [39]. The loss of neurally mediated satiety signals is probably compensated by hormonal factors.

Hormonal Mechanisms. Evidence for a hormonal mechanism of action to convey satiety signals from the peri-

phery to the central regulatory centers has been obtained in cross-perfusion experiments with rats, where blood from the fed animal reduces food intake in the fasting animal [106]. Furthermore, instillation of food into a transplanted stomach which is devoid of neural connections to the rest of the organism reduces food intake to a similar degree as does an identical nutrient load given into the natural stomach of the respective animal [107].

Anorectic Effects. This leads to the question of which hormones are responsible for the effect. Considering the gastric origin of satiety signals and the complete absence of hunger/satiety feelings in gastrectomized patients, intestinal hormones are most likely of minor or no relevance. Nevertheless, several intestinal hormones are under discussion as satiety factors. When adequate criteria of methodology were used, either by properly evaluating the doses employed or by administering a potent CCK-antagonist, there was no evidence for CCK acting as a physiological hormonal satiety factor in lean and obese human subjects [39, 108, 109]. A critical consideration of the so-called physiological effects [110, 111] of CCK reveals considerable discrepancies between physiological plasma levels and those seen after i.v. CCK. Furthermore, glucagon-like peptide 1(7-36) amide (GLP-1) has been shown to reduce food intake. GLP-1 plasma levels, however, were from 2.5 to more than 5 times higher than the physiological postprandial values [112–115], while an only twofold increase had no effect [116]. Other intestinal hormones located predominantly in the distal small bowel include peptide YY (PYY) and oxyntomodulin. Both peptides reduce food intake when given intravenously to normal-weight and/or obese subjects [117; 118]. Oxyntomodulin was given at a dose that led to a 600% increase over postprandial levels. The PYY infusion also increased plasma levels to clearly supraphysiological concentrations (+134% in lean and +307% in obese subjects). Although all of the aforementioned gastrointestinal hormones are extremely weak candidates as physiological regulators of feeding behavior, this does not exclude their potential usefulness as pharmacological tools in the management of obesity. Promising evidence in this direction has been reported recently [119]. Insulin has been proposed to be a regulator of energy balance [120], based mainly on studies in rats and baboons. It should be noted that very high and clearly supraphysiological levels of plasma insulin are required for small changes (~Δ 2–3 µU/ml) of CSF insulin with a lag period of more than 2 h [121]. Further arguments against a physiological role of insulin as a satiety factor in man are derived from the aforementioned studies on intestinal nutrient loads, which have no effect on satiety but profoundly stimulate insulin release [39]. In addition, the numerous studies that have compared the satiating efficacy of macronutrients did not find any difference, although it can be assumed that the carbohydrate meals employed elicited a greater insulin response compared with protein or fat [45–49, 53–58, 63]. This is illustrated in ▢ Fig. 4.5. The two meals with different quantity but an identical macronutrient ratio elicit an almost comparable insulin response, while satiety feelings are much greater in response to the high-volume load.

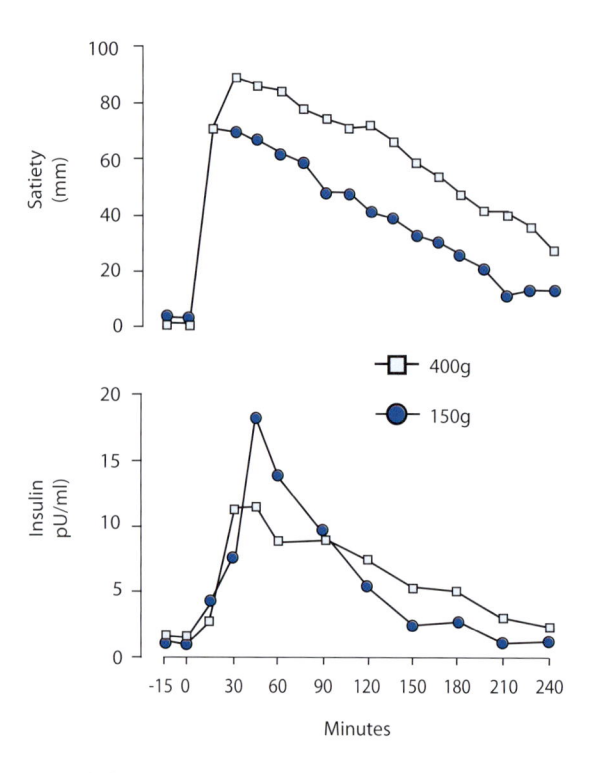

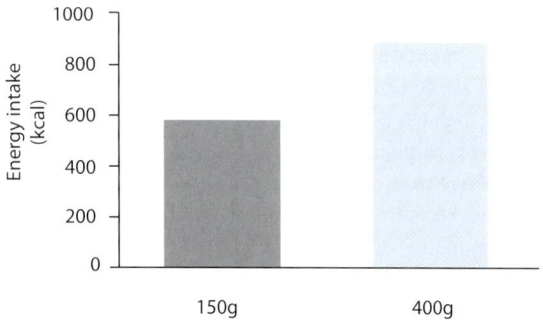

▢ **Fig. 4.5.** Ingestion of two meals with identical macronutrient ratios but different quantities of 150 g and 400 g, respectively, by ten normal-weight subjects. As expected, satiety was greater with the larger meal, while peak insulin was even lower and total integrated insulin over the 4-h period was not different

Orexigenic Effects. For two to three decades there was an intensive search for gastrointestinal hormones with anorectic properties, and ghrelin has recently been added to the list of hormonal feeding regulators [122]. Ghrelin, however, stimulates appetite and food intake following peripheral and intracerebroventricular administration [123, 124]. Plasma levels decrease following the ingestion of a meal, returning back to baseline during the later postprandial and interdigestive phase [125, 126]. The initial decrease of ghrelin could support vagally mediated initiation of satiety signals, and later on, the rise of ghrelin could stimulate appetite and food intake again. The evidence for a contribution of ghrelin to the generation of acute satiety is rather poor. First, in contrast to carbohydrate-rich meals, protein-, fat- and vegetable-rich meals can stimulate ghrelin levels [47, 49], while hunger and satiety ratings are identical. Second, trough levels of ghrelin occur approximately 60 min later than maximal satiety. Third, gastric distention, which is important for the satiating effect of a meal, does not contribute to the suppression of ghrelin [127]. The contribution of ghrelin to the recurrence of appetite and hunger in the later postprandial phase could be of greater relevance, and this is supported by correlations [47, 128, 129] which, however, do not prove a causal relationship. There is evidence for a contribution of endogenous ghrelin to the regulation of feeding behavior and body weight, since studies in mice demonstrated an attenuation of food intake and weight gain by a ghrelin receptor antagonist [130]. On the other hand, a stimulation of food intake in man has been accomplished only with i.v. ghrelin in doses that stimulate growth hormone secretion. Since growth hormone does not rise after a meal, such doses have to be considered supraphysiological and, accordingly, conclusive evidence for a physiological relevance of plasma ghrelin levels has to be obtained in further experimental studies.

4.3.3   Central Mechanisms

The hypothalamus is the integrative center of feeding behavior. Several hypothalamic loci have been identified that contribute substantially to feeding regulation. These comprise the arcuate nucleus (ARC), the ventromedial (VMN) and dorsomedial (DMN) nuclei, the paraventricular nucleus (PVN), and the lateral hypothalamic area (LH). The neuronal connections to extrahypothalamic sites provide the anatomical basis for the functionally important modification of feeding behavior by sensory cues (taste, smell, sight) and cognitive mechanisms (for a detailed review see [131–133]).

The role of individual neurotransmitters and neuropeptides as important regulators of feeding behavior has experienced a dramatic shift over the past 20 years. With the discovery of new peptides, the older "most important regulators of feeding behavior" became of minor interest. ◻ Table 4.1 summarizes the neurotransmitters and neuropeptides that are of physiological relevance for the suppression of food intake (for review see [134]). The recognition of physiological importance is based on the effect of neuropeptides exogenously administered directly into the central nervous system (CNS) and the production of the inverse effect following administration of a specific receptor antagonist or a specific secretagogue, which suggests that the respective endogenously released neuropeptides exert similar effects. Comparable to the anorectic group, there is a group of orexigenic substances with good evidence for a physiological role in stimulating food intake (◻ Table 4.1). Central Neuropeptide Interaction Prevents Overactivation of Satiety Signals. Since permanent energy expenditure is a mandatory condition for staying alive, the feeding drive is of much greater relevance for survival than are satiety signals. Thus augmentation of satiety signals should be as short as necessary and the time course of recurrent hunger and appetite sensations should be adequately balanced by a functional interaction between anorectic and orexigenic neuropeptides. This notion is supported by several lines of evidence. The release of anorectic neuropeptides prevents a too rapid recurrence of hunger and exaggerated food intake, which can be demonstrated by blockade of GLP-1 receptors [135]. Loss of orexigenic counter-regulation, on the other hand, augments feeding inhibition as shown in chronic NPY-deficient mice in whom the anorectic effect of leptin is augmented [136]. Therefore, it is not too surprising that the influence of feeding inhibitors such as GLP-1 and xenin is compensated by a prompt activation of counter-regulatory orexigenic neuropeptides such as NPY and endogenous opioids, preventing an exaggerated inhibition of food intake. When the concentration of feeding inhibitors exceeds a certain threshold, counter-regulatory mechanisms are still operative but not sufficient to maintain feeding, which finally results in interruption of food intake [137].

4.4 Adipose Tissue and Tonic Control

The acute control of food intake by the gastrointestinal tract and the hypothalamus is intended to recruit as much energy and substrate as possible for the preservation of life. In the rather unlikely evolutionary situation of a prolonged or – as nowadays – even permanent positive energy balance the magnitude of overweight could have made the organism vulnerable in terms of fight and flight. Thus, a certain feedback should exist between the nutritional state and the acute phasic feeding regulation. The fat cell mass of the adipose tissue is the mirror image of the body´s energy balance. Any relevant information about energy abundance or deficit and the ongoing tendencies in either direction should ideally originate in the adipose tissue. All factors secreted from fat cells in an amount sufficient to increase their plasma concentrations are potential candidates to modify gastrointestinal satiety signals as well as CNS neurotransmitter activity.

◻ Table 4.1. Neurotransmitters and neuropeptides with anorectic or orexigenic activity following intracerebroventricular administration or direct application into various hypothalamic loci. Substances are considered physiologically relevant when the effect of exogenously applied factors can be mimicked by specific receptor blockade or selective secretagogues to verify the role of the respective endogenous substance

Physiological relevance	
Anorectic	**Orexigenic**
Norepinephrine	Neuropeptide Y (NPY)
Serotonin	Endogenous opioid peptides (ß-endorphin, dynorphin, enkephalins)
Dopamine	Melanin-concentrating hormone (MCH)
Cholecystokinin (CCK)	Ghrelin
Glucagon-like peptide 1 (GLP-1)	Gamma aminobutyric acid (GABA)
α-Melanocyte-stimulating hormone (α-MSH)	Anandamide (= cannabinoid CB-1 receptor agonist)
Cocaine- and amphetamine-regulated transcript (CART)	Agouti-related protein (AgRP)

The existence, the importance, but also the limitations of such a tonic feedback control are demonstrated by the physiology and pathophysiology of leptin (for review see [138]. Leptin is predominantly produced in and secreted from white adipose tissue in proportion to the number of fat cells. Obese subjects show higher plasma leptin concentrations than lean subjects, and changes of body weight are associated with the respective shift of circulating leptin [139]. Circulating levels of leptin do not change acutely in response to ingested food, however, which supports the concept that leptin is a tonic rather than an acute satiety factor. Leptin plays a major role in the regulation of body weight since leptin deficiency leads to a dramatic weight gain both in animals and in man [138, 140]. Evidence from morphological and functional studies demonstrates that leptin can modulate feeding via three pathways (see ◘ Fig. 4.3). First, leptin can modulate food intake via interaction with the vagal afferent neuroendocrine signaling that originates in the stomach [141; 142]. Second, leptin interacts with a large number of neurons that are involved in the hypothalamic regulation of feeding behavior [143]. Third, leptin is a potent inhibitor of the gastric appetite-stimulating hormone ghrelin [144]. On the other hand, leptin's regulatory role seems to be limited in obesity. Mice becoming obese on a high-fat, energy-dense diet develop the expected hyperleptinemia which is associated with an up-regulation of melanocortin- 4 receptors mediating the anorectic effect of α-MSH and a reduced activity of orexigenic transmitter systems. Despite this obviously intact feedback regulation between leptin and the central transmitter system, it cannot prevent the development of obesity with an energy-dense diet [145]. Furthermore, the vast majority of obese human beings have elevated concentrations of leptin, which apparently does not function properly. This would suggest that leptin exerts an inadequate effect on the stimulation of anorectic or suppression of orexigenic signals or a combination of both. In man, the effect of leptin on vagal afferents and CNS neuropeptide activity is difficult to examine. Therefore, the interaction between leptin and ghrelin could give some more insight into this problem, provided the leptin-ghrelin interaction is the mirror image of the other regulatory pathways of leptin. In a large cohort of normal-weight and obese subjects with comparably low basal insulin concentrations there was a good inverse correlation between basal leptin and ghrelin levels [146]. The inverse relationship between ghrelin and leptin reached a plateau at basal leptin concentrations of ~10 ng/ml, corresponding to BMI 28 kg/ m², which could reflect the upper margin of the evolutionarily relevant weight range. Thus, leptin seems to be a potent regulator of feeding signals at normal body weight. It should be considered that body weight has most likely been more in the range of BMI 20 kg/m² for millions of years and there has never been a real demand for a control system at BMI levels above 30 kg/m². This might be at least one possible explanation for the apparent "leptin resistance" in the vast majority of obese subjects.

4.5   The Power of Cognitive and Sensory Mechanisms

Feeding is not only the consequence of internal neuroendocrine mechanisms; it is also a behavior. On the one hand, behavior is motivated by the physiological requirements; on the other hand, behavior can dominate neuroendocrine physiology. Behavior comprises a number of cognitive and sensory mechanisms that can modify the basic internal regulatory loop. Thus, feeding is not only a reflex mechanism that is automatically activated when hunger arises. Despite more or less intense hunger or satiety sensations, most subjects can voluntarily override such internal signals in either direction. Major factors in this context are taste, texture, portion size, palatability, novelty, and variety of food. Apart from these meal-related factors, time of the day and emotional and social influences are of great importance. The question whether cognitive or neuroendocrine regulation of appetite is more dominant has been a matter of debate for several years. In this context it is interesting to note that highly palatable fat-rich and especially sweet food items stimulate neuropeptides such as endogenous opioids and NPY [147–149], which override satiety signals and prolong food intake. From experience in daily life we know that taste is a major determinant for food selection. This includes the chemical senses of taste and olfaction, the perception of texture and the overall pleasantness. All these factors are influenced by sociocultural and economic variables, gender, age, and body weight [150]. The pleasantness of a food is relevant because it does not remain constant. Repeated or prolonged consumption of a food can lead to a decrease in its pleasantness, while other food items uneaten for some time period appear to be more pleasant. In an environment with a great selection among a variety of foods, this has great impact on overall intake [151]. Similarly, taste and smell, as well as knowledge about certain foods with regard to their nutrient composition, will affect intake [150, 152]. Portion sizes, especially those of packaged snacks, can modify intake substantially, since most items are consumed completely [153]. Social environment is another important factor that can modify food intake. Even in 24-h food-deprived subjects the hunger sensations are considerably affected by social factors [154]. And we have to keep in mind that 24-h food deprivation is an extremely rare situation. These findings thus support the concept that behavior dominates physiology. Also, the number of people present during meal ingestion is of considerable importance. Meal size increased by as much as 40% when eaten in a group compared with a meal eaten alone. This effect is due primarily to an increase in the duration of meals rather than an increase in the rate of intake of the meal [154]. Due to our hedonistic attitude, we always attempt to prolong the rewarding sensation of satiety as much as possible. The necessity of restricting energy intake in relation to the progressively decreasing energy expenditure requires a learning process that is difficult, to some degree painful, and it challenges all the positive aspects of eating. All these environmental changes are extremely new; accordingly, no regulatory systems exist to automatically cope with this challenge.

4.6   Implication for Obesity Treatment

The major reasons for an increased energy intake are: (a) food items with high energy density; (b) liquid energycontaining beverages; (c) a great variety of foodstuffs with optimally tuned taste, texture, palatability, etc.; and (d) high meal frequency. Especially these aspects have to be considered if eating behavior is to be changed successfully, and they must be combined with a satiating amount of food that matches the taste preferences of the individual patient and guarantees a hypocaloric food intake for long-term weight loss and maintenance of reduced body weight. The latter is the most crucial problem of non-surgical treatment concepts [155]. The analysis of 29 studies with either a mixed hypocaloric diet or very low calorie formula diets (VLCD) has demonstrated that a substantial amount of weight regain occurred within the first 2 years following the end of the treatment period. It must be noted that at this time point less than 50% of the patients were available for follow-up; after 5 years less than 10% were recorded. This indicates that we do not know very much about the long-term success of non-surgical weight-reduction programs. One major problem of these treatment concepts is the limited time frame during which patients can get advice. In our outpatient setting patients can come for dietary advice as long as they feel that it is advantageous. In general, the recommended time period between visits is 4 weeks. Dietary changes are based on the energy density (ED) of the va-

rious food items [68]. An ED of 1.5 kcal/g is considered the upper limit for food items that can be consumed in largely unlimited quantity. These are the food items for satiation. Food of higher ED is not forbidden but should not be consumed in satiating quantities, since this would inevitably jeopardize a hypocaloric diet for weight loss. To change their eating behavior patients should largely maintain the food quantity to feel satiated. In case snacks between main meals are consumed for reasons other than feeling hungry, they are advised to reduce snacks. If this is not possible for whatever reason they are told to reduce the ED, since most snacks have an ED well above the recommended limit of 1.5 kcal/g. Furthermore, they should avoid liquid calories as much as possible. With this concept, 467 patients were treated between 2003 and 2006; 40% of the patients had BMI ≥40 kg/ m2. They consulted the nutrition center over an average treatment period of 7.4 months. During this time they lost 4.0 +0.34 kg. For 366 patients (78.4%) follow-up information was obtained. After a mean follow-up period of 26 months weight loss was 7.0 +0.54 kg. The subgroup of 129 type-2 diabetics was treated over 10.4 +1.2 months with a weight reduction of -5.7 +0.7 kg. Of the diabetic patients, 108 (82%) were followed over 22 +1.2 months with a weight loss of -10 +0.9 kg; 25% of these patients injected 30–200 U of insulin per day. At follow-up only eight patients had insulin on demand when postprandial blood glucose exceeded 250 mg/dl. All in all, these data demonstrate that long-term weight loss is feasible even in grossly obese subjects without surgical intervention in the perspective of our modern food supply, when the shortcomings of our system of feeding regulation are counterbalanced as much as possible by adequate dietary counseling. This can lead to long-term changes in individual eating habits. Such a learning process can be supported by new strategies of food production, helping to provide less energy-dense food that is still compatible with the hedonistic expectations of overweight and obese subjects.

References

1. Bundesministerium für Ernährung, Landwirtschaft und Verbraucherschutz-Max Rubner-Institut (2008) Nationale Verzehrs-Studie II-Ergebnisbericht, Teil 1. Berlin
2. Calle EE, Thun MJ, Petrelli JM, Rodriguez C, Heath CW jr (1999) Body-mass index and mortality in a prospective cohort of US adults. N Engl J Med 341:1097–1105
3. Adams KF, Schatzkin A, Harris TB, Kipnis V, Mouw T, Ballard-Barbash R, Hollenbeck A, Leitzmann MF (2006) Overweight, obesity, and mortality in a large prospective cohort of persons 50 to 71 years old. N Engl J Med 355:763–778

4. Calle EE, Rodriquez C, Walker-Thurmond K, Thun MJ (2003) Overweight, obesity and mortality from cancer in a prospectively studied cohort of US adults. N Engl J Med 348:1625–1638

5. Van Itallie TB (1985) Health implications of overweight and obesity in the United States. Ann Intern Med 103:983–988

6. Hubert HB, Feinleib M, McNamara PM, Castelli WP (1983) Obesity as an independent risk factor for cardiovascular disease: a 26-year follow-up of participants in the Framingham Heart Study. Circulation 67:968–977

7. Jousilahti P, Tuomilehto J, Vartiainen E, Pekkanen J, Puska P (1996) Body weight, cardiovascular risk factors, and coronary mortality. 15-year follow-up of middle-aged men and women in eastern Finland. Circulation 93:1372–1379

8. Stamler R, Stamler J, Riedlinger WF, Algera G, Roberts RH (1978) .Weight and blood pressure. Findings in hypertension screening of 1 million Americans. JAMA 240:1607–1610

9. Abbott RD, Behrens GR, Sharp DS, Rodriquez BL, Burchfiel CM, Ross GW, Yano K, Curb JD (1994) Body mass index and thromboembolic stroke in nonsmoking men in older middle age. The Honolulu Heart Program. Stroke 25:2370–2376

10. Colditz GA, Willett WC, Stampfer MJ, Manson JE, Hennekens CH, Arky RA, Speizer FE (1990) Weight as a risk factor for clinical diabetes in women. Am J Epidemiol 132:501–513

11. Erdmann J, Kallabis B, Oppel U, Sypchenko O, Wagenpfeil S, Schusdziarra V (2008) Development of hyperinsulinemia and insulin resistance during the early stage of weight gain. Am J Physiol Endo Met 294:E568–E575

12. Erdmann J, Mayr M, Oppel U, Sypchenko O, Wagenpfeil S, Schusdziarra V (2009) Weight-dependent differential contribution of insulin secretion and clearance to hyperinsulinemia of obesity. Regul Pept 152:1–7

13. Fujimoto WY (2000) Background and recruitment data for the US. Diabetes Prevention Program. Diabetes Care 23 [Suppl 2]: B11–B13

14. Knowler WC, Barrett-Connor E, Fowler SE, Hamman RF, Lachin JM, Walker EA, Nathan DM (2002) Reduction in the incidence of type 2 diabetes with lifestyle intervention or metformin. N Engl J Med 346:393–403

15. Knowler WC, Hamman RF, Edelstein SL, Barrett-Connor E, Ehrmann DA, Walker EA, Fowler SE, Nathan DM, Kahn SE (2005) Prevention of type 2 diabetes with troglitazone in the Diabetes Prevention Program. Diabetes 54:1150–1156

16. Sjostrom L, Lindroos AK, Peltonen M, Torgerson J, Bouchard C, Carlsson B, Dahlgren S, Larsson B, Narbro K, Sjostrom CD, Sullivan M, Wedel H (2004) Lifestyle, diabetes, and cardiovascular risk factors 10 years after bariatric surgery. N Engl J Med 351:2683–2693

17. Adams TD, Gress RE, Smith SC, Halverson RC, Simper SC, Rosamond WD, Lamonte MJ, Stroup AM, Hunt SC (2007) Long-term mortality after gastric bypass surgery. N Engl J Med 357:753–761

18. Sjostrom L, Narbro K, Sjostrom CD, Karason K, Larsson B, Wedel H, Lystig T, Sullivan M, Bouchard C, Carlsson B, Bengtsson C, Dahlgren S, Gummesson A, Jacobson P, Karlsson J, Lindroos AK, Lonroth H, Naslund I, Olbers T, Stenlof K, Torgerson J, Agren G, Carlsson LM (2007) Effects of bariatric surgery on mortality in Swedish obese subjects. N Engl J Med 357:741–752

19. WHO (2000) Obesity: preventing and managing the global epidemic. Report of a WHO consultation. World Health Organ Tech Rep Ser 894:1–253

20. Janowitz HD, Grossman M (1948) Some factors affecting food intake of normal dogs and dogs with esophagostomy and gastric fistulas. Am J Physiol 159:143–148

21. Mook D (1963) Oral and postingestional determinants of the intake of various solutions in rats with esophageal fistulas. J Comp Physiol Psychol 56:645–659

22. Young RC, Gibbs J, Antin J, Holt J, Smith GP (1974) Absence of satiety during sham feeding in the rat. J Comp Physiol Psychol 87:795–800

23. Deutsch JA, Young WG, Kalogern TJ (1978) The stomach signals satiety. Science 201:165–167

24. Kraly FS, Smith GP (1978) Combined pregastric and gastric stimulation by food is sufficient for normal meal size. Physiol Behav 21:405–408

25. Schick RR, Schusdziarra V, Schröder B, Classen M (1991) Effect of intraduodenal or intragastric nutrient infusion on food intake in man. Z Gastroenterol 29:637–641

26. Gibbs J, Maddison SP, Rolls ET (1981) Satiety role of the small intestine examined in sham-feeding rhesus monkeys. J Comp Physiol Psychol 95:1003–1015

27. Koopmans HS (1975) Jejunal signals in hunger satiety. Behav Biol 14:309–324

28. Greenberg D, Smith GP, Gibbs J (1990) Intraduodenal infusions of fats elicit satiety in sham-feeding rats. Am J Physiol 259:R1-10–R118

29. Liebling DS, Eisner JD, Gibbs J, Smith GP (1975) Intestinal satiety in rats. J.Comp Physiol Psychol 89:955–965

30. Hill RG, Ison EC, Jones WW, Archdeacon JW (1952) The small intestine as a factor in regulation of eating. Am J Physiol 170:201–205

31. Welch IM, Saunders K, Read NW (1985) Effect of ileal and intravenous infusions of fat emulsions on feeding and satiety in human volunteers. Gastroenterology 89:1293–1297

32. Welch IM, Sepple CP, Read NW (1988) Comparisons of the effects on satiety and eating behaviour of infusion of lipid into the different regions of the small intestine. Gut 29:306–311

33. Drewe J, Gadient A, Rovati LC, Beglinger C (1992) Role of circulating cholecystokinin in control of fat-induced inhibition of food intake in humans. Gastroenterology 102:1654–1659

34. Hunt JN, Stubbs RJ (1975) The volume and energy content of meals as determinants of gastric emptying. J Physiol 245:209–225

35. McHugh PR, Moran TH (1979) Calories and gastric emptying: a regulatory capacity with implications for feeding. Am J Physiol 236:R254–R260

36. Oesch S, Degen L, Beglinger C (2005) Effect of a protein preload on food intake and satiety feelings in response to duodenal fat perfusions in healthy male subjects. Am J Physiol Regul Integr Comp Physiol 289:R1042–R1047

37. Geliebter A (1988) Gastric distention and gastric capacity in relation to food intake in humans. Physiol Behav 44:665–668

38. Geliebter A, Westreich S, Gage D (1988) Gastric distention by balloon and test-meal intake in obese and lean subjects. Am J Clin Nutr 48:592–594

39. Schick RR, Schusdziarra V (1994) Regulation of food intake. In: Ditschuneit H, Gries FA, Hauner H, Schusdziarra V, Wechsler JG (eds) Obesity in Europe 1993. John Libbey, London, pp 335–348

40. Rolls BJ, Bell EA, Thorwart ML (1999) Water incorporated into a food but not served with a food decreases energy intake in lean women. Am J Clin Nutr 70:448–455

41. Rolls BJ, Bell EA, Waugh BA (2000) Increasing the volume of a food by incorporating air affects satiety in men. Am J Clin Nutr 72:361-368

42. Rolls BJ, Castellanos VH, Halford JC, Kilara A, Panyam D, Pelkman CL, Smith GP, Thorwart ML (1998) Volume of food consumed affects satiety in men. Am J Clin Nutr 67:1170–1177

43. van Stratum P, Lussenburg RN, van Wezel LA, Vergroesen AJ, Cremer HD The effect of dietary carbohydrate:fat ratio on energy intake by adult women. Am J Clin Nutr (1978) 31:206–212

44. Stubbs RJ, van Wyk MC, Johnstone AM, Harbron CG (1996) Breakfasts high in protein, fat or carbohydrate: effect on within-day appetite and energy balance. Eur.J.Clin.Nutr 50:409–417

45. Lissner L, Levitsky DA, Strupp BJ, Kackwarf H, Roe DA (1987) Dietary fat and the regulation of energy intake in human subjects. Am J Clin Nutr 46:886–892

46. Porrini M, Crovetti R, Testolin G, Silva S (1995) Evaluation of satiety sensations and food intake after different preloads. Appetite 25:17–30

47. Erdmann J, Töpsch R, Lippl F, Gussmann P, Schusdziarra V (2004) Postprandial response of plasma ghrelin levels to various test meals in relation to food intake, plasma insulin and glucose. J Clin Endocrinol Metab 89:3048–3054

48. Blom WA, Lluch A, Stafleu A, Vinoy S, Holst JJ (2006) Effect of a high-protein breakfast on the postprandial ghrelin response. Am J Clin Nutr 84:664–665

49. Erdmann J, Leibl M, Wagenpfeil S, Lippl F, Schusdziarra V (2006) Ghrelin response to protein and carbohydrate meals in relation to food intake and glycerol levels in obese subjects. Regul Pept 135:23–29

50. Blundell JE, Burley VJ, Cotton JR, Lawton CL (1993) Dietary fat and the control of energy intake: evaluating the effects of fat on meal size and postmeal satiety. Am J Clin Nutr 57:772S–777S

51. Holt SH, Miller JC, Petocz P, Farmakalidis E (1995) A satiety index of common foods. Eur J Clin Nutr 49:675–690

52. Rolls BJ, Hetherington M, Burley VJ (1988) The specificity of satiety: the influence of foods of different macronutrient content on the development of satiety. Physiol Behav 43:145–153

53. Cecil JE, Castiglione K, French S, Francis J, Read NW (1998) Effects of intragastric infusions of fat and carbohydrate on appetite ratings and food intake from a test meal. Appetite 30:65–77

54. Shide DJ, Caballero B, Reidelberger R, Rolls BJ (1995) Accurate energy compensation for intragastric and oral nutrients in lean males. Am J Clin Nutr 61:754–764

55. Rolls BJ, Kim S, McNelis AL, Fischman MW, Foltin RW, Moran TH (1991) Time course of effects of preloads high in fat or carbohydrate on food intake and hunger ratings in humans. Am J Physiol 260:R756–R763

56. Vozzo R, Wittert G, Cocchiaro C, Tan WC, Mudge J, Fraser R, Chapman I (2003) Similar effects of foods high in protein, carbohydrate and fat on subsequent spontaneous food intake in healthy individuals. Appetite 40:101–107

57. de Graaf C, Hulshof T, Weststrate JA, Jas P (1992) Short-term effects of different amounts of protein, fats, and carbohydrates on satiety. Am J Clin Nutr 55:33–38

58. Driver CJ (1988) The effect of meal composition on the degree of satiation following a test meal and possible mechanisms involved. Br J Nutr 60:441–449

59. Hill AJ, Blundell JE (1986) Macronutrients and satiety: the effects of a high-protein or high carbohydrate meal on subjective motivation to eat and food preferences. Nutr Behav 3:133–144

60. Latner JD, Schwartz M (1999) The effects of a high-carbohydrate, high-protein or balanced lunch upon later food intake and hunger ratings. Appetite 33:119–128

61. Poppitt SD, McCormack D, Buffenstein R (1998) Short-term effects of macronutrient preloads on appetite and energy intake in lean women. Physiol Behav 64:279–285

62. Marmonier C, Chapelot D, Fantino M, Louis-Sylvestre J (2002) Snacks consumed in a non-hungry state have poor satiating efficiency: influence of snack composition on substrate utilization and hunger. Am J Clin Nutr 76:518–528

63. Geliebter AA (1979) Effects of equicaloric loads of protein, fat, and carbohydrate on food intake in the rat and man. Physiol Behav 22:267–273

64. Melanson KL, Westerterp MS, Saris WHM, Campfield A (1997) Meal initiation in human isolated from time cues: role of plasma glucose, macronutrient ingestion and dietary restraint. Int J Obes Relat Metab Disord 21:S77

65. Erdmann J, Hebeisen Y, Lippl F, Schusdziarra V (2007) Inverse plasma ghrelin response to potatoes does not impair its beneficial effect on energy intake and insulin release compared to rice and pasta. Eur J Nutr 46:196–203

66. Ball SD, Keller KR, Moyer-Mileur LJ, Ding YW, Donaldson D, Jackson WD (2003) Prolongation of satiety after low versus moderately high glycemic index meals in obese adolescents. Pediatrics 111:488–494

67. Stubbs RJ, Johnstone AM, O'Reilly LM, Barton K, Reid C (1998) The effect of covertly manipulating the energy density of mixed diets on ad libitum food intake in ,pseudo free-living' humans. Int J Obes Relat Metab Disord 22:980–987

68. Schusdziarra V, Hausmann M (2007)Satt essen und abnehmen. MMI-Verlag, Neuisenburg

69. Stubbs RJ, Johnstone AM, Harbron CG, Reid C (1998) Covert manipulation of energy density of high carbohydrate diets in 'pseudo free-living' humans. Int J Obes Relat Metab Disord 22:885–892

70. Stubbs RJ, Ritz P, Coward WA, Prentice AM (1995) Covert manipulation of the ratio of dietary fat to carbohydrate and energy density: effect on food intake and energy balance in free-living men eating ad libitum. Am J Clin Nutr 62:330–337

71. Stubbs RJ, Harbron CG, Murgatroyd PR, Prentice AM (1995) Covert manipulation of dietary fat and energy density: effect on substrate flux and food intake in men eating ad libitum. Am J Clin Nutr 62:316–329

72. Poppitt SD, Prentice AM (1996) Energy density and its role in the control of food intake: evidence from metabolic and community studies. Appetite 26:153–174

73. Rolls BJ, Bell EA (1999) Intake of fat and carbohydrate: role of energy density. Eur J Clin Nutr 53 [Suppl 1]:S166–S173

74. Rolls BJ, Roe LS, Meengs JS (2004) Salad and satiety: energy density and portion size of a first-course salad affect energy intake at lunch. J Am Diet Assoc 104:1570–1576

75. Kral TV, Rolls BJ (2004) Energy density and portion size: their independent and combined effects on energy intake. Physiol Behav 82:131–138

76. Spiegel TA (1973) Caloric regulation of food intake in man. J Comp Physiol Psychol 84:24–37

77. Duncan KH, Bacon JA, Weinsier RL (1983) The effects of high and low energy density diets on satiety, energy intake, and eating time of obese and nonobese subjects. Am J Clin Nutr 37:763–767

78. Campbell RG, Hashim SA, Van Itallie TB (1971) Studies of food intake regulation in man: responses to variations in nutritive density in lean and obese subjects. N Engl J Med 285:1402–1407

79. Devitt AA, Mattes RD (2004) Effects of food unit size and energy density on intake in humans. Appetite 42:213–220

80. Porikos KP, Booth G, Van Itallie TB (1977) Effect of covert nutritive dilution on the spontaneous food intake of obese individuals: a pilot study. Am J Clin Nutr 30:1638–1644

81. Tordoff MG, Alleva AM (1990) Effect of drinking soda sweetened with aspartame or high-fructose corn syrup on food intake and body weight. Am J Clin Nutr 51:963–969

82. Himaya A, Fantino M, Antoine JM, Brondel L, Louis-Sylvestre J (1997) Satiety power of dietary fat: a new appraisal. Am J Clin Nutr 65:1410–1418

83. Malagelada JR (1977) Quantification of gastric solid-liquid discrimination during digestion of ordinary meals. Gastroenterology 72:1264–1267

84. Green SM, Burley VJ, Blundell JE (1994) Effect of fat- and sucrose-containing foods on the size of eating episodes and energy intake in lean males: potential for causing overconsumption. Eur J Clin Nutr 48:547–555

85. Malagelada JR, Go VLW, Summerskill WHL (1979) Different gastric, pancreatic, and biliary responses to solid-liquid or homogenized meals. Dig Dis Sci 24:101–110

86. Hunt JN, Smith JL, Liang C (1985) Effect of meal volume and energy density on the gastric emptying of carbohydrates. Gastroenterology 89:1326–1330

87. Gray R, French S, Robinson T, Yeomans M (2002) Dissociation of the effects of preload volume and energy content on subjective appetite and food intake. Physiol Behav 76:57–64

88. Mattes RD (1996) Dietary compensation by humans for supplemental energy provided as ethanol or carbohydrate in fluids. Physiol Behav 59:179–187

89. Anderson GH, Catherine NL, Woodend DM, Wolever TM (2002) Inverse association between the effect of carbohydrates on blood glucose and subsequent short-term food intake in young men. Am J Clin Nutr 76:1023–1030

90. Himaya A, Louis-Sylvestre J (1998) The effect of soup on satiation. Appetite 30:199–210

91. Mattes RD, Rothacker D (2001) Beverage viscosity is inversely related to postprandial hunger in humans. Physiol Behav 74:551–557

92. Tournier A, Louis-Sylvestre J (1991) Effect of the physical state of a food on subsequent intake in human subjects. Appetite 16:17–24

93. Haber GB, Heaton KW, Murphy D, Burroughs LF (1977) Depletion and disruption of dietary fibre. Effects on satiety, plasma-glucose, and serum-insulin. Lancet 2:679–682

94. Hulshof T, de Graaf C, Weststrate JA (1993) The effects of preloads varying in physical state and fat content on satiety and energy intake. Appetite 21:273–286

95. Porrini M, Corvetti R, Riso P, Santangelo A, Testolin G (1995) Effects of physical and chemical characteristics of food on specific and general satiety. Physiol Behav 57:461–468

96. Di Meglio DP, Mattes (2000) RD Liquid versus solid carbohydrate: effects on food intake and body weight. Int J Obes 24:794–800

97. De Castro JM (1993) The effects of the spontaneous ingestion of particular foods or beverages on the meal pattern and overall nutrient intake of humans. Physiol Behav 53:1133–1144

98. Rose D, Murphy SP, Hudes M, Viteri FE (1995) Food energy remains constant with increasing alcohol intake. J Am Diet Assoc 95:698–700

99. Harnack L, Stang J, Story M (1999) Soft drink consumption among US children and adolescents: nutritional consequences. J.Am Diet Assoc 99:436–441

100. Bray GA, Nielsen SJ, Popkin BM (2004) Consumption of high-fructose corn syrup in beverages may play a role in the epidemic of obesity. Am J Clin Nutr 79:537–543

101. Gonzalez MF, Deutsch JA(1978) Vagotomy abolishes cues of satiety produced by gastric distension. Science 1283–1284

102. Schwartz GJ, McHugh PR, Moran TH (1991) Integration of vagal afferent responses to gastric loads and cholecystokinin in rats. Am J Physiol 261:R64–R69

103. Schick RR, Yasksh TL, Go VLW (1986) An intragastric meal releases the putative satiety factor cholecystokinin from hypothalamic neurons in cats. Brain Res 370:349–353

104. Schick RR, Reilly WM, Yasksh TL, Roddy DR, Go VLW (1987) Neuronal cholecystokinin-like immunoreactivity is postprandially released from primate hypothalamus. Brain Res 418:20–26

105. Schick RR, Yaksh TL, Roddy DR, Go VL (1989) Release of hypothalamic cholecystokinin in cats: effects of nutrient and volume loading. Am J Physiol 256:R248–R254

106. Davis JD, Gallagher RJ, Ladove RF (1967) Food intake controlled by a blood factor. Science 157:1247–1248

107. Koopmans HS (1983) A stomach hormone that inhibits food intake. J Auton Nerv System 9:157–171

108. Schick RR, Schusdziarra V, Mössner J, Neuberger J, Schröder B, Segmüller R, Maier V, Classen M (1991) Effect of CCK on food intake in man: physiological or pharmacological effect? Z Gastroenterol 29:53–58

109. Pi-Sunyer X, Kissileff HR, Thornton J, Smith GP (1982) C-terminal octapeptide of cholecystokinin decreases food intake in obese men. Physiol Behav 29:627–630

110. Ballinger A, McLoughlin L, Medbak S, Clark M (1995) Cholecystokinin is a satiety hormone in humans at physiological postprandial plasma concentrations. Clin Sci (Lond) 89:375–381

111. Lieverse RJ, Jansen JBMJ, Masclee AAM, Lamers CBHW (1995) Satiety effects of a physiological dose of cholecystokinin in humans. Gut 36:176–179

112. Flint A, Raben A, Astrup A, Holst JJ (1998) Glucagon-like peptide 1 promotes satiety and suppresses energy intake in humans. J Clin Invest 101:515–520

113. Flint A, Raben A, Ersboll AK, Holst JJ, Astrup A (2001) The effect of physiological levels of glucagon-like peptide 1 on appetite, gastric emptying, energy and substrate metabolism in obesity. Int J Obes Relat Metab Disord 25:781–792

114. Gutzwiller JP, Goke B, Drewe J, Hildebrand P, Ketterer S, Handschin D, Winterhalder R, Conen D, Beglinger C (1999) Glucagon-like peptide-1: a potent regulator of food intake in humans. Gut 44:81–86

115. Näslund E, Gutniak M, Skogar S, Rössner S, Hellström PM (1998) Glucagon-like peptide 1increases the period of postprandial satiety and slows gastric empting in obese men. Am J Clin Nutr 68:525–530

116. Long SJ, Sutton JA, Amaee WB, Giouvanoudi A, Spyrou NM, Rogers PJ, Morgan LM (1999) No effect of glucagon-like peptide-1 on short-term satiety and energy intake in man. Br J Nutr 81:273–279

117. Cohen MA, Ellis SM, Le RC, Batterham RL, Park A, Patterson M, Frost GS, Ghatei MA, Bloom SR (2003) Oxyntomodulin suppresses appetite and reduces food intake in humans. J Clin Endocrinol Metab 88:4696–4701

118. Batterham RL, Cohen MA, Ellis SM, Le RC, Withers DJ, Frost GS, Ghatei MA, Bloom SR (2003) Inhibition of food intake in obese subjects by peptide YY3-36. N Engl J Med 349:941–948

119. Holst JJ (2002) Therapy of type 2 diabetes mellitus based on the actions of glucagon-like peptide-1. Diabetes Metab Res Rev 18:430–441

120. Schwartz MW, Figlewicz DP, Baskin DG, Woods SC, Porte D jr (1992) Insulin in the brain: a hormonal regulator of energy balance. Endocr Rev 13:387–414

121. Wallum BJ, Taborsky GJ, Jr., Porte D, Jr., Figlewicz DP, Jacobson L, Beard JC, Ward WK, Dorsa D (1987) Cerebrospinal fluid insulin levels increase during intravenous insulin infusions in man. J Clin Endocrinol Metab 64:190–194

References

45   4

122. Kojima M, Hosoda H, Date Y, Nakazato M, Matsuo H, Kangawa K (1999) Ghrelin is a growth-hormone-releasing acylated peptide from stomach. Nature 402:656–660

123. Tschop M, Smiley DL, Heiman ML (2000) Ghrelin induces adiposity in rodents. Nature 407:908–913

124. Wren AM, Small CJ, Ward HL, Murphy KG, Dakin CL, Taheri S, Kennedy AR, Roberts GH, Morgan DG, Ghatei MA, Bloom SR (2000) The novel hypothalamic peptide ghrelin stimulates food intake and growth hormone secretion. Endocrinology 141:4325–4328

125. Wren AM, Seal LJ, Cohen JA, Brynes AE, Frost GS, Murphy KG, Dhillo WS, Ghatei MA, Bloom SR (2001) Ghrelin enhances appetite and increases food intake in humans. J Clin Endocrinol Metab 86:5992–5995

126. Cummings DE, Purnell JQ, Frayo RS, Schmidova K, Wisse BE, Weigle DS (2001) A preprandial rise in plasma ghrelin levels suggests a role in meal initiation in humans. Diabetes 50:1714–1719

127. Erdmann J, Lippl F, Schusdziarra V (2003) Differential effect of protein and fat on plasma ghrelin levels in man. Regul Pept 116:101–107

128. Cummings DE, Frayo RS, Marmonier C, Aubert R, Chapelot D (2004) Plasma ghrelin levels and hunger scores in humans initiating meals voluntarily without time- and food-related cues. Am J Physiol Endocrinol Metab 287:E297–E304

129. Monteleone P, Bencivenga R, Longobardi N, Serritella C, Maj M (2003) Differential responses of circulating ghrelin to high-fat or high-carbohydrate meal in healthy women. J Clin Endocrinol Metab 88:5510–5514

130. Asakawa A, Inui A, Kaga T, Katsuura G, Fujimiya M, Fujino MA, Kasuga M (2003) Antagonism of ghrelin receptor reduces food intake and body weight gain in mice. Gut 52:947–952

131. Luiten PG, ter Horst GJ, Steffens AB (1987) The hypothalamus, intrinsic connections and outflow pathways to the endocrine system in relation to the control of feeding and metabolism. Prog Neurobiol 28:1–54

132. Kalra S, Dube MG, Pu S, Xu B, Horvath TL, Kalra PS (1999) Interacting appetite-regulating pathways in the hypothalamic regulation of body weight. Endocrine Rev 20:68–100

133. Schwartz MW, Woods SC, Porte D jr, Seeley RJ, Baskin DG (2000) Central nervous system control of food intake. Nature 404:661–671

134. Schusdziarra V, Erdmann J, Schick RR (2008) Neuroendocrine feeding regulation in the perspective of modern food supply – lessons for obesity treatment. In: Columbus F (ed) New research in obesity. Nova Science, New York

135. Schick RR, Zimmermann JP, vorm Walde T, Schusdziarra V (2003) Peptides that regulate food intake: glucagon-like peptide 1-(7-36) amide acts at lateral and medial hypothalamic sites to suppress feeding in rats. Am J Physiol Regul Integr.Comp Physiol 284:R1427–R1435

136. Hollopeter G, Erickson JC, Seeley RJ, Marsh DJ, Palmiter RD (1998) Response of neuropeptide Y-deficient mice to feeding effectors. Regul Pept 75-76:383–389

137. Schusdziarra V, Zimmermann JP, Schick RR (2004) Importance of orexigenic counter-regulation for multiple targeted feeding inhibition. Obes Res 12:627–632

138. Friedman JM, Halaas J (1998) Leptin and the regulation of body weight. Nature 395:763–770

139. Cone RD, Cowley MA, Butler AA, Fan W, Marks DL, Low MJ (2001) The arcuate nucleus as a conduit for diverse signals relevant to energy homeostasis. Int J Obes Relat.Metab Disord 25:S63–S67

140. Zhang Y, Proenca R, Maffei M, Barone M, Leopold L, Friedman JM (1994) Positional cloning of the mouse obese gene and its human homologue. Nature 372:425–432

141. Wang HY, Tache Y, Sheibel AB, Go VLW, Wei JY (1997) Two types of leptin-responsive gastric vagal afferents terminals: an in vitro single-unit study in rats. Am J Physiol 273:R833–R837

142. Trayhurn P, Hoggard N, Mercer JG, Rayner DV (1999) Leptin: fundamental aspects. Int J Obes Relat Metab Disord 23 [Suppl 19]: 22–28

143. Schwartz MW, Seeley RJ, Campfield LA, Burn P, Baskin BG (1996) Identification of tagets of leptin action in rat hypothalamus. J Clin Invest 98:1101–1106

144. Lippl F, Erdmann J, Atmatzidis S, Schusdziarra V (2005) Direct effect of leptin on gastric ghrelin secretion. Horm Metab Res 37:123–125

145. Huang XF, Han M, South T, Stzorlien L (2003) Altered levels of POMC, AgRP and MC4-R mRNA expression in the hypothalamus and other parts of the limbic system of mice prone or resistant to chronic high-energy diet-induced obesity. Brain Res 992:9–19

146. Erdmann J, Lippl F, Wagenpfeil S, Schusdziarra V (2005) Differential association of basal and postprandial plasma ghrelin with leptin, insulin, and type 2 diabetes. Diabetes 54:1371–1378

147. Apfelbaum M, Mandenoff A (1981) Naltrexone suppresses hyperphagia induced in the rat by a highly palatable diet. Pharmacol Biochem Behav 15:89–91

148. Drewnowski A, Krahn DD, Demitrack MA, Nairn K, Gosnell BA (1992) Taste responses and preferences for sweet high-fat foods: evidence for opioid involvement. Physiol Behav 51:371–379

149. Welch CC, Kim EM, Grace MK, Billington CJ, Levine AS (1996) Palatability-induced hyperphagia increases hypothalamic Dynorphin peptide and mRNA levels. Brain Res 721:126–131

150. Drewnowski A (1997) Taste preferences and food intake. Annu Rev Nutr 17:237–253

151. Rolls BJ, Rowe EA, Rolls ET (1982) How sensory properties of foods affect human feeding behavior. Physiol Behav 29:409–417

152. Mela DJ, Sacchetti DA (1991) Sensory preferences for fats: relationships with diet and body composition. Am J Clin Nutr 53:908–915

153. Rolls BJ, Roe LS, Kral TV, Meengs JS, Wall DE (2004) Increasing the portion size of a packaged snack increases energy intake in men and women. Appetite 42:63–69

154. De Castro JM (2000) Eating behavior: lessons from the real world of humans. Nutrition 16:800–813

155. Anderson JW, Konz EC, Frederich RC, Wood CL (2001) Long-term weight-loss maintenance: a meta-analysis of US studies. Am J Clin Nutr 74:579–584

Physical Activity as A Significant Factor in The Therapy of Obesity

Aloys Berg, MD, Daniel König, MD

5.1 Conventional Therapeutic Approach

According to the guidelines of the German Obesity Society (Deutsche Adipositas Gesellschaft: www.adipositasgesellschaft.de), obesity is a state characterized by an excessive accumulation of fatty tissue in the body. It is based on the polygenetic disposition to store triglycerides as energetic substrates in fat cells, and is to be understood as a chronic health disorder that also requires chronic treatment. To promise success, this therapy should be integrated into a comprehensive health-care concept, including lifestyle changes and increased leisure-time physical activity. Although therapeutic lifestyle changes (TLC) are recommended for overweight people in general, the feasibility and success of TLC are focused on pre-obesity (BMI 25–30 kg/m²) and obesity grades I and II (grade I: BMI 30–<35 kg/m², grade II: BMI >35–<40 kg m²). Data about TLC results in obesity grade III (BMI >40 kg/m²) are still rare. Obesity involves a phenomenon that is difficult to treat and highly complex; it is usually not experienced by the patient as a health disorder or disease until the advanced stage. Indispensable for the treatment of obesity are a patient's change in lifestyle and cooperation with a health professional. Therefore, obesity therapy must be planned right from the beginning on a long-term basis. Generally,

- Obese patients frequently decide on a therapy for cosmetic-aesthetic reasons and not for health reasons.
- A patient can maintain long-term high motivation only if the target level is not set unrealistically high.
- Reaching interim targets and having a sense of achievement are decisive factors in supporting and maintaining patient motivation; this concept applies in principle for both diet and behavioral strategies, as well as for programs to increase activity.
- Fasting and monitoring must not remain the focus of the therapy as time progresses.

Germany is meanwhile being flood by a wave of weight-reduction programs; more than 200 are currently offered by a variety of institutions. However, few programs offer reliable success. Similarly, only few have been evaluated and fulfill the criterion of continuous quality management. However, without a doubt the only lasting success can come from a permanent change in dietary and physical activity to an energetically balanced lifestyle and simultaneous improvement in diet quality, mediated and accompanied by a behavioral psychological concept. Details of a successful lifestyle concept for obese adults were recently published by the authors. It was shown that it is possible to lose body weight at an average of about 5–6 kg after participation in a 1-year lifestyle program and, with good response to the program, even more than 15 kg body weight within 1 year. There is agreement that for a successful health-care regimen, the following lifestyle changes must be applied to treat obese adults:

- Adjustment of the energy balance to the reduced body weight and altered baseline turnover
- Adjustment of the diet towards a reduction in the intake of fat and carbohydrates with a high glycemic index
- Increase in everyday activity and selective physical activity
- Continuation of behavioral psychological support with guidance in selfmanage-ment and weight monitoring
- Integration into a self-help group

5.2 Pathophysiology and Diagnostics

In principle, the BMI value gives only a person's weight-length ratio and does not indicate the proportion of fat mass to body weight; the BMI value, therefore, does not make a direct statement concerning the body's composition and does not discriminate between fatty and fat-free body mass in regard to a person's fitness and activity behavior. However, like an increasing BMI value, the body fat mass is responsible for an increase in weight. In the normal individual, for a BMI value of over 30 kg/m² an elevated proportion of body fat may be assumed (in men over 25% and in women over 35% of body weight). Also helpful in assessing the body's composition and in estimating the amount of abdominal and visceral fat is the measurement of the abdominal circumference. Values over 102 cm in men and over 88 cm in women have been identified as being considerably elevated. The amount of visceral fat closely correlates with the increased risk of metabolic and cardiovascular complications.

Contrary to what is generally assumed, however, the health-specific statement of an elevated BMI value, as well as of the excess amount of fat, is unsatisfactory. Thus, on the one hand, the proportion of fat with the same BMI value can show extreme diversity in men and women (◘ Fig. 5.1). On the other hand, there are often also only small differences in the classical atherogenic and inflammatory risk factors even when there are significant differences in BMI, percentage of body fat, or abdominal circumference. Thus, anthropometric parameters such as BMI, fat mass, and abdominal circumference act only as indicators of an increased probability of the presence of metabolic and cardiovascular risk factors; they do not replace the further clinical diagnostic tests and the necessity of determining the concomitant risk factors regarding blood pressure regulation, fat metabolism profile, glucose regulation, and, when possible, vascular morphology using carotid sonography and endothelium function tests. From a physiological viewpoint, not only does fatty tissue, or the adipocytes, serve as an energy storage organ for lipids (triglycerides); it is also of outstanding significance for the regulation of the energy balance. On the one hand, adipocytes themselves possess the ability to form and selectively release hormone-like messenger substances (adipokines); on the other hand, they are furnished with specific receptors, so that they can respond directly to signals from the other organs. In this way, there is close communication between the fat cells and all other body organs and a complex interactive coordination of energy utilization, e.g., by physical activity, and storage from fats. As the result of an excessive availability of fat, whether due to increased intake (diet) or to insufficient utilization (physical activity), with a genetic predisposition a disturbance of this cellular competence may occur. The "dysfunctional" fat cell, overloaded with fat, is then no longer able to control the balance between fat storage and fat utilization (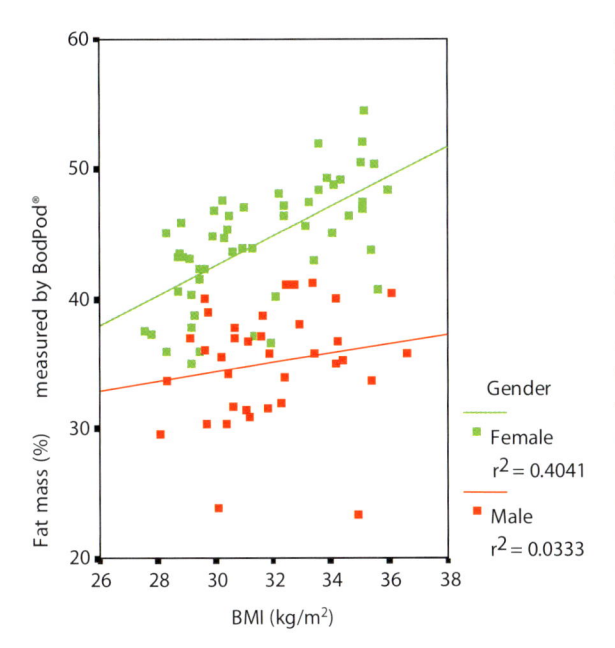 Fig. 5.2). Fat and its metabolic products are now also stored in the cells of other organs (e.g., cardiac muscle, pancreas, kidneys, and neurons); as a result, they disturb their specific functions and pave the way for organ-specific sequelae. Subcutaneous and visceral adipocytes differ in their metabolic activity and in the pattern of their adipokine and cytokine expression. Meanwhile, it has also been deduced that truncal (android) and/or abdominal obesity with a high proportion of visceral fat is accompanied by a greater health risk than gynecoid obesity.

The pathological form of obesity presents with an abundance of alarming symptoms. Although there is primarily a visible increase in body weight due to an increase in fat mass, more decisive for health are the physiological and biochemical changes in the entire

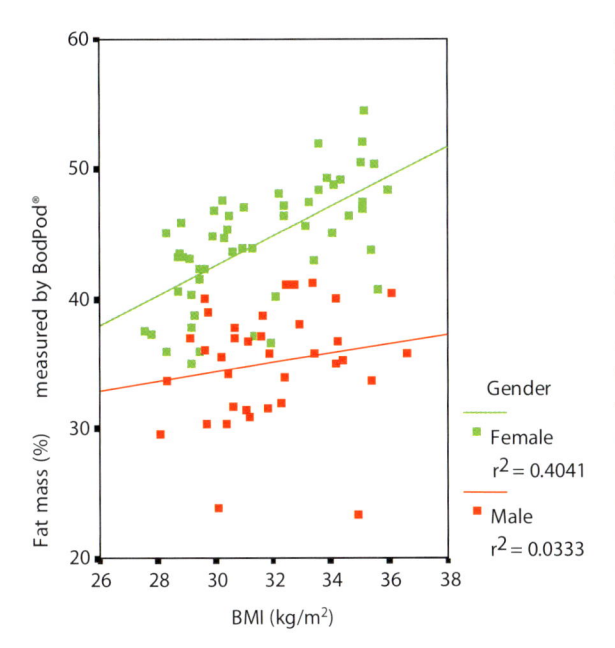

Fig. 5.1. Correlation between BMI and fat mass. Despite identical BMI values there is a significant difference in the individual percentage of fat mass between overweight and obese women and men

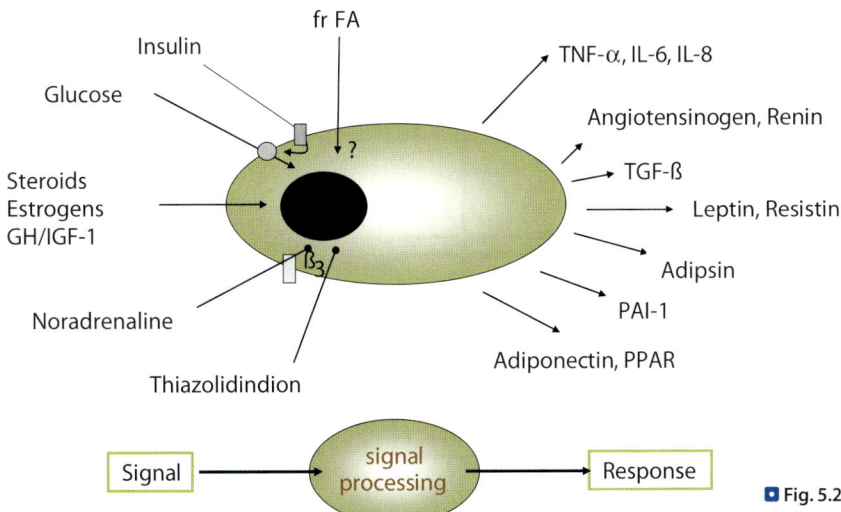

Fig. 5.2. The adipocyte as an intelligent organ in the regulation of energy balance

body, which, however, initially remain unnoticed for the person concerned. In most cases, combined with low fitness and a low activity level, there are shifts in the adipokines measured in the blood (elevated leptin, lowered adiponectin), including inflammatory factors (CRP and interleukin-6), elevated insulin efficacy, and metabolic fitness. Additionally, blood flow properties and vascular reaction show pronounced deterioration. As a result of increased fatness and decreased fitness, the risks of type-2 diabetes, cardiac infarction, and tumors increase. Furthermore, the rate of the aging process of the entire body, and the associated probability of becoming prematurely chronically ill in all organ systems, is accelerated.

5.3 Significance of Inactivity for the Clinical and Physiological Picture

Corresponding to the existing motor utilization and the goal of increased leisure activity, respectively, it is essential to differentiate between power-oriented training, with its benefits regarding muscle mass, and endurance-oriented training, with its benefits for energy balance. Undisputed in this context are the relationships between body composition, percentage fat mass, and energy balance.

Good physical fitness and motor competence contribute decisively to being active in everyday life – a fundamental prerequisite to maintaining the energy balance in a stable state and not worsening the body's composition by an increase in fat mass (◨ Fig. 5.3). Thus, good physical fitness and good motor competence generally increase the amount of everyday activity and correlate directly with the activity-induced energy expenditure (AEE). As a result, directly via the AEE, the daily total energy expenditure (TEE) can be varied positively by enhanced activity. Because the resting metabolic rate (resting energy expenditure, REE) correlates closely with age and with fat-free body mass, i.e., muscle mass, the history of activity and movement behavior also has an indirect effect on the daily TEE. Frequent uncritical calorie intake and concomitant lack of physical activity leads to an imbalance in the TEE and to an increase in weight. On average, middle-aged men increase their BMI by 0.8 units and women by 1.2 units in every decade of their life. The unit MET (metabolic equivalents of task) is used to describe activity behavior in the literature of applied sports medicine. The unit MET reflects the energy consumption of human beings per time unit by physical activity; 1 MET is defined as being equivalent to the O_2 consumption under resting conditions and for healthy adult organisms is given as 3.5 ml O_2/kg body weight per minute.

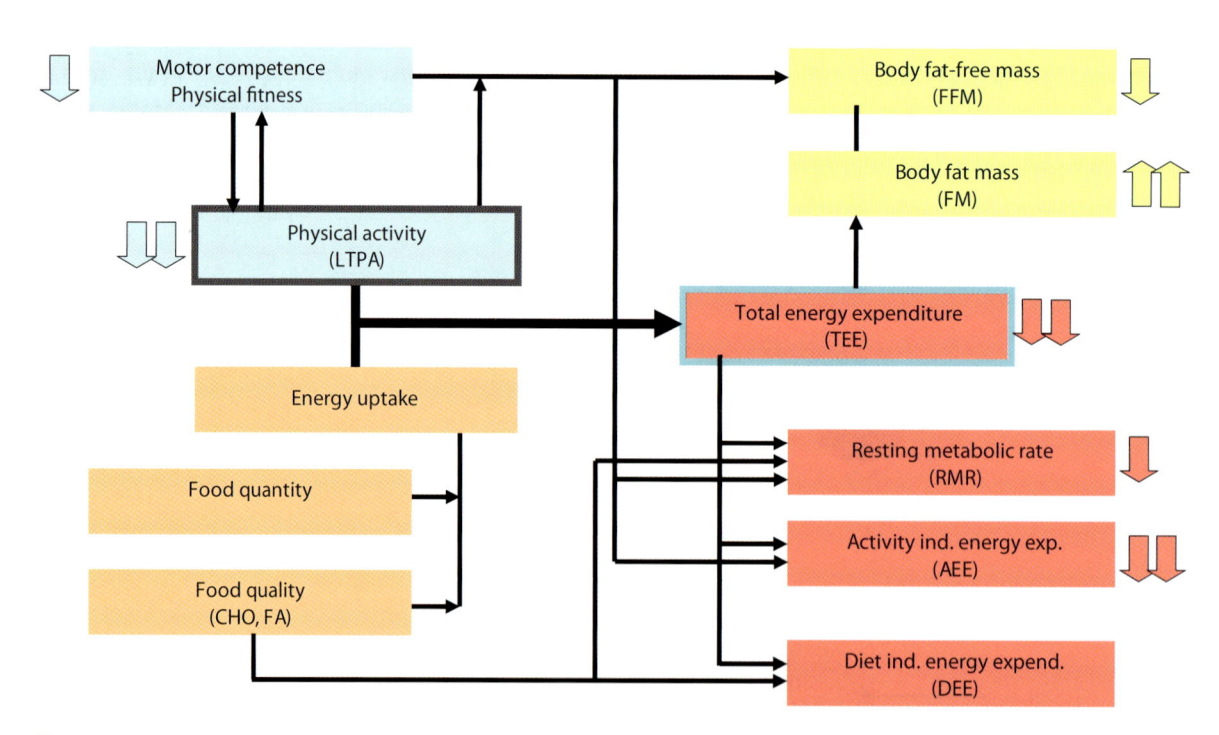

◨ **Fig. 5.3.** Activity behavior and its influence on energy expenditure and body composition

The specification as MET-hour (METh) thus gives the energy expenditure per hour during physical activity as a multiple of the resting energy expenditure. The following calculations can serve as practical examples for reference: 2 MET for walking at 3 km/h, 5 MET for walking at 6 km/h, and 8 MET for jogging at 10 km/h, in each case over a period of 60 min. During aerobic utilization of the energy carriers glucose and fatty acids, per consumed liter of oxygen 5 kcal are released as energy equivalent (EE). Comparing the standardized oxygen consumption during ergometry permits the calculation of the watt-related energy content. In addition to the resting turnover of 0.25–0.30 l O_2/ min, for every watt produced in physical activity an average of 11.5 ml O_2/min is required. From this it can be derived that, dependent on intensity, for 100 watts/h approximately 350 kcal (60 min x 1.15 l O_2 x 5 kcal EE), and for 200 watts/h approximately 700 kcal (60 min x 2.3 l O_2 x 5 kcal EE) are expended in addition to the resting turnover.

These data are required for discussions about the value of leisure activities in kcal/week or about negative energy expenditures in kcal/day, with regard to obesity prevention. However, physical activity does not only include sports. For normal persons, activities such as working in the garden or the house, climbing steps, hiking, going on walks, or shopping on foot or by bike contribute towards activity turnover. The data on adult activity history show impressively that these everyday activities can achieve therapeutic and preventive effective energy expenditures without any problems. Everyday activities also help to stabilize body weight and fitness in old age. Considering the activity recommendations for the prevention of chronic degenerative disorders, according to current data, only 46% of West German and even only 30% of East German men aged 18–19 years fulfill these recommendations. Already after the age of 30, this percentage drops to under 20% in both West and East Germany. In 18- to 19-year-old women it is also less than 20%; after 30 years of age the percentage of women who fulfill this recommendation is even less than 10%. One current reports that the prevalence of physical inactivity in the entire German population is about 30%; 45% play no sports and only 13% of the entire population move enough to achieve a preventative effect. This information is largely in accordance with the results of the data collected at the beginning of the 1990s by the Giessen Nutrition and Food Consumption Study (representative sample for 18- to 55-year-old, healthy adults in our population) and explains why the prevalence of excess weight (BMI>25) and obesity (BMI>30) in Germany has almost doubled in the past three decades.

5.4 Practical Sport Therapy

Compared with the sport unit in each case, the caloric content of the physical activity and its percentage of the daily calorie expenditure are often overestimated. Nevertheless, for the evaluation of the energy balance it is important that during endurance exercise the energy expenditure can be maintained at a multiple factor of the resting expenditure: in normal individuals, around four- to fivefold, whereas in those with endurance training even increased eight- to tenfold. It is reasonable that by combating excess weight with increased physical activity, one can successfully reduce weight in the long term, if not in the short term as well. To derive the energy provided by 1000 g of body fat, one would have to walk 20 h at a speed of about 6 km/h or to run 11 h at 12 km/h in order to convert this fat mass into energy. On the other hand, even small daily additional expenditure on a regular basis, e.g., walking a distance of 2 km per day, corresponding to an energy content of approximately 140 kcal, already leads to a considerable sum of energy per year, in this case to 51,000 kcal, corresponding to a fat tissue mass of approximately 8 kg. These examples make it easy to understand why a small expenditure of fat and energy can lead to a considerable disturbance in weight development and an increase in fat deposit over the years. To achieve adequate weight reduction in persons with a pronounced elevated body weight (BMI >30 kg/m^2) within a time frame of 6–12 months, a change in activity behavior alone is generally insufficient. Nevertheless, from a physical viewpoint, the energy content of greater calorie consumption as a result of greater activity and the calorie saving by restricting calorie intake should be rated as being of equal importance. Accordingly, under conditions of a standardized energy balance, an identical loss in weight can be observed with reduced calorie intake or with increased calorie consumption.

5.5 Contraindications and Complications for Sport Therapy

Absolute as well as relative contraindications to initiating sports therapy or participation in a sports medicine-oriented training program for obese adults, e.g., the M.O.B.I.L.I.S. program, are in accordance with the comments of the ACSM and the current guidelines of the German Cardiological Society on ergometry. To conduct an adequate training program, participants in sports medicineoriented programs should achieve a symptom-free performance of 75 watts over a period of at least 2 min.

An indication restriction may also result from inadequate motor competence or reduced ability of the skeletal and locomotor system to cope with the exercise. Patients with psychiatric disorders and fixated eating disorders (e.g., binge eating disorder) are generally unsuitable for sports therapy within a group and require permanent expert medical monitoring. Also to be excluded from sports therapies are type-2 DM patients, in whom a diabetic foot syndrome, polyneuropathy, or severe diabetic retinopathy has been diagnosed. Special complications due to sports therapy are not to be expected; no negative experiences regarding adverse effects have been observed with patients treated so far.

5.6 Conclusions in Practice

With an identical intensity of movement, more energy is required for a greater body weight. This idea is reflected in measurable terms in the absolute values for oxygen consumption per work unit and the related calorie expenditure (◘ Table 5.1). With increasing body weight, the same work intensity thus requires more energy and is experienced as being more physically taxing. Overweight persons should thus select a lower work intensity than those of normal weight, so they do not tire prematurely and discontinue their training program in frustration. Thus, work intensity cannot be selected randomly, but should be determined only according to the individual level of fitness. It is neither motivating nor does it lead to the desired goal when untrained and overweight patients make comparisons to the endurance exercise performance and the energy expenditure of persons trained in endurance or even in competitive sports.

Accordingly, the fundamental principle "start slowly, increase gradually, and continue over the long-term" is important for successful weight management propagated with the practically oriented "50+50 Point Program" in current movement-oriented sports-medicine training programs such as M.O.B.I.L.I.S. and M.O.B.I.L.I.S. light (www.mobilis-programm.de). One-year results in sports medicine training programs for obese adults warrant the statement that with a lifestyle-oriented training program, a person can significantly reduce body weight and body fat mass by more than 0.25 kg/week over a period of 6 months. The weight reduction leads to an improvement in body composition and to a reduction in visceral body fat mass. Correspondingly, the weight reduction is accompanied by increased physical fitness and positive adjustments in metabolism as well as in atherogenic risk factors. With evidence that such results are reproducible and that the participants' assessment of the programs prove positive, it appears prudent to recommend sports-medicine intervention programs such as the M.O.B.I.L.I.S. program for obesity therapy.

References

1. Kyle UG, Genton L, Pichard C (2002) Body composition: what's new? Curr Opin Clin Nutr Metab Care 5:427–433
2. Lollgen H (2003) Primarpravention kardialer Erkrankungen: Stellenwert der korperlichen Aktivitat. Deutsch Arztebl 100:A987–A996
3. Mayer F, Gollhofer A, Berg A (2003) Krafttraining mit Alteren und chronisch Kranken. Deutsch Z Sportmed 54:88–94
4. Mensink M, Blaak EE, Corpeleijn E, Saris WH, de Bruin TW, Feskens EJ (2003) Lifestyle intervention according to general recommendations improves glucose tolerance. Obes Res 11:1588–1596
5. Mokdad AH, Bowman BA, Ford ES, Vinicor F, Marks JS, Koplan JP (2001) The continuing epidemics of obesity and diabetes in the United States. JAMA 286:1195–1200
6. Ravussin E, Smith SR (2002) Increased fat intake, impaired fat oxidation, and failure of fat cell proliferation result in ectopic fat storage, insulin resistance, and type 2 diabetes mellitus. Ann NY Acad Sci 967:363–378
7. Ross R, Dagnone D, Jones PJ et al (2000) Reduction in obesity and related comorbid conditions after diet-induced weight loss or exercise-induced weight loss in men. A randomized, controlled trial. Ann Intern Med 133:92–103

◘ Table 5.1 Calculated increased energy expenditure at a walking speed of 6 km/h (intensity 5 MET) dependent on body weight

	Body weight (kg)								
	60	70	80	90	100	110	120	130	140
O_2 consumption (l/min)	1.0 5	1.23	1.40	1.58	1.75	1.93	2.10	2.28	2.45
Energy expenditure:									
– per min (kcal/min)	5.25	6.15	7.00	7.90	8.75	9.65	10.50	11.40	12.25
– per h (kcal/h)	315	369	420	474	525	579	630	684	735

The Role of Adipokines and Gastrointestinal Tract Hormones in Obesity

Julian Swierczynski, MD, Tomasz Sledzinski, MD

The chapter briefly reviewed the environmental and genetic risk factors for obesity and the impact of obesity on several disorders. It is focused on some adipokines (leptin, adiponectin, resistin), endocannabinoids, steroid hormones (estrogens, androgens, glucocorticosteroids) and fatty acids. We discussed the role of some adipokines (leptin, adiponectin), inflammation (TNFα, IL-6, MCP-1, MIF), insulin resistance (adiponectin, proinflammatory adipokines, retinol binding protein-4), cardiovascular diseases (adiponectin, angiotensinogen, PAI-1, leptin), and cancer (leptin, adiponectin) in obesity. It would be answered how gastrointestinal tract hormones, such as ghrelin, obestatin, cholecystokinin (CCK), peptide YY (PYY), pancreatic peptide (PP), glucagon-like peptide-1 (GLP-1), oxyntomodulin, and gastric inhibitory polypeptide (GIP) can contribute to obesity

6.1 Introduction

In the past three decades, obesity has reached epidemic proportions in industrialized countries. In general, obesity as a multifactorial and heterogeneous state results from alterations of socioeconomic status, from environmental factors including overeating, physical inactivity, and smoking cessation [1; 2], and from alterations of

various genes, each having a partial and additive effect. As the net result of excessive energy intake compared with energy usage, an excessive accumulation of triacylglycerols in adipose tissue occurs. Due to hyperplasia and hypertrophy of adipocytes the mass of adipose tissue varies enormously (from 10 kg in lean subjects to more than 100 kg in morbidly obese subjects) between individuals.

Genetic factors are currently estimated to account for 40–70% of the variance in human obesity [3]. In most subjects, the genetic basis for obesity is very complex and involves the interaction of multiple genes as well as of genes and the environment. Among genetic factors, there are rare examples of monogenic causes for obesity, presented in ◘ Table 6.1.

Monogenic obesity serves as a good model for understanding hormonal and neuronal interactions that regulate adiposity. Moreover, it provides an insight into pathways that contribute to obesity and possible targets for therapeutic intervention. This is why we pay more attention to this problem in this chapter. It is obvious that genetic changes cannot account for the recent trends toward increased obesity, because human genes have not changed substantially during the past three decades. The epidemic obesity observed in the past 30 years is due mainly to socioeconomic and environ-

◘ **Table 6.1** Classification of obesity according to genetic etiology

Classification of human genetic linkage to obesity	Characteristic features	Ref
I. Monogenic obesity	Obesity itself is the predominant presenting feature. Usually no mental retardation and developmental abnormalities are observed. Results from alteration of a single gene, mainly from the disruption of the hypothalamic leptin-melanocortin signaling pathway.	[4–7]
1. Leptin gene (*LEP*) mutation: *LEP* maps to human chromosome 7q31.3, comprises 3 exons separated by 2 introns	Different *LEP* mutation was detected in severe obese children and adults. Subjects produce very small quantity of leptin and have very low (in heterozygotes) or undetectable serum leptin concentration (homozygotes). Clinical features include: hyperphagia, severe obesity, hypogonadism, and impaired T-cell-mediated immunity (profound abnormalities of T-cell number and function). Obesity caused by *LEP* mutation can be treated by recombinant leptin. Up to 2007, 12 subjects with a mutation in the gene encoding leptin have been described.	[5–7]
2. Leptin receptor gene (*LEPR*) mutation: *LEPR* maps to human chromosome 1p31. *LEPR* encodes 5 protein isoforms. The prevalence of pathogenic *LEPR* mutation in a cohort of 300 subjects with severe, early-onset obesity is approximately 3% ▼	Mutation in *LEPR* results in early-onset morbid obesity, lack of pubertal development, alteration in immune function (similarities with leptin-deficient subjects – see above). Surprisingly (considering that leptin is the only known agonist of leptin receptor), clinical features were less severe than those of subjects with congenital leptin deficiency. Serum leptin and insulin concentrations were elevated but within the range predicted by fat mass in these subjects.	[8]

◘ **Table 6.1** *Continued*

Classification of human genetic linkage to obesity	Characteristic features	Ref
3. Pro-opiomelanocortin gene (*POMC*) mutation: *POMC* maps to human chromosome 2p22 and encodes: ACTH (predominant peptide produced by pituitary corticotrophes), MSH α,β, and γ (all produced by hypothalamus) and β-endorphin	The genetic defects in *POMC* resulted in hyperphagia, early-onset obesity, adrenal insufficiency, and altered (pale) skin) and hair pigmentation (red) due to the lack of MSH function at melanocortin receptor 1 (MC1-R) in the skin.	[9, 10]
4. Melanocortin 4 receptor gene (*MC4R*) mutation: The melanocortin 4 receptor (MC4-R) is a G-protein-coupled receptor present in the hypothalamus, and stimulated by α-MSH binding. Animal studies showed that (a) selective blockage of the MC4-R stimulates food intake, and (b) MC4-R is involved in mediation of the inhibitory effect of leptin on food intake.	Heterozygous mutation in *MC4-R* is related to hyperphagia, severe hyperinsulinemia, and morbid obesity. This syndrome is characterized by an increase in lean body mass and bone mineral density. Moreover, increased linear growth throughout childhood was observed. It seems that MCR4 deficiency is the most common obesity syndrome described so far and one of the most common monogenic diseases.	[11, 12]
5. Prohormone convertase 1 gene (*PC1*) mutation: *PC1* encodes neuroendocrine (present in neuroendocrine tissues) prohormone convertase (PC1), which belongs to the family of serine proteases. It acts on many substrates including: proinsulin, proglucagon and pro-opiomelanocortin (POMC)	*PC1* mutation (heterozygous missense mutation, Gly⬛Arg483 prevents processing of proPC1 and leads to its retention in endoplasmic reticulum) resulted in severe early-onset obesity, hypogonadotrophic hypogonadism, hypocortisolism, abnormal glucose homeostasis, increased plasma concentrations of proinsulin and pro-POMC, and very low plasma insulin concentration.	[13,14]
6. Single-minded, drosophila homologue of 1 gene (*SIM1*) mutation: *SIM1* encodes a human homologue of Drosophila Sim (single-minded), transcription factor regulating neurogenesis. It is likely that the transcription factor, SIM1, plays an important role in the regulation of food intake in humans.	Balanced translocation between chromosome 1p22.1 and 6q16.2 disrupts *SIM1* gene function and results in early-onset obesity caused by excessive food intake.	[15]
7. Neurotropic tyrosine kinase receptor type 2 gene (*NTRK2*) mutation: *NTRK2* encodes tyrosine receptor kinase B (TrkB), which binds (with high affinity) to brain-derived neurotrophic factor (BDNF). BDNF regulates the development, survival, and differentiation of neurons and contributes to the regulation of body weight and food intake.	Mutation of *NTRK2* (heterozygous missense mutation Tyr722Cys) results in impairment of receptor autophosphorylation and signaling to mitogen-activated protein kinase, leading to a hyperphagic obesity, associated with impairment of memory, learning, and nociception.	[16]
II. Polygenic obesity. Two main approaches have been suggested to find the genetics variants that affect obesity: 1. Linkage analysis 2. Association studies	Results from several gene alterations. Different genes and gene combinations are responsible for the pathogenesis of obesity in different populations.	[4–7]
III. Pleiotropic obesity syndrome (syndromic obesity). Syndrome arises from discrete genetic defects or chromosomal abnormalities. Can be either autosomal (dominant or recessive) or X-linked disorders. Approximately 25 genetic obesity syndromes have been described so far.	Obesity associated with a disease such as mental retardation, dysmorphic features, or organ-specific developmental abnormalities For instance: Prader-Willi syndrome (PWS). PWS is an autosomal dominant disorder caused by lack of the paternal segment 15q11.2-q12. Characterized by hyperphagia, obesity, hypogonadotropic hypogonadism, hypotonia, mental retardation, and short stature. Moreover, patients with PWS have a fasting plasma ghrelin concentration several times higher than that of equally obese subjects without PWS. It is likely, therefore, that ghrelin plays some role in the pathogenesis of hyperphagia in these patients.	[4–7]

6

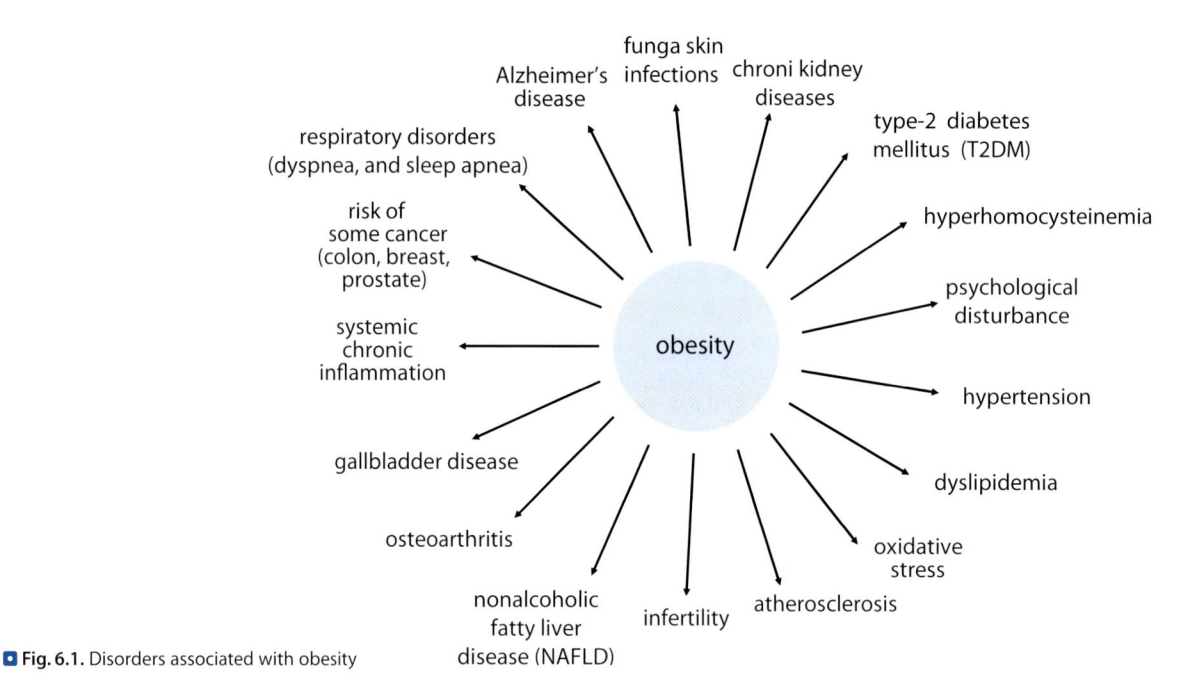

■ **Fig. 6.1.** Disorders associated with obesity

mental factors that promote excessive food ingestion. In rich countries this phenomenon results from an unlimited supply of high energy-dense foods and discourages physical activity [1].

In general, overweight is disadvantageous for human beings because it is usually associated with several disorders (and abnormalities), presented in ■ Fig. 6.1.

However, overweight can also be associated with some benefits, for instance, an increase in bone density and consequently a lower prevalence of osteoporosis and hip facture [17].

Growing evidence suggests that molecules synthesized and secreted by adipose tissue play an active, important role in the development of several disorders associated with obesity (see ■ Fig. 6.1). Adipose tissue produces and secretes into circulation three groups of substances: (a) fatty acids, (b) adipokines, and (c) miscellaneous substances including estrogens, androgens, prostaglandins, nitric oxide (NO), and endocannabinoids [18–25] (see ■ Fig. 6.2), which appear to have different implications for human health.

6.2 Free Fatty Acids

Quantitatively, free fatty acids (FFA) are the major substances released from adipose tissue, which is the main site of energy storage in man. It seems that hormones

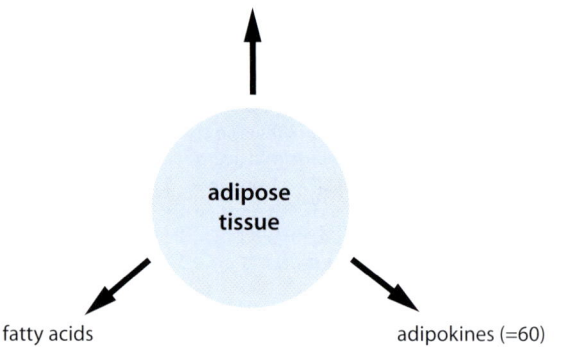

■ **Fig. 6.2.** Three main groups of substances produced and released by adipose tissue

such as insulin and sympathetic activation in adipose tissue are the chief factors contributing to regulation of lipolysis (triacylglycerol hydrolysis into glycerol and FFA) and consequently to FFA release from adipose tissue. In the fasting state, when insulin concentration is low, lipolysis is greatly activated. Increased adipose tissue fat is stored and disturbs insulin-mediated regulation of lipolysis in obese subjects, increasing the circulating FFA concentration. Elevated serum FFA concentration leads to several abnormalities including insulin resistance [26, 27] and inflammatory responses [28]. A high concentration of circulating FFA is associated with lipid accumulation (specifically triacylglycerols) in several organs including skeletal muscle, heart, liver, and pancreatic β-cells. Lipid accumulation in cardiomyocytes produces cellular damage and ventricular dysfunction [27]. Skeletal muscle insulin resistance correlates with intracellular lipid accumulation and decreased mitochondrial function [26]. FFA may also induce insulin resistance in skeletal muscle and in liver by reduction of insulin receptor substrates [27]. The excess of circulating FFA can also lead to diminished function and/or to apoptosis of pancreatic β-cells (so-called pancreatic lipotoxicity) [29]. Collectively, the excess of circulating FFA can act both to decrease the responsiveness of peripheral tissue to insulin and to decrease the insulin supply. In addition to insulin resistance and inflammation, the elevated circulating FFA concentration leads to impairment of endothelium-dependent and insulin-mediated vasodilatation as a result of a decrease in NO production [30, 31].

6.3 Adipokines

Adipose tissue is not only a storage tissue for triacylglycerols; it also acts as an endocrine organ, releasing many biologically active substances that communicate with and affect other tissue/organs. Adipose tissue secretes a multiplicity of proteins (or peptides), generally called adipokines [18–24, 32–35]. The diversity of the adipokines in terms of structure and function is considerable [18–24, 32–35]. ◘ Figure 6.3 gives examples of the best-known adipokines. The main functions of adipokines are presented in ◘ Fig. 6.4.

6.3.1 Obesity, Inflammation, and Cardiovascular Disease

As already mentioned, altered circulating concentrations of adipokines secreted from excess adipose tissue (as a consequence of body weight gain in obese subjects) may be pathogenically involved in the risk for many disorders. For instance, serum leptin concentration was found to be associated with the white blood cell count [36], a possible marker for future cardiovascular mortality. Blood pressure level was also related to serum leptin concentration independent of insulin concentration [37]. On the

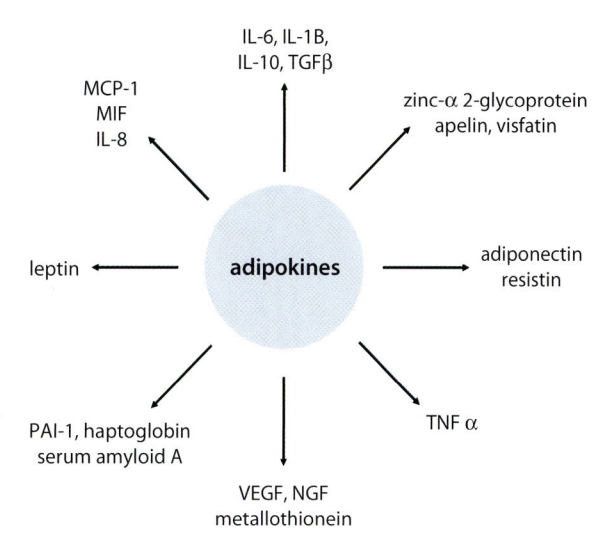

◘ **Fig. 6.3.** The best-known adipokines. Nerve growth factor (*NGF*), vascular endothelial growth factor (*VEGF*), monocyte chemotactic protein-1 (*MCP-1*), serum amyloid A (*SSA*), tumor necrosis factor α (*TNFα*), transforming growth factor β (*TGFβ*), macrophage migration inhibitory factor β (*MIFβ*), and interleukins (*IL-1β, IL-6, IL-8, IL-10*)

other hand, circulating adiponectin concentration was inversely associated with serum CRP concentration in healthy subjects, suggesting its anti-inflammatory and anti-atherosclerotic properties [38].

In obese subjects, hypertrophic adipocytes produce more proinflammatory adipokines (sometimes called adipocytokines) such as TNFα, IL-6, MCP-1 than are found in non-obese individuals. Moreover, hypertrophic adipocytes produce less adiponectin (anti-inflammatory and anti-atherosclerotic adipokines) than normal adipocytes. The changes in production of adipokines in obese subjects may have systemic and/or local effects. Due to less production of adiponectin and more production of proinflammatory adipokines in obese subjects, the latter group of substances enter the circulation to promote insulin resistance and atherosclerosis [39]. Changes in the production of adipokines also have local effects, for instance on the endothelium. The action of proinflammatory cytokines on endothelium causes overproduction of adhesion molecules. Moreover, proinflammatory cytokines cause an increase in vascular permeability, monocyte recruitment and differentiation, macrophage infiltration, and cytokine production. Thus, the crosstalk among adipocytes, endothelial cells and monocytes/macrophages contributes to insulin resistance (and associated pathologies such as metabolic syndrome) and atherosclerosis [39].

The key question is why the production and secretion of adipocytokines and other proinflammatory substances

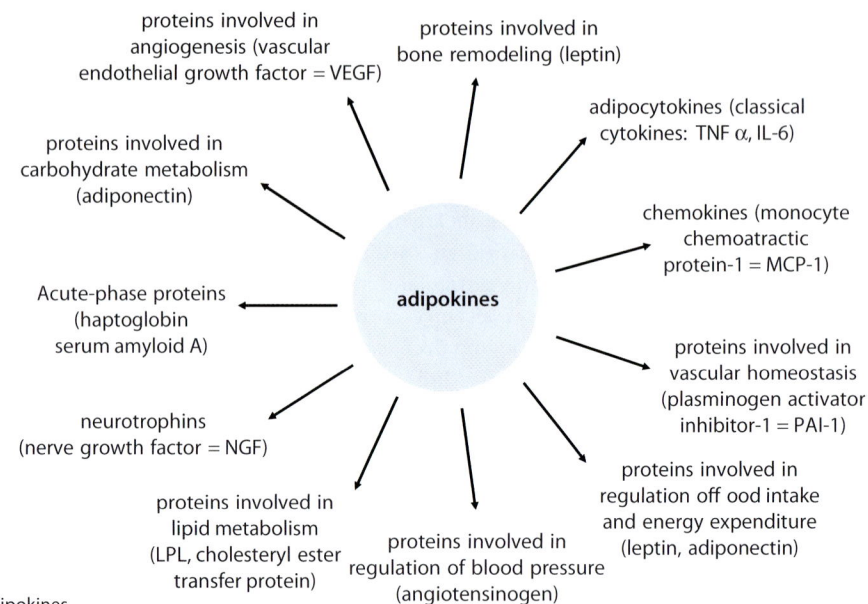

■ **Fig. 6.4.** The main functions of adipokines

by adipose tissue rise in obesity. Recent data indicate that hypoxia-inducible factor–1 (HIF-1α) plays a key role in regulating the production of proinflammatory substances in adipose tissue. The expansion of adipose tissue mass (the characteristic feature of obese subjects) causes relative hypoxia within clusters of adipocytes remote from the blood vessels. Hypoxia leads to an increase in the HIF-1α level. In turn, the HIF-1α combines with hypoxia-inducible factor-1β (also known as ARNT = aryl hydrocarbon receptor nuclear translocator) to form the transcription factor called hypoxia-inducible factor-1. The transcription of many genes, including genes encoded by proinflammatory (IL-6, MIF, PAI-1, leptin) and anti-inflammatory (adiponectin) substances, is regulated by hypoxia-inducible factor-1 (similar to the *EPO* gene in the kidneys). Interestingly, gene-encoded TNFα is not affected by HIF-1α (■ Fig. 6.5) [40, 41]. In this way, relative hypoxia caused by the expansion of adipose tissue (in obese subjects) may underlie the development of the inflammatory response in adipocytes, leading to obesity-related diseases [41].

6.3.2 Obesity and Cancer

There is growing evidence that obesity greatly influences the risk and prognosis of many common forms of cancer [42, 43]. For instance, obese breast cancer patients exhibit a higher risk for lymph-node metastasis, a larger tumor burden, and higher mortality when compared with non-

obese breast cancer patients [44]. The biological activities of some adipokines suggest an important role of the substances in cancer proliferation, invasion, and metastasis. Leptin, the best-known adipokine (see below), seems to play the major role in growth stimulation [45], promotion of invasion, and migration [46] of some carcinoma cells. Leptin exerts its biological actions through its specific receptors localized in the cell membranes of a variety of tissues [47]. The leptin signaling is transmitted by the tyrosine kinase named Janus-activated kinase (JAK) and by the signal transducers and activators of transcription (STAT) pathway [48]. Binding of leptin to leptin receptor results in its dimerization, in the autophosphorylation of JAK, and in the phosphorylation of the cytoplasmic domain of the leptin receptor and the STAT. The activated (phosphorylated) STAT translocates into the nucleus and activates target genes. The gene activation by transcription factors (for instance STAT) involves the recruitment of different co-activator complexes contributing to the regulation of gene transcription. Many STAT target genes are key components of the regulation of cell-cycle progression from G1 to S phase [49]. Recent data suggest that *CYCLIN D1* may be a target gene for leptin-mediated growth stimulation of breast cancer, and STAT 3 plays a key role in this process [45]. The binding of leptin to its receptor may also stimulate other intracellular signaling pathways which may be involved in the growth/survival process, cell migration and invasion, and angiogenesis [50–52]. A potential mechanism for obesity-induced cancer is presented in ■ Fig. 6.6.

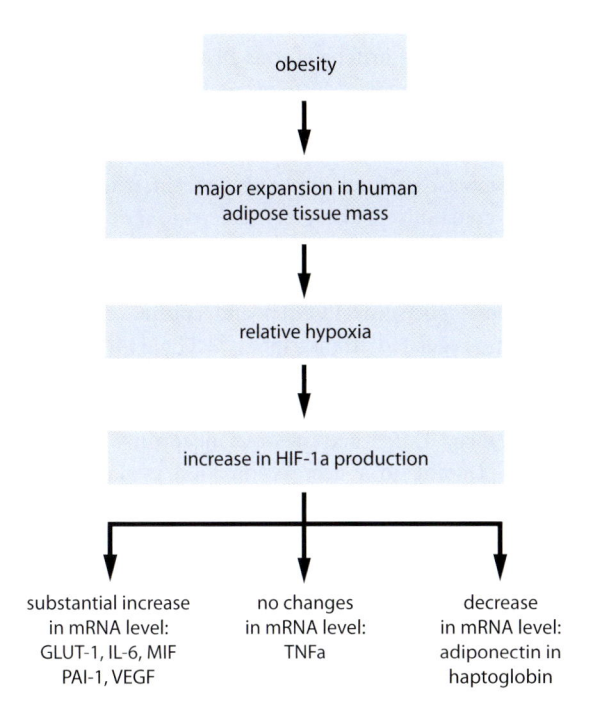

Fig. 6.5. Potential mechanism for obesity-dependent regulation of adipokine production

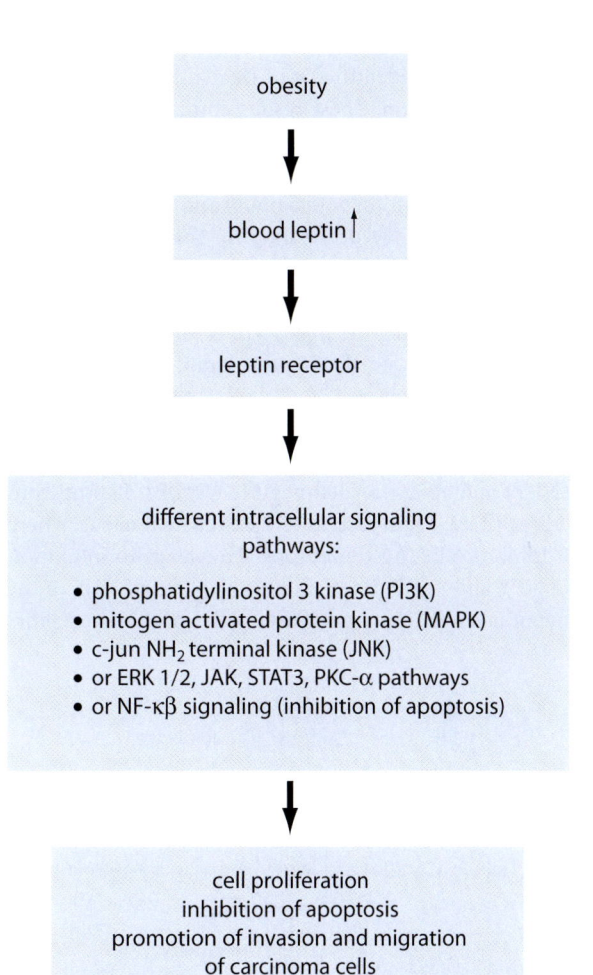

Fig. 6.6. Potential mechanism for obesity-induced cancer

Briefly, expansion of adipose tissue leads to overproduction and over-secretion of leptin. Consequently, the concentration of circulating leptin increases. Leptin binds to its receptor present in the membrane of many cells and activates different intracellular signaling pathways. These events lead to cell proliferation, inhibition of apoptosis, promotion of invasion, and migration of cancer cells. Indeed, the association between serum leptin concentration and breast cancer, colorectal cancer, prostate cancer, pancreatic cancer, lung cancer, and endometrial cancer has been reported [50, 53, 54]. Interestingly, in vitro studies indicate that adiponectin, acting via adiponectin receptor, inhibits leptin-stimulated esophageal adenocarcinoma cell proliferation [55]. However, some studies do not support a role for hyperleptinemia in intestinal carcinogenesis [56].

6.3.3 The Adipokines

Leptin. Leptin is a 16-kDa protein encoded by the *leptin* gene, named after the Greek word *leptos*, meaning thin [20, 34, 35, 48, 57]. This protein (hormone) is produced predominantly by adipocytes [57]. Much less leptin is also produced by the placenta, the ovaries, the stomach, skeletal muscle, the pituitary, and the liver [57]. There is a strong positive correlation in human beings between plasma leptin concentration and BMI [32, 34]. Obese subjects have higher plasma leptin concentrations than non-obese subjects [32, 34]. Weight reduction in obese patients leads to a decrease in plasma leptin concentration [32, 34]. Women have higher circulating leptin concentrations than men [32, 34]. In general, leptin acts as an afferent satiety signal, regulating appetite and body weight [20, 34]. Leptin suppresses food intake and stimulates energy expenditure [20, 34, 35, 48, 57]. In this way leptin plays a key role in the control of body fat stores through coordinated regulation of feeding behavior, metabolism, autonomic nervous system, and body energy balance. In obese (*ob/ob*) mice, a nonsense mutation in the *ob* (*leptin*) gene inhibits the synthesis of biologically active protein [35]. Administration of leptin to *ob/ob* mice reduced food intake and body weight [35]. Similarly (see ▪ Table 6.1), human beings with severe obesity caused by *leptin gene* mutation and circulating leptin deficiency were identified and treated successfully with recombinant leptin. These results confirmed the significance of leptin for the regulation of body weight. The current view is that leptin is an adipose tissue-derived signal to the brain (hypothalamus) and other tissue, and acts as a negative feedback loop for the maintenance of energy homeostasis [34, 35, 48, 57]. The major effects of leptin are mediated by a direct activation or inhibition of neurons possessing the long form of the leptin receptor (OB-Rb), mainly in the hypothalamic arcuate nucleus regulating food intake [34, 35, 48]. The arcuate nucleus contains two distinct populations of leptin-responsive neurons [34]. One population produces neuropeptide Y (NPY) and agouti-related peptide (AgRP). Leptin from adipose tissue gains access to the arcuate nucleus, where it inhibits NPY/AgRP neurons. This leads to inhibition of NPY and AgRP production. A low level of NPY in the hypothalamus limits activation of Y1 and Y5 receptors

present in second-order neurons of the hypothalamus. This leads to a decrease in food intake and an increase in peripheral metabolism and thermogenesis. Collectively, the action of leptin on NPY/AgRP neurons results in the decrease in food intake and the increase in peripheral metabolism. These events lead to a decrease in body weight (☐ Fig. 6.7).

The second population of arcuate neurons produces pro-opiomelanocortin (POMC) and cocaine- and amphetamine-regulated transcript (CART) [34]. Leptin activates POMC/CART neurons, leading to stimulation of α-melanocyte-stimulating hormone (α-MSH) production. In turn, αMSH activates melanocortin receptor 4 (MC4R), leading to a decrease in food intake and an increase in peripheral metabolism and thermogenesis (☐ Fig. 6.8). The decrease in food intake and the increase in peripheral metabolism and thermogenesis lead to a decrease in body weight (☐ Fig. 6.8).

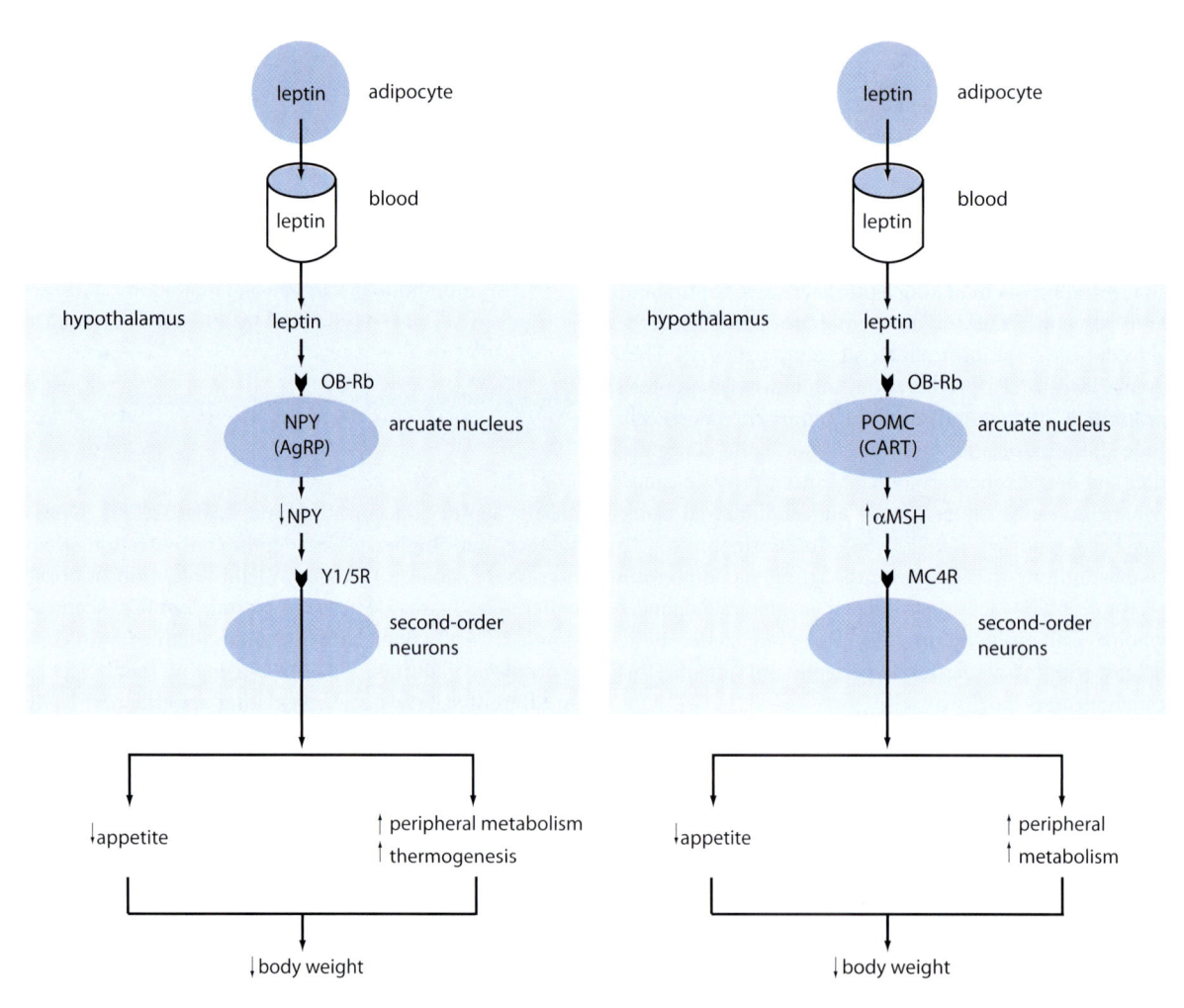

☐ **Fig. 6.7.** Molecular mechanism of leptin action via inhibition of NPY production in hypothalamus on body mass

☐ **Fig. 6.8.** Molecular mechanism of leptin action via stimulation of αMSH production in hypothalamus on body mass

Collectively, the action of leptin on NPY/AgRP and POMC/CART neurons leads to the decrease in body weight (Figs. 1.6.7, 1.6.8). The best-known orexigenic and anorexigenic pathways in the hypothalamus affected by leptin are presented in ◘ Fig. 6.9. In general, orexigenic pathways are inhibited by leptin, whereas anorexigenic pathways are stimulated by leptin. These combined effects of leptin lead to a significant inhibition of food intake and consequently to body weight loss. Indeed, in genetically obese human beings who have a mutation in the *leptin* gene such that biologically active leptin is not synthesized (see ◘ Table 6.1), administration of recombinant leptin results in a significant reduction of body weight caused by reduced hyperphagia and fat mass loss (see ◘ Table 6.1). It should be noted that in most cases the syndrome of leptin deficiency (see ◘ Table 6.1) improved following recombinant leptin administration.

Leptin receptors belong to the cytokine receptor class I superfamily and are present in brain and peripheral tissue/organs [57]. Deletion of the leptin receptors in *db/db* mice leads to obesity and diabetes. In human beings nonsense and missense mutation in leptin receptors also has been found (see ◘ Table 6.1). In general, leptin deficiency and a defect of leptin receptor lead to severe obesity (see ◘ Table 6.1).

As already mentioned, the JAK/STAT pathway is a key mediator of intracellular signaling from the leptin receptor [34, 35, 48, 57]. When leptin binds to leptin receptor, JAK2 is activated. The JAK2 phosphorylates a number of sites in the intracellular domain of leptin receptor, including tyrosine (Tyr) 1138. Phosphorylation of Tyr 1138 recruits the STAT3, which subsequently is phosphorylated. Phosphorylated STAT3 dimerizes and translocates into the nucleus to regulate transcription of a number of genes including those encoding target neuropeptides (regulating food intake). Consequently, an increase of anorexigenic neuropeptides and a decrease of orexigenic neuropeptides take place. These events lead to a decrease in body weight (◘ Fig. 6.9).

Leptin Resistance. A major question is why the molecular mechanisms described above do not work in obese subjects, who have significantly higher (sometimes several-fold higher) circulating leptin concentrations than non-obese subjects. In other words, why are human beings with a high circulating leptin concentration obese, or why does a high circulating leptin concentration not prevent obesity? This phenomenon can be explained by so-called leptin resistance (similar to insulin resistance). The molecular basis for leptin resistance can be explained as follows: Activated (phosphorylated and dimerized) STAT3, besides regulating gene transcription as mentioned above (genes encoding orexigenic and anorexigenic peptides), induces gene-encoded SOCS3 (suppressor of cytokine signaling). When SOCS3 binds to phosphorylated moieties on the intracellular domain of leptin receptor, leptin intracellular signaling is disrupted (inhibited). Simply put, SOCS3 produced in excess inhibits the action of leptin via the so-called feedback inhibition of leptin receptor/JAK2 signaling [58; 59] (◘ Fig. 6.10). This regulatory mechanism is known as a system of intracellular feedback, whereby activated STAT3 induces expression of SOCS3, a potential mediator of neuronal leptin resistance [34]. Protein-tyrosine phosphatase-1b (PTP1B) is held to be another potential mediator of neuronal leptin resistance [34]. This enzyme catalyzes dephosphorylation of some phosphorylated proteins, including phosphorylated moieties of the intracellular domain of leptin receptor. Since phosphorylation of leptin receptor catalyzed by JAK plays a key role in intracellular signaling, dephosphorylation catalyzed by PTP1B leads to disruption of this process and consequently to leptin resistance (◘ Fig. 6.10). It is tempting to speculate that PTP1B-selective or -specific inhibitors might prevent, at least in part, leptin resistance.

Besides the above-mentioned neuroendocrine effects of leptin in the control of food intake and energy expenditure, this hormone affects the metabolism of carbohydrates and lipids in peripheral tissues [57, 60]. For instance, leptin inhibits lipogenesis in adipocytes, preventing over-accumulation of triacylglycerols in the cells [60]. In this way, leptin could protect against a further increase of the fat mass [60]. Leptin is also involved

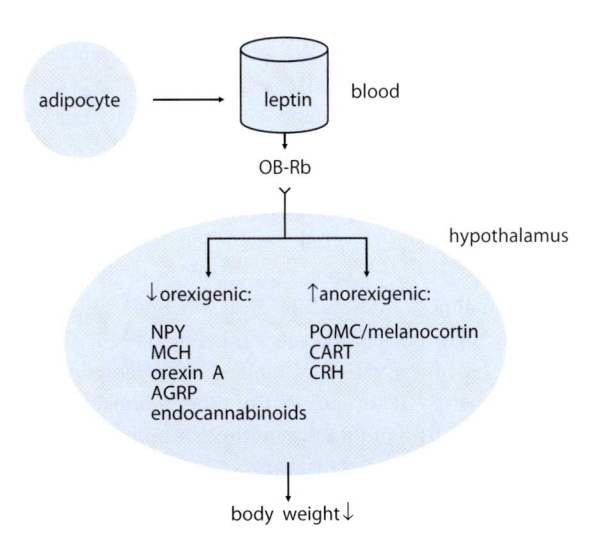

◘ **Fig. 6.9.** Effect of circulating leptin on body weight via inhibition of orexigenic and stimulation of anorexigenic pathways

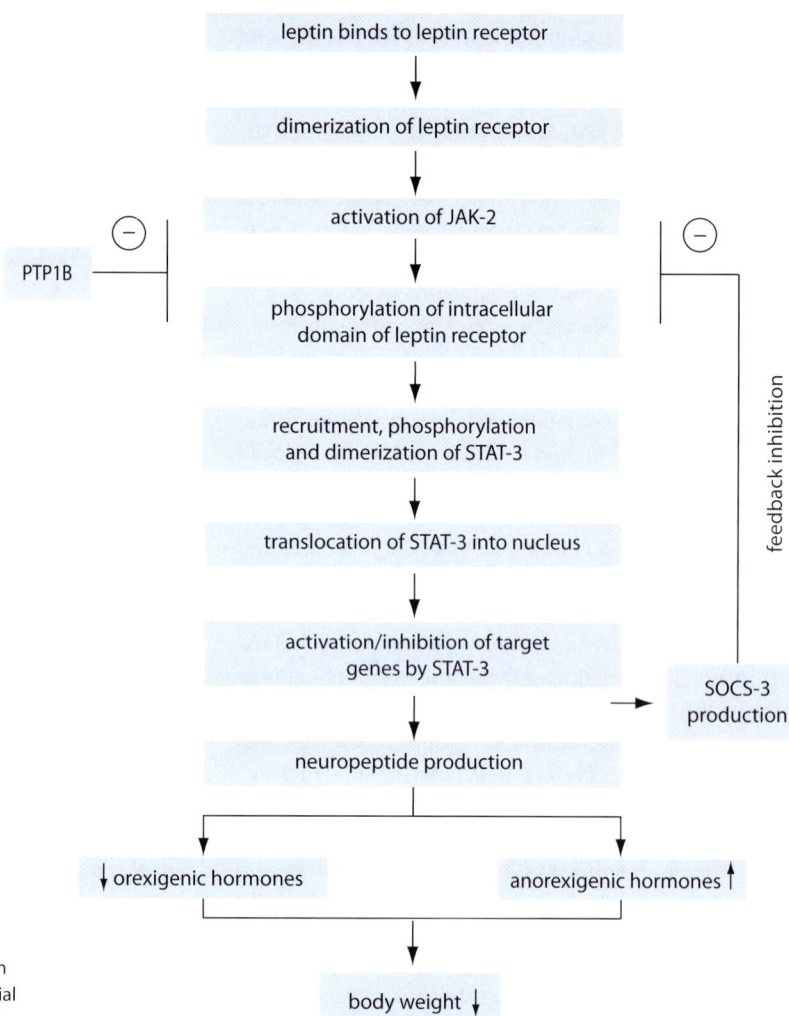

■ **Fig. 1.6.10.** Possible molecular mechanism of leptin action on body weight. The potential roles of SOCS3 and PTP1B in leptin resistance

in such diverse physiological functions as reproduction, hematopoiesis, angiogenesis, immune responsiveness, blood pressure control, bone remodeling, and regulation of some hormone synthesis and release (for instance: LH, FSH, growth hormone, ghrelin, prolactin) [48, 57]. Recently, evidence has been presented implicating an important role for leptin in modulating hippocampal synaptic plasticity [61]. Moreover, some studies have linked changes in plasma leptin concentration to neurodegenerative disorders such as Alzheimer's disease [61].

Adiponectin. Adiponectin (also termed Acrp30, GBP28, or AdipoQ) is secreted by mature adipocytes, with increasing synthesis and secretion during adipocyte differentiation [20, 32, 34]. Structurally, adiponectin displays homology with collagen and complement factor [20]. Monomeric subunits (30 kDa) form trimers, which further associate to form polymeric complexes of higher structure, including low-molecular-weight (LMW) hexamers (approximately 180 kDa) and high-molecular-weight (HMW) polymers containing 16–18 monomeric subunits (approximately 400–600 kDa) [20, 34]. These complexes are the predominant forms of adiponectin in human blood [20, 34]. It seems that oligomerization of adiponectin is essential for some biological effects of this protein [20, 34]. Besides its structural properties, adiponectin differs from other adipokines in almost all of its biological functions and in an unusually high concentration in human blood [20, 32, 34, 62–65]. The concentration of human serum adiponectin is approximately 1000 times that of other adipokines, accounting for 0.01% of total serum protein [62]. Moreover, in contrast to leptin, there is a strong negative correlation in human beings between plasma concentration and BMI [20, 32, 34]. Obese subjects have lower plasma adiponectin concentrations (despite higher fat mass) than non-obese subjects [20, 34]. Weight reduction in obese patients leads to an increase in plasma adiponectin concentration [20]. Men have significantly lower plasma adiponectin concentrations than women [20]. In human beings, the circulating concentration of adiponectin can be increased by treatment with thiazolidinediones [34, 62]. Experimental and clinical studies suggest that adiponectin contributes to the pathogenesis of diabetes, metabolic syndrome, and cardiovascular disease [20, 32, 34, 62–65]. Low circulating adiponectin concentrations are associated with obesity, insulin resistance, dyslipidemia, atherosclerosis, cardiovascular disease, essential hypertension, metabolic syndrome, and type-2 diabetes [20, 32, 34, 62–65]. Collectively, it can be said that a low concentration of circulating adiponectin may be disadvantageous, whereas a high concentration could be beneficial to human health. The administration of adiponectin to rodents decreases fat mass by stimulation of fatty acid oxidation in muscle. Moreover, chronically elevated serum adiponectin concentration leads to reduced food intake and amelioration of obesity and glycemic and lipid parameters in obese rats. In man missense mutations have been identified in the adiponectin gene which are associated with hypoadiponectinemia and type-2 diabetes [34]. Two adiponectin receptors (named adipoR1 and adipoR2) exist in animal tissue. It seems that adipoR1 has a higher affinity for HMW forms of adiponectin, whereas adipoR2 has equal affinity for all forms of adiponectin. AdipoR is found in many tissues including brain. In mice, adipoR1 is located predominantly in muscle, whereas adipoR2 is present in the liver. In man, both adipoR1 and adipoR2 are present in muscle. Adiponectin appears to exert its beneficial effects through action in both skeletal muscle and liver (◘ Fig. 6.11). When adiponectin binds to adipoR, AMPK (adenosine monophosphate-activated protein kinase) is activated (phosphorylated). Active APMK phosphorylates other enzymes such as acetyl-CoA carboxylase (ACC). Phosphorylated ACC is inactive; consequently, intracellular concentration of malonyl-CoA (product of ACC) is diminished. This leads to the inhibition of fatty acid synthesis (the rate of lipogenesis is low because malonyl-CoA is one of the substrates in this process) and stimulates fatty acid oxidation. A low intracellular concentration of malonyl-CoA is associated with stimulation of fatty acid oxidation, because a high malonyl-CoA level inhibits the transport of fatty acids into mitochondria. A decrease of fatty acid synthesis and an increase in fatty acid oxidation lead to the decrease in serum fatty acid concentration (◘ Fig. 6.11). Adiponectin also lowered the plasma glucose concentration by inhibiting glucose production (gluconeogenesis) in liver and by stimulating glucose uptake by skeletal muscle [62]. It seems that AMPK is involved in these processes. As already mentioned, adiponectin also has anti-atherosclerotic and anti-inflammatory effects [63–65].

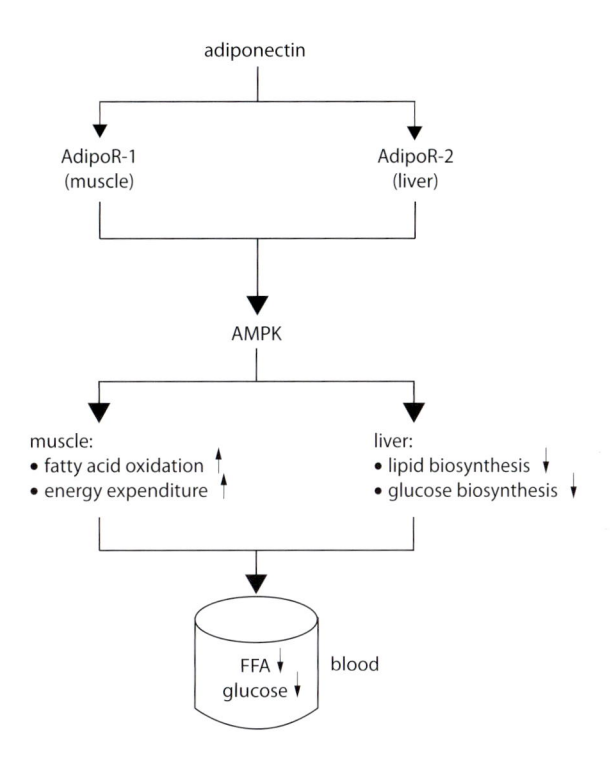

◘ **Fig. 6.11.** Potential molecular mechanism of adiponectin action on lipid and carbohydrate metabolism in liver and skeletal muscle

Resistin. Resistin is a member of the proinflammatory protein family known as resistin-like molecules (RELMs) [66]. This protein family is characterized by a highly conserved, cysteine-rich C-terminus [67]. Four members of the mouse RELMs family have been described: resistin, RELMα, RELMβ, and RELMγ [68]. In human beings, only two RELMs have been found: resistin and RELMβ [68]. Mouse resistin is produced mainly in adipose tissue, whereas human resistin is expressed at a high level in the bone marrow and lung [68]. Human resistin mRNA has also been found in placenta [69], pancreatic islet cells [70], whole blood cells [71], and adipose tissue [71]. In contrast to the mouse, the expression of resistin in human adipocytes is very low, even undetectable under some conditions [68]. It seems that adipose tissue macrophages are the predominant source of human adipose tissue resistin [71]. Based on animal and cell line studies, three physiological roles have been postulated for resistin: (a) regulation of carbohydrate and lipid metabolism in the liver, muscle, and adipose tissue; (b) inhibition of adipogenesis; (c) proinflammatory action [68, 71–73]. It has been shown that resistin mRNA abundance was strongly increased by TNFα in human peripheral blood mononuclear cells [74] and by endotoxin in primary culture of human macrophages

[72]. Moreover, it has been shown that resistin up-regulates IL-6 and TNFα in human peripheral blood mononuclear cells [75] and IL-12 and TNFα in human macrophages via the NF-κB pathway [76]. The involvement of resistin in the development of atherosclerosis [77], diabetes mellitus [78], non-alcoholic fatty liver disease [79], and inflammatory bowel disease [80] has also been proposed. Collectively, these data suggest that resistin could be involved in obesity, inflammation, insulin resistance, and in some other disorders. However, epidemiological studies in human beings have not provided a clear link between circulating resistin concentration and obesity or insulin resistance [62]. Recently, Schaffler et al. [81] reported elevated serum resistin concentrations in patients with severe acute pancreatitis and suggested that resistin may be a potential marker for severity of acute pancreatitis.

Visfatin. Visfatin is a 52-kDa adipokine produced mainly in adipose tissue, bone marrow, liver, and muscle [20]. The adipokine was initially identified in human leukocytes as a protein which facilitates the development of early-stage B cells (called pre-B cell colony-enhancing factor, PBEF) [20]. Moreover, this protein displayed activity of nicotinamide 5-phosphoribosyl-1-pyrophosphate transferase (NAMPT, EC 2.4.2.12), an enzyme that catalyzes the rate-limiting step in NAD biosynthesis [20]. In general, visfatin exerts an insulin-like effect on plasma glucose concentration [34, 35]. However, in contrast to insulin, plasma visfatin concentration does not change upon feeding or fasting in rodents. The possible molecular mechanism of vifatin action is as follows: Visfatin binds to the insulin receptor (probably at different sites than insulin; thus no competition with insulin is observed) with an affinity comparable to that of insulin. The binding of visfatin to the insulin receptor causes phosphorylation of the insulin receptor and of insulin receptor substrates (IRS-1 and IRS-2), binding of phosphatidylinositol 3-kinase to insulin receptors, and the phoshorylation of Akt kinase and mitogen-activated protein kinase (MAPK) in adipocytes, myocytes and hepatocytes [34, 35]. Administration of visfatin to diabetic rodents caused a rapid decrease in plasma glucose concentration without changing plasma insulin concentrations. However, the effect of visfatin on glucose metabolism and insulin resistance is not clear [20]. Similarly, controversial reports have been published concerning the relationship between circulating visfatin concentration and obesity [20].

Retinol-binding Protein 4. Retinol-binding protein 4 (RBP4), a 21-kDa protein, is synthesized mainly in the liver and is associated with insulin resistance. Serum RBP4 is elevated in mice models of obesity and diabetes. Similarly, an elevated serum RBP4 concentration is present in diabetic patients. Moreover, the serum RBP4 concentration in human beings correlates positively with obesity (abdominal obesity) and with plasma insulin concentration and negatively with insulin sensitivity. Although the role of RBP4 in human beings has not been supported by all studies, some data indicate that noncoding variants located close to *RBP4* may contribute to impaired insulin sensitivity and insulin secretion. A significant decrease in serum RBP4 following weight loss was observed [34, 35]. Both experimental and clinical studies indicate that RBP4 may contribute to the pathogenesis of insulin resistance. Although the molecular mechanism by which RBP4 causes insulin resistance is not clear, it seems that impaired insulin signaling in muscle and the increase in *PEPCK* (PEP carboxykinase or phosphoenolpyruvate carboxykinase) gene expression, and consequently the increase in glucose production in liver, play important roles in RBP4 action [34, 35].

Vaspin. Vaspin belongs to the superfamily of 45- to 50-kDa proteins called serpins. Serpins are a group of structurally related molecules which display serine protease inhibitor activity. It should be noted that α1-antitrypsin is the best known serpin. In human beings vaspin is produced mainly in visceral adipose tissue; however, vaspin mRNA was also found in subcutaneous adipose tissue. Vaspin synthesis is associated strongly with adiposity and is rarely detected in lean subjects. The administration of recombinant vaspin improves insulin sensitivity and glucose tolerance in a mice model of dietary-induced obesity. However, a direct effect of vaspin on adipocyte in vitro has not been confirmed. It is likely that vaspin improves insulin sensitivity and glucose tolerance indirectly, probably by inhibiting the local inflammatory milieu within adipose tissue [34].

Fasting-induced Adipose Factor. Fasting-induced adipose factor (FIAF), also known as angiopoietin-like peptide 4 (ANGPTL4), a 35-kDa protein, belongs to the fibrinogen/angiopoietin-like protein family. Synthesis of FIAF is induced by fasting and by activation of PPARγ in adipose tissue and by activation of PPARα in liver [18, 34]. FIAF associates with circulating lipoproteins. Administration of FIAF to rodents causes an increase in plasma triacylglycerol concentration, which could be the result of inhibition of lipoprotein lipase and/or altered function of mitochondria [34].

Angiotensinogen. Angiotensinogen is the substrate for renin in the renin-angiotensin-aldosterone system, which plays a key role in blood pressure regulation. Adipose tissue is important with respect to the synthesis and secretion of angiotensinogen [18, 34]. The plasma angiotensinogen concentration is elevated in obesity [18], and it seems that this elevation is a consequence of the increase of adipose tissue mass [18]. Consequently, hypertension in the obese subjects may result from the increased synthesis and secretion of angiotensinogen in adipose tissue [18]. Moreover, adipose tissue expresses the genes encoding angiotensin-converting enzyme (ACE) and type-1 angiotensin receptor, which suggests that a local renin-angiotensin system is present in adipose tissue. Angiotensin II (a product formed from angiotensinogen), besides affecting blood pressure, is able to stimulate the synthesis and release of prostacyclin, which in turn can stimulate differentiation of preadipocytes to adipocytes [18, 34].

Plasminogen Activator Inhibitor 1. Plasminogen activator inhibitor-1 (PAI-1) – an 85-kDa protein, is another member of the serpin superfamily. PAI-1 is synthesized in different cell types within adipose tissue, mainly in visceral adipose tissue. Primarily, PAI-1 is an inhibitor of fibrinolysis. It inactivates urokinase-type and tissue-type plasminogen activator and thereby inhibits fibrinolysis. Moreover, PAI-1 may also be involved in angiogenesis and atherogenesis. The circulating PAI-1 concentration is higher in subjects with visceral adiposity and in the metabolic syndrome [18, 32, 34]. Improvement in insulin sensitivity by weight loss or treatment with metformin or thiazoladinediones (insulin sensitizers) significantly decreases plasma PAI-1 concentration. Elevated circulating concentration of PAI-1 is observed in subjects with myocardial infarction, deep-vein thrombosis, type-2 diabetes, and obesity. The increase of incidence of cardiovascular disease in obese subjects has been linked to the elevated circulating concentration of PAI1 [18]. Moreover, it is suggested that PAI-1 could be a marker for metabolic syndrome and visceral obesity [32, 34]. PAI-1 null mice have increased energy expenditure, enhanced insulin sensitivity, and are resistant to diet-or genetically induced obesity [18, 32].

Acylation-stimulating Protein. Acylation-stimulating protein (ASP, also named C3ades-Arg) is derived from the C3 complex through the action of adipsin (called complement factor D, which is a serine protease of the alternative complement pathway), factor B, and a carboxypeptidase. Studies on transgenic mice suggest that ASP is important in the postprandial clearance of triacylglycerols. It stimulates the uptake of fatty acids by adipocytes and their estrification, increasing triacylglycerol synthesis in the cells [18, 32].

Metallothionein. Metallothionein is a stress-response and metal-binding protein. The protein is synthesized mainly in liver, kidney, and other tissue, including adipose tissue (in adipocytes). Gene expression and protein secretion are stimulated by dexamethasone and by the compounds increasing cAMP concentration. It has been suggested that an antioxidant property, protecting fatty acids from oxidative damage, is the main function of metallothionein in adipose tissue. This action of metallothionein could be beneficial because human obesity is associated with increased oxidative stress [18].

6.4 Cytokines, Chemokines and Growth Factors

The association between serum "classical" proinflammatory cytokine concentration and obesity has long been recognized. Recently, the contribution of adipose tissue cytokines to metabolic syndrome and diabetes has been suggested. This is based on the fact that several cytokines, chemokines, and growth factors are synthesized and secreted in adipose tissue. TNFα, interleukin 6 (IL-6), and TGFβ are the most widely studied of these cytokines. TNFα synthesis in adipose tissue and the circulating concentration of TNFα is higher in obese than in lean subjects. An important observation was that TNFα may play a role in the development of insulin resistance. However, suppression of plasma TNFα concentration by immunoneutralization fails to ameliorate insulin resistance. TGFβ gene expression in adipose tissue is higher in genetically obese rodents (both *ob/ob* and *db/db* mice). Interestingly, TGFβ gene expression is stimulated by TNFα. The synthesis of IL-6 in adipose tissue and the plasma IL-6 concentration are higher in obese subjects than in lean individuals. In human beings, IL-6 may originate both from adipocytes and from stromovascular cells within adipose tissue. Adipose tissue produces and secretes several other cytokines (e.g., IL-1 and IL-18) and chemokines such as monocyte chemotactic protein-1. The plasma concentration of this chemokine is increased in obesity. Recent studies suggest that adipose-specific overproduction of monocyte chemotactic protein-1 leads to macrophage accumulation in adipose tissue [18, 22, 23, 32, 34, 39].

6.5 Other Adipokines

The most important adipokines are described above. However, it must be kept in mind that approximately 60 adipokines have been described so far including (besides those mentioned above): nerve growth factor (NGF),

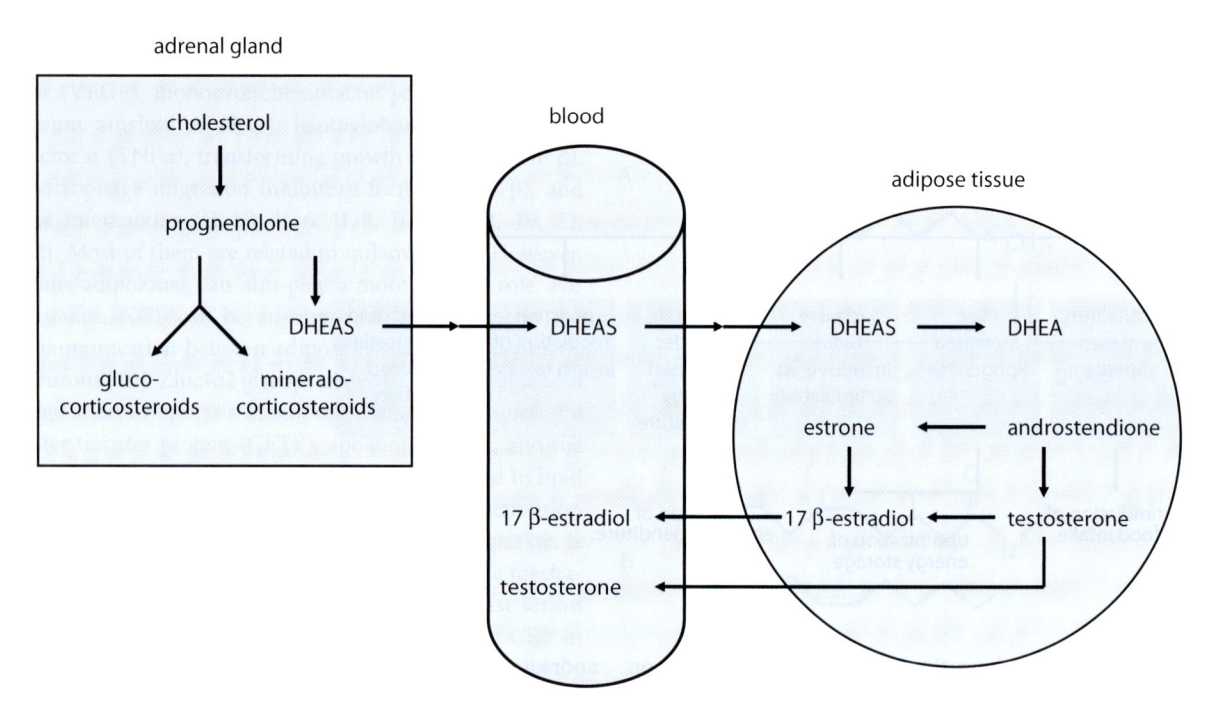

Fig. 6.14. Role of adipose tissue in estrogen (17β-estradiol) and androgen (testosterone) biosynthesis

cortisol concentration. Interestingly, 11β-HSD1 is present predominantly in visceral adipose tissue. 11β-HSD1 activity was higher in the adipose tissue of obese human subjects than in that of lean subjects. Up-regulation of the 11β-HSD1 mRNA level by estrogen in preadipocytes of women has been observed. The tissue-specific regulation of 11β-HSD1 has been implicated in obesity, diabetes, hypertension, dyslipidemia, cardiovascular diseases, metabolic syndrome, and polycystic ovarian syndrome. Moreover, pharmacological inhibition of 11β-HSD1 increases insulin sensitivity. In general, many observations (mentioned above) made in man have been confirmed in experimental animals. Thus, it can be said that 11β-HSD1 and its role in glucocorticosteroid metabolism might play some role in the pathogenesis of visceral obesity and metabolic syndrome [32, 87].

Obesity is also associated with hyperaldosteronism, which can contribute to elevated blood pressure in obese subjects. On the other hand, weight loss is associated with a decrease in circulating aldosterone concentrations and blood pressure. However, the mechanism by which an excess of fat mass might increase the serum aldosterone concentration is not clear. Lack of aldosterone synthase in adipose tissue, a key enzyme in the aldosterone synthesis pathway, suggests that synthesis of aldosterone in this tissue does not occur. Recent data suggest that adipose tissue can synthesize 11-deoxycorticosterone (DOC), which displayed mineralocorticoid activity [85].

6.8 The Gastrointestinal Tract Hormones and Obesity

In addition to adipose tissue and the pancreas, the gastrointestinal tract produces hormones which influence the appetite through their action via the hypothalamus, the brain steam, and the autonomic nervous system [87–90]. Gastrointestinal tract hormones also regulate the metabolism. Changes in circulating gastrointestinal hormones might lead to the development of obesity.

Ghrelin. Ghrelin is a 28-amino acid peptide derived from preproghrelin, a 117-amino acid prohormone [87, 88]. Data reported so far suggest a role for ghrelin as a meal initiator (hunger signal). The peptide is synthesized (approximately 70%) and secreted by stomach cells (named X/A-like cells and sometimes called ghrelin cells) localized particularly in the gastric fundus. Much less (approximately 30%) ghrelin is produced by the duodenum and the small intestine (Fig. 6.15) [88]. In addition to the stomach and proximal small intestine, ghrelin may be produced within the brain in amounts that do not affect the circulating concentration of the hormone (ghrelin). The functional role of ghrelin produced within the brain is not clear [88]. Ghrelin synthesis and secretion by the gastrointestinal tract are increased by fasting, weight loss, and insulin-induced hypoglycemia (Fig. 6.15) [88]. Ghrelin undergoes acylation by covalent binding of oc-

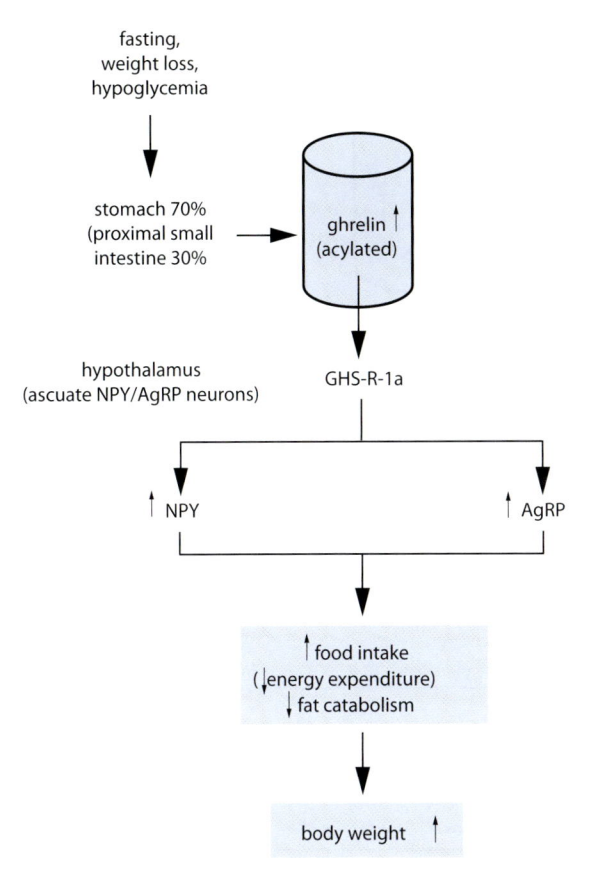

Fig. 6.15. Regulation of ghrelin secretion and potential mechanism of ghrelin

exogenous ghrelin have been observed including regulation of glucose homeostasis, gut motility, pancreatic exocrine secretion, cardiovascular function, and immunity. However, the physiological significance of the action of ghrelin on these organs remains to be determined. In human beings, serum ghrelin concentration is inversely correlated with adiposity, being low in the obese subject and high in subjects who are cachectic due to diverse diseases, including cancer [88]. However, in one patient with a malignant gastric cancer (ghrelinoma), a high serum ghrelin concentration was observed [92]. Moreover, this patient remained obese with preserved appetite despite advanced disease. Several data indicate that ghrelin can be used as a drug. For instance, ghrelin administration (by intravenous infusion) results in weight gain in patients with cardiac cachexia and chronic obstructive pulmonary disease. Moreover, ghrelin is also effective when given by subcutaneous injection to malnourished patients on peritoneal dialysis. Several active agonists for GHS-R1a have been synthesized, and this may have therapeutic potential for cachectic patients [88].

Obestatin. Obestatin is a 23-amino acid peptide derived from preproghrelin (note that ghrelin is also formed from preproghrelin) [88, 93]. This peptide is synthesized in the stomach and secreted into the blood [88, 93]. In contrast to ghrelin, obestatin suppressed food intake, inhibited jejunal contraction, and decreased body weight. This implies that two antagonistic hormones (ghrelin and obestatin) are derived from the same gene, as the results of different post-translational modification of preproghrelin [88, 93]. Obestatin binds to the orphan receptor named GPR39. GPR39 is a G-protein-coupled receptor found in the stomach, in the intestine, and within the hypothalamus [93]. However, the true physiological role of obestatin requires further investigation. It has been reported recently that obestatin had no effect on food intake in rodents [94].

Cholecystokinin. Cholecystokinin (CCK) is a gastrointestinal peptide which acts as a postprandial satiety signal [87, 88]. It is synthesized and released into the blood and the surrounding tissue from endocrine cells of the duodenum and jejunum (in small amounts also from other parts of the gastrointestinal tract) in response to lipid- and protein-rich meals [87, 88] (■ Fig. 6.16). CCK acts at two distinct G protein-coupled receptors: CCK-A (also named CCK-1) and CCK-B [88]. CCK-A is found in the pancreas, on vagal afferent neurons, enteric neurons, and in the brain (nucleus of the solitary tract, area postrema, dorsomedial hypothalamus) [88]. CCK-B is present in the stomach, the afferent vagus nerve, and the

tanoic acid (or other medium-chain fatty acids) [88]. Only acylated ghrelin can bind and activate GHS-R1a receptor, present in brain areas involved in the regulation of appetite and energy balance, including arcuate NPY/AgRP neurons [88]. When ghrelin binds to GHS-R1a the levels of NPY and AgRP are enhanced (■ Fig. 6.15) [88]. Consequently, food intake increases and energy expenditure decreases. This can lead to an increase in body weight (■ Fig. 6.15). It should be noted that ghrelin is the only known peripheral appetite-stimulating hormone (also called orexigenic or hunger hormone).

The increase in body weight was observed after chronic administration of ghrelin to rodents. The weight gain was greater than expected for the degree of hyperphagia [88]. This phenomenon might reflect stimulation of adipogenesis, inhibition of apoptosis, transfer from fatty acid oxidation to glucose utilization, and inhibition of sympathetic nervous system activity [88]. GHS-R1a receptor is widely distributed and is found in the stomach, the colon, pancreatic adipose tissue, liver, heart, kidney, placenta, and T cells [88]. Accordingly, diverse biological actions of

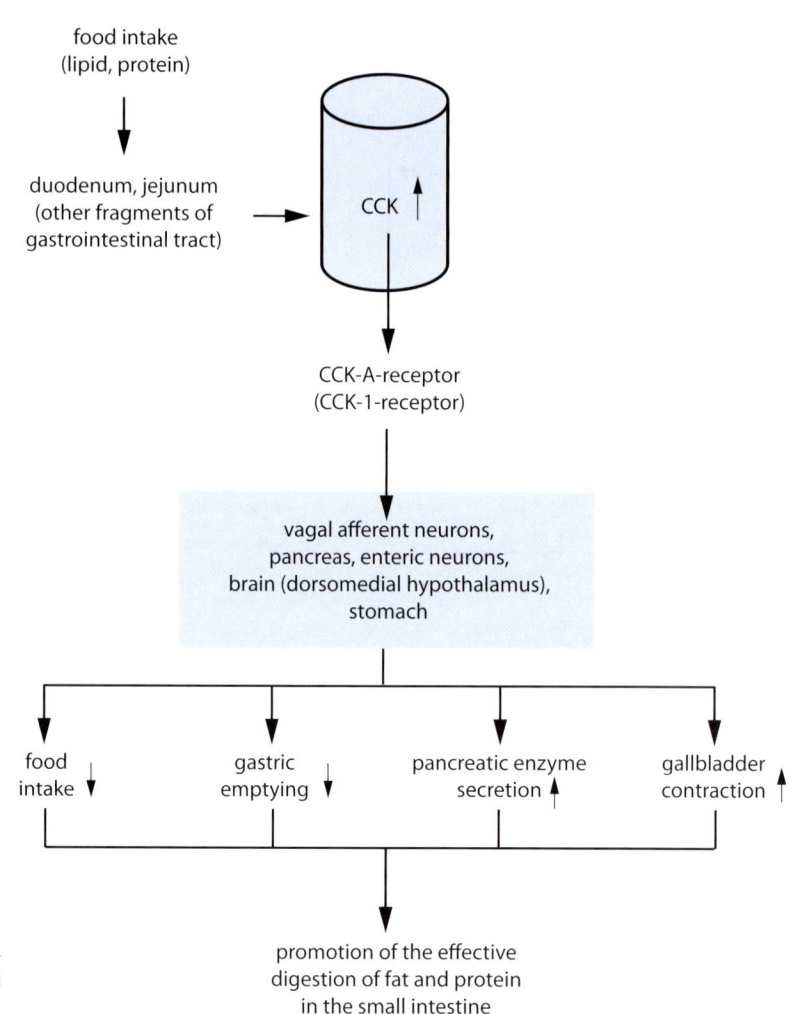

food intake
(lipid, protein)

duodenum, jejunum
(other fragments of
gastrointestinal tract)

CCK ↑

CCK-A-receptor
(CCK-1-receptor)

vagal afferent neurons,
pancreas, enteric neurons,
brain (dorsomedial hypothalamus),
stomach

food
intake ▼

gastric
emptying ▼

pancreatic enzyme
secretion ▲

gallbladder
contraction ▲

promotion of the effective
digestion of fat and protein
in the small intestine

◘ Fig. 6.16. Cholecystokinin secretion, potential mechanism of cholecystokinin action, and main physiological effect

brain. When CCK binds to its receptor, several events occur: decrease of food intake, delayed gastric emptying, stimulation of pancreatic enzyme, and stimulation of gall bladder contraction. Collectively, these actions promote the effective digestion of fat and protein in the small intestine [87, 88] (Fig. 1.6.16).

Peptide YY. Peptide YY (PYY) occurs in two forms: as PYY_{1-36} (consisting of 36 amino acids) and PYY_{3-36} (consisting of 34 amino acids) [88; 89]. PYY_{3-36} is the major circulating form. It is created from PYY_{1-36} by cleavage of the N-terminal Tyr-Pro (a dipeptide consisting of tyrosine-proline residues) catalyzed by dipeptidyl peptidase IV (DPPIV) according to the reaction: $PYY_{1-36} + H_2O \rightarrow PYY_{3-36} + Tyr\text{-}Pro$ [89]. PYY is synthesized and secreted from the endocrine L-cells of the entire gastrointestinal tract, particularly in the distal portion. Blood PYY concentration is low in the fasting state [88; 89]. Food intake

causes a significant increase of PYY_{1-36} and PYY_{3-36} in circulation [88; 89]. PYY_{1-36} binds with similar affinity to all known G protein-coupled Y receptors. PYY_{3-36} shows selectivity for Y2 receptor and lower affinity for Y1 and Y5 [89]. These receptors are present in the hypothalamus, the gastrointestinal tract, and other organs [89]. When PYY binds to Y receptor in the gastrointestinal tract it increases the absorption of fluids and electrolytes from the ileum after a meal, inhibits pancreatic and gastric secretions, inhibits gastric emptying, and inhibits gall bladder contraction [89] (◘ Fig. 6.17).

Several data suggest that PYY_{3-36} inhibits food intake both in rodents and in man; however, the mechanism whereby this peptide inhibits appetite and food intake is not clear [89]. It is probable that the anorectic effect of PYY is associated with activation of POMC neurons and inhibition of NPY neurons in the arcuate nucleus. In human beings, a lower postprandial circulating PYY_{3-36}

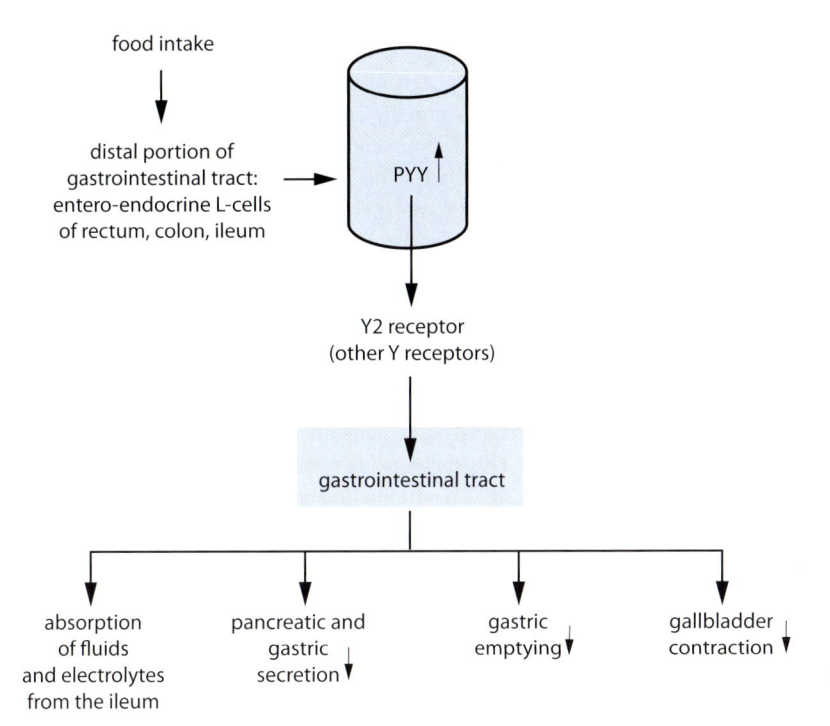

food intake

distal portion of gastrointestinal tract: entero-endocrine L-cells of rectum, colon, ileum

PYY

Y2 receptor (other Y receptors)

gastrointestinal tract

absorption of fluids and electrolytes from the ileum

pancreatic and gastric secretion

gastric emptying

gallbladder contraction

Fig. 6.17. Secretion and main physiological effects of PPY

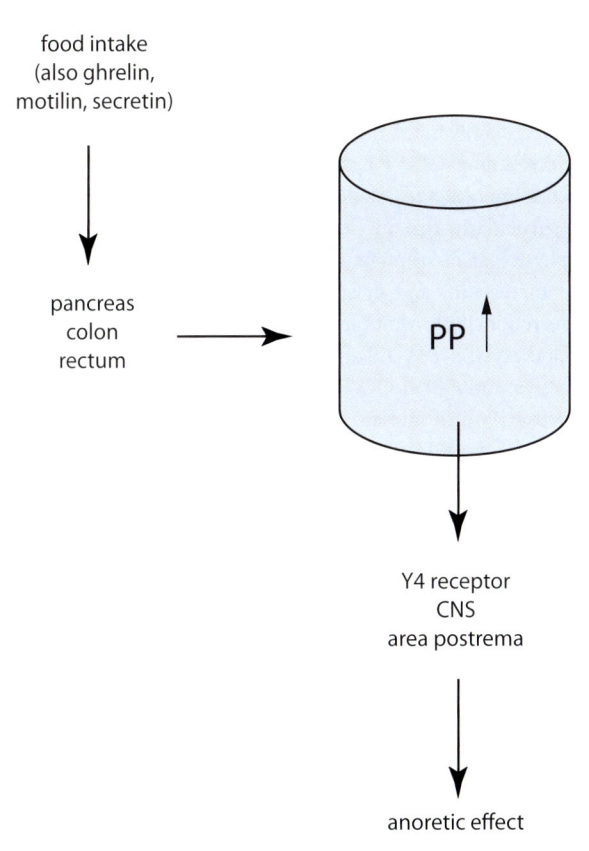

food intake (also ghrelin, motilin, secretin)

pancreas colon rectum

PP

Y4 receptor CNS area postrema

anoretic effect

Fig. 6.18. Regulation of PP secretion and its main physiological effects

concentration has been reported [89]. Bariatric surgery (RYGB) results an increase of the postprandial serum PYY concentration [95].

Pancreatic Polypeptide. Pancreatic polypeptide (PP) is another circulating satiety factor. It is produced and secreted by the pancreas (both endocrine and exocrine), the colon, and the rectum [89]. PP is released in response to food (especially containing lipids) intake (like other satiety signal hormones) [89]. Circulating PP concentration is also regulated by gastrointestinal hormones. Ghrelin, motilin, and secretin increase, whereas the circulating PP concentration of somatostatin decreases [89] (Fig. 6.18).

Circulating PP acts on the CNS via areas that have a deficient blood-brain barrier, such as the area postrema. PP binds with high affinity to Y4 (and Y5 receptors) and has an anorectic effect [89] (Fig. 6.18). In general, PP is considered a long-term appetite suppressor.

Oxyntomodulin. Oxyntomodulin (OXM), is a 37-amino acid peptide that, like GLP-1 (see below), is a product of the preproglucagon gene. Thus, it combines the 29 amino acids of glucagon with an 8 amino acid C-terminal extension [89]. It is released from intestinal L-cells in response to food intake (similar to other satiety signals) [89]. In general, it acts as a satiety signal. Some data indicate that OXM participates in long-term body weight regulation [89]. It reduces gastric motility and gastric secretion

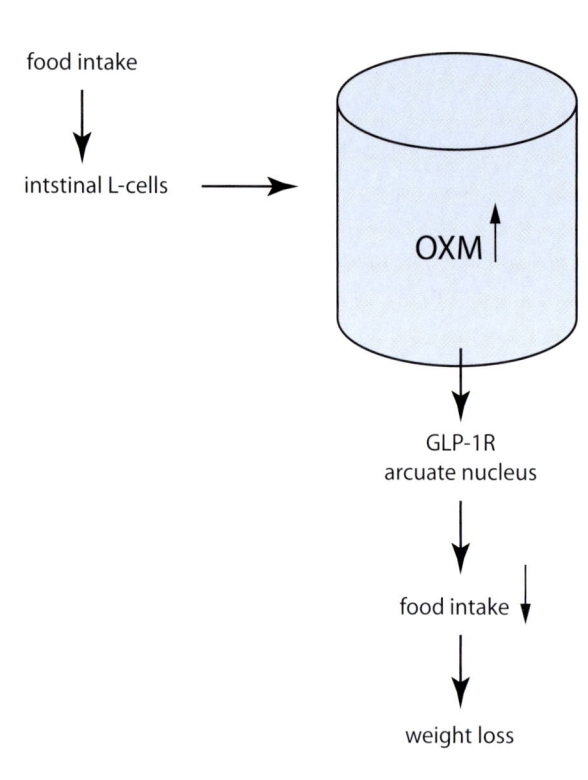

Fig. 6.19. Oxyntomodulin secretion and its action

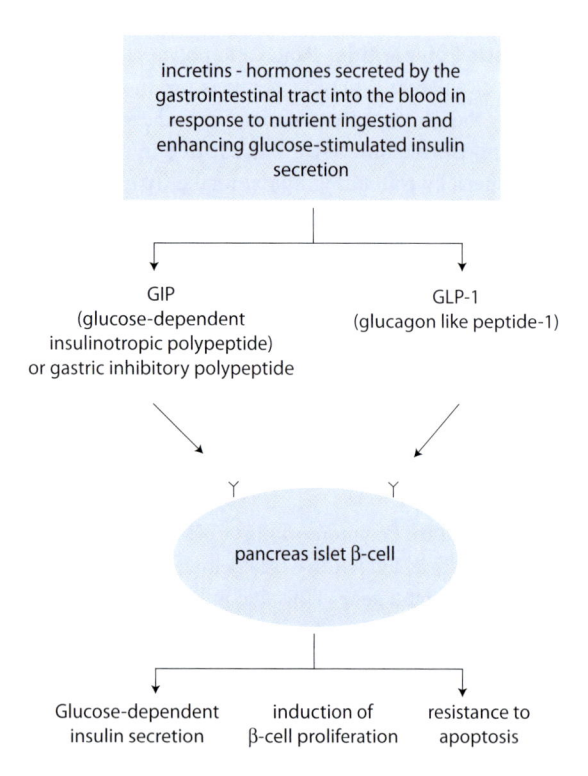

Fig. 6.20. Action of incretins on islet β-cells

[89]. In human beings OXM is an effective anorectic peptide [89]. Part of this effect may be via a decrease of the plasma ghrelin concentration [89]. Administration of OXM to overweight subjects resulted in significant weight loss [89]. This may be due to inhibition of caloric intake and to an increase of energy expenditure. OXM exerts its effect probably via the GLP-1 receptor (GLP-1R), which is present in the brain, including the arcuate nucleus (Fig. 6.19) [89]. It cannot be excluded that OXM has its own receptor; however, the putative receptor has not been cloned. The effect of OXM on food intake following peptide administration is brief. Significant weight loss requires subcutaneous injection of OXM three times daily. This may be due to the rapid degradation of OXM by DDPIV, mentioned earlier [89].

Incretin Peptide. Glucose-dependent insulinotropic polypeptide (GIP) and glucagon-like peptide-1 (GLP-1) are produced and secreted by the gastrointestinal tract within minutes of food ingestion [90]. They act on islet β-cells via the structurally different incretin receptor. The activation of incretin receptors by GIP or GLP-1 leads to glucose-dependent insulin secretion, induction of β-cells proliferation, and enhanced resistance of β-cells to apoptosis [90] (Fig. 6.20).

GLP-1. GLP-1 is secreted by intestinal endocrine L-cells, located mainly in the distal ileum and colon [90] (Fig. 6.21). Secretion of GLP-1 is stimulated by nutrient, neural, and endocrine factors, including leptin [90]. Food ingestion (particularly rich in carbohydrates and fats) is the main physiological stimulus for GLP-1 secretion [90]. Insulin, somatostatin, and galanin (neuropeptide) inhibit GLP-1 secretion [90]. Multiple forms of GLP-1 are secreted, including GLP-1 (1-37) and GLP-1 (1-36) NH_2 which are inactive, and GLP-1 (7-37) and GLP-1 (7-36) NH_2 which are active [90]. In human beings, the main form of GLP-1 in the blood is GLP-1 (7-36) NH_2. Active forms are produced from their full-length precursor. For instance, GLP-1 (7-36) NH2 is formed from GLP-1 (1-36) NH_2 according to the reaction: GLP-1 (1-36) NH_2 + H_2O → GLP-1 (7-36) NH2 + hexapeptide. The presence of an amide group (-NH_2) in GLP-1 (7-36) NH_2 increases the half-life of the peptide in the blood, which is less than 2 min [90]. Rapid inactivation of GLP-1 (7-36) NH_2 is catalyzed by proteolytic enzyme dipetidyl peptidase-4 [90] (Fig. 6.21). Interestingly, dipeptidyl peptidase-4 is elevated in obese subjects, and this does not change after bariatric surgery [96].

DPP-4. The inhibition of DPP-4 can prolong the half-life of biologically active GLP-1. This suggests a potential clinical role of selective or specific inhibitors of DPP-4.

Experiments performed on rodents indicate that DPP-4 inhibitors lower blood glucose concentration in normal and in diabetic animals [91]. Moreover, animals with a mutation in the DPP-4 gene exhibit enhanced glucose-stimulated insulin secretion and improved glucose clearance [91]. A beneficial effect of vildagliptin (inhibitor of DPP-4) on the blood glucose concentration also was observed in diabetic patients [91]. Postprandial blood concentrations of biologically active GLP-1 are lower in obese and type-2 diabetic subjects. The active form of GLP-1 acts via GLP-1 receptor (GLP-1R), which belongs to the family of G-protein coupled receptors. GLP-1R is present in several tissues including pancreas, lung, heart, kidney, stomach, intestine, pituitary, skin, vagus nerve, and in several regions of the brain including the hypothalamus. It is not excluded that GLP-1R is also present in adipose tissue, skeletal muscle, and liver. Exenatide and liraglutide are known GLP-1 receptor agonists and have been approved for use in patients with type-2 diabetes. GLP-1 activates neurons in the hypothalamus to increase satiety and decrease hunger. Several biological actions of the active form of GLP-1 are presented in ◘ Fig. 6.22 [90].

GIP. GIP is a 42-amino acid peptide synthesized and released from intestinal K-cells located mainly in the duodenum and the jejunum (◘ Fig. 6.23); however, cells that produce and secrete GIP can be found throughout the entire small intestine (similarly L-cells producing GLP-1) [90, 91]. In human beings GIP is secreted in response to the ingestion of food, particularly food containing lipids (in rodents, carbohydrates). More precisely, the rate of nutrient absorption rather than the presence of nutrients in the intestine stimulates GIP release [90]. Consequently, GIP secretion is lower in subjects with intestinal malabsorption. The half-life of biologically active human GIP is approximately 5 min [90]. Similar to GLP-1, GIP is inactivated by DPP-4 [90] (◘ Fig. 6.23).

GIP acts via G-protein-coupled receptor (GIPR), localized in the pancreas, stomach, small intestine, adipose tissue, adrenal cortex, pituitary, heart, testes, endothelial cells, bone, trachea, spleen, thymus, lung, kidney, thyroid, and several regions of the brain [90]. The biological actions of GIP are presented in ◘ Fig. 6.24.

Amylin. Amylin is a 37-amino acid peptide (co-secreted with insulin), which affects food intake and body weight. Amylin is also produced in the stomach, duodenum, jejunum, colon, and rectum; however, pancreatic β-cells appear to be the predominant source of circulating amylin

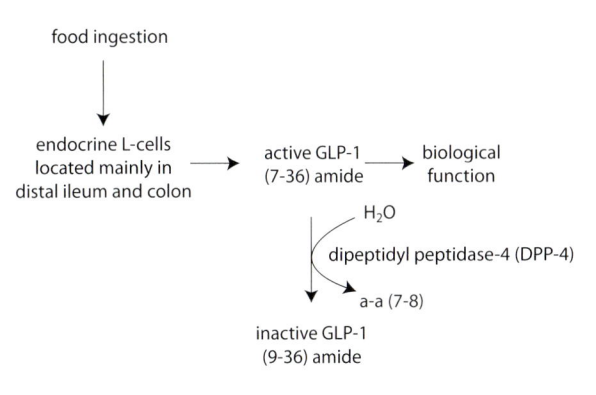

◘ **Fig. 6.21.** Secretion and degradation of biologically active GLP-1

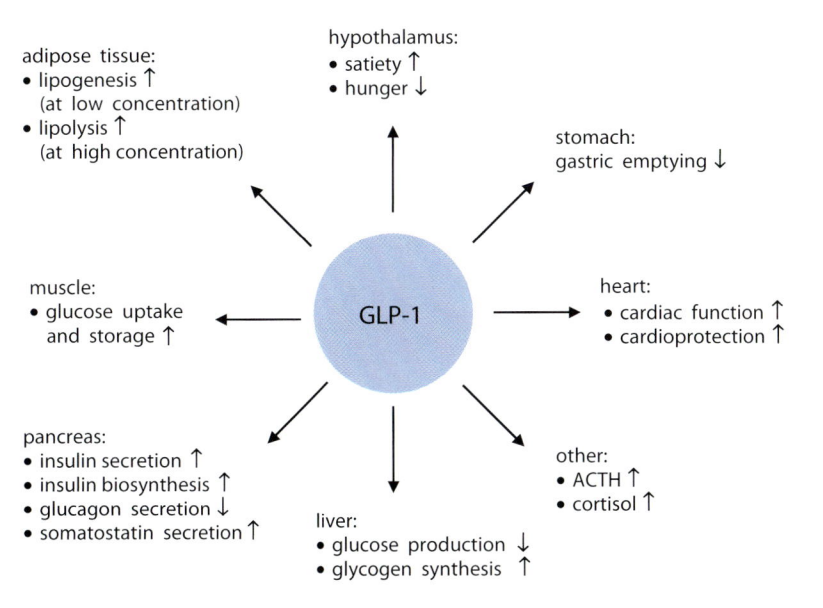

◘ **Fig. 6.22.** Biological action of GLP-1

[91]. Nutritional stimuli play a key role in the regulation of blood amylin concentration. Amylin secretion is inhibited by insulin and somatostatin and stimulated by glucagon, GLP-1, and cholinergic agonist [91]. It is believed that endogenous amylin contributes to the long-term control of satiety and body weight [91]. Exogenous amylin reduces short-term food intake and inhibits gastric emptying and gastric acid secretion [91]. Sustained amylin administration causes weight loss [91]. The acute glucoregulatory actions of amylin result from inhibition of gastric emptying and inhibition of glucagon secretion [91]. Finally, it should be noted that the amylin analog pramlintide has been approved for the treatment of diabetes [91].

In conclusion, a great deal of progress has been made in identifying the hormonal and neural mechanisms involved in the regulation of food intake and energy balance.

The hypothalamus, gastrointestinal tract hormones, and substances released by adipose tissue (including adipokines and endocannabinoids) play crucial roles in the regulation of food intake and energy expenditure. The dysregulation of this remarkable regulatory system is probably important role in the development of obesity. However, it is far from clear what specific neuro-hormonal systems and mechanisms are affected mainly by changes in environment and lifestyle, leading to the development of obesity.

6.9 Circulating Adipokines and Gastrointestinal Tract Hormones in Obese Subjects Prior to and Following Bariatric Surgery

It is generally accepted that weight loss following bariatric surgery is due mainly to diminished food intake. However, there is strong evidence that bariatric surgery has a direct impact on appetite and satiety independent of the amount of food ingested, because (a) bariatric surgery is a more effective inductor of weight loss than non-surgical procedures, (b) a decrease in appetite is evident within days of bariatric surgery being performed, and (c) following bariatric surgery patients report reduced hunger long before substantial weight loss occurs. Moreover, in animal models, many beneficial effects of bariatric surgery can be mimicked by gastrointestinal tract hormone administration [95]. It is likely, therefore, that gastrointestinal tract hormones contribute to a regulation of appetite leading to weight loss following bariatric surgery. As dis-

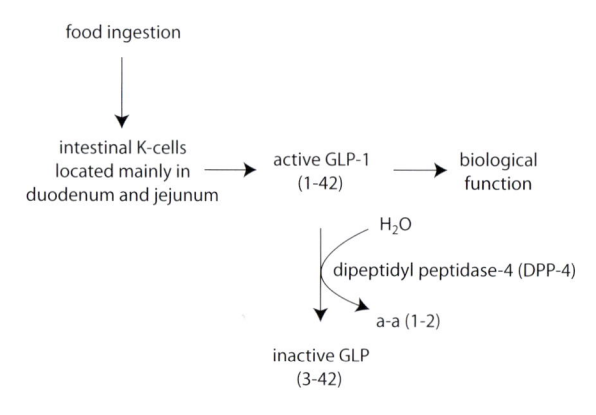

Fig. 6.23. Secretion and degradation of biologically active GIP

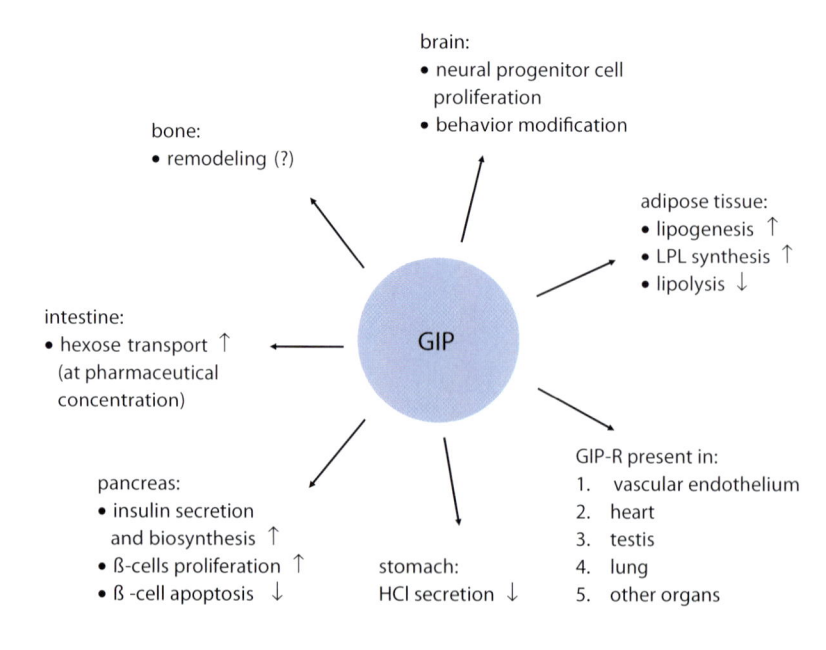

Fig. 6.24. Biological action of GIP

cussed above, some gastrointestinal tract hormones increase food intake (ghrelin), whereas others decrease food intake (obestatin, cholecystokinin, peptide YY, GLP-1). Moreover, these hormones are synthesized and released by different parts of the gastrointestinal tract. Ghrelin is produced mainly by the stomach, whereas cholecystokinin and other appetite suppressants (PYY, YY, GLP-1) are released chiefly from the distal intestine. Due to anatomical changes (rearrangement of the intestine) and less food ingestion the synthesis and secretion of gastrointestinal tract hormones might significantly change following bariatric surgery. Accordingly, the circulating concentrations of four gastrointestinal tract hormones – PYY, GLP-1, CCK, and oxyntomodulin (hormones which cause a decrease in food intake) – are higher, whereas the circulating concentration of ghrelin (a hormone which causes an increase of food intake) is lower (but not in all studies) following bariatric surgery (◘ Table 6.2). This supports

◘ **Table 6.2** Circulating adipokines and gastrointestinal tract hormones in obese patients prior to and following bariatric surgery

Adipokine or gastro-intestinal tract hormones	Obese patients		Type of surgery	Reference
	Prior to surgery*	Following surgery#		
leptin	↑	↓	VBG, LAGB, RYGBP	[101]*#
adiponectin	↓	↑	VBG, RYGBP, JIB, EGS.	[101]*#
resistin	↑ (NC?)	NC	RYGBP	[101]*#
IL-8	↑	NC	LAGB 2 days after surg.	[102]* [103]#
IL-6	↑	↑	LNAGB 3 days after surg.	[22]* [104]#
IL-1B	↑	NC	LNAGB 3 days after surg.	[105]* [104]#
IL-10	↑	unknown	–	[106]*
TGFβ	↑	unknown	–	[105]*
apelin	↑	unknown	–	[107]*
visfatin	↑	↓	LAGB	[108]*#
MCP-1	↑	NC	RYGBP	[109]*#
MIF	↓(↑?)	↑	VBG, LAGB	[22,110]* [110]#
TNFα	↑	NC	RYGBP	[109]*#
VEGF	↑	↑	LAGB 3 days after surg.	[111]* [112]#
NGF	↑	unknown	–	[113]*
metallothionein	unknown	↑	JIBP in rats	[114]#
PAI-1	↑	↓	LAGB	[115]*#
haptoglobin	↑	unknown	–	[22]*
serum amyloid A	↑	↓	RYGBP	[109]*#
ghrelin	↓	conflicting results (↓, NC, ↑?)	VBG, RYGBP, LAGB	[95,116]*#
PYY	↓	↑	VBG, RYGBP, JIB	[117,119]*#
PP	↓ (not all studies)	unknown	–	[119]*
CCK	↑ (not all studies)	↑	JIB	[119]* [120]#
GLP-1	↓	↑	RYGBP	[98,118,119]*#
oxyntomodulin	unknown	↑	–	[89]#

EGS elective gastric surgery, *JIB* jejunoileal bypass, *LAGB* laparoscopic adjustable gastric banding, *LNAGB* laparoscopic non-adjustable gastric banding, *RYGBP* Roux-en-Y gastric bypass, *VBG* vertical banded gastroplasty, ↓ decrease, ↑ increase, *NC* no changes

the hypothesis that gastrointestinal tract hormones may play an important role in the regulation (specifically, the inhibition) of food intake and consequently in weight loss following bariatric surgery. In another words, the success of bariatric surgery might, at least in part, be the result of the increase in circulating PYY, oxyntomodulin, and GLP-1 and/or the decrease in circulating ghrelin. However, the magnitude of this effect has to be determined. Moreover, the role of the circulating gastrointestinal tract hormone concentrations in obesity remains to be established. ◘ Table 6.2 shows circulating gastrointestinal tract hormones prior to and following different types of bariatric surgery. Data regarding circulating gastrointestinal tract hormone concentrations in obese patients (compared with non-obese) and in patients following bariatric surgery are still incomplete. The major problem with precise determination of gastrointestinal tract hormones is their very short half-life. Therefore, no clear-cut conclusion can be drawn from the results presented in ◘ Table 6.2. Thus, future work is required to understand the role of gastrointestinal tract hormones and other signals regulating appetite and body weight changes following bariatric surgery. Considering that a significant reduction in circulating ghrelin concentration was found following gastric bypass [97] but not gastric banding [98], the effects of different types of bariatric surgery on circulating gastrointestinal tract hormones should be evaluated and compared. Recently published data provide further evidence that gastrointestinal tract hormones (PYY and GLP-1) play important roles in weight loss following bariatric surgery [99, 100].

◘ Table 6.2 also shows the circulating concentration of some adipokines in obese patients prior to and following bariatric surgery. Obese patients displayed higher circulating concentrations of almost all adipokines studied. Only the circulating adiponectin concentration was lower in obese patients. Bariatric surgery resulted in significant decreases in circulating leptin, PAI-1, serum amyloid A, and visfatin concentrations. The circulating concentration of adiponectin significantly increased after bariatric surgery. Other adipokines studied were not changed or increased following bariatric surgery. The physiological significance of these changes remains to be established. It is unlikely that changes in circulating leptin and adiponectin concentrations influence food intake following bariatric surgery. However, the decrease in circulating leptin concentration and the increase in adiponectin concentration may be beneficial (particularly the significant increase in the adiponectin/leptin ratio) in terms of obesity-associated disorders such as insulin resistance, dyslipidemia, atherosclerosis, cardiovascular disease, essential hypertension, metabolic syndrome, and type-2 diabetes.

References

1. Hill JO, Peters JC (1998) Environmental contributions to the obesity epidemic. Science 280:1371–1374
2. Klesges RC, Meyers AW, Klesges LM et al (1989) Smoking, body weight, and their effect on smoking behavior: a comprehensive review of the literature. Psychol Bull 1006:204–230
3. Allison DB et al (1996) Risch's λ values for human obesity. Int J Obes Relat Metab Disorder 20:990–999
4. Rankinen T, Zuberi A, Chagnon A et al (2006) The human obesity gene map: the 2005 update. Obesity 14:529–644
5. Farooqi S, O'Rahilly S (2005) Monogenic obesity in humans. Annu Rev Med 56:443–458
6. Ichihara S, Yamada Y (2008) Genetic factors for human obesity. Cell Mol Life Sci 65:1086–1098
7. O'Rahilly S, Farooqi S (2006) Genetics of obesity. Phil Trans R Soc B 361:1095–1105
8. Farooqi S, Wangensteen T, Collins S et al (2007) Clinical and molecular genetic spectrum of congenital deficiency of the leptin receptor. N Engl J Med 356:237–247
9. Krude H, Biebermann H, Schnabel D et al (2003) Obesity due to proopiomelanocortin deficiency: Three new cases and treatment trials with thyroid hormone and ACTH4-10. J Clin Endocrinol Metab 88:4633–4640
10. Farooqi S, Drop S, Clements A et al (2006) Heterozygosity for POMC-null mutation and increased obesity risk in humans, Diabetes 55:2549–2553
11. Vaisse B, Clement K, Guy-Grand B et al (1998) A frameshift mutation in human MC4R is associated with a dominant form of obesity. Nature Genetics 20:113–114
12. Mergen M, Mergen H, Ozata M et al (2001) A novel melanocortin 4 receptor (MCR4) gene mutation associated with morbid obesity. J Clin Endocrinol Metab 86:3448–3451
13. Jackson R S, Creemers JWM, Ohagi S et al (1997) Obesity and impired prohormone processing associated with mutations in the human prohormone convertase 1gene. Nature Genetics 16:303–306
14. Jackson RS, Creemers JWM, Farooqi S et al (2003) Small-intestine dysfunction accompanies the complex endocrinopathy of human proprotein convertase 1 deficiency. J Clin Invest 112:1550–1560
15. Holder JL jr, Butte NF, Zinn AR (2000) Profound obesity associated with a balanced translocation that disrupts the *SIM1* gene. Human Mol Genet 9:101–108
16. Yeo GSH, Hung Ch-Ch C, Rochford J et al (2004) A de novo mutation affecting human TrkB associated with severe obesity and developmental delay. Nature Neurosci 7:1187–1189
17. Norgan NG (1997) The beneficial effects of body fat tissue in humans. Int I Obes Relat Metab Disord 21:738–746
18. Trayhurn P, Beattie JH (2001) Physiological role of adipose tissue: white adipose tissue as an endocrine secretory organ. Proc Nutr Soc 60:329–339
19. Trayhurn O (2005) The biology of obesity Proc Nutr Soc 64:31–38
20. Kiess W, Petzold S, Topfer M et al (2008) Adipocyte and adipose tissue. Best Practice Res Clin Endocrinol Metab 22:135–153
21 Trayhurn P, Bing C (2006) Appetite and energy balance signals from adipocytes. Philos Trans R Soc Lond B Biol Sci 361:1237–1249
22. Trayhurn P, Wood IS (2005) Signalling role of adipose tissue: adipokines and inflammation in obesity. Bioch Soc Trans 33:1078–1081
23. Trayhurn P (2005) Endocrine and signaling role of adipose tissue: new perspective on fat. Acta Physiol Scand 184:285–293

24. Trayhurn P, Bing C, Wood S (2006) Adipose tissue and adipok-ines-energy regulation from the human perspective. J Nutr 136:1935S–1939S

25. Matias I, Cristino L, Di Marzo V (2008) Endocannabinoids: Some like it fat (and sweet too). J Neuroendocrinol 20 [Suppl]: 100–109

26. Petersen KF, Befroy D, Dufour S et al (2003) Mitochondrial dys-function in the elderly: possible role in insulin resistance. Science 300:1140–1142

27. Schaffer JE (2003) Lipotoxicity: when tissue overeat. Curr Opin Lipidol 14:281–287

28. Tripathy D, Mohanty P, Dhindsa S, et al(2003) Elevation of free fatty acids induces inflammation and impairs vascular reactivity in healthy subject. Diabetes 52:2882–2887

29. Lupi R, Dotta F, Marselli L, et al (2002) Prolonged exposure to free fatty acid has cytostatic and proapoptotic effects on human pan-creatic islets; evidence that beta cell death is caspase mediated, partially dependent on ceramide pathway, and Bcl-2 regulated. Diabetes 51:1437–1442

30. Steinberg HO, Tarshoby M, Monestel R et al (1997) Elevated circulating free fatty acids levels impair endothelium dependent vasodilatation. J Clin Invest 100:1230–1239

31. Steinberg HO, Paradisi G, Hook G et al (2000) Free fatty acids ele-vation impairs insulin-mediated vasodilatation and nitric oxide production. Diabetes 49:1231–1238

32. Kershaw EE, Flier JS (2004) Adipose tissue as an endocrine organ. J Clin Endocrinol Metab 89:2548–2556

33. Sikaris KA (2004) The clinical biochemistry of obesity. Clin Bio-chem Rev 25:165–181

34. Flier JS (2007) The adipocytes as an active participant in energy balance and metabolism. Gastroenterology 132:2103–2115

35. Waki H, Tontonoz P (2007) Endocrine function of adipose tissue Annu Rev Pathol Mech Dis 2:31–56

36. Mabuchi T, Yatsuya H, Tamakoshi K et al (2005) Association bet-ween serum leptin concentration and white blood cell counts in middle-aged Japanese men and women. Diabetes Metab Res Rev 21:441–447

37. Wada K, Yatsuya H, Tamakoshi K et al (2006) A positive associ-ation between leptin and blood pressure of normal range in Japanese men Hypertens Res 29:485–492

38. Matsushita K, Yatsuya H, Tamakoshi K et al (2006) Inverse associa-tion between adiponectin and C-reactive protein in substantially healthy Japanese men. Atherosclerosis 188:184–189

39. Shoelson SE, Herrero L, Nazz A (2007) Obesity, inflammation, and insulin resistance. Gastroenterology 132:2169–2180

40. Trayhurn P, Wood IS (2004) Adipokines: inflammation and the pleiotropic role of white adipose tissue. Br J Nutr 92:347–355

41. Wang B, Wood S, Trayhurn P (2007) Dysregulation of the expres-sion and secretion of inflammation-related adipokines by hypo-xia in human adipocytes. Pflugers Arch-Eur J Physiol 455:479–492

42. Abu-Abid S, Szold A, Klausner J (2002) Obesity and cancer. J Med 33:73–86

43. Calle EE, Rodriguez C, Walker-Thurmond K et al (2003) Over-weight, obesity, and mortality from cancer in a prospectively studied cohort of U.S. adults. N Engl J Med 348:1625–1638

44. Berclaz G, Li S, Price K et al (2004) Body mass index as a prog-nostic feature in operable breast cancer: the International Breast Cancer Study Group experience. Ann Oncol 15: 875–884

45. Saxena NK, Vertino PM, Anania FA, Sharma D (2007) Leptin-induced growth stimulation of breast cancer cells involves recruitment of histone acetyltransferase and mediator complex to CYCLIN D1 promoter via activation of stat3. J Biol Chem 282:13316–13325

46. Saxena NK, Sharma D, Ding X et al (2007) Concomitant activation of the JAK/STAT, PI3K/AKT and ERK signaling is involved in leptin-mediated promotion of invasion and migration of hepatocellular carcinoma cells. Cancer Res 67:2497–2507

47. Bjorbaek C, Uotani S, da Silva B, Flier JS (1997) Divergent signal-ing capacities of the long and short isoform of the leptin recep-tor. J Biol Chem 272:32686–32695

48. Ahima RS, Osei SY(2004) Leptin signaling. Physiol Behav 81:223–241

49. Bowman T, Garcia R, Turkson J et al (2000) STATs in oncogenesis. Oncogene 19: 2474–2488

50. Garofalo C, Surmacz E (2006) Leptin and cancer. J Cell Physiol 2007:12–22

51. Ogunwobi O, Mutungi G, Beales ILP (2006) Leptin stimulates proliferation and inhibits apoptosis in Barrett's oesophageal adenocarcinoma cells by COX-2 dependent, PGE2 mediated transactivation of EFF receptor and JNK activation. Endocrinol-ogy 147:4505–4516

52. Gonzalez RR, Cherfils S, Escobar S et al (2006) Leptin signaling promotes the growth of mammary tumors and increases of vascular endothelial growth factor (VEGF) and its receptor type two (VEGF-R2). J Biol Chem 281:26320–26328

53. Baillargeon J, Rose DP (2006) Obesity, adipokines, and prostate cancer. Int J Oncol 28:737–745

54. Vona-Davis L, Rose DP (2007) Adipokines as endocrine, paracrine and autocrine factors in breast cancer risk and progression. Endocr Rel Cancer 14:189–206

55. Ogunwobi OO, Beales ILP (2008) Globular adiponectin, acting via adiponectin receptor-1, inhibits leptin-stimulated oesophageal adenocarcinoma cell proliferation. Mol Cell Endocronol 285:43–50

56. Aparicio T, Kotelevets L, Tsocas A et al (2005) Leptin stimulates the proliferation of human colon cancer cells in vitro but does not promote the growth of colon cancer xenografts in nude mice or intestinal tumorigenesis in Apc$^{Min/+}$ mice. Gut 54:1136–1145

57. Fruhbeck G (2001) A heliocentric view of leptin. Proc Nutr Soc 60:301–318

58. Dunn SL, Bjornholm M, Bates SH et al (2005) Feedback inhibi-tion of leptin receptor/JAK2 signaling via Tyr 1138 of the leptin receptor and suppressor of cytokine signaling 3. Mol Endocrinol 19:925–938

59. Zhang Y, Scarpace PJ (2006) The role of leptin in leptin resistance and obesity. Physiol Behav 88:249–256

60. Swierczynski J (2006) Leptin and age-related down-regulation of lipogenic enzymes genes expression in rat white adipose tissue. J Physiol Pharmacol 57 [Suppl 6]:85–102

61. Harvey J, Solovyova N, Irving A (2006) Leptin and its role in hipocampal synaptic plasticity. Prog Lipid Res 45:369–378

62. Meier U, Gressner AM (2004) Endocrine regulation of energy metabolism: Review of pathobiochemical and clinical chemical aspects of leptin, ghrelin, adiponectin, and resistin. Clin Chem 50:1511–1525

63. Matsuzawa Y (2006) The metabolic syndrome and adipocytok-ines. FEBS Lett 580:2917–2921

64. Kobayashi K, Onoguchi T (2005) Adipokines: therapeutic targets for metabolic syndrome. Curr Drug Targets 6:525–529

65. Diez JJ, Iglesias P (2003) The role of the novel adipocyte-derived hormone adiponectin in human disease. Eur J Endocrinol 148:293–300

66. Steppan CM, Lazar MA (2002) Resistin and obesity-associated insulin resistance. Trends Endocrinol Metab 1:18–23

Diabetological Assessment of Metabolic Surgery

Janusz Gumprecht, MD, Katarzyna Nabrdalik, MD

The prevalence of diabetes is epidemic, with more than 170 million people affected worldwide in the year 2000, and it is estimated that the number will exceed 366 million by 2030 [1-3]. The recently discussed idea to promote surgical treatment for type-2 diabetes that is not necessarily linked to obesity has astonished many scientist and clinicians, who have so far interpreted the anti-diabetic effect of surgery as an isolated result of surgically induced weight loss and decreased caloric intake [4-7]. Surprisingly, complete remission of diabetes is often observed within days after surgery, before weight loss occurs, which suggests a direct effect of surgical intervention by mechanisms independent of weight loss that most likely involve changes in the gastrointestinal hormones that are engaged in the regulation of glucose metabolism [8, 9]. The idea emerged from the large amount of published material concerning unintentional disease remission following conventional gastrointestinal operations for morbid obesity and is linked to a novel concept suggesting that type-2 diabetes may be an intestinal disease that is possible to control with the use of surgical methods [10]. Because the disease is so widespread, one of the most important and urgent goals of twenty-first-century medicine is to find a new approach to understanding the mechanisms of diabetes and to develop a method to treat it successfully. Type-2 diabetes has always been considered a chronic, progressive, and irreversible disease; however, the revolutionary idea of surgical treatment now presents the possibility of achieving complete, long-term, medication-free remission.

7.1   Role of Foregut in Diabetes

Type-2 diabetes is a heterogeneous disorder. It results from both insulin insensitivity and progressive β-cell dysfunction. However, there is mounting evidence indicating that gastrointestinal factors may also be of essential importance. Since many gut hormones are involved in the regulation of glucose homeostasis, the gastrointestinal tract is thought to play an important role in energy balance [11]. There is a hypothesis that type-2 diabetes may be caused by an over stimulation of the foregut by food in vulnerable patients, resulting in excess islet-cell stimulation by incretins, intestinal hormones, the two most important of which are glucagon-like peptide-1 (GLP-1) and glucose-dependent insulinotropic polypeptide (GIP) [12]. These two main incretins are released in response to food ingestion, and both potentiate glucose-dependent insulin response, accounting for 50–60% of insulin secretion; this is referred to as the incretin effect, which is blunted in type-2 diabetes [13–15]. GLP-1 is sec-

reted from endocrine L-cells of intestinal mucosa located predominantly in the distal small intestine and colon, and GIP is released by endocrine K-cells found in the entire small intestine mucosa but with the highest density in the duodenum and proximal jejunum [16, 17]. It is of great interest that in type-2 diabetes the GLP-1 response to glucose or a mixed meal is diminished but its insulinotropic action is preserved, while the secretion of GIP is unaffected, whereas the β-cell response to GIP is greatly impaired. This has raised the hypothesis that β-cell incompetence contributes to the impaired incretin effect. The mechanism of impaired GLP-1 secretion as well as impaired GIP function in diabetes has been not elucidated so far [13, 14, 18, 19]. GLP-1 has the capacity to inhibit gastrointestinal secretion and motility, especially gastric emptying, which is of special importance in type-2 diabetes because it potentially reduces postprandial glucose excursions and provides the sensation of fullness following a meal [20, 21]. Additionally, unlike GIP, GLP-1 physiologically inhibits glucagon secretion, taking part in the regulation of elevated blood glucose [22]. There is also a defective amplification of the late-phase insulin response to glucose by GIP [23]. The incretin theory has been strengthened by clinical data showing that the use of GLP-1 receptor agonists in diabetic patients leads to normalization of glycemia [15]. New experimental studies indicate that a primary aspect of type-2 diabetes control through metabolic surgery is the rearrangement of gastrointestinal anatomy. Gastrointestinal bypass operations may counteract the dysfunctional intestinal pathway responsible for abnormalities of glucose homeostasis, although the exact mechanism is not yet known [24]. It is supposed that each surgical procedure that specifically changes the intestinal anatomy may interfere with glucose metabolism.

Ileal transposition (IT) is a type of gastrointestinal rearrangement where an isolated segment of the ileum is transposed to the jejunum, with preserved gastroduodenal continuity and nutrients emptying directly into the ileum; this causes an increase in the synthesis and secretion of gastrointestinal regulatory peptides [25]. It was shown that IT resulted in the elevation of GLP-1 levels and improved glucose control independent of weight loss in studies of rodent models as well as in human beings [26, 27]. Following both malabsorptive/restrictive Roux-en- Y gastric bypass (RYGB) and biliopancreatic diversion (BPD) GLP-1 levels increase early. However, it remains unclear how the anatomical rearrangements, via either bypassing the duodenum and upper jejunum (RYGB) or excluding the larger part of the entire gastrointestinal tract from food transit (BPD), improve GLP-1 release [28–30]. Additionally, the early phase of insulin secretion as a response to glucose stimuli regulated by GIP is reduced in type-2 diabetes and reverses to normal after RYGB, which suggests that GIP functions might also return to normal [31–33].

To explain which anatomical rearrangement of the small intestine exerts the most important impact on glucose homeostasis, several hypotheses have been introduced. The hindgut hypothesis proposes that nutrients that have been rapidly delivered to the distal intestine may result in enhanced glucose metabolism by strengthening a physiological signal that improves glucose metabolism, potentially mediated via GLP1 or other distal gut-active peptides [26, 27]. In contrast, the foregut hypothesis, supported by studies in non-obese rats, assumes that the positive influence on glucose metabolism may be an effect of excluding the duodenum and proximal jejunum from the nutrient flow, which probably prevents secretion of a putative signal that promotes insulin resistance and type-2 diabetes [29, 34].

Although no such signal has been identified to date, Rubino et al. developed the "anti-incretin" theory, supporting the foregut hypothesis in trying to explain how duodenal exclusion improves diabetes and the possible contribution of the proximal small bowel to the pathophysiology of this disease. They postulate the existence of a counter-regulatory mechanism with an action opposite to that of the incretins [34]. The presumed existence of an unknown diabetogenic signal (hormonal and/or neural) that might be generated by the contact of nutrients with the duodenal mucosa was also proposed by Ferrannini et al. in their very lucid review of mechanisms involved in the amelioration of type-2 diabetes following bariatric surgery. [35]. Additionally, a very interesting study was recently performed by Salinari et al. comparing obese with non-obese type-2 diabetic patients to test the hypothesis that insulin resistance can be determined by an imbalance in the release of intestinal hormones, and that secretion of those hormones is reduced after BPD, resulting in normalization of insulin sensitivity and subsequent improvement in the glucose sensitivity of β-cells. The study was designed to obtain the most reliable outcomes using carefully chosen experimental methods of β-cell function and peripheral insulin sensitivity assessment. Restoration of first-phase insulin secretion and full normalization of insulin sensitivity were observed, but the authors underline that the latter effect cannot be explained by the increase in GLP-1 and GIP plasma concentrations, suggesting that another, still unrecognized, intestinal factor (or factors) takes part in the control of insulin activity in peripheral tissues which is inhibited in the presence of nutrient diversion following surgery [36]. Considering the existing evidence, it is reasonable to

suppose that an excessive production of anti-incretin can take part in the pathophysiology of type-2 diabetes.

On the other hand, impaired anti-incretin production following gastrointestinal bypass surgery could explain the rare occurrence of such complications as postprandial hypoglycemia and dumping syndrome that are sometimes observed after gastrectomy with duodenal exclusion or nesidioblastosis [37].

7.2 Bariatric Surgery Studies

Animal Model. The study performed by Rubino and Marescaux in Goto-Kakizaki (GK) rats that served as a non-obese, spontaneous model of type-2 diabetes revealed improvement of fasting glycemia and glucose tolerance, independent of weight loss and/or decreased caloric intake following duodeno-jejunal bypass (DJB). The authors concluded that the proximal jejunum is primarily responsible for the hormonal influences controlling glucose metabolism, and suspected that the resection of segments of the small intestine in human non-obese diabetics might be a revolutionary new approach to diabetes management [24]. A further study performed by Rubino et al. on the same animal model confirmed that exclusion of the duodenal passage for nutrients improves glucose tolerance. They noticed that, conversely, restoration of the duodenal passage leads to impaired glucose tolerance [38]. Based on studies in rats, Strader et al. described that effects similar to those of duodenal exclusion could be obtained by transposing an ileal segment into the upper intestine [26].

Clinical Studies in Human Beings. With their pioneering research into the effect of bariatric surgery on type-2 diabetes, Ackerman and Pories et al. [10, 39] were the first to notice the phenomenon of early improvement or normalization of carbohydrate metabolism following bariatric surgery. Ackerman supposed that diabetes improvement may occur due to a complex mechanism combining glucose malabsorption and changes in gut hormone regulation. In contrast, Pories et al. thought that the primary mechanism was food exclusion from a hormonally active antrum, duodenum, and proximal jejunum, delayed transit time, and presentation of the mid-jejunum with undigested food directly from the stomach [39, 40]. In their studies, Cohen et al. focused on diabetes control, with no attempt at weight loss. In one of the early studies performed in two not-morbidly-obese patients who underwent DJB to treat diabetes a complete resolution of the disease without any significant changes in body mass index (BMI) was observed [41]. Other types of bariatric operations, namely RYGB and BPD, performed in not-morbidly-obese patients were also found to result in amelioration of type-2 diabetes [42–44]. De Paula et al. studied 39 type-2 diabetic patients (BMI <35 kg/m2) undergoing laparoscopic ileal transposition into the proximal jejunum via sleeve or diverted sleeve gastrectomy. In 87% of these the surgery resulted in discontinuation of all preoperative diabetes-related medications. Additionally, the HbA1c value decreased from 8.8% to 6.3%, and the authors came to the conclusion that either one of the mentioned surgical procedures appears to be promising for controlling diabetes and metabolic syndrome [45].

Since there is much evidence that type-2 diabetes can be improved following gastric bypass surgery for morbid obesity, while evidence regarding its power to improve or resolve the disease, especially in non-obese patients who have undergone DJB, is scarce, Ferzli et al. recently performed a 12-month prospective study aiming to evaluate the clinical effects of DJB on glucose metabolism in seven patients with diabetes and BMI <35 kg/m2. At the end of the study almost all patients had decreased requirements for their diabetic medications. HbA1c values and fasting blood glucose were improved, although none of the outcomes were statistically significant. What is important is that all patients experienced relief from preoperative symptoms such as fatigue, pain in their extremities, polyuria, and polydipsia. In contrast to the study by De Paula et al., no gastric resection was performed in these patients, but similar diabetic control was achieved [46]. The first randomized, controlled trial in the medical literature demonstrating superior efficacy of bariatric surgery compared with conventional medical therapy for the treatment of type-2 diabetes was the study performed recently by Dixon et al. among 60 obese patients (BMI >30 but <40 kg/m2) who were randomized either to a group undergoing lifestyle modification or to a group undergoing laparoscopic adjustable gastric banding. Diabetes remission was seen in 73% of the patients allocated to surgical treatment but in only 27% of those in the conventional therapy group [47]. The outcome suggests that bariatric surgery may be considered a treatment option for patients with type-2 diabetes and mild to moderate obesity. However, due to the follow-up of only 2 years, caution is required in interpreting the longer-term advantages. Buchwald et al. have performed a meta-analysis of 136 studies regarding 22 094 patients undergoing bariatric surgery, showing that weight loss is long-lasting in 50–60% of patients who undergo RYGB. It is interesting, however, that total remission of type-2 diabetes was obtained in >40% of patients who underwent laparoscopic adjustable gastric banding, in >80% of patients who underwent RYGB, and in >90% of those who had malabsorptive BPD [48]. There is evidence that remission of diabetes following RYGB and BPD is prolonged, and the recurrence of diabetes after more than 10 years following surgery is rare [49].

In a recent, consecutive meta-analysis performed by Buchwald et al., 135 246 patients from 621 studies conducted from 1990 to 2006 were analyzed. It was found that as the result of bariatric surgery 78.1% of diabetic patients showed complete resolution of the disease and in 86.6% of the patients diabetes was improved or resolved; 3188 patients reported resolution of the clinical and laboratory manifestations of type-2 diabetes. Nineteen studies including 11 175 patients evaluated weight loss and diabetes resolution outcomes separately in 4070 diabetic patients. Researchers observed a progressive relationship of diabetes resolution and weight loss as a function of the operation performed: laparoscopic adjustable gastric banding, gastroplasty, gastric bypass, and BPD/duodenal switch (DS). Resolution of diabetes was seen in 56.7% following gastric banding, in 79.7% following gastroplasty, in 80.3% following gastric bypass, and in 95.1% following BPD/DS. More than 2 years postoperatively, the corresponding findings were 58.3%, 77.5%, 70.9%, and 95.9%. The excess weight loss was 46.2%, 55.5%, 59.7%, and 63.6%, respectively, for the type of surgery performed. The meta-analysis outcomes indicate that bariatric surgery performed in morbidly obese patients with type-2 diabetes provides a powerful treatment effect [50].

7.3 Interventional Diabetology

The patient selection process for metabolic surgery should focus less on BMI, and the diabetes-specific criteria should be defined. BMI is not a good parameter for evaluating the risk:benefit ratio. As studies in rodents have shown, DJB was related to diabetes improvement both in type-2 diabetic rats that were obese (Zucker fa/ fa) and in lean ones (GK) [24, 51]. The animal studies are consistent with clinical observations of diabetes remission following RYGB and BPD operation in moderately obese or lean patients [42–44]. There is evidence from large clinical trials that patients who had suffered from diabetes for >8–10 years and required high doses of insulin to control glycemia did not experience complete diabetes remission following bariatric surgery; therefore, it is suggested that long-lasting type-2 diabetes linked to end-stage β-cell failure may be the reason for irreversibility of the disease [10, 52]. This finding is in accordance with the one reported by Schauer et al. and Torqueti et al., whereby shorter duration and lesser severity of type-2 diabetes were linked to higher rates of postoperative remission [8,

53]. These outcomes lead to the conclusion that surgical intervention should be offered early rather than late in the natural course of type-2 diabetes mellitus for those who are eligible. There is no need to be afraid of excessive weight loss because the evidence from both animal and clinical studies proves that gastrointestinal bypass procedures have no significant effect on weight loss when performed in subjects with normal body weight. No weight reduction was observed in either normal (Wistar) or diabetic (GK) lean rats, while the effect was seen in obese (Zucker fa/fa) rodents [24, 51]. Surgical intervention for diabetes management may become a new milestone treatment. RYGB and BPD seem to have a greater potential to treat diabetes than other types of surgery. However, the question of which of the bariatric operations is the best to treat diabetes remains unanswered, and future research is expected to solve the problem.

In March 2007, a first multidisciplinary consensus conference on gastrointestinal surgery to treat type-2 diabetes was held in Rome, where over 50 international authorities in diabetes and bariatric surgery prepared guidelines for clinical practice and research.

7.4 Conclusions

Although the meta-analysis presented by Buchwald et al. suggested that gastric banding results in lower rates of diabetes remission than RYGB or BPD, a recent randomized trial conducted by Dixon et al. found that this surgical procedure results in dramatically better control of diabetes compared with standard medical treatment, even in patients with BMI between 30 and 35 kg/m2 [47, 48]. This study confirmed, however, that the control of diabetes after gastric banding, unlike after GJB, requires substantial weight loss and no additional mechanisms are involved. While gastrointestinal procedures for diabetes treatment are being studied, new operations and devices are being developed and tested. These are based on the notion that changing the anatomy of the small intestine alters the way nutrients stimulate the intestinal mucosa and may result in modification of gut hormone secretion with beneficial effects on diabetes [27, 54]. One such procedure is ileal transposition, a surgical operation whereby a segment of distal small bowel (lower ileum) is transposed into the upper intestine. The procedure has been shown to increase satiety and GLP1 levels in rats and has been employed to treat diabetes in obese and non-obese human beings [45]. The multiplicity of evidence allows us to assume that metabolic surgery may be appropriate for normal-weight or slightly overweight diabetic patients. Taking into account the current epidemic growth of diabetes, there is an urgent need to promote the scientific development of interventional diabetology, as it has been noted that metabolic surgery can lead to remission of diabetes.

In order to increase the rate of success and diminish the rate of complications of this intervention, metabolic surgery for diabetes should be based on the multidisciplinary collaboration of endocrinologists, surgeons, physicians, and scientists. However, it ought to be remembered that a weak point of bariatric surgery – the long-term anti-diabetic effect – is not yet known. Since a bariatric operation is not without risk, the question arises, in view of a progressive loss of β-cell function after diabetes is diagnosed, whether the disease can be cured or might relapse with further, significant loss of β-cell function. This is the issue with almost all current medications for diabetes, and there is no reason to suppose that anything differentiates surgery from the other treatment methods in this regard. To support the above notion, the 1st World Congress on Interventional Therapies for Type-2 Diabetes took place in New York on September 15–16, 2008, where a multidisciplinary forum of world health leaders, endocrinologists and surgeons, diabetes and obesity specialists, and basic scientists and policy makers focused on the possibility of new interventional therapies inducing long-term remission of type-2 diabetes following bariatric and gastrointestinal surgery [55].

References

1. James WPT, Rigby N, Leach R (2004) The obesity epidemic, metabolic syndrome and future prevention strategies. Eur J Cardiovasc Prev Rehabil 11:3–8
2. Hossain P, Kawar B, El Nahas M (2007) Obesity and diabetes in the developing world – a growing challenge. N Engl J Med 356:213–215
3. Wild S, Roglic G, Green A, Sicree R, King H (2004) Global prevalence of diabetes: estimates for the year 2000 and projections for 2030. Diabetes Care 27:1047–1053
4. Anderson JW, Grant L, Gotthelf L, Stifler LT (2006) Weight loss and long-term follow-up of severely obese individuals treated with an intense behavioral program. Int J Obes (Lond) 31:488–493
5. MacDonald KG, Long SD, Swanson MS et al (1997) The gastric bypass operation reduces the progression and mortality of NIDDM. J Gastrointest Surg 1:213–220
6. Lee WJ, Huang MT, Wang W, Lin CM, Chen TC, Lai IR (2004) Effects of obesity surgery on the metabolic syndrome. Arch Surg 139:1088–-1092
7. Ballantyne GH, Gumbs A, Modlin IM (2005) Changes in insulin resistance followin bariatric surgery and adipoinsular axis:role of the adipocytokines, leptin, adiponectin and resistin. Obes Surg 15:692–699
8. Torquati A, Lutfi R, Abumrad N, Richards WO (2005) Is Roux-en-Y gastric bypass surgery the most effective treatment for type 2

diabetes mellitus in morbidly obese patients? J Gastrointest Surg 9:1112–1116, discussion 1117–1118

9. Clements RH, Gonzalez QH, Long CI et al (2004) Hormonal changes after Roux-en-Y gastric bypass for morbid obesity and the control of type II diabetes mellitus. Ann Surg 70:1–4

10. Pories WJ, Swanson MS, MacDonald KG, Long SB, Morris PG, Brown BM et al (1995) Who would have thought it? An operation proves to be the most effective therapy for adult-onset diabetes mellitus. Ann Surg 222:339–350, discussion 350–352

11. Ferrannini E (1998) Insulin resistance versus insulin deficiency in non-insulin-dependent diabetes mellitus:problems and prospects. Endocr Rev 19:477–490

12. Creutzfeldt W, Nauck M (1992) Gut hormones and diabetes mellitus. Diabetes Metab Rev 8:149–177

13. Vilsboll T, Holst JJ (2004) Incretins, insulin secretion and type 2 diabetes mellitus. Diabetologia 47:357–366

14. Nauck M, Stockmann F, Ebert R, Creutzfeldt W (1986) Reduced incretin effect in Type 2 (non-insulin-dependent) diabetes. Diabetologia 29:46–52

15. Gautier JF, Fetita S, Sobngwi E, Salaun-Martin C (2005) Biological actions of the incretins GIP and GLP-1 and therapeutic perspectives in patients with type 2 diabetes. Diabetes Metab 31:233–242

16. Mojsov S, Heinrich G, Wilson IB, Ravazzola M, Orci L, Habener JF (1986) Preproglucagon gene expression in pancreas and intestine diversifies at the level of post-translational processing. J Biol Chem 261:11880–11889

17. Mortensen K, Petersen LL, Orskov C (2000) Colocalization of GLP-1 and GIP in human and porcine intestine. Ann N Y Acad Sci 921:469–472

18. Kieffer TJ, Pederson RA Defective glucose- dependent insulinotropic polypeptide receptor expression(2001) in diabetic fatty Zucker rats. Diabetes 50:1004–1011

19. Muscelli E, Mari A, Casolaro A, Camastra S, Seghieri G, Gastaldelli A et al (2008) Separate impact of obesity and glucose tolerance on the incretin effect in normal subjects and type 2 diabetic patients. Diabetes 57:1340–1348

20. Holst JJ (2002) Therapy of type 2 diabetes mellitus based on the actions of glucagon-like peptide-1. Diabetes Metab Res Rev 18:430–441

21. Nauck MA, Niedereichholz U, Ettler R, Holst JJ, Orskov C, Ritzel R et al (1997) Glucagon-like peptide 1 inhibition of gastric emptying outweighs its insulinotropic effects in healthy humans. Am J Physiol 273:E981–E988

22. Creutzfeldt WO, Kleine N, Willms B, Orskov C, Holst JJ, Nauck MA (1996) Glucagonostatic actions and reduction of fasting hyperglycemia by exogenous glucagon-like peptide I(7-36) amide in type I diabetic patients. Diabetes Care 19:580–586

23. Vilsboll T, Knop FK, Krarup T, Johansen A, Madsbad S, Larsen S et al (2003) The pathophysiology of diabetes involves a defective amplification of the late-phase insulin response to glucose by glucose-dependent insulinotropic polypeptide-regardless of etiology and phenotype. J Clin Endocrinol Metab 88:4897–4903

24. Rubino F, Marescaux J (2004) Effect of duodenal-jejunal exclusion in a non-obese animal model of type 2 diabetes. A new perspective for an old disease. Ann Surg 2:1–11

25. Layer P, Holst JJ, Grandt D, Goebell H (1995) Ileal release of glucagon-like peptide-1 (GLP-1). Association with inhibition of gastric acid secretion in humans. Dig Dis Sci 40:1074–1082

26. Strader AD, Vahl TP, Jandacek RJ, Woods SC, D'Alessio DA, Seeley RJ (2005) Weight loss through ileal transposition is accompanied by increased ileal hormone secretion and synthesis in rats. Am J Physiol Endocrinol Metab 288:E447–E453

27. DePaula AL, Macedo AL, Rassi N, Vencio S, Machado CA, Mota BR et al (2008) Laparoscopic treatment of metabolic syndrome in patients with type 2 diabetes mellitus. Surg Endosc 22:2670–2678

28. Laferrere B, Teixeira J, McGinty J, Tran H, Egger JR, Colarusso A et al (2008) Effect of weight loss by gastric bypass surgery versus hypocaloric diet on glucose and incretin levels in patients with type 2 diabetes. J Clin Endocrinol Metab 93:2479–2485

29. Guidone C, Manco M, Valera-Mora E, Iaconelli A, Gniuli D, Mari A et al (2006) Mechanisms of recovery from type 2 diabetes after malabsorptive bariatric surgery. Diabetes 55:2025–2031

30. Rubino F, Gagner M, Gentileschi P, Kini S, Fukuyama S, Feng J et al (2004) The early effect of the Roux-en-Y gastric bypass on hormones involved in body weight regulation and glucose metabolism. Ann Surg 240:236–242

31. Lewis JT, Dayanandan B, Habener JF, Kieffer TJ (2000) Glucose-dependent insulinotropic polypeptide confers early phase insulin release to oral glucose in rats: demonstration by a receptor antagonist. Endocrinology 141:3710–3716

32. Ostenson CG (2001) The pathophysiology of type 2 diabetes mellitus: an overview. Acta Physiol Scand 171:241–247

33. Polyzogopoulou EV, Kalfarentzos F, Vagenakis AG, Alexandrides TK (2003) Restoration of euglycemia and normal acute insulin response to glucose in obese subjects with type 2 diabetes following bariatric surgery. Diabetes 52:1098–1103

34. Rubino F (2008) Is type 2 diabetes an operable intestinal disease? A provocative yet reasonable hypothesis. Diabetes Care 31 [Suppl 29]:S290–S296

35. Ferrannini E, Mingrone G (2009) Impact of different bariatric surgical procedures on insulin action and β-cell function in type 2 diabetes. Diabetes Care 32:514–520

36. Salinari S, Bertuzzi A, Asnaghi S, Guidone C, Manco M, Mingrone G (2009) First-phase insulin secretion restoration and differential response to glucose load depending on the route of administration in type 2 diabetic subjects after bariatric surgery. Diabetes Care 32:375–380

37. Service GJ, Thompson GB, Service FJ, Andrews JC, Collazo-Clavell ML, Lloyd RV (2005) Hyperinsulinemic hypoglycemia with nesidioblastosis after gastric-bypass surgery. N Engl J Med 353:249–254

38. Rubino F, Forgione A, Cummings DE, Vix M, Gnuli D, Mingrone G et al (2006) The mechanism of diabetes control after gastrointestinal bypass surgery reveals a role of the proximal small intestine in the pathophysiology of type 2 diabetes. Ann Surg 244:741–749

39. Ackermann NB (1990) Physiologic approaches to the control of obesity. Ann Surg. 211:107

40. Pories WJ, Albrecht RJ (2001) Etiology of type II diabetes mellitus: role of the foregut. World J Surg 25:527–531

41. Cohen RV et al (2007) Duodenal-jejunal bypass for the treatment of type 2 diabetes in patients with BMI 22-34: a report of two cases. Surg Obes Relat Dis :195–197

42. Noya G, Cossu ML et al (1998)Biliopancreative diversion preserving the stomach and pylorus in the treatment of hypercholesterolemia and diabetes type II:results in the first 10 cases. Obes Surg:67–72

43. Cohen R, Pinheiro JS et al (2006) Roux-en-Y gastric bypass for BMI <35 kg/m²: a tailored approach. Surg Obes Relat Dis 2:401–404

44. Castagneto M, De Gaetano A, Mingrone G, Capristo E, Benedetti G, Tacchino RM et al (1998) A surgical option for familial chylomicronemia associated with insulin-resistant diabetes mellitus. Obes Surg 8:191–198

45. de Paula AL, Macedo AL, Prudente AS, Queiroz L, Schraibman V, Pinus J (2006) Laparoscopic sleeve gastrectomy with ileal inter-

position ("neuroendocrine brake") – pilot study of a new operation. Surg Obes Relat Dis 2:464–467

46. Ferzli GS, Dominique E, Ciaglia M, Bluth MH, Gonzalez A, Fingerhut A (2009) Clinical Improvement after duodenojejunal bypass for nonobese type 2 diabetes despite minimal improvement in glycemic homeostasis. World J Surg 33:972–979

47. Dixon JB, O'Brien PE, Playfair J, Chapman L, Schachter LM, Skinner S et al (2008) Adjustable gastric banding and conventional therapy for type 2 diabetes: a randomized controlled trial. JAMA 299:316–323

48. Buchwald H, Avidor Y, Braunwald E, Jensen MD, Pories W, Fahrbach K et al (2004) Bariatric surgery: a systematic review and meta-analysis. JAMA 292:1724–1737

49. Scopinaro N, Marinari GM, Camerini GB, Papadia FS, Adami GF (2005) Specific effects of biliopancreatic diversion on the major components of metabolic syndrome: a long-term follow-up study. Diabetes Care 28:2406–2411

50. Buchwald H, Estok R, Fahrbach K, Banel D, Jensen MD, Pories WJ et al (2009) Weight and type 2 diabetes after bariatric surgery: systematic review and meta-analysis. Am J Med 122:248–256

51. Rubino F, Zizzari P, Tomasetto C, Bluet-Pajot MT, Forgione A, Vix M et al (2005) The role of the small bowel in the regulation of circulating ghrelin levels and food intake in the obese Zucker rat. Endocrinology 146:1745–1751

52. Schauer PR, Ikramuddin S, Gourash W, Ramanathan R, Luketich J (2000) Outcomes after laparoscopic Roux-en-Y gastric bypass for morbid obesity. Ann Surg 232:515–529

53. Schauer PR, Burguera B, Ikramuddin S, Cottam D, Gourash W, Hamad G et al (2003) Effect of laparoscopic Roux-en Y gastric bypass on type 2 diabetes mellitus. Ann Surg 238:467–484, discussion 484–485

54. Depaula AL, Macedo AL, Schraibman V, Mota BR, Vencio S (2008) Hormonal evaluation following laparoscopic treatment of type 2 diabetes mellitus patients with BMI 20–34. Surg Endosc 2:2

55. www.interventionaldiabetology.org

Lipids and Bariatric Surgery

Tina Schewe MD, Karl Winkler MD

Lipids are either resorbed with food or produced by the body itself. All animal cells are able to produce cholesterol, but cholesterol cannot be degraded by the human body. A considerable characteristic of lipids is their poor water solubility. In aqueous solution free fatty acids are transported by binding to albumin, while all other lipids are bound to lipid-protein complexes, the so-called lipoproteins. Depending on their function, lipoproteins are of variable composition: Water-insoluble triglycerides and cholesterol esters are located in the core, whereas better water-soluble apolipoproteins, phospholipids, and free cholesterol are transported in the outer shell. Lipoproteins are defined by their density, depending on their triglyceride content:

- Lipoproteins of very low density have a high content of triglycerides, chylomicrons, and very low density lipoproteins (VLDL).
- Low-density lipoproteins (LDL)
- Intermediate-density lipoproteins (IDL)
- High-density lipoproteins (HDL) hold an increasingly lower fraction of triglycerides and therefore have an increased density.

Lipid-binding proteins (apolipoproteins) serve as structural proteins:

- Apolipoprotein B (ApoB48 and ApoB100) for chylomicrons, VLDL, IDL, and LDL
- Apolipoprotein A-I (ApoA-I) for HDL

They are involved in receptor-mediated absorption into the cell (ApoB100 and ApoE) and affect the activity of lipid-metabolism-relevant enzymes.

8.1   Metabolism of Lipids

Three pathways of lipid metabolism may be distinguished:

- Exogenous lipid metabolism
- Endogenous lipid metabolism
- Reverse cholesterol transport

8.1.1   Exogenous Lipid Metabolism

Resorption and metabolization of nutritional fat is referred to as exogenous lipid metabolism. Fat has to be brought into solution before being absorbed. For this purpose bile acids with cholesterol as the main component are synthesized by the liver as emulgents. Dietary fat is hydrolyzed by pancreatic lipase. Bile acids, as well as nutritional fat, are then absorbed by the small intestines; bile acids are re-delivered to the liver. This "recycling" of bile acids may be inhibited by bile acid sequestrants such as colesevelam or colestyramine. The absorbed fat is reassembled to form chylomicrons, which are delivered to the thoracic duct, thus bypassing the liver. In blood vessels chylomicrons are quickly delipidated – mainly by lipoproteinlipase (LPL) – to chylomicron remnants with higher cholesterol content. LPL is produced mainly by adipose tissue and muscle cells and is transported to the surfaces of the endothelium. It binds to proteoglycans on the luminal side of these endothelial cells, where it interacts with triglyceride-rich lipoproteins and, in the presence of apolipoprotein C-II (Apo C-II), hydrolyzes triglycerides. Apolipoprotein CIII inhibits the hydrolysis of triglycerides, and the ratio of ApoC-II to ApoC-III may be critical in the regulation of delivery of triglycerides to adipose tissue [1]. Insulin is a major regulator of LPL synthesis and activity in adipose tissue: It up-regulates the expression of LPL and stimulates intracellular lipogenic enzymes such as acetyl-CoA-carboxylase and fatty acid synthase. Fatty acids (FA) that are released by the hydrolysis of triglycerides need to be trapped by adipose tissue to prevent high FA flux to tissues that do not require fatty acids as an energy source at that moment. Approximately 90– 100% of LPL-released FA are trapped by adipose tissue after feeding [2]. The efficiency of this FA entrapment after postprandial hydrolysis of triglycerides in healthy individuals is best illustrated by the fact that postprandial FA levels are actually lower than fasting levels.

8.1.2   Endogenous Lipid Metabolism

This metabolism serves as a supplier for high-energy triglycerides and cholesterol in the fasting state. The reserves for this are stored mainly in visceral adipose tissue with the liver as a turntable, which receives FA as a substrate for the assembly of triglyceride-rich lipoproteins (VLDL). These are delipidated in the periphery, mainly by LPL with LDL as the end product. In the fasting state insulin levels are low and catecholamine-stimulated lipolysis in adipocytes by the hormone-sensitive lipase (HSL) is unopposed.

8.1.3   Reverse Cholesterol Transport

The cholesterol deposited in the vessel wall may be neutralized only by backhaul to the liver. Initially, HDLs serve as agents for this backhaul; due to the action of the enzyme cholesterol ester transfer protein (CETP), IDL and LDL are involved, too. Low HDL cholesterol is an independent cardiovascular risk factor.

8.2 Laboratory Methods of Lipid Analysis and Their Clinical Utility

Lipoproteins may be defined by density. Usually, however, lipoproteins are not separated and defined by density, but rather by other unique properties. In the most common method total cholesterol and triglyceride are measured, and this is followed by a precipitation of all ApoB-containing lipoproteins (in the fasting state usually LDL, IDL, and VLDL). Following precipitation, the cholesterol content of the remaining plasma (which is identical with the HDL cholesterol concentration) is measured, and LDL cholesterol is calculated with the Friedewald equation [3]: Using this method IDL is included in the LDL. It has been shown that when LDL and IDL are individually determined, the natural history of coronary artery disease is related to IDL and inversely to HDL [4]. However, LDLs are a heterogeneous class of lipoproteins that may convey different risk for cardiovascular disease. Using different techniques they can be further divided by charge, size, and density. Data concerning the atherogenicity of different "LDL qualities" remains controversial: Epidemiological data showing that small LDL particles are more atherogenic than large ones are derived from studies that found that small LDL size was associated with higher cardiovascular risk [5], but not all studies found this association to be independent of other risk factors such as triglycerides or ApoB, with which small LDL particles are strongly associated, since every LDL particle carries just one ApoB [6, 7]. The question remains whether small LDL particles are actually more atherogenic or whether it is rather the number of LDL particles that conveys an increased risk [8]. Similar to LDL subclasses, HDLs may be separated on the basis of their differing density: The most dense, relatively cholesterol-poor form is termed HDL3. Following interaction with other lipoproteins and certain enzymes, namely lecithin-cholesterol-acyltransferase (LCAT) and hepatic triglyceride lipase (HTGL), their cholesterol ester content is increased and the particle becomes less dense and larger. This relatively cholesterol-rich form is termed HDL2 [9]. The cardioprotective aspects of high HDL-c appear to be related to differences in HDL subclasses [10]. The progression of atherosclerosis has been linked to differences in HDL subclass distribution independent of the effect of triglycerides [11].

8.3 Clinical Impact of Hyperlipidemia

As a general rule, the various types of hyperlipidemia do not have clinical relevance per se; rather there is an increased risk for certain diseases depending on the type of hyperlipidemia. Principally, three hyperlipidemias may be distinguished:
- Hypercholesterolemia
- Hypertriglyceridemia
- Combined hyperlipidemia: hypertriglyceridemia and hypercholesterolemia

8.3.1 Hypercholesterolemia

When the LDL-cholesterol level is very high ($\geq$190 mg/dl) this type of hyperlipidemia usually is inherited (cf. NCEP, ATP III, Full Report, VII-I). Without concomitant hypertriglyceridemia, about 30% of total cholesterol and LDL cholesterol can be accounted for by nutrition. About 60–70% of total cholesterol in plasma is usually carried by LDL. Patients with hypercholesterolemia alone are usually not overweight; very often they are quite slender. Their cardiovascular risk depends for the most part on the severity of LDL-cholesterol elevation and an eventually decreased HDL-c. The more effective LDL cholesterol is lowered, the greater the cardiovascular risk can be reduced: A decrease in LDL cholesterol by about 30% can reduce the risk for CAD by about 30%. In addition to the relatively simple measurement of the cholesterol content of LDL, further information about cardiovascular risk and – to some extent – about treatment strategies can be gathered by measurement of ApoB and subfractionation of LDL.

8.3.2 Hypertriglyceridemia

In hypertriglyceridemia without hypercholesterolemia either VLDL or chylomicrons and VLDL are increased. Due to the fact that especially VLDL do carry a certain fraction of cholesterol in addition to their triglyceride content, depending on the severity of triglyceride elevation and therefore on the number and type of circulating VLDL, total cholesterol is also increased. This elevation does not necessarily imply that LDL cholesterol is increased as well. For clinical purposes hypertriglyceridemia can be distinguished using the gravity of triglyceride elevation as a cut-off point [12]:
- Borderline high triglycerides 150–199 mg/dl: common component of the metabolic syndrome
- High triglycerides 200–499 mg/dl: also a common component of metabolic syndrome with a stronger genetic component

— Very high triglycerides ≥500 mg/dl: strong genetic component, may also be a component of the metabolic syndrome

In patients with excessive triglycerides (≥1000 mg/ dl/11.3 mmol/l) LDL-cholesterol levels are usually low, the hypertriglyceridemia has a strong genetic component, and the patients have an increasing risk of acute pancreatitis. Patients with such high levels of triglycerides are, because of the genetic cause, not necessarily overweight. Nevertheless, they have to be treated with lifestyle intervention (dietary counseling, physical training) and triglyceride-lowering drugs (fibrates or nicotinic acid). The first priority for these patients is to prevent acute pancreatitis. The second goal of therapy is to reduce cardiovascular risk, in case this risk is increased. The atherogenic risk of high triglycerides depends on the kind and quality of lipoproteins that are elevated and on the accompanying changes in LDL quality. Large VLDL with high triglyceride content and a low cholesterol content convey a much smaller atherogenic risk than VLDL remnants with a relatively large cholesterol fraction. In fact, these VLDL remnants seem to have an atherogenic potential similar to that of LDL. These remnants are usually present when triglycerides are between 200 and 500 mg/dl (2.26–3.4 mmol/l). In case that triglyceride serum levels are higher than 500 mg/dl (5.65 mmol/l), a part of the cholesterol may be present in the triglyceriderich lipoproteins. They are non-atherogenic triglycerides (f.i. large VLDL and chylomicrons). Therefore, extensive lipoprotein testing and subfractionation may sometimes be necessary to make a good prediction of the cardiovascular risk related to a certain type of hypertriglyceridemia.

8.3.3 Combined Hyperlipidemia

A combination of hypercholesterolemia with elevation of total and LDL cholesterol and hypertriglyceridemia is the most common form of hyperlipidemia. Its causes are diverse: Elevation of LDL cholesterol may have a genetic background, but it may also very well be a transient elevation caused by delipidation of VLDL to LDL after resolution of a more severe hypertriglyceridemia. Thus, laboratory-analyzed findings should be judged in a timedependent context.

8.4 Atherogenic Dyslipidemia and the Metabolic Syndrome

Atherogenic dyslipidemia is defined by low HDL levels (<40 mg/dl), elevation of triglycerides (≥150 mg/dl), and the presence of small, dense LDL. Characteristics of patients with atherogenic dyslipidemia are obesity (abdominal obesity), insulin resistance, and physical inactivity. Several investigators have demonstrated that insulin resistance is associated with increased small LDL particle numbers [13, 14]. Additionally, patients often show an accumulation of cholesterol-rich remnants. In the Framingham heart study, a community-based longitudinal study, patients with the metabolic syndrome as defined by the ATPIII had a high number of small LDL particles proportional to the number of components of the metabolic syndrome, while LDL cholesterol remained stable [15].

8.5 Therapeutic Considerations

Besides reducing the risk of acute pancreatitis when triglycerides are ≥1000 mg/dl, the main therapeutic goal for all hyperlipidemic patients is the reduction of cardiovascular risk. The Adult Treatment Panel III (ATPIII) of the National Cholesterol Education Program (NCEP) has defined targets of therapy:

— Due to the strong causal relationship between LDL cholesterol and CHD, LDL-c is considered the primary target of lipid-lowering therapy.
— Since VLDL cholesterol is correlated with highly atherogenic remnant lipoproteins, it can be reasonably combined with LDL cholesterol to improve risk prediction.
  This "non-HDL-c" contains all lipoproteins with ApoB (VLDL + LDL) and should be considered a secondary target in patients with high triglycerides (200–400 mg/dl in the fasting state).
— For the inverse relationship between HDL cholesterol and CHD no threshold relationship has been found. Non-drug and drug therapies that increase HDL cholesterol should be considered, even though no specific HDL cholesterol goal has been defined.
— Atherogenic dyslipidemia: Most therapies – drug or non-drug – targeting low HDL cholesterol and high triglycerides actually modify all components of the atherogenic dyslipidemia.

There are two general approaches to treatment of atherogenic dyslipidemia and the generally accompanying metabolic syndrome: The first strategy treats the metabolic risk factors (hypertension, atherogenic dyslipidemia, insulin resistance, and prothrombotic state) directly with pharmacotherapy. The second approach aims at the causes: overweight/obesity, physical inactivity, and the associated insulin resistance. Physical activity and weight reduction lower insulin resistance and mitigate the other metabolic risk factors

8.6   Pathophysiology of Hyperlipidemia in Obese Patients

Virtually all morbidly obese patients have a measurably impaired glucose tolerance, and 36% of these patients will progress to type-2 diabetes within 10 years [16]. Insulin sensitivity traditionally is assessed by its ability to promote normal glucose metabolism. Besides maintenance of glucose homeostasis, its physiological role encompasses lipid and protein metabolism. As described above, insulin promotes anabolism through up-regulation of LPL and lipogenic enzymes and inhibits catabolism by inhibition of hormone-sensitive lipase, the rate-limiting enzyme in lipolysis in adipocytes [17, 18]. In the insulinresistant state the responses of both LPL and HSL are blunted: Because of absent up-regulation of LPL and the resulting decreased hydrolysis of triglycerides in triglyceride- rich lipoproteins (chylomicrons and VLDL), as well as ineffective inhibition of HSL-mediated lipolysis in adipocytes, dietary energy cannot be effectively trapped. Postprandial lipemia and elevated plasma levels of fatty acids are well-known abnormalities in obesity and insulin resistance. The reduced uptake of triglycerides and fatty acids by adipose tissue results in a greater partitioning to non-adipose tissues including muscle and liver. Increased secretion of ApoB was first shown in diabetic patients [19], in whom an increased flux of fatty acids was linked to an increased secretion of VLDL triglycerides and ApoB [20]. Increased free fatty acid release from adipose tissue with increased flux to the liver by the portal vein can increase VLDL, triglycerides, and ApoBsecretion [21]. Insulin-resistant states are associated not only with the release of larger quantities of free fatty acids from the increased mass of circulating lipoproteins but also with reduced free fatty acid uptake by peripheral tissues. Thus a vicious cycle is set up in insulin-resistant states involving free fatty acids and hypertriglyceridemia: Despite the ability of the liver to assemble and secrete triglycerides in the form of VLDL, fatty liver is a common consequence of inappropriate flux of plasma fatty acids and lipoprotein remnants to that organ. Obesity is the most common cause of non-alcoholic fatty liver disease (NAFLD), which represents a spectrum of liver disease that spans from steatosis to non-alcoholic steatohepatitis (NASH) and then to fibrosis and cirrhosis. NAFLD is associated with obesity, hyperinsulinemia, hyperlipidemia, type-2 diabetes mellitus, and hypertension. Reports evaluating this relationship have shown the prevalence of NAFLD in morbidly obese patients undergoing bariatric surgery to range from 84% to 93% [22]. Also, the severity of liver histopathology seems to correlate with the degree of impaired glycemic status [23]. Patients with hyperlipidemia and greater BMI seem to have more advanced liver disease.

8.7   Lipids after Bariatric Surgery

8.7.1   Restrictive Procedures

In the prospective, controlled Swedish Obese Subjects Study (SOS), surgically treated patients (either gastric bypass, banding, or vertical banded gastroplasty) had a greater weight loss and showed more favorable recovery rates from hypertriglyceridemia, diabetes, and hyperuricemia than control subjects. Recovery from hypercholesterolemia did not differ between the groups. The mean changes in risk factors were more favorable among the patients treated with gastric bypass than among those treated by banding or vertical banded gastroplasty [24]. In a study by Zambon et al. [25], 14 patients with a BMI ≥40 kg/m2 were treated with laparoscopic gastric banding (LAGB): After 12 months BMI was significantly reduced, with an average weight loss of 34 kg (25% of initial body weight). Similar to results in the SOS study, total cholesterol and LDL cholesterol levels were not modified when compared with baseline, whereas plasma triglycerides (TG) significantly decreased and HDL cholesterol significantly increased and normalized. Although the amount of LDL cholesterol was not modified, LDL quality as assessed with a single vertical spin density gradient ultracentrifugation did show a shift to a presumably less atherogenic profile with larger, more buoyant LDL particles. Nevertheless, this, as well as an increase in HDL cholesterol, was not reflected in apolipoproteins: ApoB (the major protein constituent of LDL and VLDL particles) as well as Apo AI and AII (HDL particles), CII and CIII did not show any variation 12 months after surgery. After purely restrictive surgery total and LDL cholesterol were mostly unchanged, usually in combination with a postoperative increase in HDL-c. The atherogenic ratio of total cholesterol to HDL-c therefore decreased [26, 27].

8.7.2   Malabsorptive Procedures

The Program on the Surgical Control of the Hyperlipidemias (POSCH), a randomized clinical trial, was designed to test whether cholesterol lowering induced by the partial ileal bypass operation would favorably affect overall mortality or mortality specifically due to coronary heart disease. Between 1975 and 1983, 838 survivors of a single myocardial infarction who had plasma cholesterol levels >220 mg/dl or >200 mg/dl in combination with LDL cholesterol >140 mg/dl were assigned either to dietary treatment (control group) or to dietary treatment plus partial ileal bypass (intervention group). In this procedure the last 2 m of the small intestine is bypassed. The majority of cholesterol absorption and re-absorption and bile acid reabsorption takes place in this part of the intestine. Partial ileal bypass effected a 23.3% decrease in total plasma cholesterol, a 37.7% decrease in LDL cholesterol, and a 4% increase in HDL-c at 5 years post randomization. The HDL/TC and HDL/LDL ratios were significantly increased in the surgery group as compared either with baseline values or with the control group. Unlike cholesterol, plasma triglyceride levels increased up to 22% in the surgery group as compared with controls. These findings were accompanied by a reduction of mortality from ACHD (nonfatal myocardial infarction, coronary artery bypass grafting, percutaneous transluminal coronary angioplasty) and a consistent decrease in the rate of disease progression [28]. Today's popular malabsorptive procedures for treatment of obesity are the biliopancreatic diversion and the duodenal switch. In a study by Vila et al. [29], changes in lipid parameters, glucose, insulin, and insulin resistance before and 3, 6, 12, 18, and 24 months after surgery were studied in 115 obese patients divided into two groups based on the criteria by the ADA: non-diabetics and diabetics. In both groups BMI, glucose, insulin, and HOMA were significantly reduced: BMI reduction was 35% in diabetics and 8% in non-diabetics. Levels of total cholesterol and LDL cholesterol decreased significantly from the third month post surgery and triglyceride levels decreased from the 6-month follow-up in diabetics and from 1 year in non-diabetics. HDL cholesterol levels were similar in both groups; they showed an early decrease, possibly due to rapid weight loss. HDL cholesterol did not increase until the sixth month after surgery, but this increase was not significant. In a trial by Lubrano et al. 45 morbidly obese patients (BMI >40 kg/m2) were treated with a jejunoileal bypass with a large gall bladder-jejunum anastomosis at the excluded jejunum, which induces a constant reflux of most bile in the defunctionalized intestinal loop. Body weight, lipid profile (fasting), glucose, and insulin blood levels during fasting and 120 min after an oral glucose tolerance test were evaluated every 3 months in the first year and every 6 months thereafter until the end of the 3-year follow-up [30]. A significant and persistent weight loss was present in all patients at the end of the 3-year follow-up period (p<0.001). Parallel to this, a significant reduction in systolic (p<0.001) and diastolic (p<0.001) blood pressure was observed. Total and LDL cholesterol were significantly reduced (p<0.001), while HDL showed no modifications; triglycerides declined progressively during the 3-year follow-up (p<0.001). Fasting glucose levels and glucose levels 120 min after an oral glucose tolerance test were reduced from 95.1+/-20.3 mg/dl to 78.6+/-9.1 mg/ dl (p<0.001) and from 116.9+/-34.7 mg/ dl to 77.6+/- 15.5 mg/dl (p<0.001), respectively, at baseline and at the end of the study. Moreover, fasting insulin decreased from 30.0+/-20.4 µU/ml to 8.6+/-2.9 µU/ml (p<0.001) after 3 years, while insulin levels after (120 min) oral glucose load decreased from 105.5+/-61.5 µU/ml to 12.0+/- 6.0 µU/ml (p<0.001). Therefore, in this study all patients who underwent surgery achieved a normalization of glycemic and insulinemic values as well as successful control of blood pressure after significant weight loss. In a study by Brizzi et al., 29 patients with morbid obesity (17 patients with type-2 diabetes mellitus and 12 non-diabetics) were treated with biliopancreatic diversion [31]. Before and 6 months after surgery plasma lipids and LDL composition in particular were studied and compared with those of a control group of non-diabetic and non-obese subjects. LDL composition was determined by measuring cholesterol, triglycerides, ApoB, and phospholipids following LDL separation from plasma. For LDL preparation density gradient ultracentrifugation was used. The lipid profile in the diabetic group was typical, with significantly higher total and LDL cholesterol and triglycerides and significantly lower HDL cholesterol as compared with non-diabetics and the control group. Six months after surgery a highly significant reduction of BMI and all measured variables (total cholesterol, LDL cholesterol, HDL cholesterol, triglycerides, and ApoB after LDL separation from plasma) was present in all subjects regardless of whether they were diabetics or not. Notably, the homeostatic model assessment (HOMA-IR: glucose (mmol/l) x insulin (µU/ml)/22.5)) as a measure of insulin sensitivity after surgery was similar in both groups. After surgery all lipid parameters decreased significantly to the same degree in diabetics and in non-diabetics. LDL composition was changed after surgery, showing a significant increase in the triglyceride percentage. These triglyceride-rich LDLs seem to be correlated with severity and rate of progression of coronary atherosclerosis assessed by angiography, as discussed above. The ApoB/LDL cholesterol ratio increased in both groups significantly (non-diabetics from 0.98 to 1.09, diabetics from 0.9 to 1.09), which would also correlate with a greater number of LDL particles at a given cholesterol concentration in LDL. The seemingly greater atherogenicity of LDL particles might be compensated by improvement in the general metabolic condition.

8.7.3 Combined Procedures: Malabsorptive and Restrictive

Garcia-Dias et al. [32] subjected 58 patients with morbid obesity (mean BMI 49.4 kg/m^2) to subtotal gastrectomy in combination with biliopancreatic diversion with a jejunoileostomy 50 cm proximal to the ileocecal valve. Serum lipoproteins, apolipoprotein B, and AI were assessed. At baseline 25.9% of patients were diabetics. Only a minority were on hypolipidemic medication and lipid parameters were normal or slightly elevated in the majority of the patients, including triglycerides, but these showed a great variability. Mean HDL-c was 52.3 mg/dl. Follow-up ranged from 12 to 72 months and was routinely carried out every 6 months. After 18 months no additional significant changes were observed. Regarding lipid parameters, early and significant changes were observed up to the first postoperative year, which stabilized from then on with the exception of HDL-c. After surgery there was a remarkable and significant reduction in lipid parameters: the mean changes after 1 year were total cholesterol -69.1 mg/dl, LDL-C -57.9 mg/dl, triglycerides -52.0 mg/dl, ApoB -44.0 mg/dl, and ApoAI -13.4 mg/dl (not significant). Mean HDL-c was decreased (-1.4 mg/dl), but this reduction was not significant. The ratio of total cholesterol/HDL-c as an indicator of cardiovascular risk decreased significantly. All benefits persisted for at least 5 years after BPD.

Nguyen et al. reviewed retrospectively [33] the charts of 95 morbidly obese patients with documented hyperlipidemia who underwent laparoscopic Roux-en-Y gastric bypass. The mean duration of hyperlipidemia was 44+/-56 months. Hyperlipidemia was defined as an elevated level of triglycerides (>150 mg/dl) or total cholesterol (>200 mg/dl). Changes in the lipid profile of a subset of patients with subnormal levels of HDL cholesterol (≤40 mg/dl) and high levels of LDL cholesterol (>130 mg/dl) and VLDL cholesterol (>40 mg/dl) were also examined. Fasting lipid profiles were measured preoperatively and at 3-month intervals. The mean body mass index was 47+/-5 kg/m^2. The mean percentage of excess body weight loss at 12 months postoperatively was 66%. One year following gastric bypass, mean total cholesterol levels decreased by 16%, triglyceride levels decreased by 63%, LDL cholesterol levels decreased by 31%, VLDL cholesterol decreased by 74%, total cholesterol/HDL-c risk ratio decreased by 60%, and HDL-c levels increased by 39%. Also, within 1 year, 23 of 28 (82%) patients who had required lipid-lowering medications preoperatively were able to discontinue their medications. This improvement in lipid profiles was observed as early as 3 months postoperatively and was sustained at 1 year.

In a trial by Corradini et al. [34] a malabsorptive procedure was compared with a restrictive procedure. The effects on blood lipids of biliointestinal bypass (BI-bypass) with a wide cholecystojejunal anastomosis or adjustable gastric banding (LAGB) were investigated in obese patients. For clarification of the hypocholesterolemic effect of BI-bypass daily fecal sterol excretion was measured by gas-liquid chromatography (GLC). At 1 year after BI-bypass compared with baseline, the hypercholesterolemic (n=18) and the normocholesterolemic (n=19) patients showed significantly reduced total (-38% and -27%, respectively), LDL (-47% and -24%, respectively), and HDL (-11% and -13%, respectively) cholesterol and total/HDL cholesterol ratio (-25% and -13%, respectively). At 1 year after AGB, the total/HDL cholesterol ratio was significantly decreased (-11%) compared with baseline in hypercholesterolemic (n=12) but not in normocholesterolemic (n=6) patients, while total and LDL cholesterol were not affected in either group. At 3 years after BI-bypass compared with baseline, the hypercholesterolemic (n=9) and the normocholesterolemic (n=11) patients significantly showed reduced total (-43% and -28%, respectively) and LDL (-53% and -29%, respectively) cholesterol and total/HDL cholesterol ratio (-38% and -21%, respectively). The BI-bypass induced a significant (p<0.005; n=7) sixfold increase in mean fecal cholesterol output. At 1 year after AGB, the total/HDL cholesterol ratio was significantly decreased (-11%) compared with baseline in hypercholesterolemic (n=12) but not in normocholesterolemic (n=6) patients, while total and LDL cholesterol were not affected in either group.

8.8 Conclusion

In a meta-analysis by Buchwald et al. including 136 studies of bariatric surgery performed on a total of 22,094 patients, a significant decrease in total cholesterol, LDL-c, and triglycerides without a significant increase in HDL-c [35] was observed. In this analysis restrictive, malabsorptive, and combined procedures were included. Nevertheless, in choosing the bariatric procedure for an obese patient from a "lipidologic viewpoint", several things should be taken into account:

- A reduction in total cholesterol has to be perceived in context: Is this reduction based on a triglyceride reduction? A thereby resulting reduction in triglyceride- rich VLDL particles also decreases total cholesterol, since in addition to triglycerides VLDL particles always carry a certain fraction of cholesterol as well.
- Restrictive surgery does have beneficial effects on BMI, triglycerides, HDL cholesterol and, probablyre-

lated to weight loss and loss of truncal fat, glucose metabolism. Total cholesterol and LDL cholesterol are not significantly decreased independent of a reduction in triglycerides. Whether the "quality" of LDL shifts to a less atherogenic profile needs to be further evaluated [34].

▬ Both malabsorptive procedures and combined procedures (malabsorptive + restrictive) induce significant reductions of BMI, as well as of triglycerides. In addition they decrease total and LDL cholesterol. Hypercholesterolemia should be considered a criterion for selecting a malabsorptive rather than a purely restrictive surgical procedure.

References

1. Shachter NS (2001) Apolipoproteins C-I and C-III as important modulators of lipoprotein metabolism. Curr Opin Lipidol 12:297–304
2. Evans K, Burdge GC, et al (2002) Regulation of dietary fatty acid entrapment in subcutaneous adipose tissue and skeletal muscle. Diabetes 51:2684–2690
3. Friedewald WT, Levy RI, et al (1972) Estimation of the concentration of low-density lipoprotein cholesterol in plasma, without use of the preparative ultracentrifuge. Clin Chem 18:499–502
4. Phillips NR, Waters D, Havel RJ (1993) Plasma lipoproteins and progression of coronary artery disease evaluated by angiography and clinical events. Circulation 88:2762–2770
5. Gardne, CD, Fortmann SP, et al (1996) Association of small low-density lipoprotein particles with the incidence of coronary artery disease in men and women. JAMA 276:875–881
6. Stampfer MJ, Krauss RM, et al (1996) A prospective study of triglyceride level, low-density lipoprotein particle diameter, and risk of myocardial infarction. JAMA 276:882–888
7. St-Pierre AC, Cantin B, et al (2005) Low-density lipoprotein subfractions and the long-term risk of ischemic heart disease in men: 13-year follow-up data from the Quebec Cardiovascular Study. Arterioscler Thromb Vasc Biol 25:553–559
8. Mora S (2009) Advanced lipoprotein testing and subfractionation are not (yet) ready for routine clinical use. Circulation 119:2396–2404
9. Lindgren FT, Jensen LT, Hatch FT (1972) The isolation and quantitative analysis of serum lipoproteins. In: Nelson GJ (ed) Blood lipids and lipoproteins: quantitation, composition and metabolism.
10. Sich D, Saidi Y, et al (1998) Hyperalphalipoproteinemia: characterization of a cardioprotective profile associating increased high-density lipoprotein 2 levels and decreased hepatic lipase activity. Metabolism 47:965–973
11. Miller NE, Hammett F, et al (1981) Relation of angiographically defined coronary artery disease to plasma lipoprotein subfractions and apolipoproteins. Br Med J (Clin Res Ed) 282:1741–1744
12. Grundy SM, Cleeman JI, et al (2004) Implications of recent clinical trials for the National Cholesterol Education Program Adult Treatment Panel III guidelines. Circulation 110:227–239
13. Goff DC jr, D'Agostino RB jr, et al (2005) Insulin resistance and adiposity influence lipoprotein size and subclass concentrations. Results from the Insulin Resistance Atherosclerosis Study. Metabolism 54: 264–270
14. Garvey WT, Kwon S, et al (2003) Effects of insulin resistance and type 2 diabetes on lipoprotein subclass particle size and concentration determined by nuclear magnetic resonance. Diabetes 52:453–462
15. Kathiresan S, Otvos JD, et al (2006) Increased small low-density lipoprotein particle number: a prominent feature of the metabolic syndrome in the Framingham Heart Study. Circulation 113:20–29
16. Burstein R, Epstein Y, et al (1995) Glucose utilization in morbidly obese subjects before and after weight loss by gastric bypass operation. Int J Obes Relat Metab Disord 19:558–561
17. Kersten S (2001. Mechanisms of nutritional and hormonal regulation of lipogenesis. EMBO Rep 2:282–286
18. Anthonsen MW, Ronnstrand L, et al (1998) Identification of novel phosphorylation sites in hormone-sensitive lipase that are phosphorylated in response to isoproterenol and govern activation properties in vitro. J Biol Chem 273:215-–221
19. Kissebah AH, Alfarsi S, et al (1976) The metabolic fate of plasma lipoproteins in normal subjects and in patients with insulin resistance and endogenous hypertriglyceridaemia. Diabetologia 12:501-–509
20. Kissebah AH, Alfarsi S, et al (1976) Transport kinetics of plasma free fatty acid, very low density lipoprotein triglycerides and apoprotein in patients with endogenous hypertriglyceridaemia: effects of 2,2-dimethyl, 5(2, 5-xylyoxy) valeric acid therapy. Atherosclerosis 24:199–218
21. Lewis GF (1997) Fatty acid regulation of very low density lipoprotein production. Curr Opin Lipidol 8:146–153
22. Gholam PM, Kotler DP, et al (2002) Liver pathology in morbidly obese patients undergoing Roux-en-Y gastric bypass surgery. Obes Surg 12:49–51
23. Silverman JF, O'Brien KF, et al (1990) Liver pathology in morbidly obese patients with and without diabetes. Am J Gastroenterol 85:1349–1355
24. Sjostrom L, Lindroos AK, et al (2004) Lifestyle, diabetes, and cardiovascular risk factors 10 years after bariatric surgery. N Engl J Med 351:2683–2693
25. Zambon S, Romanato G, et al (2009) Bariatric surgery improves atherogenic LDL profile by triglyceride reduction. Obes Surg 19:190–195
26. Wolf AM, Beisiegel U, et al (1998) Does gastric restriction surgery reduce the risks of metabolic diseases? Obes Surg 8:9–13
27. Busetto L, Pisent C, et al (2000) Variation in lipid levels in morbidly obese patients operated with the LAP-BAND adjustable gastric banding system: effects of different levels of weight loss. Obes Surg 10:569–577
28. Buchwald, H., S. E. Williams, et al. (2002). „Overall mortality in the program on the surgical control of the hyperlipidemias." J Am Coll Surg 195:327–331
29. Vila M, Ruiz O, et al (2009) Changes in lipid profile and insulin resistance in obese patients after Scopinaro biliopancreatic diversion. Obes Surg 19:299–306
79. Lubrano C, Cornoldi A, et al (2004) Reduction of risk factors for cardiovascular diseases in morbid-obese patients following biliary-intestinal bypass: 3 years' follow-up. Int J Obes Relat Metab Disord 28:1600–1606
30. Brizzi P, Angius MF, et al (2003) Plasma lipids and lipoprotein changes after biliopancreatic diversion for morbid obesity. Dig Surg 20:18–23
31. Garcia-Diaz J, Lozano DO, et al (2003) Changes in lipid profile after biliopancreatic diversion. Obes Surg 13:756–760

32. Nguyen NT, Varela E, et al (2006) Resolution of hyperlipidemia after laparoscopic Roux-en-Y gastric bypass. J Am Coll Surg 203:24–29
33. Corradini SG, Eramo A, Lubrano C, Spera G, Cornoldi A, Grossi A, Liguori F, Siciliano M, Pisanelli MC, Salen G, Batta AK, Attili AF, Badiali M (2005) Obes Surg 15:367–377
34. Buchwald H, Avidor Y, et al (2004) Bariatric surgery: a systematic review and meta-analysis. JAMA 292:1724–1737

The Border of Internal Medicine and Metabolic Surgery

Iwon Karcz-Socha, MD

>140 mmHg and the index of diastolic arterial pressure is >90 mmHg; 120/80 mmHg is regarded as the optimum index. There is overall agreement that non-pharmacological methods of arterial hypertension treatment should already be undertaken in the stage of high-appropriate pressure, that is, when the values are within the range of 130–139/85–89 mmHg [53]. Such an undertaking is vital, since arterial hypertension poses one of the most significant factors in the risk of incidental cardiovascular events such as stroke, coronary disease, and myocardial infarction. In 2009, the National Heart, Lung, and Blood Institute published JNC 8 (Eighth Report of the Joint National Committee on Prevention, Detection, Evaluation, and Treatment of High Blood Pressure), which contains new guidelines concerning the definition, classification, presence or lack of risk factors, early markers of the disease, and damage to inner organs in relation to the arterial blood pressure index [54]. According to the WHO, arterial hypertension and its complications are one of the most important factors in the risk of death worldwide. Almost 1 billion people all over the world are affected by hypertension; 37.5% in developed countries and 22% in developing countries suffer from this disease [55]. In Poland, research by NATPOL PLUS in 2002 provided an expertise on the subject of the prevalence of arterial hypertension: Twenty-nine percent of adults in the population meet the criteria of hypertension and 30% have high-normal pressure. Only 12% of patients were appropriately treated [56]. It is thought that as many as 80% of cases of spontaneous arterial hypertension in Poland are associated with obesity [57]. Obesity is classified as one of the most important factors in the risk of arterial hypertension and ischemic heart disease. In the Framingham study, it was concluded that an increase in body mass index correlates with an increase in the arterial pressure index. It was demonstrated that 70% of men and 61% of women with arterial hypertension are obese [58, 59]. The risk of arterial hypertension is three times higher in obese persons than in those with a correct body mass index [60]. Arterial hypertension results in numerous organ complications, such as left ventricular hypertrophy (LVH), or the development of structural changes within vascular walls. Myocardial hypertrophy occurs in about 30% of patients with mild and moderate hypertension (1st and 2nd degree, according to the European Society of Cardiology), and in almost 90% of patients with severe hypertension (3rd degree, according to the ESC). There are many factors which influence the left ventricular mass index. They are, among others: age, sex, race, body mass index, the content of sodium in the diet, and genetic factors. Endogenic factors such as angiotensin II, noradrenaline, endothelin, or insulin in pathological conditions might be co-responsible for generating left ventricular hypertrophy [61]. Adipokines (i.e., leptin, and adiponectin) [62, 63] and ghrelin have cardioprotective effects [64, 65]. In obese persons, there are changes in echocardiographic parameters in the form of an increase in end-diastolic capacity of the left ventricle and an increase in thickness of the end-diastolic septum and the back wall of the left ventricle. It is suggested that the above-mentioned changes are caused by proinflammatory factors, among others CRP, TNF-α, and IL-6 [66]. Apart from arterial hypertension, obesity is also regarded as the most essential etiological factor in the development of left ventricular hypertrophy [67]. Kuch and associates indicate that the fat mass index is the main factor determining left ventricular hypertrophy in postmenopausal women with glucose intolerance [68]. Ischemic heart disease is the main cause of mortality worldwide, being responsible for half of all deaths [69]. As shown in the HOPE (Heart Outcomes Protection Evaluation) research, the consequence of abdominal obesity is an increase in the risk of death due to myocardial infarction, cardiovascular diseases, and death independent of its cause [70]. The probability of myocardial infarction increases by 20% in persons with abdominal obesity (the INTERHEART study) [71] and the number of people suffering from ischemic heart disease increases independent of BMI, age, and other risk factors [72].

9.4 Diagnosis, and Then What?

Patients who are under specialized ambulatory cardiological care belong to the group at increased cardiovascular risk. Incorrect body mass index (BMI >25 kg/m^2) occurs in about 80% of these patients (our own observation). Considering the risk of the cardiovascular complications which are the consequence of obesity, it is becoming a priority to struggle for the correct body mass index. Nowadays, the treatment of obesity includes:
1. Behavioral therapy
2. Pharmacological therapy
3. Surgical intervention.

Modification of behavioral factors is currently thought to be the most necessary and effective method of obesity treatment. Through this, the reduction of body mass index lowers arterial blood pressure, improves the function of the vascular endothelium, and decreases the frequency of diabetes and insulin resistance development [73]. Maintaining the correct body mass index by introducing healthy nutrition, increasing the level of physical activity (systematic physical exercise: 30–45 min of exercise daily on 3–5 days per week), quitting cigarette smoking, and moderate intake of alcohol all decrease cardiovascular risk [74]. Unfortunately, the percentage of patients who follow these guidelines is small [72]. Pharmacological obesity treatment is indicated when there is no loss of body mass index within 6 months of beginning behavioral therapy and the BMI is ≥30 kg/m², or BMI ≥27 kg/m² in patients with cardiovascular risk factors [75]. The purpose of pharmacotherapy is help in reducing body mass index, maintaining reduced body mass index, and reducing cardiovascular risk. Medicines currently used to treat obesity include sibutramine, orlistat, and rimonabant [75, 76]. Orlistat is a lipase inhibitor. It reduces absorption of fat from the digestive system. Taking this medicine regularly results in body mass index reduction by 5–10% in 50–60% of patients, and a characteristic reduction of risk factors positively influences lipid metabolism and insulin sensitivity. Undesirable symptoms most often include digestive system disorders [77]. Sibutramine inhibits the reuptake of noradrenaline and serotonin and results in a feeling of satiety. It also reduces body mass index by 5–10% in 60–70% of patients. It improves the monitoring of glycemia independent of the influence on the body mass index. It might cause undesirable symptoms concerning the circulatory system, such as an increase of arterial blood pressure and tachycardia. Hence, sibutramine should be administered with great caution to patients with arterial hypertension, coronary disease, or arrhythmia [75]. Rimonabant is the antagonist of the cannabinoid-1 receptor, which results in restriction of appetite. The reducing influence of this medicine on body mass index is comparable to that of the two previous ones. Rimonabant decreases the frequency of metabolic syndrome by about 50% [76]. The improvement of the cardiometabolic profile might reduce cardiovascular risk, although this requires further clinical research [78]. In the case of rimonabant, the most essential side effect is its pro-depression effect. Psychological disorders limit the use of this medicine [76, 78]. Surgical treatment is considered for patients in whom the above-mentioned methods of obesity treatment are disappointing, and whose BMI is ≥40 kg/m², or ≥35 kg/ m² with co-existing risk factors (arterial hypertension, diabetes). Surgical treatment is considered to be the most effective means of reducing body mass index and risk factors [79].

9.5   Summary

Obesity poses an ever-greater clinical problem. It is a challenge for modern medicine to find an effective method of obesity treatment. Appropriate treatment and care for an obese patient involves the cooperation of an internist, a diabetologist, a cardiologist, and a metabolic surgeon. The effectiveness and progress of obesity therapy depend on integrity and cooperation among representatives of these medical disciplines. In light of the insufficient success of behavioral therapy and the obstacles connected with pharmacotherapy (side effects of medicines reducing body mass index, polipharmacotherapy in the group of obese patients, lack of discipline in drug intake), it might be worth considering patients with a BMI ≥30 kg/m² and significant cardiological risk as qualifying for surgical treatment (a task for the internist, diabetologist, and cardiologist), particularly because contemporary laparoscopic surgical techniques applied in metabolic surgery are becoming less and less invasive and offer the highest effectiveness in treating obesity and its complications. Surgical therapy of diabetes type 2 and metabolic syndrome seems to be a real consideration. Parallel to searching for clinical solutions to obesity treatment, prohealthy education and obesity prevention are still very important and necessary.

References

1. WHO Expert Committee (1995) Physical status: the use and interpretation of anthropometry; report of WHO Expert Committee. WHO Technical Report Series: WHO Geneva, pp 312–340
2. World Health Organization (1997) Obesity: preventing and managing the global epidemic. Report of a WHO Consultation presented at: the World Health Organization. June 3–5, 1997. Geneva
3. Hedley AA, Ogden CL, Johnson CL, Carroll MD, Curtin LR, Flegal KM (2004) Prevalence of overweight and obesity among US children, adolescents and adults, 1999–2002. JAMA 291:2847–2850
4. Tackling obesity In England (2001) Report by the Comptroller and Auditor General HC 220 Session 2000–2001, 15 Feb 2001 London. The Stationary Office
5. Bendixen H, Holst C, Sorensen TI, et al (2004) Major increase in prevalence of overweight and obesity between 1987 and 2001 among Danish adults. Obes Res 12:1464-1472
6. Maillard G, Charles MA, Thibult M, et al (1999) Trends in prevalence of obesity in the French adult population between 1980 and 1991. Int J Obes Relat Metab Disord 23:389-394
7. Program POL-MONICA BIS Warszawa. Stan zdrowia ludności Warszawy w roku 2001. Część 1. Podstawowe wyniki badania przekrojowego. Biblioteka Kardiologiczna nr79. Warszawa 2002
8. Program POL-MONICA BIS Kraków (2002) Heath disorders of Tarnobrzeg area in the year 2001. Cardiologic Library nr. 82., Warsaw
9. Zdrojewski T, Babińska Z, Bandosz P, et al (2002) Connection of overweight and morbid obesity with hypertention in polisch population in 1997 and 2002 (NATPOL II, NATPOL III). Metabolic Medicine, 4:32
10. Zdrojewski T, Bandosz P, Szpakowski P, et al (2004) Expantion of Cardiological risk factors in Poland NATPOL PLUS. Kardiol Pol 61[Suppl 4]:1–26

11. Trayhum P, Wood IS (2004) Adipokines: inflammation and the pleiotropic role of white adipose tissue. Br J Nutr 92:374–355

12. Cancello R, Tounian A, Poitou Ch, Clement K (2004) Adiposity signals, genetic and body weight regulation in humans. Diab Metab 30:215–227

13. Zhang Y, Proenca R, Maffei M, et al (1994) Positional cloning of the mouse obese gene and its human homologue. Nature 372:425–432

14. Meler U, Gressner AM (2004) Endocrine regulation of energy metabolism: review of pathobiochemical and clinical chemical aspects of lepton, ghrelin, adiponectin, and resistin. Clin Chem 50:1511–1525

15. Kershaw EE, Flier JS (2004) Adipose tissue as an endocrine organ. J Colin Endocrinol Metab 89:2548–2556

16. Rajala MW, Scherer PE (2003) Minireview: The adipocyte – at the crossroads of energy. Endocrinology. 144, No. 9: 3765-3773

17. Boucher J, Masri B, Daviaud D, et al (2005) Apeiin, a newly identified adipokine up-regulated by insulin and obesity. Endocrinology 146:1764–1771

18. Fukuhara A, Matsuda M, Nishizawa M, et al (2005) Visfatin: protein secreted by visceral fat that mimics the effects of insulin. Science 307:426–430

19. Messeguer A, Puche C, Cabero A (2002) Sex steroid biosynthesis in white adipose tissue. Horm Metab Res 34:731–736

20. Ruan H, Lodish HF (2003) Insulin resistance in adipose tissue: direct and indirect effects of tumor necrosis factor alfa. Cytokine Growth Factor Rev 14:447–455

21. Weisberg SP, McCann D, Desai M, Rosenbaum M, Leibel RL, Ferrante AW jr (2003) Obesity Is associated with macrophage accumulation in adipose tissue. J Clin Invest 112:1796–1808

22. Skurk T, Hauner H (2004) Obesity and impaired fibrinolisis: role of adipose production of plasminogen activator inhibitor-1. Int J Obes Relat Metab Disord 28:1357–1364

23. Engeli S, Schling P, Gorzelniak K et al (2003) The adipose-tissue rennin-angiotensin-aldosterone system; role in the metabolic syndrome? Int J Biochem Cell Biol 35:807–825

24. Barsh GS, Farooqi IS, O'Rahilly S (2000) Genetics of body-weight regulation. Nature 404:644–651

25. Jaworowska A, Bazylak G (2006) Viral infections in Obesity etiology. Postêpy Higieny i Medycyny Docewiadczalnej 60:227–236

26. Jensen MD (2006) Potential role of new therapies in modifying cardiovascular risk in overweight patients with metabolic risk factors. Obesity 14 [Suppl]:143–149

27. Hou Z, Miao Y, Gao L,Pan H, Zhu S (2006) Ghrelin-containing neuron in cerebral cortex and hypothalamus linked with the DVC of brain stern in rat. Regul Pept 134:126–131

28. Konturek SJ, Konturek JW, Pawlik T, Brzozowski T (2004) Brain-gut axis and its role in the control of food intake. J Physiol Pharmacol 55:137–154

29. Park AJ, Bloom SR (2005) Neuroendocrine control of food intake. Curr Opin Gastroenterol 21:228–233

30. Small CJ, Bloom SR (2004) Gut hormones and the controle of appetite. Trends Endocrinol Metab 15:259–263

31. Higgins SC, Gueorguiev M, Korbonitis M (2007) Ghrelin, the peripheral hunger hormone. Ann Med 39:116–136

32. Popovic V, Miljic D, Damjanovic S, Arvat E, Ghigo E, et al (2003) Ghrelin's main action on the regulation of growth hormone release is exerted at hypothalamic level. J Clin Endocrinol Metab 88:3450–3453

33. Qader SS, Hakanson R, Rehfeld JF, Lundquist I, Salehi A (2007) Proghrelin-derived peptides influence the secretion of insulin, glucagon, pancreatic polypeptide and somatostatin: study on isolated islets from mouse and rat pancreas. Regul Pept 146:230–237

34. Date Y, Murakami N, Toshinai K et al (2002) The role of the gastric afferent vagal nerve in ghrelin-induced feeding and growth hormone secretion in rats. Gastroenterology 123:1120–1128

35. Hardie DG (2005) New roles for the LKB1-AMPK pathway. Curr Opin Cell Biol 17:167–173

36. WHO (1999) Report of WHO Consultation, Geneva

37. Yang-Woo Park et al (2003) The metabolic syndrome. Prevalence and associated risk factors findings in the US population from the Third National Health and Nutrition Examination Survey 1988–1994. Arch Intern Med 163:427

38. Reaven GM (2005) The metabolic syndrome, requiescat in pace. Clin Chem 51:931–938

39. Ogden CL, Carroll MD, Curtin LR, McDowell MA, Tabak CJ, Flegal KM (2006) Prevalence of overweight and obesity in the United States, 1999–2004. JAMA 295:1549–1555

40. Meigs JM (2006) Definition and mechanisms of the metabolic syndrome. Curr Opin Endocrinol Diabetes 13:103–110

41. Klein B, Klein R, Lee KE (2002) Components of the metabolic syndrome and risk of cardiovascular disease and diabetes in Beaver Dam. Diabetes Care 25:1790–1794

42. Wilson PW, D'Agostino RB, Parise H, et al(2005) Metabolic syndrome as a precursor of cardiovascular diseases and type 2 diabetes mellitus. Circulation 112:3066–3072

43. Gami AS, Witt BJ, Howard DF, et al (2007) Metabolic syndrome and risk of incident cardiovascular events and death. Am Coll Cardiol 49:404–414

44. Kahn AM, Seidel CL, Allen JC, Oneil RG, Shelat H, Song T (1993) Insulin reduces contraction and intracellular calcium concentration in vascular smooth muscle. Hypertension 22:735–742

45. De Fronzo RA, Cooke CR, Andres R, Faloona GR, Davis PJ (1975) The effect of insulin on renal handing of sodium, potassium, calcium and phosphate in man. J Clin Invest 55:845–847

46. Schonsjans K, Staels B, Auverax J (1996) The peroxisome proliferator activated receptors (PPARs) and their effects on lipid metabolism and adipocyte differentiation. Biochem Biophys Acta 1302:93–109

47. Pan DA (1997) Skeletal muscle triglyceride levels are inversely related to insulin action. Diabetes 46:983–988

48. Szulińska M, Pupek -Musialik D, Bogdański P, Miczke A, Bryl W (2006) Estimation of Insulin resistance with euglicaemic metabolic clamping in patients with simple obesity. Endokrynologia, Oty³oœæ, Zaburzenia Przemiany Materii 2:5–11

49. Reaven GM (1988) Role of insulin resistance in human disease. Diabetes 37:1595–1607

50. Mertens I, Van Gaal FL (2002) Obesity, haemostasis and the fibrinolytic system. Obes Rev 3:85–101

51. Garcia EA, Karbonitis M Ghrelin and cardiovascular health. Current Opinion in Pharmacology 2006 6:142–147

52. Reaven GM (2003) Insulin resistance/compensatory hiperinsulinemia, essential hypertension, and cardiovascular disease. J Clin Endocrinol Metab 88:2399–2403

53. Mancia G, De Backer, Dominiczak A, et al (2007) Guidelines for the management of arterial hypertension: The Task Force for the Management of Arterial Hypertension of the European Society of Hypertension (ESH) and of the European Society of Cardiology (ESC). J Hypertension 25:1105–1187

54. Małyszko J, Małyszko J, Bachórzewska-Gajewska H (2008) Hypertention whats new in the last year? Kardiodiabetologia 3:39–44

55. Wysocka M (2006) Hypertention: challange XXI century. Puls Medycyny 11:

56. Zdrojewski T, Wyrzykowski B, Szczęch R, Wierucki L, Naruszewicz M, Narkiewicz K, Zarzeczna-Baran M (2005) Epidemiology and prevention of arterial hypertension in Poland. Blood Press 14 [Suppl 2]:10–16

57. Szczęch R, et al (2000) Estimation of concious, frequence and effctivity of hypertension therapy in action „do meassure your blood pressure". Nadciśnienie Tętnicze 4:27–37

58. Kannel WB, Garrison RJ, Dannenberg AL (1993) Secular blood pressure trends in normotensive persons: the Framingham Study. Am Heart J 125:1154–1158

59. Higgins M, Kannel WB, Garrison R, Pinsky J, Stokes JI (1988) Hazards of obesity: the Framingham experience. Acta Med Scand 10:267–273

60. Van Itallie TB (1985) The problem of obesity: health implications of overweight and obesity. Ann Inter Med 103:963–988

61. Januszewicz A (1999) Organ complication of Hypertension – influence of hypotensive treatment. Medipress Kardiologia 6:

62. Matsumura K, Tsuchihashi T, Fujii K, Iida M (2003) Neural regulation of blood pressure by leptin and the related peptides. Regul Pept 114:79–86

63. Ebinç H, Ebinç FA, Özkurt ZN et al(2008) Impact of adiponectin on left ventricular mass index in non-complicated obese subjects. Endocrine J 55:523–528

64. Baessler A et al (2006) Association of ghrelin receptor gene region with ventricular hypertrophy in the general population: result of the MONICA/KORA Augsburg Echocardiographic Substudy. Hypertension 47:920–927

65. Jodła-Mydłowska B, Kobusiak-Prokopowicz, Przewłocka-Kosmala M, Witkowska M (2006) Urotensin II and Grelin – complication in primary hypertension. Arterial Hypert 10:128–135

66. Malavazos AE, Corsi MM, Ermetice F, et al (2007) Proinflammatory cytokines and cardiac abnormalities in uncomplicated obesity: Relationship with abdominal fat deposition. Nutr Metab Cardiovasc Dis 17:294–302

67. de Simone G, Devereux RB, Chinali M, et al (2009) Metabolic syndrome and left ventricular hypertrophy in the prediction of cardiovascular events: the strong heart study. Nutr Metab Cardiovasc Dis 19:98–104

68. Kuch B, Scheidt WS, Peter W, et al (2007) Sex-specific determinants of left ventricular mass in pre-diabetic and type 2 diabetic subjects. Diabetes Care 30:946–952

69. Mackay J, Mensah G (2004) The atlas of heart disease and stroke. World Health Organization, Geneva

70. Dagenais GR, Yi Q, Mann J, et al (2005) Prognostic impact of body weight and abdominal obesity in woman and men with cardiovascular disease. Am Heart J 149:54–60

71. Yusuf S, Hawken S, Ounpuu S (2004) Effect of potentially modifiable risk factors associated with myocardial infarction in 52 countries (the INTERHEART study): case-control study. Lancet 364:937–952

72. Carey V, Walters E, Colditz G, et al (1997) Body fat distribution and risk of non-insulin-dependent diabetes mellitus in women. The Nurses' Health Study. Am J Epidemiol 145:614–619

73. Gill J, Malkova D (2006) Physical activity, fitness and cardiovascular disease risk in adults: interactions with insulin resistance and obesity. Clin Sci 110:409–425

74. Lean M, Lara J, Hill JO (2006) ABC of obesity. Strategies for preventing obesity. BMJ 333:959–962

75. Joannides-Demos LL, Proietto J, McNeil JJ. (2005) Pharmacotherapy for obesity. Drugs 65:1391–1418

76. Pi-Sunyer FX, Arron JL, Heshamati HM, et al (2006) Effect of Rimonabant, a cannabinoid 1 receptor blocker on weight and cardio-metabolic risk factors in overweight or obese patients: Rio-North America: a randomized controlled trial. JAMA 295:761–775

77. Torgerson JS, Hauptman J, Boldrin MN, Sjöströmm L (2004) Xenical in the prevention of diabetes in obese subjects (XENDOS study): a randomized study of orlistat as an adjunct to lifestyle changes for the prevention of type 2 diabetes in obese patients. Diabetes Care 27:155–161

78. Nissen S, Nicholls S, Wolski K, et al (2008) Effect of rimonabant on progression of atherosclerosis in patients with abdominal obesity and coronary disease: the STRADIVARIUS randomized controlled trial. JAMA 299:1547–1560

79. Sjöstrom L, Lindroos AK, Peltonen M, et al (2004) The Swedish Obese Subjects Study Scientific Group. Lifestyle, diabetes and cardiovascular risk factors 10 years after bariatric surgery. N Engl J Med 351:2683–2693

Innovative Approach to Treatment of the Metabolic Syndrome

Joel Ricci MD, Michael Timoney MD, George Ferzli MD

In recent decades, we have seen a massive increase in the incidence of the metabolic syndrome. With the advent of bariatric surgery as the most effective method to achieve and maintain weight loss, multiple changes have also been discovered regarding its role in the management of diabetes and the metabolic syndrome. There is now extensive evidence to support metabolic surgery as a treatment not only for obesity but also for the well documented metabolic derangements that accompany it. The site of nutrient delivery in the gastrointestinal tract, malabsorption, and gut hormone secretion are all believed to play important roles in the proposed mechanism of action of metabolic surgery. Although the mechanisms of the long-term remission of diabetes and other obesity-associated co-morbidites are still being outlined, novel techniques and surgical innovations have provided very promising results in select groups of patients. This chapter deals with the history of metabolic surgery and its effects on diabetes and the metabolic syndrome. An overview of several hypotheses and theories behind the surgically induced changes that may lead to sustained remission of this disease is given, along with a discussion of the ongoing trials, to create a better understanding of the future role of surgery in the management of this patient population.

10.1 Background

The sky-rocketing rise in morbid obesity and associated complications in the United States is alarming and is a well-recognized problem worldwide [1]. The constellations of conditions associated with morbid obesity are numerous and include high blood pressure, dyslipidemia, insulin resistance, and visceral adiposity, and, combined, they lead to the metabolic syndrome. This syndrome is proven to be a risk factor for development of cardiovascular disease. The presence of insulin resistance in patients with metabolic syndrome confers an increased risk for type-2 diabetes, further increasing the risk for cardiovascular disease [2]. Obesity is a modifiable component of this syndrome and therefore the primary target for intervention [3, 4]. This intervention has traditionally been medical; however, with increasing surgical expertise in bariatric procedures, surgery has taken on a pivotal role in the management of the obese patient. Lifestyle modifications have been recommended as first-line therapy for weight reduction, resulting in lower serum cholesterol and triglyceride levels, higher serum HDL cholesterol, lower blood pressure and glucose levels, and reduced insulin resistance [3]. Pharmacological agents that treat specific components of the metabolic syndrome have also been successful in selective patients.

These include statins, antihypertensive drugs, anti-platelet therapy, anti-obesity agents (such as lipase inhibitors and appetite suppressants), and insulin sensitizers or hypoglycemic agents when diabetes ensues. These therapies have proven to play important roles in the treatment of this disease. However, in the majority of obese patients with metabolic syndrome, medical therapy has not been sufficient as a long-term treatment to achieve sustained weight loss and glucose control [5]. In recent years, surgery has emerged as a promising alternative therapy for these morbidly obese patients with poor response to less invasive intervention. Gastric bypass surgery and other associated procedures have been proven to facilitate weight loss and ameliorate or resolve conditions associated with obesity, particularly type-2 diabetes mellitus [6–8]. Complete resolution of diabetes can be achieved not only in the morbidly obese but also in the semi-obese patient following bariatric surgery. This chapter provides an overview of the benefits of surgery as therapy for the metabolic changes associated with obesity, diabetes, and the metabolic syndrome.

10.2 Diabetes and the Metabolic Syndrome

10.2.1 Public Health and Economic Crisis

Diabetes is the fifth leading cause of death in the United States [9]. There are approximately 20 million people in the United States (7% of the population) who have diabetes. In 2005, one and a half million new cases of diabetes were diagnosed in people 20 years or older [10]. It is of even more concern that, despite a decrease in the death rate related to heart disease, stroke, and cancer, the death rate due to diabetes has increased by 45% during the past 20 years [9]. It is projected that by 2012, the diabetic population will be an estimated 22.7 million in the United States and 226 million outside of the US [11]. Type-2 diabetes mellitus (T2DM) is estimated to constitute up to 90% of all diabetes cases [12]. Diabetes is now the most costly disease in the United States. In 2002, diabetes was accountable for cost amounting to 138 billion dollars between medical expenses and lost wages and productivity. By 2020, the overall cost associated with DM is expected to be close to 200 billion dollars per year [11].

10.2.2 Success and Failure of Medical Management of Diabetes

Insulin resistance is central to the pathophysiology of T2DM. In its earlier phase, insulin levels rise to counteract the peripheral effects of resistance within the muscle, liver, and adipose tissues, and thus, normal glucose levels are maintained. This leads to hypertrophy of the pancreatic β-cells. Eventually, the β-cells are unable to produce adequate levels of insulin. Unopposed insulin resistance and decreased levels of insulin production promote glucose intolerance, which ultimately progresses to diabetes [13]. Obesity has been defined as the primary predictor of diabetes [14]. A BMI greater than 40 kg/m^2 exponentially increases the risk of developing T2DM [15]. Around 40% of these patients have altered levels of fasting glucose or impaired glucose tolerance, and 20% of them develop T2DM [16]. Management of T2DM is complicated. Not only must it focus on the amelioration of symptoms; it must also achieve long-term remission in order to delay or prevent the complications of the disease. Lifestyle modifications for weight reduction, along with the use of glucose control medications and antihypertensive and antilipidemic agents, have been the mainstay of treatment of obesity and its associated complications for the past 20 years [17–22]. The success of medical management has been associated mostly with well-motivated semi-obese patients, but there has been limited effectiveness for morbidly obese patients. This might be due in part to the complicated task of managing advanced insulin resistance associated with these types of patients. Glycosylated hemoglobin (HbA1c) is an excellent indicator of plasma glucose concentrations over extended time periods. The United Kingdom Diabetes Prospective Study (UKPDS) demonstrated that mortality risk is decreased if HbA1c is maintained within normal values [23–25]. However, even intensive multifactorial therapy has not yielded complete resolution of diabetes or elimination of cardiovascular- and microvascular-associated mortality. The Steno 2 Trial reported that patients treated with intensive multipharmaceutical therapy and behavior modification had a 20% reduction in incidence of cardiovascular events compared with patients treated conventionally [26]. Similarly, there was a 50% decrease in development of nephropathy, retinopathy, and autonomic neuropathy. Although these results provided improved outcomes from medical management, a significant number of patients remained with poor glycemic control and long-term diabetes-related risk. This highlights the need for more aggressive therapy in these patients, introducing the potential benefit from "metabolic surgery".

10.3   What Is the Metabolic Syndrome?

The clustering of abnormalities that compose the metabolic syndrome has been widely studied during the past 30 years. In 1977, Haller used the term "metabolic syndrome" to describe the additive effects of risk factors for atherosclerosis: obesity, diabetes mellitus, hyperlipoproteinemia, hyperuricemia, and hepatic steatosis [27]. That same year, Phillips proposed obesity as the linking factor among its components for predisposition to myocardial infarction [28, 29]. A decade later, Reaven reported insulin resistance as a common etiological factor for the convergence of impaired glucose intolerance (IGT), hyperinsulinemia, high levels of very low density lipoprotein (VLDL), hypertriglyceridemia, low levels of highdensity lipoprotein (HDL), cholesterol, and hypertension [30]. He named this coalition of symptoms "syndrome X". The "deadly quartet" was introduced by Kaplan a year later, adding central adiposity to IGT, hyperlipidemia, and hypertension as the main components that increase risk of cardiovascular disease [31]. Following these findings, more evidence implicated insulin resistance as the cause for development of the syndrome and DeFronzo and Ferrannini therefore named it "insulin resistance syndrome" [32]. In the past 10 years multiple efforts have been made to define the metabolic syndrome. The World Health Organization (WHO) [33], the European Group for the study of Insulin Resistance (EGIR) [34], the National Cholesterol Education Program/Adult Treatment Panel III (NCEP/ATP III) [35], and the American Association of Clinical Endocrinologists (AACE) [36] have all provided definitions (see ▢ Table 10.1). Although no definition has been universally accepted, the aforementioned consensus groups agree that for a person to be diagnosed as having metabolic syndrome he or she must have central obesity plus any two of the following: raised triglyceride levels, reduced HDL cholesterol, increased blood pressure, and elevated fasting plasma glucose. An estimated 47 million US residents have the metabolic syndrome. The age-adjusted prevalence for both men and women is 23.7%. Prevalence increases dramatically with age, from 6.7% among people ages 20–29 to 43.5% for people older than 60 years [37]. Metabolic syndrome increases the risk for development of CVD and diabetes. According to the Framingham study, the presence of metabolic syndrome predicted about 25% of all new cases of CVD and almost 50% of cases of new-onset diabetes [38]. Non-diabetic patients with metabolic syndrome had a 10–20% increase in the 10-year risk for CHD. However, when diabetes was pres ent, the 10-year risk for CHD increased to >20% in men and to almost 20% in women. Obesity and insulin resistance are closely linked to the pathogenesis of metabolic syndrome. Therapeutic measures to achieve weight loss and glucose homeostasis include multifactorial approaches; surgery has

and glucose use but also decreases monocyte adhesion and promotes nitric oxide production in endothelial cells. This acts as a protective mechanism for the vascular wall [68]. Hence, adiponectin stands out among the adipocyte-related cytokines, as it counters the progress of diabetes and suppresses atherogenesis. Resistin is a hormone secreted by adipose tissue. Serum resistin levels increase with increased adiposity, particularly at the level of the waistline in the presence of so-called android obesity [69, 70]. Given the well-documented association between central obesity and insulin resistance, it is believed that resistin may in fact contribute to impairment of insulin action by impairing glucose tolerance [71, 72]. Serum levels of resistin are increased in obese rodent models. This connection is also found in human beings, but the correlation is not as clear [73, 74]. It also plays a role in the inflammatory response and increases production of IL-6 and TNF-α [75, 76]. These cytokines worsen insulin resistance by inhibiting muscle glucose uptake. IL-6 increases C-reactive protein, which is strongly associated with vascular disease. TNF-α activates serial serine kinases that phosphorylate insulin receptor substrates, impairing insulin action. Ghrelin is an orexigenic hormone that is produced mainly by the oxyntic cells lining the fundus of the stomach [77, 78]. It is also known as the "hunger hormone", as its injection has been proven to stimulate food intake in rodents and humans [79]. Ghrelin increases the hypothalamic expression of neuropeptide Y, which also stimulates food intake and promotes weight gain by increasing the proportion of energy stored as fat. Ghrelin stimulates appetite, reduces fat utilization, and increases gastric motility and acid secretion. Preprandial increase and postprandial decrease of ghrelin levels have been extensively studied in relation to obesity and weight loss [80]. Obese persons have decreased levels of ghrelin [81].

10.5.3   The Enteroinsular Axis

The enteroinsular axis presupposes that a signaling pathway between the pancreas and the instestines promotes insulin secretion in response to meals. Insulin secretagogues known as incretins include glucagon like peptide-1(GLP-1) and glucose-dependent insulinotropic peptide (GIP). GLP-1 is secreted mainly by the L-cells of the terminal ileum and colon [82], and GIP is produced by the K-cells in the duodenum [83]. Both hormones are secreted in response to the presence of nutrients in the lumen of the intestine. They increase insulin secretion from the pancreas [84, 85], decrease glucagon secretion [86], increase β-cell mass and insulin gene expression,

inhibit acid secretion and gastric emptying in the stomach [87], and decrease food intake by increasing satiety [87, 88]. Alterations in the enteroinsular axis can lead to hyperinsulinism and T2DM [89]. Decreased expression of glucose-dependent insulinotropic polypeptide receptor (GIPR), which binds GIP, in type-2 diabetics leads to defective signaling pathways and attenuation of the incretin effect from GIP [90, 91]. Peptide YY (PYY) is a peptide produced in the distal gastrointestinal tract at the level of the ileum and the colon. It is secreted in response to food intake and it inhibits the release of neuropeptide Y, slows gastric emptying, and prolongs intestinal transit [92, 93]. This mechanism of action leads to satiety. Morbidly obese individuals have been shown to have diminished response of PYY release and decreased levels compared with lean controls [94, 95].

10.6   Metabolic Effects of Gastrointestinal Surgery

Metabolic changes associated with bariatric surgery have been the subject of intensive investigation during the past decade (see ◘ Table 10.3). The most dramatic effect observed has been in the remission of T2DM, and its most promising feature is that the improved glycemic control occurs independently of weight loss. Often this occurs in the immediate postoperative period. In 1995, Pories reported long-term control of T2DM in 83% of patients 10 years after Roux-en-Y gastric bypass (RYGB) [7]. The study also noted that 98% of patients with preoperative impaired glucose tolerance did not progress to T2DM following surgery and eventually returned to the euglycemic status. Hickey reported significant reduction in fasting plasma glucose, insulin, and serum leptin after RYGB compared with a group of patients treated nonsurgically [96]. In 2003, Schauer concluded that RYGBP resulted in resolution of T2DM in 82% of patients, and those patients with the mildest and earlier-phase T2DM had a higher rate of resolution after surgery [97]. In what is perhaps the landmark study about changes associated with metabolic surgery, the Swedish Obese Subjects Study (SOSS) determined that surgically treated patients had more favorable 2- and 10-year recovery rates from hypertension, diabetes, hypertriglyceridemia, HDL cholesterol, and hyperuricemia than control subjects [98]. One year later, a meta-analysis conducted by Buchwald compared the efficacy of four variations of bariatric procedures for improvement of diabetes [99]. The study reported a 98% remission rate after biliopancreatic diversion (BPD) or duodenal switch, an 84% rate after RYGB, and 68% and 48% for gastroplasty and gastric ban-

▣ **Table 10.3** Effect of bariatric procedures in obese type-2 diabetic patients [103]

Author/Study	Procedure	n	BMI	Years	Result
SOS Study [98]	VBG (70%) RYGBP (24%)	1029	42	2	R = 47%
Dixon et al. [54, 118]	LAGB	500	48	1	R = 64%
Pories et al. [7]	RYGB	608		10	R = 89%
Schauer et al. [97, 102, 103]	LRYGB	1160	48	4	R = 82%
Sugerman [103]	LRYGB RYGB	1025	51	1-10	R = 86%
Scopinaro et al. [101, 121–123]	BPD	2241		1-21	R = 100%
Marceau et al. [125–127]	BPD/DS	465	47	4	R = 96%

BMI body mass index, *BPD* biliopancreatic diversion, *DS* BPD with duodenal switch, *LAGB* laparoscopic adjustable gastric banding, *LRYGBP* laparoscopic roux-en-Y gastric bypass, *R* resolved, *RYGBP* open Roux-en-Y gastric bypass, *VBG* vertical banded gastroplasty

▣ **Table 10.4** Effect of bariatric procedures on obesity-related co-morbidities

Study	Type and size	Effect on weight	Effect on co-morbidities
Swedish Obese Subject trial (SOS) [98]	Prospective matched cohort (n=4047)	At 10 years: Medical: 1.6% gain Surgical: 16% loss	Resolution of: Diabetes Lipid profile Hypertension Hyperuricemia
Buchwald et al. [99]	Meta-analysis (n=22 094)	Mean excess weight loss: 61%	Resolution of: Diabetes: 70% Hypertension: 62% Sleep apnea: 86%

ding, respectively or recovery from hypertension, sleep apnea, and hypertriglyceridemia was also reported (see ▣ Table 10.4). Nguyen described substantially improved lipid profiles after RYGBP, with 75% decrease in VLDL cholesterol levels, 31% decrease in LDL cholesterol, 39% increase in HDL cholesterol, and 63% decrease in triglyceride levels [100]. These findings confirm that bariatric surgery not only accomplishes long-term weight loss but also ameliorates the components of the metabolic syndrome and can lead to resolution of T2DM. Improvement in T2DM results from all the variations of bariatric surgery but is particularly marked following RYGB and BPD. These procedures lead to postoperative normalization of glucose and insulin levels along with HbA1c in morbidly obese patients with diabetes [7, 101–103]. They prevent the progression to diabetes by promoting the recovery of β-cell function and reduce the morbidities associated with this condition in the nondiabetic

patient with impaired glucose tolerance. The normalization of glucose and insulin levels after gastric bypass was attributed for years to the changes following weight loss. However, these changes occur early in the postoperative period, long before the patients start losing weight. In 1998, Scopinaro reported normal glucose levels in 100% of morbidly obese patients after BPD 1 month following the surgery [101]. The excess average weight of these patients had been more than 80%, and they did not require any medication or diet restriction. These findings strongly suggest that RYGB and BPD have a direct impact on glucose homeostasis.

10.6.1 Intestinal Malabsorption

Weight loss is induced after postoperative intestinal malabsorption. This may lead to reduced insulin resistance.

Malabsorption of glucose is believed to reduce the stress on β-cells and fat malabsorption, leading to decreased numbers of circulating free fatty acids. This improves insulin sensitivity through its effect on the adipoinsular axis. A full discussion of the variables involved in malabsorptive surgery is beyond the scope of this chapter but they include the length and region of the GI tract that is bypassed.

10.6.2 Hormonal Regulation

It has been proposed that changes in the route of food through the gastrointestinal tract may in fact alter the secretion of gut hormones in response to meal stimuli (see ◘ Table 10.5). Markedly suppressed ghrelin levels following RYGB were first reported by Cummings in 2002, leading him to propose that this hormone contributes to the weight-reduction effect of the procedure by reducing hunger [49]. He stated that chronic isolation of the enterocytes from nutrient stimulation suppresses ghrelin production versus increased production, with acute hunger and starvation. Other studies have shown conflicting effects on ghrelin following RYGB. Its role in satiety and weight loss following bariatric and metabolic surgery has yet to be completely elucidated [104, 105]. More recent data have associated other peptides and hormones with postoperative effects on glucose metabolism. Decreased levels of leptin, glucose, and insulin, along with increased levels of GLP-1, PYY, and adiponectin, have been reported following metabolic surgery [106–111]. Leptin, which is produced by adipocytes, suppresses neuropeptide Y production and thus reduces appetite and increases the metabolic rate. Leptin also decreases lipogenesis [112]. Hickey found leptin reduction in post-RYGB patients compared with non-bypassed, BMI-matched obese patients. Rubino and Hickey both feel that this seemingly paradoxical decrease in leptin levels is actually the result of increased leptin sensitivity, leading to a decreased need for leptin production. The mechanism by which this is accomplished remains unknown [96, 106]. Adiponectin, which increases insulin sensitivity and is vasoprotective, is decreased in the obese state. Weight loss following bariatric surgery is associated with increased levels of adiponectin, theoretically increasing insulin sensitivity and decreasing atherogeneis [73, 74, 106]. The roles of PYY and GLP-1 are discussed later in this chapter. Thus, mechanisms of weight loss and improved glucose metabolism have been attributed to a combination of appetite suppression, increased metabolic rate, amelioration of insulin resistance, and improved β-cell function – all mediated by induced changes in hormonal regulation after metabolic surgery.

10.6.3 The Gut Hypothesis

Recently, Rubino reported that regulation of ghrelin levels and appetite suppression can be achieved, without stomach resection, after DJB in Zucker ZDF obese rats with diabetes [113]. These findings suggest that restriction of gastric volume is not necessarily primarily responsible for changes in glucose homeostasis, and that

◘ Table 10.5 Hormones involved in the enteroinsular axis			
Hormone	**Site of secretion/production**	**Action**	**Surgically induced effect**
Ghrelin	Oxyntic cells, stomach (fundus)	Stimulate appetite, food intake	↑↓ RYGB ↑ BPD
GIP	K-cells (duodenum-foregut)	↑Insulin secretion ↑β-cell mass ↑Satiety ↓Glucagon secretion ↓Acid secretion	↓ RYGB ↓ BPD
GLP-1	L-cells (ileum, colon-hindgut)	↑Insulin secretion ↑β-cell mass ↑Satiety ↓Gastric emptying ↓ Glucagon secretion ↓Acid secretion	↑ RYGB ↑ BPD
PYY	L-cells (ileum, colon-hindgut)	↓Gastric emptying ↑Intestinal transit	↑ RYGB

re-arrangement of anatomy after DJB and RYGB alters hormone signaling and secretion. Hence, this raises the question of portion of the gut needs to be re-arranged for surgery to have an effect on diabetes. There are two hypotheses regarding the role of the gut in the anti-diabetic effects of surgery. The two proposed mechanisms are (a) lack of stimulation of the foregut due to absence of food and (b) over-stimulation of the hindgut because of rapid exposure to partially digested food. The "foregut hypothesis" holds that exclusion of the duodenum and proximal part of the jejunum from digestion of nutrients is the determining factor for the effects of metabolic surgery [114]. A recent study by Rubino and associates supports this hypothesis [114, 115]. They isolated Goto-Kakizaki rats, a spontaneous non-obese model of T2DM, into two groups. One group received a DJB, a variation of the RYGB that preserves the stomach while bypassing the duodenum. The other group received a sham gastrojejunostomy without exclusion of the proximal GI tract. DJB-treated rats were found to have better oral glucose tolerance, lower fasting glucose levels, and lower glucose nadir after insulin injection than the control group. Furthermore, when duodenum continuity was restored, impaired glucose tolerance was re-exhibited. The pathophysiology of this mechanism remains uncertain. The authors hypothesize that alterations in gut hormones, especially incretins secreted by the proximal intestine in response to meals, play a crucial role in glucose metabolism. Several studies have reported decreased levels of the foregut-produced incretin, GIP, following RYGB and DJB, particularly in diabetic individuals. This strengthens the case for a role of the foregut in regulation of glucose homeostasis. A counter-regulatory signal with anti-insulinemic effects has been proposed which is thought to counteract the known effects of incretins on insulin secretion. This effect has been dubbed the "anti-incretin" signal, and it is believed to prevent hypoglycemia. Disregulation of this signal in predisposed individuals may lead to insulin resistance and T2DM by promoting imbalances between incretins and anti-incretins. These proposed "anti-incretins" are thought to be produced in the foregut, so foregut bypass may indeed eliminate signal disparity in these individuals and re-establish normal glucose metabolism [114, 115]. The "hindgut hypothesis" was first described by Mason in 1999 [116]. It proposes that stimulation of the distal intestine by early exposure to undigested nutrients improves glucose homeostasis after metabolic surgery. This is a common pathway for both RYGB and BPD. Increased secretion of GLP-1 is thought to mediate this mechanism [110, 116, 117]. An anorectic hormone response with increased levels of PYY and GLP-1 has

been associated with ileal transposition (IT). Patriti performed IT in Goto-Kakizaki type-2 diabetic rats and in euglycemic Sprague-Dawley rats. Results revealed markedly improved glucose tolerance, insulin sensitivity, and acute insulin response in the GK rats [110]. GLP-1 secretion in this group was associated with better sustained oral glucose tolerance than non-treated rats. No effect on GLP- 1-dependent glucose metabolism was observed in euglycemic rats. These findings suggest that the hindgut may regulate glucose metabolism and resolution of diabetes after RYGB, IT, and BPD by upgrading gastrointestinal peptide secretion.

10.7 Established Surgical Techniques

Metabolic surgical procedures can be categorized into three different types: restrictive, malabsorptive, and mixed. This classification is based on the suggested mechanisms by which they induce weight loss.

10.7.1 Restrictive Procedures

Restrictive procedures combine the creation of a small gastric pouch and a small luminal diameter to limit the amount of food ingested, promoting early satiety. The laparoscopic adjustable gastric band (LAGB) and the vertical banded gastroplasty (VBG), which is no longer performed, are examples of restrictive procedures. Neither of these procedures involves exclusion of any part of the gastrointestinal tract or re-direction of food transit through the intestines. Only LAGB has been associated with remission of T2DM and metabolic syndrome. Recently, in a randomized controlled trial, Dixon reported remission of T2DM in 73% of patients 2 years after undergoing LAGB [118]. More interestingly, only 4% of the patients in the group that was treated conventionally showed remission of T2DM. HbA1c levels were significantly lower in the surgically treated group. Improvements in the co-morbidities associated with weight loss were also reported. Ninety-seven percent of the patients who underwent LAGB fulfilled the criteria for metabolic syndrome. Of these, 70% did not meet the requirements for metabolic syndrome 2 years after surgery. These findings are an improvement over the less than 50% remission of symptoms following LAGB previously reported by Buchwald in 2004 [99]. Although gastroplasties have been reported to improve glucose metabolism [119], there is no evidence of long-term remission of diabetes associated with this technique. Compared with RYGB, the VBG achieves less reduction of hyperglycemia and hyperinsulinemia [120].

10.7.2 Malabsorptive Procedures

Malabsorptive procedures promote weight loss by re-routing nutrients away from the proximal small bowel and directing them to its distal portion. The jejunoileal bypass (JIB) was the first procedure of this kind. JIB promoted weight loss by bypassing the proximal intestine while keeping the stomach intact. Although it achieved excellent weight loss, too many patients developed complications such as severe diarrhea, electrolyte imbalances, night blindness (from vitamin-A deficiency), osteoporosis (from vitamin-D deficiency), protein-calorie malnutrition, interstitial nephritis, enteritis, and nephrocalcinosis. Severe complications were associated with bacterial overgrowth that led to cirrhosis. Consequently, surgeons abandoned the practice of JIB and it is no longer a recommended option for weight loss. The BPD was developed by Scopinaro in Italy in an attempt to obtain better results than with previous operations [121]. The surgical technique includes a partial gastrectomy that creates a 200- to 500-ml gastric pouch. The "alimentary channel" is re-established by connecting the stomach to the distal small bowel. The bypassed intestine, which contains the biliopancreatic secretions, is re-connected at 50 cm proximal to the ileocecal valve. The "common channel" is the segment of terminal ileum that mixes food and bile and is where most of the fat absorption takes place. Scopinaro reported a series of 312 patients; serum glucose concentration was reduced to normal values in all but two members of the group soon after they had undergone BPD [122]. Long-term follow-up revealed maintenance of euglycemia in all but six of the patients up to 10 years after surgery. He recently reported normalization of glucose, cholesterol, and triglyceride levels in seven patients with BMI <35 kg/m^2 5 years following BPD [123]. These findings imply that intervention in semi-obese patients can be as effective in resolving diabetes as it is in the morbidly obese. The duodenal switch is an alternative to BPD first described concomitantly by Hess and Hess and by Marceau [124, 125]. A sleeve vertical gastrectomy is performed, leaving a tube-shaped gastric reservoir of 150–200 ml. The duodenum is transected 2–4 cm from the pyloric valve and a duodeno- ileal switch is completed. This creates a longer common channel (100 cm) than the 50-cm common channel of the BPD. Advantages of the DS include pyloric preservation, which maintains physiological digestion and decreases the risk of dumping syndrome and ulcer development, and decreased hypocalcemia due to vitamin-D malabsorption [126]. Marceau et al have reported resolution of diabetes with discontinuation of medications in 92% of patients as long as 15 years

after DS [127]. The Roux-en-Y gastric bypass (RYGB) remains the standard treatment for morbid obesity. This procedure was first described by Mason in 1967 [128]. It has both restrictive and malabsorptive features. A small vertical gastric pouch of 30 ml is created and anastomosed to the jejunal roux limb of at least 100–150 cm in length, located 150 cm from the ligament of Treitz. A jejuno-jejunal anastomosis is used to re-establish bowel continuity and forms the common channel. Multiple studies have documented the beneficial effects of RYGB in the resolution of diabetes and metabolic complications associated with morbid obesity. Sixty to seventy percent excess weight loss can be achieved with RYGB and effectively maintained in the long term.

10.7.3 Novel Techniques

Several alternative approaches to the known bariatric techniques have been developed during the past decade. Laparoscopic sleeve gastrectomy (LSG), initially used as part of the BPD, has recently been performed as a sole procedure to achieve weight loss. It has a solely restrictive effect. Karamanakos reported markedly decreased weight loss in patients undergoing LSG compared with RYGB [109]. Increased PYY and decreased ghrelin levels were observed after sleeve gastrectomy, suggesting that the restrictive actions of this procedure can be associated with appetite suppression and effective weight loss. Some authors recommend LSG over RYGB because the former spares the patient rare complications such as intestinal malabsorption and dumping syndrome, as there is no intestinal bypass and the pylorus is preserved. Vidal has described a similar amount of weight loss and comparable rates of resolution of T2DM and MS among patients undergoing LSG and RYGB [129]. LSG has also been recommended as a first-stage procedure for super-super obese patients with BMI >60 kg/ m2. Several studies have reported that this population of patients has a better outcome after LSG, as they achieve significant weight loss and improvement of associated co-morbidities in route to becoming better surgical candidates for intestinal bypass [130–133]. Ileal transposition has been advocated by Strader [107] and Patriti [110], among others, as an effective method for weight loss and improved glucose metabolism in animal models. A 10-cm segment of ileum located 5–15 cm proximal to the ileocecal valve is transected and transposed at 5–10 cm distal to the ligament of Treitz via two end-to-end anastomoses. Improved weight loss and decreased food intake were observed in rats that underwent IT compared with a group that had a sham operation. Patriti reported improved glucose tolerance and insulin response after ileal transposition [110]. Both authors found that synthesis and release of GLP-1 and PYY were significantly increased after IT. This association suggests that stimulation of gastrointestinal endocrine function promotes weight loss and improved glucose homeostasis via an anorectic hormonal response in the distal intestine. Variants of IT have been utilized by De Paula and associates with short-term results favoring resolution of T2DM and MS in semi-obese patients with BMI <35 kg/m² [134]. At 7.4 months' mean postoperative follow-up, 52 of 60 patients (86.7%) achieved outstanding reduction in BMI and adequate glycemic control. Up to 90% of the patients demonstrated normalization of triglyceride levels, increased high-density lipoprotein levels, control of hypertension, and decreased abdominal circumference. Enthusiasm for duodeno-jejunal bypass (DJB) has increased lately due to the promising results observed in animal studies performed by Rubino and associates [114, 115]. The stomach is left intact, and exclusion of the duodenum from transit of food is obtained by transecting the gut just distal to the pylorus. Early delivery of food occurs distal to the ligament of Treitz via a gastrojejunostomy. The common channel is re-established in the mid jejunum. Rats treated with DJB demonstrated improved glucose tolerance without significant changes in weight compared with sham-operated rats that underwent gastrojejunostomy [114]. These findings support the hypothesis that remission of diabetes after surgery is independent of weight loss or decreased food intake. Exclusion of the duodenum from early delivery of nutrients supports the "foregut hypothesis" as the mechanism of glucose control. Our early experience with DJB supports findings similar to those demonstrated by Rubino and colleagues. Our technique for DJB is as follows: Trocar placement resembles that of conventional laparoscopic RYGB. The duodenum is divided just below the pylorus with a GIA stapler. Both the biliary and the alimentary limb are 75 cm in length. The gastro-jejunal anastomosis is half hand-sewn and half stapled. The duodeno-jejunal anastomosis is hand-sewn with 3-0 silk sutures (see Fig. 10.1). Our 12-month data, which we report below, suggests that this surgical intervention may become a valuable tool in the armamentarium against morbid obesity, metabolic syndrome, and poor subsequent glycemic control [135].

10.8   Ongoing Trials

The newest techniques and variations of metabolic surgery, although still in their early phases of development,

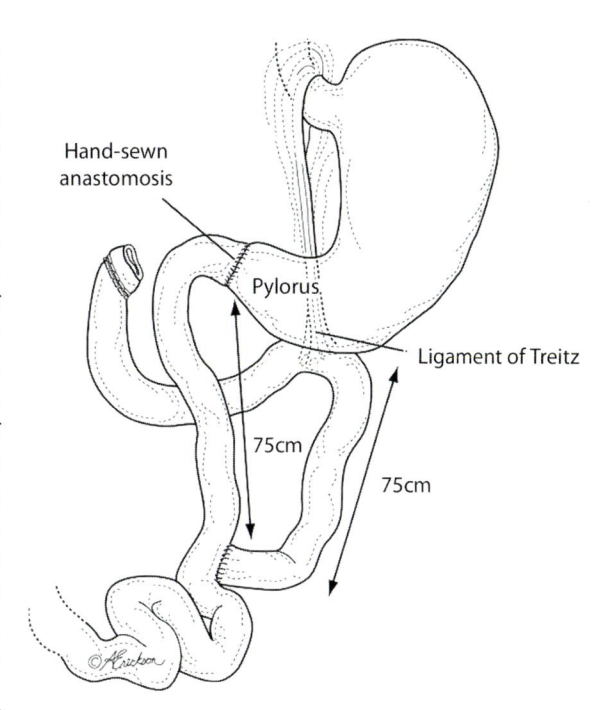

Fig. 10.1. Duodeno-jejunal bypass

have shown promising results. Findings after DJB and IT in non-obese diabetic animal models have shown that long-term glucose control and resolution of T2DM can be achieved independent of weight loss [110, 114, 115]. This anti-diabetic effect of surgery in semi-obese patients with BMI of 22–34 has not yet been reported in randomized human trials. Several clinical trials involving voluntary non-obese diabetic patients are underway. Cohen and colleagues, in Sao Paulo, Brazil, have reported early results at 6-month follow-up in 20 diabetic patients following laparoscopic DJB [136]. Significant improvements in fasting plasma glucose, HbA1c, and insulin resistance (HOMA-IR) are documented, while the excess weight loss at this time is essentially unchanged. Most of the insulin-dependent patients have not required insulin for 6 months following surgery. Hypertensive medications have been discontinued in 73% of the patients, as their blood pressure has been effectively controlled with diet and exercise. We have had exciting early results in our series of semi-obese diabetic patients with BMI <35 kg/m2 who underwent DJB [135]. We conducted a 12-month prospective study on the changes in glucose homeostasis and the metabolic syndrome in seven non-obese patients with T2DM undergoing laparoscopic duodenal-jejunal bypass (LDJB), matched for duration of DM, type of DM treatment, and glycemic control. Laboratory values inluding HbA1c, fasting plasma glucose, cholesterol, triglyceride, and C-peptide levels were measured throughout the 12 months, at different time intervals. Serum levels of gastro-inhibitory peptide (GIP) and ghrelin were followed for 1 month. Serum levels of gastrin and GLP were followed for 3 months. At 12 months, subjects felt relief from fatigue and decreased extremity pain and numbness. They also reported decreased polyuria and polydipsia. Fasting plasma glucose, HbA1c levels, and postprandial blood sugar levels, as well as insulin requirements, were considerably reduced 12 months after surgery. Subjects demonstrated an overall improved HbA1c from 9.6 to 8.5 and a fasting plasma glucose level decrease from 209 mg/ dl to 154 mg/dl. C-peptide was slightly decreased at 3 months. Cholesterol and triglycerides increased slightly, however. Although improvements in homeostasis did not achieve statistical significance in our patients, all of them experienced relief from their diabetes-associated symptoms and all stated that they would recommend the surgery to others. We stand poised at the forefront of a new era in surgery for the treatment of diabetes and the metabolic syndrome. It is clearly established that Roux-en Y gastric bypass has long-term beneficial effects on diabetic control and control of obesity-associated hypertension and hyperlipidemia. The interaction between gut hormones and control of diabetes and the metabolic syndrome is slowly being elucidated. Animal studies have shown resolution of diabetes after DJB in non-obese diabetic mice. Other surgical models have also shown promise. The results of DJB in diabetic patients in Cohen's study and in our cohort are very encouraging, but large studies are still needed to determine the interplay between these hormones and glycemic and adipose homeostasis, and to determine the best surgical options for the non-obese diabetic patient and the patient with metabolic syndrome.

References

1. Flegal, KM, Caroll MD, Ogden CL et al (2002) Prevalence and trends in obesity among US adults, 1999–2000. JAMA 288:1723–1727
2. Ford ES (2005) Risks for all cause mortality, cardiovascular disease, and diabetes associated with the metabolic syndrome: a summary of the evidence. Diabetes Care 28:769–1778
3. Brown SA, Upchwich S, Anding R et al (1996) Promoting weight loss in type II diabetes. Diabetes Care 19:613–624
4. Field AE, Coakley EH, Must A et al (2001) Impact of overweight on the risk of developing common chronic diseases during a 10-year period. Arch Intern Med 161:1581–1586
5. Zimet P, Shaw J, Alberti KG (2003) Preventing type 2 diabetes and the dysmetabolic syndrome in the real world: a realistic view. Diabetes Med 20:693–702
6. Buchwald H, Avidor Y, Braumwald E, Jensen MD, Pories W, Fahrbach K et al (2004) Bariatric surgery: a systematic review and meta-analysis. JAMA 292:1724–1737
7. Pories WJ, Swanson MS, MacDonald KG et al (1995) Who would have thought it? An operation proves to be the most effective therapy for adult-onset diabetes mellitus. Ann Surg 222:339–350
8. Schauer PR, Ikramuddin S, Gourash W et al (2000) Outcomes after laparoscopic Roux-en-Y gastric bypass for morbid obesity. Ann Surg 232:515–529
9. American Diabetes Association, The dangerous toll of diabetes. http://www.diabetes.org/diabetes-statistics/dangerous-toll.jsp
10. American Diabetes Association, Diabetes Statistics. http://www.diabetes.org/diabetes-statistics/prevalence.jsp
11. American Diabetes Association, Direct and indirect cost of diabetes in the United States. http://www.diabetes.org/diabetes-statistics/cost-of-diabetes-in-us.jsp
12. Zimmet P, Alberti KG, Shaw J (2001) Global and societal implications of the diabetes epidemic. Nature 414:782–787
13. Rattarasan C (2006) Physiological and pathophysiological regulation of regional adipose tissue in the development of insulin resistance and type 2 diabetes. Acta Physiol 186:87–101
14. Hu FB, Manson JE, Stampfer MJ et al (2001) Diet, lifestyle, and the risk of type 2 diabetes mellitus in women. N Engl J Med 345:790–797
15. Mokdad AH, Ford ES, Bowman BA et al (2003) Prevalence of obesity, diabetes, and obesity-related health risk factors, 2001. JAMA 289:76–79
16. Willet WC, Dietz WH, Colditz GA (1999) Guidelines for healthy weight. N Engl J Med 141:427–434
17. Prospective Diabetes Study UK (1998) Group Intensive blood glucose control with sulphonylureas or insulin compared with conventional treatment and risks of complications in patients with type 2 diabetes (UKPPS 33). Lancet 352:837–853
18. Anon (2002) The Antihypertensive and Lipid-lowering Treatment to Prevent Heart Attack Trial (ALLHAT). JAMA 288: 2981–2997
19. Knowler WC, Barrett-Connor E, Fowler SE et al (2002) Diabetes Prevention Program Reserved Group. Reduction in the incidence of type 2 diabetes with lifestyle intervention or metformin. N Engl J Med 346:393–403
20. Padwal R, Li SK, Lau DCW (2004) Long-term pharmacotherapy for obesity and overweight (Cochrane Review). The Cochrane Library 3:C0004094
21. Norris SL, Zhang X, Avenell A et al (2004) Efficacy of pharmacotherapy for weight loss in adults with type 2 diabetes mellitus: a meta-analysis. Arch Intern Med 164:1395–1404
22. Chiasson JL, Josse RG, Gomes R et al (2003) STOP-NIDDM Trial Research Group. Acarbose treatment and the risk of cardiovascular disease and hypertension in patients with impaired glucose tolerance: the STOP-NIDDM trial. JAMA 290:486–494
23. UK Prospective Diabetes Study Group (1996) UK Prospective Diabetes Study (UKPDS) 17. A 9-year update of a randomized controlled trial on the effect of improved metabolic control on complications in non-insulin dependent diabetes mellitus. Ann Intern Med 124:132–145
24. Chalmers J, Cooper ME (2008) UKPDS and the legacy effect. N Engl J Med 359:1618–1620
25. Holman RR, Paul SK, Bethel MA et al (2008) 10-Year follow-up of intensive glucose control in type 2 diabetes. N Engl J Med 359:1577–1589
26. Pedersen O, Gaede P (2003) Intensified multifactorial intervention and cardiovascular outcome in type 2 diabetes. The Steno-2 study. Metabolism 52 [Suppl 1]:19–23

27. Haller H (1977) Epidemiology and associated risk factors of hyperlipoproteinemia. Z Gesamte Inn Med 32:124–128

28. Phillips GB (1978) Sex hormones, risk factors and cardiovascular disease. Am J Med 65:7–11

29. Phillips GB (1977) Relationship between serum sex hormones and glucose, insulin, and lipid abnormalities in men with myocardial infarction. Proc Natl Acad Sci USA 74:1729–1733

30. Reaven GM (1988) Banting lecture 1988. Role of insulin resistance in human disease. Diabetes 37:1595–1607

31. Kaplan NM(1989) The deadly quartet. Upper body obesity, glucose intolerance, hypertriglyceridemia and hypertension. Arch Intern Med 149:1514–1520

32. De Fronzo RA, Ferranini E (1991) Insulin resistance: a multifaceted syndrome responsible for NIDDM, obesity, hypertension, dyslipidemia and atherosclerotic cardiovascular disease. Diabetes Care 14:173–194

33. Alberti KG, Zimmet PZ (1998) Definition, diagnosis and classification of diabetes mellitus and its complications. I: Diagnosis and classification of diabetes mellitus: provisional report of a WHO consultation. Diabetes Med 15:539–553

34. Hills SA, Backau B, Coppads SW et al (2004) The EGIR-RISC study (the European Group for the study of Insulin Resistance: relationship between insulin sensitivity and cardiovascular disease risk). I: Methodology and objectives. Diabetología 47:566–570

35. National Cholesterol Education Program (2002) Third Report of the National Cholesterol Education Program (NCEP) expert panel on detection, evaluation, and treatment of high blood cholesterol in adults (Adult Treatment Panel III). Final report. Circulation 106:3143–3421

36. Eihorn D, Reaven GM, Cobin RH et a(2003) I American College of Endocrinology position statement on the insulin resistance syndrome. Endocr Pract 9:237–252

37. Ford ES, Giles WH, Dietz WH (2002) Prevalence of the metabolic syndrome among US adults. Findings from the Third National Health and Nutrition Examination Survey. JAMA 287:356–359

38. Meigs JB, D'Agostino RB Sr, Wilson PW, Cupples LA, Nathan DM, Singer DE (1997) Risk variable clustering in the insulin resistance syndrome: the Framingham Offspring Study. Diabetes 46:1594–1600

39. National Institute of Health Consensus Development Panel (1991) Gastrointestinal surgery for severe obesity. Ann Intern Med 115:956–961

40. Flint JM (1912) The effect of extensive resections of the small intestine. Bull Johns Hopkins Hosp 255:127

41. Weckesser EC, Clinn AB, Scott MW jr, Price JW (1949) Extensive resection of the small intestine. Am J Surg 78:706

42. Cattell RB (1945) Massive resection of the small intestine. Lahey Clin Bull 4:167

43. Thoroughman JC, Walker LG jr, Raft D (1964) A review of 504 patients with peptic ulcer treated by hemigastrectomy and vagotomy. Surg Gynecol Obstet 119:257

44. Price WE, Grizzle JE, Postlethwait RW, Johnson WD, Grabichi P (1970) Results of operation for duodenal ulcer. Surg Gynecol Obstet 131:233

45. Friedman NM, Sancetta AJ, Magovern GJ (1955) The amelioration of diabetes mellitus following subtotal gastrectomy. Surg Gynecol Obstet 100:201–204

46. Bittner R, Bittner B, Beger HG (1981) Homeostasis of glucose and gastric resection: the influence of food passage through the duodenum. Z Gastroenterology 19:698–707

47. Sjöström CD, Lissner L, Wedel H, Sjöström L (1999) Reduction in incidence of diabetes, hypertension and lipid disturbances after intentional weight loss induced by bariatric surgery: the SOS interventional study. Obes Res 7:477–484

48. Cummings DE, Overduin J, Foster-Schubert KE (2003) Gastric bypass for obesity: mechanisms of weight loss and diabetes resolution. J Clin Endocrinol Metab 89:2608–2615

49. Cummings DE, Shannon MH (2003) Ghrelin and gastric bypass. Is there a hormonal contribution to surgical weight loss? J Clin Endocrinol Metab 88:2999–3002

50. Chen J, Muntner P, Hamm LH et al (2004) The metabolic syndrome and chronic kidney disease in US adults. Ann Intern Med 140:167–174

51. Vinik AI, Erbas T, Park TS et al (2001) Dermal neurovascular dysfunction in type 2 diabetes. Diabetes Care 24:1468–1475

52. Haffner S, Taegtmeyer H (2003) Epidemic obesity and the metabolic syndrome. Circulation 108:1541–1545

53. Richardson DW, Vinik AI (2005) Metabolic implications of obesity: before and after gastric bypass. Gastroenterol Clin N Am 34:9–24

54. Dixon JB, Bhathal PS, O'Brien PE (2001) Non-alcoholic fatty liver disease: predictors of non-alcoholic steatohepatitis and liver fibrosis in the severely obese. Gastroenterology 121:91–100

55. Saltiel AR, Kahn CR (2001) Insulin signaling and the regulation of glucose and lipid metabolism. Nature 414: 799–806

56. Almind K, Bjorback C, Vestergaard H et al (1993) Amino acid polymorphisms of insulin receptor substrate-1 in non insulin dependent diabetes mellitus. Lancet 342:828–832

57. North KE, Williams K, Williams JT et al (2003) Evidence for genetic factors underlying the insulin resistance syndrome in American Indians. Obes Res 11:1444–1448

58. Moller N, Gormsen L, Fugisan J et al(2003) Effects of aging on insulin secretion and action. Horm Res 60 [Suppl 1]:102–104

59. Morino K, Petersen KF, Shulman GI (2006) Molecular mechanisms of insulin resistance in humans and their potential links with mitochondrial dysfunction. Diabetes 55 [Suppl 2]:S9–S15

60. Machann J, Haring H, Schick F et al (2004) Intramyocellular lipis and insulin resistance. Diabetes Obes Metab 6:239–248

61. Kim JK, Gimeno RE, Higashimori T et al (2004) Inactivation of fatty acid transport protein 1 prevents fat-induced insulin resistance in skeletal muscle. J Clin Invest 113:756–763

62. Wellen KE, Hotamisligil GS (2005) Inflammation, stress, and diabetes. J Clin Invest 115:1111–1119

63. Yamada T, Katagirl H, Ishigaki Y et al (2006) Signals from intra-abdominal fat modúlate insulin and leptin sensitivity through different mechanisms: neuronal involvement in food-intake regulation. Cell Metab 3:223–229

64. Gabriely I, Ma XH, Yang XM, Atzmon G, Rajala MN, Berg AH et al (2002) Removal of visceral fat prevents insulin resistance and glucose intolerance of aging: an adipokine-mediated process? Diabetes 51:2591–2598

65. Hanley AJ, Bowden D, Wagenknecht LE, Balasubramanyam A, Langfeld C, Saad MF et al (2007) Associations of adiponectin with body fat distribution and insulin sensitivity in non-diabetic Hispanics and African-Americans. J Clin Endocrinol Metab 92:2665–2671

66. Kadowaki T, Yamauchi T, Kubota N, Hara K, Ueki K, Tobe LC (2006) Adiponectin and adiponectin receptors in insulin resistance, diabetes, and the metabolic syndrome. J Clin Invest 116:1784–1792

67. Furler SM, Gan SK, Poynter AM et al (2006) Relationship of adiponectin with insulin sensitivity in humans, independent of lipid availability. Obesity 14:228–234

68. Hopkins TA, Ouchi N, Shibata R, Walsh K A(2007) diponectin actions in the cardiovascular system. Cardiovasc Res 74:11–18

69. McTernan CL, Mcternan PG, Harte AL, Levick PL, Barnett AH, Kumar S (2002) Resistin, antral obesity, and type 2 diabetes. Lancet 359:46–47

70. McTernan PG, Mcternan CL, Chetty R, Jenner K, Fisher FM, Laner MN et al (2002) Increased resistin gene and protein expression in human abdominal adipose tissue. J Clin Endocrinol Metab 87:2407

71. Hirosumi J, Tuncman G, Chang L, Gorgun CZ, Uysal KT, Maeda K et al (2002) A central role for JNK in obesity and insulin resistance. Nature 420:333–336

72. Rajala MW, Qi Y, Patel HR, Takahashi N, Banerjee R, Pajvani UB et al (2001) Regulation of resistin expression in circulating levels in obesity, diabetes, and fasting. Diabetes 50:2199–2202

73. Rasouli N, Kern PA (2008) Adipocytokines and the Metabolic Complications of Obesity. J Clin Endocrinol Metab 93:S64–S73

74. Hivert M, Sullivan LM, Fox CS et al A(2008) ssociations of adiponectin, resistin, and tumor necrosis factor-α with insulin resistance. J Clin Endocrinol Metab 93:3165–3172

75. Milan G, Granzotto M, Scanda A, Calcagno A, Paguno C, Federspil G et al (2002) Regional adipose tissue differences of resistin and adiponectin expression in genetically obese rats: effects of weight loss. Obes Res 10:1095–1103

76. Silswal N, Singh AK, Aruna B, Mukhopadyay S, Ghosh S, Ehtensham NZ (2005) Human resistin stimulates the pro-inflammatory cytokines TNF-alpha and IL-12 in macrophages by NF-kappa B dependent pathway. Biochem Biochys Res Commun 334:1092–1101

77. Kojima M, Hosoda H, Date Y, Nakazato M, Matsuo H, Kangawa K (1999) Ghrelin is a growth hormone-releasing acylated peptide from stomach. Nature 402:656-660

78. Date Y, Kojima M, Hosoda H, Sawaguchi A, Mondal MS, Suganuma T et al (2000) Ghrelin, a novel growth hormone-releasing acylated peptide, is synthesized in a distinct endocrine cell type in the gastrointestinal tracts of rats and humans. Endocrinology 141:4255-4261

79. Cummings DE, Shannon MH(2003) Roles for ghrelin in the regulation of appetite and body weight. Arch Surg 138:389-396

80. Cummings DE, Purnel JQ, Frayo RS et al (2001) A preprandial rise in plasma ghrelin levels suggests a role in meal initiaiton in humans. Diabetes 50:1714-1719.

81. Aylin S (2005) Gastrointestinal surgery and gut hormones. Curr Opin Endocrinol Diabetes 12:89-98

82. Kreyman B, Williams G, Ghatei MA, Bloom SR (1987) Glucagon-like peptide-1 (7-36): a physiological incretin in man. Lancet 2:1300-1304

83. Bloom SR, Polak JM (1980) Gut hormones. Adv Clin Chem 21:177–244

84. Perley MJ, Kipnis DM (1967) Plasma insulin responses to oral and intravenous glucose studies in normal and diabetic subjects. J Clin Invest 46:1954–1962

85. Preitner F, Iberson M, Franklin I et al (2004) Gluco-incretins control insulin secretion at multiple levels as revealed in mice lacking GLP-1 and GIP receptors. J Clin Invest 113:635–645

86. Drucker DJ (2002) Biological actions therapeutic potential of the glucagon-like peptides. Gastroenterology 122:531–544

87. Flint A, Raben A, Ersboll AK, Holst JJ, Astrup A (2001) The effect of physiological levels of glucagon-like peptide-1 on appetite, gastric emptying, energy and substrate metabolism in obesity. Int J Obes Relat Metab Disord 25:781–792

88. Gutzwiller JP, Drewe J, Goke B, Schmidt H et al (1999) Glucagon-like peptide-1 promotes satiety and reduces food intake in patients with diabetes mellitus type 2. Am J Physiol 276:R1541–R1544

89. Nauck M, Stockman F, Ebert R, Creutzfeldt W (1986) Reduced incretin effect in type 2 (non-insulin-dependent) diabetes. Diabetología 29:46–52

90. Nauck MA, Heimesaat MM, Orksov C, Holst JJ, Ebert R, Creutzfeldt W (1993) Preserved incretin activity of glucagon-like (7-36 amide) but not of synthetic human gastrin inhibitory polypeptide in patients with type 2 diabetes mellitus. J Clin Invest 91:301–307

91. Elahi D, McAloon-Dyke M, Fukagawa NK et al (1994) The insulinotropic actions of glucose-dependent insulinotropic polypeptide (GIP) and glucagon-like peptide-2 (7-37) in normal and diabetic subjects. Regul Pept 51:63–74

92. Batterham RL, Cohen MA, Small CJ et al (2002) Gut hormone PYY 3-36 physiologically inhibits food intake. Nature 418:650–654

93. Batterham RL, Cohen MA, Ellis SM et al (2003) Inhibition of food intake in obese subjects by peptide YY 3-36. N Engl J Med 349:941–948

94. Stok S, Leichner P, Wong ACK et al (2005) Ghrelin, peptide YY, glucose-dependent insulinotropic polypeptide, and hunger responses to a mixed meal in anorexic, obese, and control female adolescents. J Clin Endocrinol Metab 90:2161–2168

95. Le Roux CW, Batterham RL, Aylwin SJ et al (2006) Attenuated peptide YY release in obese subjects is associated with reduced satiety. Endocrinology 147:3–8

96. Hickey MS, Pories WJ, MacDonald KG et al (1998) A new paradigm for type 2 diabetes mellitus: could it be a disease of the foregut? Ann Surg 227:637–644

97. Schauer PR, Burguera B, Ikramuddin S et al (1995) Effect of laparoscopic Roux-en-Y gastric bypass on type 2 diabetes mellitus. Ann Surg 222:339–352

98. Sjöstrom L, Lindroos AK, Peltonen M et al (2004) Lifestyle, Diabetes, and Cardiovascular Risk Factors 10 years after Bariatric Surgery: The Swedish Obese Subjects Study Scientific Group for Swedish Obese Surbjects Trial. N Engl J Med 351:2683–2693

99. Buchwald H, Avidor Y, Braunwald E, Jensen MD, Pories W, Fahrbach K et al (2004) Bariatric surgery: a systematic review and meta-analysis. JAMA 292:1724–1737

100. Nguyen NT, Goldman C, Rosenquist CJ et al (2001) Laparoscopic versus open gastric bypass: a randomized study of outcomes, quality of life, and costs. Ann Surg 234:279–289

101. Scopinaro N, Adami GF, Marinari GM et al (1998) Biliopancreatic diversion. World J Surg 22:936–946

102. Schauer PR, Ikramuddin S, Gourash W et al (2000) Outcomes after laparoscopic roux-en-Y gastric bypass for morbid obesity. Ann Surg 232:515–529

103. Schauer PR, Burguera B, Ikramudin S, Cottam D et al (2003) Effect of laparoscopic Roux-en Y gastric bypass on type 2 diabetes mellitus. Ann Surg 238:467–485

104. Holdstock C, Engstrom BE, Obrvall M et al (2003) Ghrelin and adipose tissue regulatory peptides: effects of gastric bypass surgery in obese humans. J Clin Endocrinol Metab 88:3177–3183

105. Geloneze B, Tambascia MA, Pilla VF et al (2003) Ghrelin: a gut-brain hormone: effect of gastric bypass surgery. Obes Surg 13:17–22

106. Rubino, F, Gagner M, Gentileschi P, Kini S, Fukuyama S, Feng J et al (2004) The Early Effects of the Roux-en-Y Gastric Bypass on hormones involved in body weight regulation on glucose metabolism. Ann Surg 240:236–242

107. Strader AD, Torsten PV, Jandacek RJ, Woods SC, Alessio DA, Seeley RJ (2005) Weight loss through ileal transposition is accompanied by increased ileal hormone secretion and synthesis in rats. Am J Physiol Endocrinol Metab 288:E447–E453

108. Pacheco D, De Luis DA, Romero A, González Sagrado M et al (2007) The effects of duodenal-jejunal exclusion on hormonal regulation of glucose metabolism in Goto-Kakizaki rats. Am J Surg 194:221–224

109. Karamanakos SN, Vagenas K, Kalfarentzos F, Alexandrides TK (2008) Weight loss, appetite suppression, and changes in fasting and post-prandial ghrelin and peptide-YY levels after Roux-en-Y gastric bypass and sleeve gastrectomy. A prospective, double blind study. Ann Surg 247:401–407

110. Patriti A, Aisa MC, Annetti C, Sidoni A et al (2007) How the hindgut can cure type 2 diabetes. Ileal transposition improves glucose metabolism and beta-cell function in Goto-kakizaki rats through an enhanced proglucagon gene expression and L-cell number. Surgery 142:74–85

111. le Roux CW, Aylwin SJ, Batterham RL et al (2006) Gut hormone profiles following bariatric surgery favor an anorectic state, facilitate weight loss, and improve metabolic parameters. Ann Surg 243:108–114

112. Buettner C, Muse ED, Cheng A et al (2008) Leptin controls adipose tissue lipogenesis via central, STAT3-independent mechanisms. Nat Med 14:667–675

113. Rubino F, Zizzari P, Tomassetto C et al (2005) The role of the small bowel in the regulation of circulating ghrelin levels and food intake in the obese Zucker rat. Endocrinology 146:1745–1751

114. Rubino F, Forgione A, Cummings DE, Vix M, Gnuli D, Mingrone G et al (2006) The mechanism of diabetes control after gastrointestinal bypass surgery reveals a role of the proximal small intestine in the pathophysiology of type 2 diabetes. Ann Surg 244:741–749

115. Rubino F, Marescaux J (2004) Effects of duodenal-jejunal exclusion in a non-obese animal model of type 2 diabetes. A new perspective for an old disease. Ann Surg 239:1–11

116. Mason EE (1999) Ileal transposition and enteroglucagon/GLP-1 in obesity and diabetic surgery. Obes Surg 9:223–228

117. Mason EE (2005) The mechanism of surgical treatment of type 2 diabetes. Obes Surg 15:459–461

118. Dixon JB, O'Brien PE, Playfair J et al (2008) Adjustable gastric banding and conventional therapy for type 2 diabetes: a randomized controlled trial. JAMA 299:316–323

119. Bourdages H, Goldenberg F, Nguyen P et al (1994) Improvement in obesity-associated medical conditions following vertical banded gastroplasty and gastrointestinal bypass. Obes Surg 4:227–231

120. Kellum JM, Kuemmerle JF, O'Dorisio RM et al (1990) GI hormone response to meals before and after gastric bypass and vertical banded gastroplasty. Ann Surg 211:763–771

121. Scopinaro N, Gianetta E, Civalleri D et al (1979) Bilio-pancreatic bypass for obesity. II: Initial experience in a man. Br J Surg 66:618–620

122. Scopinaro N, Marinari GM, Camerini GB et al (2005) Specific effects of biliopancreatic diversión on the major components of metabolic síndrome: a long-term follow-up study. Diabetes Care 28:2406–2411

123. Scopinaro N, Papadia F, Marinari G, Camerini G, Adami G (2007) Long-term control of type 2 diabetes mellitus and the other major components of the metabolic syndrome after biliopancreatic diversion in patients with BMI <35 kg/m². Obes Surg 17:193–194

124. Hess DS, Hess DW (1998) Biliopancreatic diversion with a duodenal switch. Obes Surg 8:267–282

125. Marceau P, Hould FS, Simard S et al (1998) Biliopancreatic diversion with duodenal switch. World J Surg 22:947–954

126. Marceau P, Biron S, Hould FS, Lebel S, Marceau S, Lescelleur O et al (2008) Duodenal switch improved standard biliopancreatic diversion: a retrospective study. Surg Obes Relat Dis 5:43–7

127. Marceau P, Biron S, Hould FS, Lebel S, Marceau S, Lescelleur O et al (2007) Duodenal switch: long-term results. Obes Surg 17:1421–1430

128. Mason EE, Ito C (1967) Gastric bypass in obesity. Surg Clin North Am 47:1345–1351

129. Vidal J, Ibarzabal A, Romero F, Delgado S, Momblán D, Flores L et al (2008) Type 2 diabetes mellitus and the metabolic syndrome following sleeve gastrectomy in severely obese subjects. Obes Surg 18:1077–1082

130. Gagner M, Gumbs AA, Milone L, Yung E, Goldenberg L, Pomp A (2008) Laparoscopic sleeve gastrectomy for the super-super-obese (body mass index >60 kg/m2). Surg Today 38:399–403

131. Milone L, Strong V, Gagner M (2005) Laparoscopic sleeve gastrectomy is superior to endoscopic intragastric balloon as a first stage procedure for super-obese patients (BMI > or =50). Obes Surg 15:612–617

132. Silecchia G, Boru C, Pecchia A, Rizzello M, Casella G, Leonetti F et al (2006) Effectiveness of laparoscopic sleeve gastrectomy (first stage of biliopancreatic diversion with duodenal switch) on co-morbidities in super-obese high-risk patients. Obes Surg 16:1138–1144

133. Regan JP, Inabnet WB, Gagner M, Pomp A (2003) Early experience with two-stage laparoscopic Roux-en-Y gastric bypass as an alternative in the super-super obese patient. Obes Surg 13:861–864

134. DePaula AL et al (2008) Laparoscopic treatment of type 2 diabetes mellitus for patients with a body mass index less than 35. Surg Endosc 22:706-716

135. Ferzli GS, Dominique E, Ciaglia M (2009) Clinical evaluation of the effect of the duodenal-jejunal bypass on type 2 diabetes. World J Surg 33:972–979

136. Cohen R (2008) Duodenojejunal bypass for the treatment of type 2 diabetes mellitus in patients with BMI from 22 to 34. Presented at the first United States Metabolic Surgery Summit; Miami Beach, Florida; January 12

Venous Thromboembolism – Prophylaxis and Treatment

Stefan Utzolino MD, Magnus Kaffarnik MD

Venous thromboembolism has long been identified as a major concern in surgical patients. In general surgery, the rate of deep vein thrombosis is about 25% without prophylaxis. In high-risk groups such as patients undergoing knee or hip surgery, the rate of thrombosis without prophylaxis is proven to be around 50%. In patients with spinal cord injury or complicated fracture of the pelvis, rates of up to 75% are reported. In the past few years, accumulating evidence has shown an increased risk of venous thromboembolism also in acutely ill medical patients, with rates being around 20%. These data refer to the detection of thrombosis by technical means and not to clinically overt thrombosis. In prospective studies, rates of venous thromboembolism detected by suitable diagnostic tools are always much higher than rates of thrombosis detected clinically. This finding is simply due to the fact that only a minor fraction of thromboses and even pulmonary embolisms lead to clinical symptoms. If symptoms are present, they are unspecific and possibly related to an alternate underlying cause in most cases. Nevertheless, the sequelae of major concern occur at the same rate in symptomatic and non-symptomatic cases: life-threatening pulmonary embolism, chronic thromboembolic pulmonary hypertension, and post-thrombotic syndrome.

11.1   Risk Factors for Venous Thromboembolism

Several risk factors go along with an elevated risk of venous thromboembolism (◘ Table 11.1). Among these, elevated body weight is often mentioned, but the data are not quite clear. Of course, a high BMI often correlates with low physical activity and a diet rich in carbohydrates and fat, both factors by themselves correlated with an elevated risk of venous thromboembolism. Physiological considerations reveal plausible connections between lipid-related hormone activity and risk of thrombosis, but to date it is unclear whether these are clinically relevant. If venous thromboembolism is a concern in visceral surgery, it is even more of a concern in bariatric surgery, where we are dealing with a group of moderateto high-risk patients. According to the American College of Chest Physicians (ACCP) [1] and other national guidelines, patients at moderate or high risk of venous thromboembolism undergoing general surgery should receive pharmacological thromboprophylaxis. Additionally, mechanical measures such as calf-compression stockings, intermittent pneumatic calf compression, and not least early ambulation are encouraged. Nevertheless, following years of research and numerous guidelines from ap-

◘ Table 11.1 Risk factors for venous thromboembolism

Acquired factors
Reduced mobility
Advanced age
Cancer
Acute medical illness
Major surgery
Trauma
Spinal cord injury
Pregnancy and postpartum period
Polycythemia vera
Antiphospholipid antibody syndrome
Oral contraceptives
Hormone-replacement therapy
Heparins
Chemotherapy
Obesity
Central venous catheteriz ation
Immobilizer or cast

Hereditary factors
Antithrombin deficiency
Protein C deficiency
Protein S deficiency
Factor V Leiden
Activated protein C resistance without factor V Leiden
Prothrombin gene mutation
Dysfibrinogenemia
Plasminogen deficiency

Probable factors
Elevated levels of lipoprotein A
Low levels of tissue factor-pathway inhibitor (TFPI)
Elevated levels of:
homocysteine; factors VIII, IX, XI
fibrinogen; and thrombin-activated fibrinolysis inhibitor (TAFI)

proved international boards, there is still a tremendous underuse of recommended prophylaxis. The ENDORSE (Epidemiologic International Day for the Evaluation of Patients at Risk for Venous Thromboembolism in the Acute Hospital Care Setting) study [2] enrolled 68 183 patients, with 45% categorized as surgical. Only 58.5% of these surgical patients, and no more than 39.5% of the medical patients, received adequate thromboprophylaxis according to ACCP guidelines. What is the evidence? Edmonds et al. [3] identified seven studies investigating the association between obesity and postoperative deep vein thrombosis (evidence level 2+). Five of the seven studies found a significant association between an increase in obesity and risk of deep vein thrombosis and two found no significant difference. A pooled estimate was not possible because of different definitions for obesity used across the studies. There is convincing evidence that obesity is a risk factor for venous thromboembolism. In general surgery, the rate of thrombosis is ca. 25% without and ca. 2% with prophylaxis by low-molecular-weight heparins. In bariatric surgery, therefore, rates of venous thromboembolism should be considerably higher than 2% even with adequate prophylaxis. In the past 10 years, extensive work has been done on metabolic changes, hormonal differences, and alterations in the excretion of pharmaceutical agents in morbid obesity. Several aspects suggest a direct link between morbid obesity and the risk for venous thromboembolism from a physiological point of view. Thus the leptin receptor is expressed in platelets, and leptin potentiates platelet aggregation by agonists [4].

11.2 Clinical Signs of Thromboembolism

Clinical signs and symptoms of venous thromboembolism are often unspecific or even lacking. If present, they may be highly suggestive but are neither sensitive nor specific. Clinical scores have been developed that allow the identification of patients in whom further testing must be considered. One of the clinical prediction scores most often used for suspected acute pulmonary embolism and for deep vein thrombosis is that by Wells (◘ Tables 11.2 and 11.3). Depending on the probability of having pulmonary embolism as predicted by the score, a diagnostic algorithm of further testing should be instituted in each hospital. The local algorithm must include considerations about the availability of testing methods and of skilled staff to perform tests (e.g., duplex sonography, CT scanning, radionuclide scanning).

11.2.1 D-Dimer Test

To rule out venous thromboembolism, a D-dimer test (which measures plasma levels of a specific derivative of cross-linked fibrin) is appropriate. The enzyme-linked immunosorbent assay (ELISA)-based D-dimer tests have superior sensitivity (96–98%) and are available in most institutions today. A positive D-dimer test gives proof of an activation of coagulation with enhanced turnover of coagulation factors and thus indicates that venous thrombosis and pulmonary embolism are possible diagnoses. Unfortunately, this test is nonspecific, since it may be positive in patients with infection, cancer, trauma, and other inflammatory states, as well as after surgery. Thus, a negative D-dimer test along with a low or intermediate clinical probability of venous

◘ **Table 11.2** Clinical scoring system for deep vein thrombosis (DVT)

Variable	Signs and symptoms	Score
Cancer	in past 6 months	1
Paralysis	or plaster cast (leg)	1
Immobilization	>3 days or OP <4 weeks	1
Pain	along veins, sign of Payr	1
Swelling of limb	calf and thigh	1
Edema	mold forming	1
Collateral veins	visible	1
Alternative diagnosis available		-2
Pretest probability for DVT		
High	ca. 85%	>3
Modest	ca. 33%	1–3
Low	ca. 5%	0

◘ **Table 11.3** Clinical scoring system for pulmonary embolism (PE) [49]

Variable		Score
DVT symptoms and signs		3
PE as likely as or more likely than alternative diagnosis		3
Heart rate >100 beats/min		1.5
Immobilization or surgery in previous 4 weeks		1.5
Previous DVT or PE		1.5
Hemoptysis		1
Cancer		1
Pretest probability according to score		
Low	(PE in 5–10%)	<2.0
Modest	(PE in 25–45%)	2.0–6.0
High	(PE in 70–90%)	>6.0

thromboembolism makes it possible to reliably rule out this diagnosis. A positive D-dimer test in the presence of a high or intermediate clinical prediction score warrants further testing.

11.2.2 Imaging Studies

Formerly, standard pulmonary arteriography was considered the diagnostic gold standard for pulmonary embolism. Today, this invasive, risky, and expensive maneuver is rarely performed, given the ever-improving accuracy of CT scanning for this indication. Modern multislice contrast-enhanced computed tomographic (CT) arteriography allows excellent visualization of subsegment pulmonary arteries. Pulmonary embolism in more peripheral arteries is hardly related to important clinical findings. Systematic reviews and prospective randomized trials suggest that outpatients with suspected pulmonary embolism and negative CT arteriographic studies have excellent outcomes without therapy. CT scanning provides other information in addition to confirming or excluding pulmonary embolism. Given the uncertainty of clinical signs and the nearly always high probability of an alternative diagnosis, clinicians appreciate the ability of CT scanning to find pneumonia, pneumothorax, abscesses, mediastinitis, aortic aneurysm, hemothorax, rib fractures, sternum osteomyelitis, and much more. For classic as well as for CT arteriography, intravenous contrast agents are needed. If a patient has either acute or chronic renal insufficiency, caution in using contrast agents is imperative, given the possibility of inducing nephropathy associated with contrast material. Allergy to contrast agents is present in approximately 1% of patients, with life-threatening allergic reactions occurring in less than 1 of 10 000 patients. In selected patients, (occult) hyperthyroidism curtails the use of iodine-containing intravenous contrast agents.

11.3 Pharmacokinetics in the Obese

The volume of distribution of a drug is dependent on a number of factors including tissue size, tissue permeability, plasma protein binding, and the affinity of the drug for a tissue compartment. Generally, lipophilic substances, based upon the octanol/water lipid-partitioning coefficients (LPC), are increasingly affected by obesity. Less lipophilic compounds, with lower LPCs, generally have little to no change in volume of distribution with obesity. Polar compounds have been shown to have several different relationships between body weight and volume of distribution, and correction factors for dosing have been developed for a wide range of individual substances. Unfortunately, there is no way to predict the pharmacodynamics or pharmacokinetics of a distinct drug in the obese, not even within a group of similar drugs [5].

In a subtle pharmacokinetic study with enoxaparin in obese patients, Green [6] demonstrated that enoxaparin is best when dosed at 100 IU/kg (1 mg/kg) based on lean body weight every 8 h in all patients, especially if total body weight exceeds 120 kg. Lean body weight (LBW) was calculated as follows:

LBW (men) = 1.1 x total body weight -120 x BMI
LBW (women) = 1.07 x total body weight -148 x BMI.

11.4 Thromboembolism in Medical Patients

Long after venous thromboembolism was identified as a burden of morbidity in surgical patients – and some kind of thromboprophylaxis is instituted for most surgical patients today, medical wards are adapting only slowly to the use of any thromboprophylaxis for their patients. There are no studies especially addressing the risk of venous thromboembolism in obese medical patients. Nevertheless, there is overwhelming evidence today that medical patients have an increased risk of venous thromboembolism (⏺ Table 11.4). The main studies with medical patients are (a) the MEDENOX trial [7] (1102 general medical patients, enoxaparin vs. placebo), showing a reduction of venous thromboembolism from 15.5% to 7.5% in the (small) subgroup of obese patients with 40 mg of enoxaparin [8]; and (b) the PREVENT trial [9] (prospective evaluation of dalteparin efficacy for prevention

⏺ **Table 11.4** Absolute risk of deep vein thrombosis in hospitalized patients [50]. Rates based on objective diagnostic testing for deep vein thrombosis in patients not receiving thromboprophylaxis

Patient group	Deep vein thrombosis (%)
Medical patients	10–20
General surgery	15–40
Major gynecological surgery	15–40
Major urological surgery	15–40
Neurosurgery	15–40
Stroke	20–50
Hip or knee arthroplasty, hip fracture	40–60
Major trauma	40–80
Spinal cord injury	60–80
Critical-care patients	10–80

of venous thromboembolism in immobilized patients), which included 3706 acutely ill medical patients. Here, the rate of venous thromboembolism was 4.96% with placebo and 2.77% with dalteparin (p=0.002). This study included 30% obese patients. In the subgroup analysis, risk reduction was similar (4.3% for placebo versus 2.8% for dalteparin), but because of the insufficient number the result did not reach statistical significance [10]. In both trials, obesity by itself was not identified as a risk factor for venous thromboembolism, but it increased the risk significantly in combination with other risk factors. This is consistent with the findings of the United States nurses' health study, which has 16 years of followup data on 112 822 female nurses aged 30–55 years. Obesity, cigarette smoking, and hypertension were all risk factors for pulmonary embolism, but women with high cholesterol concentration or diabetes were not at any higher risk. A body mass index of 29 and over was associated with a threefold increase in the incidence of pulmonary embolism [11].

11.5 Thromboembolism in Bariatric Surgery

In a study by Westling, including 116 patients with a mean BMI of 42 undergoing Roux-en-Y gastric bypass, 100 patients received 500 ml of dextran 70 as the only thromboprophylaxis. Ten patients received 20 mg enoxaparin daily. No clinically apparent thrombosis occurred. Asymptomatic calf vein thrombosis was detected by systematic duplex sonography in three patients. One patient developed pulmonary embolism 3 weeks later. The increased risk for venous thromboembolism in obese individuals has also been questioned. In prospective studies using the 125I-fibrinogen uptake test as a diagnostic tool, neither Hill et al. [12] nor Sue-Ling et al. [13] demonstrated a correlation between obesity and the incidence of postoperative deep vein thrombosis. In a postmortem study of 152 surgical patients by Cullen and Nemeskal [14], obesity did not seem to be a risk factor for pulmonary embolism, but obesity was not clearly defined. Finally, Flordal et al. [15] evaluated risk factors for thromboembolism in 2070 patients but failed to prove a correlation between obesity and postoperative thromboembolism. However, all patients underwent prophylaxis with low-molecular-weight heparin. Gonzalez et al. [16] reported only one popliteal thrombosis in 380 patients with a mean BMI of 48.5 undergoing laparoscopic Roux-en-Y gastric bypass. Intermittent pneumatic calf compression was used in this study, but no pharmacological prophylaxis. In a registry including 3097 patients undergoing bariatric surgery, 15

patients died within 6 months following surgery. Pulmonary embolism was the cause of death in 13% [17]. However, in autopsies of ten other patients who died following bariatric surgery, pulmonary embolism was the cause of death in 30% [18], and microscopic evidence of pulmonary embolism was found in eight of the ten patients, reflecting the difficulties in correctly diagnosing venous thromboembolism in any patient and even more so in the very obese. In a meticulous review, Rocha et al. found 11 studies supporting the evidence that obese patients undergoing bariatric surgery have an increased risk of venous thromboembolism and only two studies disputing this association. They came to the conclusion that the risk of venous thromboembolism exceeds the risk associated with the surgical procedure alone in these patients [19]. In a retrospective analysis of 5554 patients undergoing bariatric surgery over a period of 24 years a 0.21% rate of fatal pulmonary embolism was detected [20]. The cofactors most commonly associated with an increased risk of venous thromboembolism were venous stasis disease, a BMI of more than 60, truncal obesity, and obstructive sleep apnea. To date, eight studies have been published addressing the efficacy of venous thromboembolism prophylaxis especially in patients undergoing bariatric surgery. In a retrospective study [21] of 668 obese patients at five centers receiving 30 mg or 40 mg enoxaparin once or twice daily, six (0.9%) cases of pulmonary embolism and one of (0.1%) deep vein thrombosis were documented by objective testing. This is a low incidence, but virtually all pulmonary emboli derive from deep vein thrombosis, whereas only 25% of deep vein thromboses lead to pulmonary embolism. Thus a large number of deep vein thrombosis episodes must have been missed in this study, again demonstrating the difficulty of correctly diagnosing deep vein thrombosis in obese patients.

11.6 Dosing of Heparins in the Obese

Low-molecular-weight heparin has theoretical advantages in obese patients as a result of superior subcutaneous bioavailability. However, even low-molecular-weight heparin at standard fixed doses may not be sufficient to prevent venous thromboembolism in morbidly obese patients. Frederiksen et al. [22] demonstrated a strong negative correlation between total body weight and heparin activity (as measured by anti-Xa assay) with fixed doses of the low-molecular-weight heparin enoxaparin. Scholten et al. [23] conducted a nonrandomized retrospective study of 481 obese patients undergoing gastric bypass surgery. In addition to multimodal therapy with mechanical compression stockings, enoxaparin 40 mg every 12 h was su-

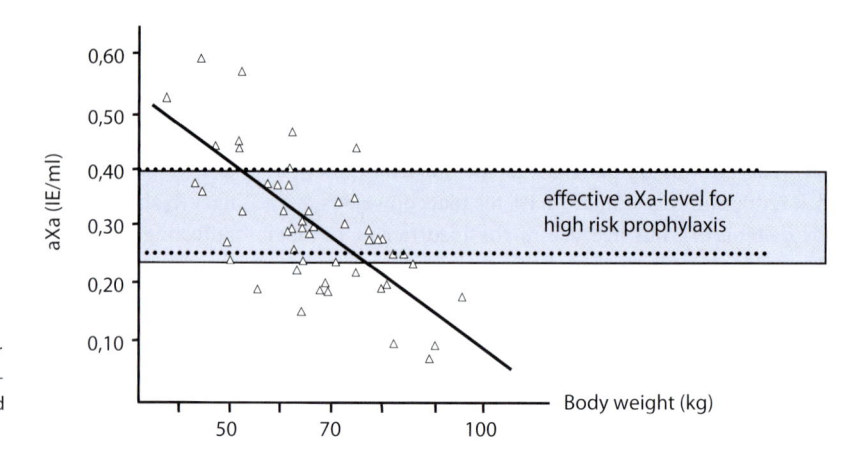

Fig. 11.1. Anti-Xa levels obtained after a fixed dose of low-molecular-weight heparin according to body weight (adapted from [26])

perior to enoxaparin 30 mg every 12 h with respect to the incidence of postoperative deep vein thrombosis (0.6% vs 5.4%; p=0.01) without an increase in bleeding complications. A different approach would be aPTT-adjusted dosing of unfractionated heparin for thromboprophylaxis. Before low-molecular-weight heparin became available, Leyvraz et al. [24] showed that aPTT adjustment is superior to fixed-dose unfractionated heparin in the prevention of venous thromboembolism in surgical patients. But measuring aPTT is very inconvenient, above all if finding the adequate dose for the individual patient requires several blood analyses per day, as is common in therapeutic anticoagulation with unfractionated heparins. All the advantages of low-molecular-weight heparins such as once-daily dosing, good correlation of dose and anti-Xa levels, and a tenfold lower risk of heparin-induced thrombocytopenia type 2, would be abandoned. Despite the lower acquisition cost of unfractionated heparins, the overall cost would be higher because of more frequent dosing and laboratory costs. Nevertheless, Shepherd et al. [25] demonstrated the feasibility of this approach in bariatric surgery patients. However, with low-molecular-weight heparin the situation is also not so easy. In the general population, anti-Xa activity achieved with a given dose of low-molecular-weight heparin correlates well with renal function – and with body weight (Fig. 11.1) [26]. This correlation has long been recognized. For therapeutic anticoagulation, package inserts and summaries of product information supplied by pharmaceutical companies contain no declaration concerning morbidly obese patients. Dosing regimens are given for body weights between 40 and 100 kg, with dosing being proportional to body weight in this range. The dose for 100 kg is the upper limit and is recommended for patients weighing more, but it is evident that dosing will be insufficient in morbidly obese patients. Several studies ascertain the fact that dosing of low-molecular-weight heparin must be much higher

than usual in morbidly obese patients to obtain adequate anti-Xa levels in prophylactic and in therapeutic anticoagulation. An open-label trial [27] evaluating two doses (75 and 175 IU/kg) of the low-molecular-weight heparin tinzaparin given to otherwise healthy obese volunteers (100–165 kg) concluded that prophylactic tinzaparin dosing should be based on actual body weight, independent of the presence of obesity, and that it need not be limited at a maximal absolute dose. It is probable that prophylactic low-molecular-weight heparin doses (like therapeutic doses) should be weight-adjusted for all patients, with or without obesity. Similarly, Al-Yaseen [28] demonstrated that full dosing according to total body weight is safe and effective in therapeutic anticoagulation with dalteparin in obese patients. On the other hand, fixed prophylactic doses of enoxaparin [29] and nadroparin [30] have been proven to be safe and effective in bariatric surgery. Dose adjustment for body weight in prophylactic indications raises concern about excessive anticoagulation and bleeding.

11.6.1 Monitoring Low-molecular-weight Heparin

Without additional data, firm recommendations are difficult to make; however, clinicians should consider escalating standard recommended doses of low-molecular-weight heparin for morbidly obese patients (i.e., 0.5 mg/kg for enoxaparin) for thromboprophylaxis with or without adjunctive use of mechanical compression devices or anti-Xa monitoring. Contemporary venous thromboembolism treatment trials of low-molecular-weight heparin have generally used weight-adjusted doses without any ceiling for obese patients. However, few patients with a total body weight greater than 150 kg and a body mass index greater than 50 kg/m^2 were actually included.

The relationship of intravascular volume and total body weight is not linear, and there is concern that dosing based on actual body weight could lead to excessive plasma concentrations of low-molecular-weight heparin. However, post hoc analysis of cardiovascular patients using full weight-adjusted doses of low-molecular-weight heparin and unfractionated heparin found no differences in hemorrhage rates between obese and normal-weight groups [31]. Similarly, anti-Xa activity is not significantly increased when low-molecular-weight heparin is administered to obese patients based on total body weight [32, 33]. Given the lack of clinical trial data for venous thromboembolism treatment with low-molecular-weight heparin in obese patients, it is still reasonable to monitor anti-Xa levels in such patients. This approach is generally recommended for patient groups with an uncertain relationship between dosing and anti-Xa levels [34]. It should not be forgotten that therapeutic target anti-Xa levels depend on the specific low-molecular-weight heparin preparation and dosing interval. In prophylaxis, it remains unclear whether anti-Xa adjusting translates into more effective reduction of venous thromboembolism. In clinical practice, anti-Xa levels are rarely measured in prophylactic dosing. In spite of the theoretical benefits of doing so, the outcome does not seem to be affected.

11.6.2 Alternatives to Heparins: Mechanical Measures

For virtually all patients undergoing any kind of surgery, mechanical measures for the prevention of deep vein thrombosis are recommended. Graduated compression stockings are often not feasible for very obese patients, simply because they do not fit. The alternative of elastic bandages is not well-tolerated by patients, and performing graduated bandaging is indeed very difficult. Usually, after a short period of time such elastic bandages tend to dislocate, resulting in strings that promote venous stasis instead of preventing it. Intermittent pneumatic compression is an often-applied and very effective means of thromboprophylaxis. Some authors even advocate the exclusive use of this method to avoid bleeding complications [16]. Inpatients undergoing surgery should be offered thigh-length graduated compression/antiembolism stockings from the time of admission to hospital unless they are contraindicated [35] (e.g., for patients with established peripheral arterial disease or diabetic neuropathy). If thigh-length stockings are inappropriate for a particular patient for reasons of compliance or fit, knee-length stockings may be used as a suitable alterna-

tive. The stocking compression profile should be equivalent to the Sigel profile and approximately 18 mm Hg at the ankle, 14 mm Hg at the mid-calf, and 8 mm Hg at the upper thigh. Patients should be encouraged to wear their stockings until they return to their usual level of mobility. Intermittent pneumatic compression or foot impulse devices may be used as alternatives or in addition to graduated compression/antiembolism stockings. According to ACCP guidelines, mechanical methods alone are adequate only for low-risk patients, but morbidly obese patients are at least at moderate risk (◘ Table 11.5). This also applies for the concept of "aggressive" early mobilization and ambulation, which today is widely accepted and practiced with surgical patients. Generally, therefore, pharmacological prophylaxis is indicated in bariatric surgery.

Danaparoid. Danaparoid has long been the only alternative to heparins. Danaparoid is a mix of heparan sulfates and is available for intravenous or subcutaneous administration. Like the unfractionated heparins, it antagonizes factor X and thrombin equally. Its main indication is thromboprophylaxis or therapy in patients with heparin-induced thrombocytopenia type 2. Unfortunately, it has 8–10% cross-reactivity, thus being able itself to induce or maintain a heparin-induced thrombocytopenia type 2. There is concern about a considerable disparity between charges of danaparoid supplied. Nowadays, there are substances that do not interfere and are less expensive, so danaparoid has been abandoned in many institutions.

Fondaparinux. Fondaparinux and its hypermethylated derivative, idraparinux, are synthetic analogues of the pentasaccharide sequence of heparin, the smallest heparin-based molecule that retains the capacity to catalyze factor Xa inhibition by antithrombin. Fondaparinux and idraparinux are too short to bridge antithrombin to thrombin and have no effect on the rate of thrombin inhibition by antithrombin. They are manufactured synthetically, in contrast to all heparins including low-molecular-weight heparin (derived from porcine mucosa). They work almost exclusively by factor Xa antagonism. Although it is theoretically possible, to date there is no convincing report of fondaparinux causing heparin-induced thrombocytopenia type 2. Fondaparinux reaches its peak level only 2 h after subcutaneous injection. Its long half-life of 16–20 h warrants a smoother anticoagulation, avoiding relatively long periods with no sufficient anti-Xa levels. The excretion is renal, so for patients with renal insufficiency (creatinine clearance lower than 20 ml/min) it is contraindicated. For therapeutic dosage, it is prudent to measure anti-Xa levels also in lesser degrees of renal insufficiency, because accu-

Risk level	Surgery	Age	Additional risk	VTE risk without prophylaxis (%)		Prevention strategies		
				Calf DVT	PE	LDUH	LMWH	Mechanical
Low	Minor	<40	No	2	0.2	None	None	Early and "aggressive" mobilization
Moderate	Minor	40–60	No	10–20	1–2	2 x 5000 U	<3400 U/day	IPC or GCS as alternative
	Minor	<40	Yes					
	Major	>40	No					
High	Minor	>60	No	20–40	2–4	3 x 5000 U	>3400 U/day	IPC or GCS alternatively if high risk of bleeding
	Minor	40–60	Yes					
	Major	40–60	No					
	Major	>40	Yes					
Highest	Major	>60	No	40–80	4–10	3 x 5000 U	>3400 U/day	IPC or GCS additionally
	Major	>40	Yes					
	Major	<40	Multiple					

☐ **Table 11.5** Levels of thromboembolism risk in surgical patients without prophylaxis. (Modified from [51])

IPC intermittent pneumatic compression, *GCS* graduated compression stockings, *DVT* deep vein thrombosis, *PE* pulmonary embolism, *LMWH* low-molecular-weight heparin, *LDUH* low-dose unfractionated heparin

mulation with the associated risk of bleeding is probable. In thromboprophylaxis, fondaparinux is given at a fixed dose of 2.5 mg subcutaneously once a day (patients without renal impairment). In four studies in orthopedic surgery, significantly fewer thromboembolic complications were observed compared with low-molecular-weight heparin. Rates of bleeding were low, but (not significantly) higher than with low-molecular-weight heparin. In general surgery, the pulmonary PEGASUS study demonstrated a non-significant reduction of proximal deep vein thrombosis from 6.1% (dalteparin) to 4.6% (fondaparinux). In the subgroup of high-risk patients operated on for cancer, the difference became significant. Major bleeding was observed in 49 (3.4%) of 1433 patients given fondaparinux and in 34 (2.4%) of 1425 given dalteparin (p=0.122). The APOLLO study of patients at increased risk undergoing major abdominal surgery, completed in 2004 but not yet published, showed an increased risk of bleeding in the fondaparinux group (versus intermittent pneumatic calf compression). An ongoing study will attempt to determine whether a fixed dose or a weight-related dose of fondaparinux is appropriate for morbidly obese subjects, and will also investigate the safety of administering weight-based doses to these individuals.

Rivaroxaban. Rivaroxaban, a new oral factor-Xa inhibitor, is a well-tolerated small molecule that binds to the active site of both free and bound factor Xa and inhibits the enzyme in a reversible and competitive manner. It proved effective in several indications. Thromboprophylaxis in surgical patients was tested with patients undergoing total hip replacement [35]. The authors concluded that 10 mg rivaroxaban showed efficacy and safety similar to enoxaparin for thromboprophylaxis after total hip replacement, with the convenience of once-daily oral dosing and without the need for coagulation monitoring. However, in abdominal surgery the oral administration is more a disadvantage, as in the first days after surgery oral intake is often disturbed or compromised by vomiting and bowel distension. , Many surgeons do not allow bariatric surgery patients to swallow tablets during the first few days. Perhaps rivaroxaban could be an alternative for prolonged thromboprophylaxis, with the adequate dosing still needed to be defined for obese patients. Rivaroxaban has been commercially available in Europe since May 2008.

Dabigatran. Dabigatran [36], an oral, direct thrombin inhibitor, is available for patients undergoing elective knee or hip joint replacement. It is given once daily in this high-risk group of patients. Dose adjustment for weight is not recommended, but severe kidney dysfunction is a contraindication. To date, dabigatran has not been approved for general surgical patients.

11.6.3 Anticoagulants under Investigation

Several innovative anticoagulants are currently under investigation [37]:

- Apixaban [38], a factor-Xa antagonist, given orally, once daily
- Idraparinux [39], a factor-Xa antagonist for subcutaneous injection, given once a week
- Recombinant nematode anticoagulant peptide (rNAPc2) [40] binds to a non-catalytic site on both factor X and factor Xa and inhibits factor VIIa within the factor VIIa/TF complex
- Recombinant thrombomodulin (ART 123) [41] binds thrombin and converts it from a procoagulant enzyme into a potent activator of protein C
- Aptamers, reversible antagonists of single coagulation factors, allowing easy stopping of the anticoagulation if needed

None of those mentioned above is commercially available today, and indications and dosing are still to be defined. The use of these new substances in special patient groups such as the morbidly obese needs further investigation. Recommendations for their use in these patients are not expected in the next few years.

Aspirin®. A word seems to be necessary about ASS (Aspirin®). There are still many people who believe that ASS is effective in venous thromboprophylaxis. It is definitely not, as found in many studies, the greatest of them being the Women's Health Study [42] with venous thromboembolism as a secondary end point. A prospective randomized trial was performed over 10 years in 39 876 women 45 years of age or more, testing 100 mg aspirin versus placebo. There was no difference in the incidence of venous thromboembolism: There were 1.18 thromboembolic events per 1000 person years in the ASS group versus 1.25 events in the placebo group (OR 0.95, p=n.s.). There was also no difference in groups at special risk such as women with previous venous thromboembolism or women with factor V or factor II mutation. Thus, in contrast to its well-documented efficacy in arterial thromboprophylaxis, there is no indication for ASS in venous prophylaxis. Following surgery, the only effect is a higher risk of bleeding.

Argatroban. Not for thromboprophylaxis, but for therapeutic anticoagulation, two additional groups of substances are available: argatroban (and successors) and the hirudins, with lepirudin being the most widely used. Argatroban is a synthetic direct thrombin inhibitor with a short half-life. Administration is by continuous infusion. There is no need for dose adaptation according to renal function, because elimination of the substance is hepatic. Thus, in cases of severe hepatic dysfunction, a dose reduction is necessary. Clinical experience shows that for critically ill patients substantially lower doses than initially recommended are appropriate (0.5 μg/kg/min instead of 2.0 μg/kg/min). Argatroban has excellent anticoagulation properties, is easily adjustable because of its short half-life, and must be monitored by measuring aPTT. Argatroban is indicated for the treatment of heparin-induced thrombocytopenia type 2.

Lepirudin. Before argatroban became available, hirudins were the alternative of choice for anticoagulation of patients with heparin-induced thrombocytopenia type 2. Hirudins are derived from leeches (*Hirudo medicinalis*). They act as direct thrombin inhibitors. They are not dependent on antithrombin and do not interfere with heparin antibodies. Unfortunately, they are allergenic by themselves, provoking allergic reactions in cases of reexposition in as many as 30% of patients. There is no way to antagonize hirudins. Excretion is renal, so in renal insufficiency they accumulate. Monitoring of aPTT is mandatory. More frequent and more serious bleeding is reported with hirudins than with other anticoagulants, and the costs of therapy are very high. Thus, all in all, hirudins are becoming less important in clinical practice, to the advantage of argatroban.

11.7 Bleeding Risk versus Thromboprophylaxis

Generally, and in each individual patient, effective thromboprophylaxis encounters increased bleeding risks even with low-dose prophylactic anticoagulation. In general surgery, the overall risk of major bleeding is estimated to be around 2%. Major bleeding is defined as life threatening, requiring more than two transfusions of packed red cells, requiring surgical intervention, or any intracerebral hemorrhage. In bariatric surgery bleeding is not a major concern, but venous thromboembolism is (◘ Table 11.5). Unfortunately, the more effective an anticoagulant drug is for thromboprophylaxis, the higher the bleeding risk following surgery (◘ Table 11.6). From this point of view, therefore, low-molecular-weight hep-

◻ Table 11.6 Events by type of in-hospital single-drug prophylaxis – general surgery patients [52]

	All DVT (%)	Symptomatic DVT (%)	Fatal PE (%)	Non-fatal symptomatic PE (%)	All major bleeding (%)	Fatal bleeding (%)	Stroke (%)
Nil	24.9	3.8	0.16	2.5	2.1	0.02	0.07
Aspirin	19.1	2.9	0.12	1.9	2.0	0.02	0.07
Danaparoid	8.8	1.3	0.06	0.9	3.7	0.04	0.13
Fondaparinux	5.4	0.8	0.03	0.5	4.7	0.05	0.16
LMWH	10.3	1.6	0.06	1.0	3.0	0.03	0.10
OAC-adj	14.6	2.2	0.09	1.4	2.7	0.03	0.09
LDUH	12.3	1.9	0.08	1.2	3.1	0.03	0.11

DVT deep vein thrombosis, *PE* pulmonary embolism, *LMWH* low-molecular-weight heparin, *OAC-adj* adjustable-dose oral anticoagulants, *LDUH* low-dose unfractionated heparin

arins in combination with mechanical prophylaxis remain the most effective and least harmful way to handle the dilemma.

11.8   Vena caval Filters

For patients at high risk for pulmonary embolism vena caval filters are a very effective means of protection. The only long-term prospective study comparing vena caval filters with anticoagulation alone [43] was disappointing: in an 8-year follow-up of 400 patients, survival was not improved by filter insertion (hazard ratio 0.97, $p=0.83$). The rate of symptomatic pulmonary embolism was reduced (hazard ratio 0.37, $p=0.008$), but inversely, there were more deep vein thromboses (hazard ratio 1.52, $p=0.042$). In the acute setting, accepted indications for vena caval filters include [44]:

- Recurrent pulmonary embolism despite adequate anticoagulation
- Pulmonary embolism when anticoagulation is contraindicated
- High mortality risk in case of pulmonary embolism (e.g., severe cor pulmonale)
- Filter placement after pulmonary thrombectomy
- Risk of paradoxical embolism in patients with deep vein thrombosis and right-left-shunt, e.g., atrial septum defect
- Floating thrombi in pelvic veins
- Prophylaxis for tumor patients with deep vein thrombosis instead of anticoagulation
- Preoperative prophylaxis for high-risk patients
- Polytrauma patients with previous pulmonary embolism

A vena caval filter can prevent pulmonary embolism with less intensive or even no anticoagulation. Therefore, on an individual basis, insertion of a vena caval filter is an option for high-risk patients also in bariatric surgery.

11.9   Timing of Prophylaxis

Most studies of low-molecular-weight heparin in surgical patients have been performed with administration of the prophylaxis 2 h before surgery. This approach is based on the consideration that most of the thrombus-generating vessel trauma and activation of the clotting system occurs during surgery. In practice, very often low-molecular-weight heparins are given the evening before surgery, making the surgeon more comfortable about the bleeding risk. Furthermore, if a peridural catheter is planned for anesthesia, commonly a 12-h interval from the last dose of low-molecular-weight heparin is required. However, this dosing regimen is not supported by studies and contradicts package insert directions. In contrast, fondaparinux prophylaxis is given 6 h following surgery. In a fondaparinux-based regimen no pharmacological prophylaxis at all is given preoperatively or during surgery. Nonetheless, rates of venous thromboembolism are remarkably lower than with low-molecular-weight heparin in very high risk patients (knee and hip surgery) [45]. In 2048 general surgery patients, including a not-specified number of obese patients, the PEGASUS [46] trial showed equivalence between the low-molecular-weight heparin dalteparin and fondaparinux for prevention of proximal deep vein thrombosis. The results of the fondaparinux studies encourage the administration also of low-molecular-weight heparin at a greater to surgery than the advised 2 h, as 2 h means that peak levels (obtained 3–4 h after subcutaneous injection) occur exactly during the operation. The evening-before or 6-h-post surgery administration was also chosen in the rivaroxaban studies. We identified one study [47] that compared low-molecular-weight heparin begun 12 h preoperatively with low-molecular-weight heparin begun 12 h postoperatively. Both groups received low-molecular- weight heparin for 14 days or until hospital discharge. There was no significant difference in the occurrence of deep vein thrombosis between the groups (RR=1.14, 95% CI: 0.74–1.76).

11.10 Duration of Prophylaxis

Generally, graduated compression stockings are recommended for surgical inpatients until they resume their usual level of activity, as mentioned above. In clinical practice, pharmacological thromboprophylaxis is given during the whole hospital stay but is stopped at discharge. For the high-risk group undergoing knee and hip replacement, several studies demonstrated the benefit of continuing pharmacological thromboprophylaxis for 4–5 weeks following surgery [25]. In a 3-year retrospective analysis of 1897 subjects with an episode of venous thromboembolism, Spencer et al. found that more venous thromboembolism was diagnosed in the 3 months following hospitalization than during hospitalization [48]. It is reasonable to consider prolonged prophylaxis in patients with a very high risk of venous thromboembolism, but patients undergoing bariatric surgery obviously do not generally belong to that group. Given that hospital stay is usually short for these patients, and presuming that staying in the hospital means that patients are not yet able to resume their usual level of activity, pharmacological thromboprophylaxis should be administered at least until hospital discharge. For selected patients more prolonged thromboprophylaxis should be considered, depending on individual risk estimation. For patients after bariatric surgery, the principal additional risk factor is prolonged immobilization.

11.11 Recommendations

11.11.1 Prophylaxis of Venous Thrombo-embolism

Morbidly obese patients undergoing abdominal surgery are a group at high risk for venous thromboembolism. "Aggressive" early mobilization and ambulation should be attempted with all patients. Graduated compression stockings should be offered, optionally only knee-long. Intermittent pneumatic compression of the calf is an alternative. All patients should receive pharmacological thromboprophylaxis at least during their hospital stay. Low-molecular-weight heparins represent the state of the art. Dosing should be adjusted to body weight. For prophylaxis, we recommend a quarter of a therapeutic dose as for non-obese patients (e.g., 0.5 mg/kg once daily for enoxaparin or nadroparin). Fondaparinux is a feasible alternative if there are contraindications to heparins. Actually, we do not have enough data to recommend higher doses for very obese patients, although this seems reasonable. For individual high-risk patients, placement of a vena caval filter is an option.

11.11.2 Therapeutic Anticoagulation

For therapeutic indications, unfractionated heparin is still the gold standard. Handling is easy and does not differ from that in non-obese patients (adjustment by aPTT). Low-molecular-weight heparins are more convenient. Dosing according to total body weight without capping is adequate and safe, but in morbidly obese patients anti-factor-Xa monitoring is mandatory. The latter also applies for danaparoid or fondaparinux. Anticoagulation is safe and easy to perform with argatroban, requiring only aPTT monitoring as with the unfractionated heparins, but it is costly. We do not recommend hirudins for this indication. Long-term anticoagulation with warfarin or phenprocoumon warrants close monitoring in patients after bariatric surgery, because the amount of enteral resorption of vitamin K and its antagonists varies considerably.

References

1. Proc. Seventh ACCP Conference on Antithrombotic and Thrombolytic Therapy (2004) Evidence-based guidelines. Chest 126 [Suppl 3]:172S–696S
2. Cohen AT, Tapson VF, Bergmann JF, Goldhaber SZ, Kakkar AK, Deslandes B, Huang W, Zayaruzny M, Emery L, Anderson FA jr, ENDORSE Investigators (2008) Venous thromboembolism risk and prophylaxis in the acute hospital care setting (ENDORSE study): a multinational cross-sectional study. Lancet 371:387–394
3. Edmonds MJR, Crichton TJH, Runciman WB, Pradhan M (2004) Evidence-based risk factors for postoperative deep vein thrombosis. ANZ J Surg 74:1082–1097
4. Nakata M, Yada T, Soejima N, Maruyama I (1999) Leptin promotes aggregation of human platelets via the long form of its receptor. Diabetes 48:426
5. Blouin RA, Warren GW (1999) Pharmacokinetic considerations in obesity. J Pharm Sci 88:1

6. Green B, Duffull SB (2003) Development of a dosing strategy for enoxaparin in obese patients. Br J Clin Pharmacol 56:96–103

7. Samama MM, Cohen AT, Darmon JY et al (1999) A comparison of enoxaparin with placebo for the prevention of VTE in acutely ill medical patients. Prophylaxis in medical patients study group. N Engl J Med 341:793

8. Alikhan R, Cohen AT, Combe S et al (2003) Prevention of VTE in medical patients with enoxaparin: a subgroup analysis of the MEDENOX study. Blood Coagul Fibrinolysis 14:341

9. Leizorovicz A, Cohen AT, Turpie AG et al (2004) Randomized placebo-controlled trial of dalteparin for the prevention of VTE in acutely ill medical patients. Circulation 110:874

10. Kucher N, Leizorovicz A, Vaitkus PT et al (2005) Efficacy and safety of fixed low dose dalteparin in preventing VTE among obese or elderly hospitalized patients: a subgroup analysis of the PREVENT trial. Arch intern Med 165:341

11. Goldhaber SZ, Grodstein F, Stampfer MJ, Manson JE, Colditz GA, Speizer FE, Willett WC, Hennekens CH (1997) A prospective study of risk factors for pulmonary embolism in women JAMA 277:642

12. Hills NH, Plug JJ, Jeyasingh K et al (1972) Prevention of deep vein thrombosis by intermittent pneumatic compression of calf. BMJ 1:131

13. Sue-Ling HM, Johnston D, McMahon MJ et al (1986) Pre-operative identification of patients at high risk of deep venous thrombosis after elective major abdominal surgery. Lancet 24:1173

14. Cullen DJ, Nemeskal AR (1986) The autopsy incidence of acute pulmonary embolism in critically ill surgical patients. Intensive Care Med 12:399

15. Flordal PA, Bergqvist D, Burmark US et al (1996) Risk factors for major thromboembolism and bleeding tendency after elective general surgical operations. Eur J Surg 162:783

16. Gonzalez QH, Tishler DS, Plata-Munoz JJ, Bondora A, Vickers SM, Leath T, Clements RH (2004) Incidence of clinically evident deep venous thrombosis after laparoscopic Roux-en-Y gastric bypass. Surg Endosc 18:1082

17. Omalu BI, Luckesevic T, Shakir AM et al (2004) Postbariatric surgery deaths, which fall under the jurisdiction of the coroner. Am J Forensic Med Pathol 25:237

18. Melinek J, Livingston E, Cortina G et al (2002) Autopsy findings following gastric bypass surgery for morbid obesity. Arch Pathol Lab Med 126:1091

19. Rocha AT, Vasconcellos AG, da Luz Neto ER et al (2006) Risk of VTE and efficacy of thromboprophylaxis in hospitalized obese medical patients and in obese patients undergoing bariatric surgery. Obesity Surg 16:1645

20. Sapala JA, Wood MH, Schuhknecht MP, Sapala MA (2003) Fatal pulmonary embolism after bariatric operations for morbid obesity: a 24-year retrospective analysis. Obes Surg 13:819

21. Hamad GG, Choban PS (2005) Enoxaparin for thromboprophylaxis in morbidly obese patients undergoing bariatric surgery. Obes Surg 15:1368

22. Frederiksen SG, Hedenbro JL, Norgren L (2003) Enoxaparin effect depends on body-weight and current doses may be inadequate in obese patients. Br J Surg 90:547

23. Scholten DJ, Hoedema RM, Scholten SE (2002) A comparison of two different prophylactic dose regimens of low-molecular-weight heparin in bariatric surgery. Obes Surg 12:19

24. Leyvraz PF, Richard J, Bachmann F et al (1983) Adjusted versus fixed-dose subcutaneous heparin in the prevention of deep-vein thrombosis after total hip replacement. N Engl J Med 309:954–958

25. Shepherd MF, Rosborough TK, Schwartz ML (2003) Heparin thromboprophylaxis in gastric bypass surgery. Obes Surg 13:249

26. Vitoux JF, Aiach M, Roncato M, Fiessinger JN (1988) Should thromboprophylactic dosage of low-molecular-weight heparin be adapted to patient's weight? Thromb Haemost 59:120

27. Hainer JW, Barrett JS, Assaid CA et al (2002) Dosing in heavy-weight/obese patients with the low molecular weight heparintinzaparin: a pharmacodynamic study. Thromb Haemost 87:817

28. AL-Yaseen E, Wells ps, Anderson J, Martin J, Kovacs MJ (2005) The safety of dosing dalteparin based on actual body weight for the treatment of acute venous thromboembolism in obese patients. J Thromb Haemost 3:100–102

29. Mismetti P, Laporte S, Darmon JY, Buchmüller A, Decousus H (2001) Meta-analysis of low-molecular-weight heparin in the prevention of venous thromboembolism in general surgery. Br J Surg 88:913

30. Kalfarentzos F, Stavropoulou F, Yarmenitis S, Kehagias I, Kara-mesini M, Dimitrakopoulos A, Maniati A (2001) Prophylaxis of venous thromboembolism using two different doses of low-molecular-weight heparin (nadroparin) in bariatric surgery: a prospective randomized trial. Obes Surg 11:670

31. Spinler SA, Inverso SM, Cohen M et al (2003) Safety and efficacy of unfractionated heparin versus enoxaparin in patients who are obese and patients with severe renal impairment: analysis from the ESSENCE and TIMI 11B studies. Am Heart J 146:33

32. Wilson SJ, Wilbur K, Burton E, Anderson DR (2001) Effect of patient weight on the anticoagulant response to adjusted therapeutic dosage of low-molecular-weight heparin for the treatment of venous thromboembolism. Haemostasis 31:42

33. Smith J, Canton EM (2003) Weight-based administration of dalteparin in obese patients. Am J Health Syst Pharm 60:683

34. Michota F, Merli G (2005) Anticoagulation in special patient populations: Are special dosing considerations required? Cleve Clin J Med 72:S37

35. Eriksson BI, Borris LC, Dahl OE, Haas S, Huisman MV, Kakkar AK, Muehlhofer E, Dierig C, Misselwitz F, Kälebo P, ODIXa-HIP Study Investigators (2006) A once-daily, oral, direct Factor Xa inhibitor, rivaroxaban (BAY 59-7939), for thromboprophylaxis after total hip replacement. Circulation 114:2313

36. Eriksson BI, Dahl OE, Buller HR et al for the BISTRO II STUDY GROUP (2005) A new oral direct thrombin inhibitor, dabigatran etexilate, compared with enoxaparin for prevention of thromboembolic events following total hip or knee replacement: the BISTRO II randomized trial. J Thromb Haemost 3:103

37. Bates SM (2007) New anticoagulants. Thromb Res 119 [Suppl 1]: S50

38. Lassen MR, Davidson BL, Gallus A, Pineo G, Ansell J, Deitchman D (2007) The efficacy and safety of apixaban, an oral, direct factor Xa inhibitor, as thromboprophylaxis in patients following total knee replacement. J Thromb Haemost 5:2368

39. van Gogh Investigators, Buller HR, Cohen AT, Davidson B, Decousus H, Gallus AS, Gent M, Pillion G, Piovella F, Prins MH, Raskob GE (2007) Idraparinux versus standard therapy for venous thromboembolic disease. N Engl J Med 357:1094

40. Lee A, Agnelli G, Buller H et al (2001) Dose response study of recombinant factor VIIa/tissue factor inhibitor recombinant nematode anticoagulant protein C2 in prevention of postoperative venous thromboembolism in patients undergoing total knee replacement. Circulation 104:74

41. Kearon C, Comp P, Douketis J, Royds R, Yamada K, Gent M (2005) Dose-response study of recombinant human soluble thrombomodulin (ART-123) in the prevention of venous thromboembolism after total hip replacement. J Thromb Haemost 3:962

42. Glynn RJ, Ridker PM, Goldhaber SZ, Buring JE (2007) Effect of low-dose aspirin on the occurrence of venous thromboembolism: a randomized trial. Ann Intern Med 147:525

43. Decousus H, Leizorovicz A, Parent F, Page Y, Tardy B, Girard P, Laporte S, Faivre R, Charbonnier B, Barral FG, Huet Y, Simonneau G (1998) A clinical trial of vena caval filters in the prevention of pulmonary embolism in patients with proximal deep-vein thrombosis. Prévention du Risque d'Embolie Pulmonaire par Interruption Cave Study Group. N Engl J Med 338:409

44. Leitlinien der Deutschen Röntgengesellschaft AWMF online ((Arbeitsgemeinschaft der Wissenschaftlichen Medizinischen Fachgesellschaften – Association of the Scientific Medical Societies in Germany). www.awmf.org

45. Lassen MR, Bauer KA, Eriksson BI, Turpie AG, European Pentasaccharide Elective Surgery Study (EPHESUS) Steering Committee (2002) Postoperative fondaparinux versus preoperative enoxaparin for prevention of venous thromboembolism in elective hip-replacement surgery: a randomised double-blind comparison. Lancet 359:1715

46. Agnelli G, Bergqvist D, Cohen AT, Gallus AS, Gent M, PEGASUS investigators (2005) Randomized clinical trial of postoperative fondaparinux versus perioperative dalteparin for prevention of venous thromboembolism in high-risk abdominal surgery. Br J Surg 92:1212

47. Palareti G, Borghi B, Coccheri S, Leali N, Golfieri R, Montebugnoli M et al (1996) Postoperative versus preoperative initiation of deep-vein thrombosis prophylaxis with a low-molecularweight heparin (Nadroparin) in elective hip replacement. Clin Appl Thromb Hemost 2:18

48. Spencer FA, Lessard D, Emery C, Reed G, Goldberg RJ (2007) Venous thromboembolism in the outpatient setting. Arch Intern Med 167:1471

49. Wells PS, Anderson DR, Rodger M et al (2001) Excluding pulmonary embolism at the bedside without diagnostic imaging: management of patients with suspected pulmonary embolism presenting to the emergency department by using a simple clinical model and D-dimer. Ann Intern Med 135:98–107

50. Geerts WH, Pineo GF, Heit JA, Bergqvist D, Lassen MR, Colwell CW, Ray JG (2004) Prevention of venous thromboembolism: the Seventh ACCP Conference on Antithrombotic and Thrombolytic Therapy. Chest 126 [Suppl 3]:338S–400S

51. Geerts WH, Heit JA, Clagett GP et al (2001) Prevention of venous thromboembolism. Chest 119:132S–175S

52. National Institute for Health and Clinical Excellence (NICE) (2007) Venous thromboembolism. Reducing the risk in surgical inpatients. Methods, evidence and guidance. National Collaborating Centre for Acute Care at The Royal College of Surgeons of England, 35-43 Lincoln's Inn Fields, London, WC2A 3PE

Principals of Nutrition after Surgical Procedure

Hartmut Bertz MD, Andrea Engelhardt MD

titis, dermatitis and neurological symptoms. Meat, fish, grains, vegetables and nuts include a great deal of vitamin B6, but cooking and long storage of the food cause a loss of >50%. Toxicity by chronic use over months (50-300mg/d) induces sensory polyneuropathy (reversible). It should be mentioned that high dose (>80mg/d) is not recommended in pregnancy. The recommended daily allowance by RDA is 1.3-1 .7mg/d; D-A-CH: 1.2 - 1.5mg/d [12,17].

Folic acid, Vitamin B9

The resorption of folate takes place mostly in the proximal part of small intestine and the whole gut. Storage is mainly in the liver. Patients have deficiencies because of reduced intake in 20% at one year after bariatric surgery [20]. The natural sources are vegetables, tomatoes, spinach, salad, cucumber, soybeans, whole-meal cereals, liver, yeast. (Folates are known as folic acid, foliacin, Pteroylpolyglutamates; dietary folate equivalents (DFE): 1DFE =1μg food folate = 0.6 μg folate from fortified food or as supplement). The recommended daily allowance by RDA is 400 μg/d; D-A-CH: 400μg /d [12,17].

Biotin

Biotin is absorbed in the proximal small intestine and in the caecum. There are low reserves, but isolated deficiency is rarely described (as dermatitis, anorexia, nausea and myalgia). Adequate blood levels are achieved through eating fruits and vegetables, milk products, liver, egg yolk, yeast and soya. In case of deficiency multivitamins are recommended. The recommended daily allowance by RDA is 30μg/d; D-A-CH: 30-60μg/d [12,17]

Cyanocobolamin, Vitamin B 12

Cyanocobolamin is absorbed in the ileum, in conjunction with the intrinsic factor, which is a glycoprotein produced by the parietal cells of the stomach; high doses of Vit B12 can be absorbed directly. Deficiency of vitamin B 12 is seen in vegan nutrition, older people, in patients with atrophic gastritis, after gastrectomy and after loss of more than 100 cm of the ileum, e.g. in short bowel syndrome. Vitamin B12 deficiency develops slowly because of longterm storage in the liver (after 1-2 years or later) and was seen in up to 2/3 of all patients after bariatric surgery. Natural sources are mainly animal products: red meat, liver, milk contain the highest amount of vitamin B12. Cyanocobalamin could be produced also by bacteria [21]. Vitamin B12 deficiency is the main cause of macroblastic anemia and neurological symptoms such as polyneuropathy or paralysis.

After bariatric surgery, long-term controls and prophylactic parenteral (subcutaneously (s.c. or i.m.) supplementation should be carried out. The recommended daily allowance by RDA is 2.4μg/d; D-A-CH: 3μg/d [12,17]

Vitamin C

Ascorbic acid is absorbed in the small intestine (jejunum and ileum). Scurvy is the main disease associated with ascorbic acid deficiency (fatigue, bleeding, impaired immune function and wound healing, swollen gingiva, depression, bone and muscle disease), which is rare in developed countries. Petechia, ecchymosis and Sjoergen syndrome have also been associated with the lack of ascorbic acid [22]. Fruits and vegetables, especially citrus fruits, tomatoes, and potatoes contain ascorbic acid. The recommended daily allowance by RDA is 60-125 mg/d [22]; D-A-CH: 100 (-150) mg/d [12]

12.2.2 Fat-soluble vitamins
(◘ Table 12.1, 12.3)

Vitamin A

There are several forms of vitamin A: retinoids, s-carotenes and carotinoides, which can be transformed to vitamin A. They require pancreatic enzymes for final absorption in the lower small intestine, optimal absorption is in association with fat [23]. Symptoms of deficiency develop gradually: night-blindness and repeated infections of the respiratory system, dry skin. Later, xerophthaImia, keratomalacia, finally blindness can occur; mucosa lesions, as well as impaired immune system leading to severe infections. First symptoms may develop before very low serum levels are detected, but the reservoir may be depleted (DACH). Children with malnutrition and patients with alcoholism or with malabsorptive surgery (e.g. after BPD) develop deficiencies. Toxicity is seen with high doses, especially if the dose exceeds 200 mg RAE (retinol equivalent) vitamin A once a day or long-term intake of more than 3mg RAE every day. Signs include fatigue, headache, and vomiting. Chronic conditions are alopecia, hepatotoxicity, and bone lesions with pain. Vitamin A accumulation is found in patients with chronic renal insufficiency. Retinols concentrations are very high in liver, and high in milk, butter, egg yolk; s-carotenes are found in plants, especially in red and orange fruits and vegetables; for beta-carotenes no toxicity is described. The recommended daily allowance by RDA is 700- 900 RAE/d; D-A-CH: 0.8-1.0 mg retinol equivalent (mg RAE) [12, 17]

Calciferol, Vitamin D

Vitamin D is not well represented in nutrition, with the exception of fish; small amounts are found in mushrooms, egg-yolk, cheese, butter. Absorption of vitamin D occurs in conjunction with fat in the lower small intestine and is reduced in impaired fat digestion. After UVA - exposition in the skin provitamin D2 = ergosterol is transferred into vitamin D2 = ergocalciferol. Provitamin D3 = dehydrocholesterol is transformed by UVB - exposition to vitamin D3 = cholecalciferol and afterwards to its active form in liver and kidney. There are multiple receptors for vitamin D in the body, however, its function is not yet fully understood. The main function is hormonal regulation of calcium and phosphor together with parathyroid hormone and calcitonin. Osteomalacia and osteoporosis are associated with low vitamin D levels; immune function [24] and others also may be impaired. Vitamin D deficiencies are described after BPD [25] and less frequently after RYGB [26]. [1µg = 40 IU vitamin D3] Recommendation of daily intake is 5µg/d; for >70y 15 µg/d (=600IU). The recommendation is considered to be too low, especially in northern countries and in the winter; daily intake of 20-25 µg (= 800-1000 IU) seems to be safe and more adequate. (25-45 IU/ml aimed level, in blood serum control) Overdoses, seen in high oral dose or parenteral application, lead to hypercalcaemia with fatigue, dehydration, abdominal cramps, somnolence and coma. Long-term toxicity may be nephrocalcinosis and renal dysfunction.

Vitamin E

The main representative of vitamin E is alpha-tocopherol; four additional tocopherols are known. For absorption pancreatic enzymes and fat is necessary. Deficiency is rare and associated with fat-malabsorption; low reserves lead to neuromuscular disorders (hyporeflexia), ataxia, and hemolysis [27]. Vitamin E is found in oil, meat, plant seeds, egg, and leafy vegetables. RDA is 15 mg TAE/d; D-A-CH: 12-15 mg/d. In the case of malabsorption 200 IU ~ 100 mg should be substituted. 100-400 IU/d are safe; high–dose supplementation is not recommended > 400 IU/d. Toxicity is seen in chronic high doses with increased risk of bleeding.

Vitamin K

Vitamin K (K1) is produced in green plants and (K2) is synthesized in microorganisms, for example, by bacteria in the colon. For the absorption of vitamin K in the small intestine pancreatic enzymes, biliary function and fat are necessary. High concentration of vitamin K can also be absorbed passively in the intestine and colon. Vitamin K is used by proteins for blood coagulation and for the bone matrix. Green vegetables (like spinach, broccoli), soya and some seeds (sunflower, rape) are the main nutritional source. No toxicity is described; deficiency shows bruises and bleeding. The recommended daily allowance by RDA 90-120 µg/d; D-A-CH: 60-80 µg/d. minimum, exact need is unclear [12,17].

12.3 Trace Elements And Electrolytes
(◘ Table 12.4)

Calcium

Calcium is mainly absorbed in the duodenum and proximal jejunum. Its deficiency leads to osteoporosis, bone loss and fractures. Milk and its products contain the most calcium, as well as some vegetables, nuts and some mineral water. Toxicity is unclear, high dose may lead to nephrolithiasis. The recommended daily allowance by RDA: 1000 mg/d. D-A-CH: 1000 mg/d [12, 17]

Potassium

Potassium is mainly absorbed in the upper small intestine, excretion is mainly renal. Potassium loss could be caused by vomiting or diarrhea, or by some medications. Both deficiency and overload of potassium are life threatening because neuromuscular dysfunction as f.e. cardiac arrest. Mainly vegetables contain lots of potassium. The exact need for daily intake is difficult to define mostly written between 2,000-5,000 mg/d. The low or controlled potassium diet is needed in patients with renal failure, who tend to accumulate potassium. The recommended daily allowance by RDA 4,700 mg/d; D-A-CH at least 2,000 mg/d [12, 17]

Iron

Iron absorption takes place predominantly in the duodenum and also in the jejunum. Deficiency is partially caused by reduced meat intake, but also by malabsorptive pathway and reduction of gastric acid secretion (which is necessary for the transformation from Fe^{3+} to Fe^{2+} as the absorbable form of iron). On average, 33% of patients have iron deficiency at 2 years after bariatric surgery [20]. Bleeding or chronic infection may be a cause of anemia in some patients. The recommended daily allowance by RDA 8-18 (females) mg/d, D-A-CH 10- 15(f) mg/d [12, 17]

Zinc

Zinc is mainly absorbed in the duodenum. The natural sources of zinc are seafood, meat and milk; grains and cereal also contain higher amounts of zinc. Lack of zinc causes hair loss, taste disturbances, increased infections and disturbances in wound healing. With high-dose supplementation copper absorption may be reduced. The recommended daily allowance by RDA for adults is 8-11 mg/d; D-A-CH: 10 mg/d [12, 17].

Iodine

Iodine is very important for the metabolism of the thyroid gland; it is absorbed in the entire gastrointestinal tract. Deficiency causes hypothyroidism, impaired mental function and in children delayed physical development. For the fetus the lack of iodine leads to abortion or is associated with cretinism, as well as psychomotor retardation. In many industrialized countries iodine is added to water, salt or bread. Germany is a country with low iodine supply. Toxicity from food is not seen, but in the case of very high-dose intake (acute) hyperthyroidism or (chronic) development of hypothyroidism with goiter is possible. Main sources of iodine are seafood and salt with iodine; in small amounts milk products also contain iodine. The recommended daily allowance by RDA is 150 ug/d; D-A-CH recommendation 200 μg/d [12, 17].

For more details, or newly adapted recommendations for micronutrients see dietary reference intakes of the Food and Nutrition Board-Institute of Medicine, USA, or D-A-CH, and chapter 26.

12.4   Common Nutritional Guidelines in Bariatric or Metabolic Surgery

Most patients who undergo bariatric surgery procedure have tried to reduce weight before and learned the rules of good eating behaviour. However, they have failed in their efforts and become frustrated. Nevertheless, they should be newly instructed before and after surgery [28] to reduce problems like vomiting and malnutrition. The patient should primarily adhere to the following common rules [29]:

- eat slowly, chew well
- separate drinking and eating
- drink between meals
- avoid sweets, avoid alcohol
- eat a lot of vitamins and protein
- 3-4 meals / day; no snacks, if the meals are big enough
- when satiated, STOP eating

12.4.1   Problems in all types of bariatric surgery

- Patients develop **intolerances** to red meat, grains, rice, bread, fruits with grains, high fat nutrition.
- A new nutrition balance has to be learned. Initially, patients tend to eat too fast, to eat big portions with risk of vomiting, or they eat very little and risk malnutrition.
- In the case of **prolonged vomiting** electrolyte disturbances, dehydration and deficiency of thiamin and folic acid may develop.
- **Dumping syndrome** may appear after gastric bypass and may cause serious nutritional problems: e.g. hypoproteinemia and dehydration [30]. To prevent symptoms like vertigo, collapse, diarrhea or hypoglycemia, in addition to common rules (eat small portions, drink between meals), patients should reduce sugar and simple carbohydrates intake and rather eat complex carbohydrates or add fibers. If necessary, they should rest after a meal.
- If the patient shows **very large weight loss** (e.g. 10kg / month), solid organ disorder may be the reason, or as well an eating disorder with very low food absorption.
- During weight loss there is a risk of **psychological instability**, including enhanced symptoms of depression.
- **Anemia**, which may affect as many as two thirds of these patients, is generally thought to be caused by iron deficiency. Chronic inflammation is presented with low iron levels. A long-term complex nutrient deficiency may also lead to anemia [31].
- **Gallstone formation** is seen in the case of very fast weight loss in up to 22% after gastric bypass; it is uncommon after gastric banding. Daily oral ursodesoxychol-acid as prophylaxis is recommended.
- **No weight loss** is due to the excessive consumption of snacks, high caloric soft or liquid foods (e.g. milk shakes), or to caloric intake exceeding the energy expenditure (very low muscle mass and activity or reduced protein intake).
- In case of **pregnancy** the micro- and macro nutrition status must be re-evaluated and the patient will require more supplementation.

12.4.2   Nutrition after bariatric surgery

Weeks 1-4:

The patient should eat 4 - 6 times / d small amounts of liquid food (protein shakes, soups, egg, yoghourt, milk, curd, puréed fruit, non-carbonated water, tea). Eating should be stopped upon feeling satiated. The increase in protein intake should prevent the loss of muscle mass. Guidelines for determining optimal caloric, protein and micronutrient requirements are lacking [32]. Recommended amount of protein is 1.0 -1.5 g/kg ideal body weight, at least ~50-75mg/d. Drinking should be stopped 30 min before eating and started 60 min after; only small amounts are recommended with the meals. Throughout the day, small portions of water or sugar-free clear fluids should be consumed at regularl intervals. Recommended intake is 2 l/d, with larger amount in the case of diarrhea (control by sufficient urine production). See ◘ Table 12.5 for an example of recommended postoperative food composition.

Weeks 4-6:

Slow, thorough chewing and 3 meals and 2-3 between very small meals are recommended. Tolerance of food should be tested by consuming mini amounts of new products.

> 6 weeks:

Normal food should be eaten during 3 meals; if these meals are small, additionally 2-3 snacks are allowed to prevent very fast weight reduction. The food should be chewed thoroughly to make it "soft" or fast fluid to prevent impaction and vomiting. Patients should be instructed to control their weight weekly and observe urine production. Complications caused by deficiencies could be avoided by regularly follow up consultations, evaluation and if necessary, adjustment and medical supplementation. The patient should be seen on a regular basis by a dietician trained and experienced in caring for obese patients after restrictive and malabsorptive surgery [9]. Noncompliance with micronutrient supplementation, as well as noncompliance with necessary dietary restrictions after surgery, may result in complications and morbidity, especially after malabsorptive procedures [32].

12.5 Nutritional Problems Associated With Specific Bariatric Surgery Procedures And Recommendations

12.5.1 Gastric Banding

Restrictive procedures such as gastric banding are unlikely to cause nutritional deficits, since none of the intestinal parts is bypassed [33]. After gastric banding,

patients should eat small portions, drink regularly, eat slowly and reduce intake of sweet and very fatty foods to reduce weight. If they reduce caloric intake to less than 1200 kcal/day or go on eating unbalanced diets, they will have deficits in micronutrients and therefore should add supplements of combined multivitamin- and trace elements (recommended dose/d see tables vitamins and trace minerals). When weight is stable, long-term need for supplementation depends on eating habits (nutrition diary) and laboratory results. Vomiting is the main cause leading to nutritional problems after gastric banding. This occurs frequently

- if the patient does not chew enough
- if the patient eats large amounts of food at once
- if bites are too big
- the band is pulled too tight

DDeficiencies of iron and vitamin B12 are rare after gastric banding [2] except in patients after vertical banding gastroplasty. Deficiencies of up to 32% of iron and up to 46% anemia have been published [34]. On the other hand, folic acid deficiency [35] caused by very fast weight loss, and deficiency of fat-soluble vitamins and thiamin [36, 37] due to gastric acid deficiency [38] appear more often, especially in the case of vomiting. Substitution/ supplementation recommended (international guidelines for supplementation are lacking):

Multivitamin: one tablet per day including all vitamins (B, C, fat-soluble) and trace minerals (see ◘ Table 12.3 and 12.5, RDA). In case of intolerance of tablets due to the pouch, liquid preparations should be introduced.

If deficiencies according blood levels are apparent following substitution should be performed, (not routinely expected after GD):

Vitamin D: up to 800-1000 IE (= 20-25µg) /day [26], (Sun exposition to the skin (summer) for 10-15min/day), or see guidelines for osteoporosis therapy

Calcium: 1000 mg / day (see RDA)

Iron: Fe (II) 100-200mg/d, until deficit is adjusted; if oral application is not tolerated i.v. application ; see guidelines for treatment of anemia

Thiamin: in case of deficiency oral 30-50mg/d; in case of severe clinical symptoms (Wernike-Korsakow): initially parenteral loading dose

Vit. B 12: up to 1-2 mg / day orally, or i.m. /s.c. 1 mg / month (=in case of malabsorption, e.g.vertical banding); 1mg every 3 months may be enough

folic acid: 0.5-1 mg / day, until deficit is adjusted (see RDA)

Recommended diagnostic (► Chapter 4.3 ▣ Table 12.5)

Month 1, 3, 6, 12 and afterwards yearly:

- weight control, evaluation of nutrition habits, psychological and physical problems: comorbidity and therapy associated
- laboratory control standards have to be found, our recommendations see ▣ Table 12.3
- in case of vomiting: special attention for potassium, vitamin B1, blood glucose, blood cell count, renal and liver function
- in case of very fast loss of weight (>10 kg) between the controls: shorten the intervals to monthly visits, magnesium and phosphor should be measured additionally.

12.5.2 Gastric Sleeve LSG

Long-term data after sleeve operation are missing; similar to gastric banding this is a mainly restrictive bariatric procedure. The size of the stomach is smaller, but it is not associated with dumping syndrome. Absorption of nutrients, minerals and drugs is not altered; there will be no problems from banding, but after a while gastric volume can partially recover and weight gain may follow [39] Sleeve resection will lead to reduced production of intrinsic factor and consequently reduced absorption of vitamin B12. Substitution/ supplementation recommended (international guidelines for supplementation are lacking):

Multivitamin: one tablet per day including all vitamins (B, C, fat-soluble) and traceminerals (see table RDA). In case of intolerance of tablets liquid preparations should be introduced.

Vit B 12: 1-2 mg / day orally or i.m. /s.c. 1 mg / month (=1000μg) or every 3 months, according blood level; life long, in case of malabsorption

If deficiencies according to blood levels are apparent, (not routinely expected), the following substitution should be performed:

Vitamin D: up to 800-1000 IE (= 20-25μg) /day [26], (sun exposition to the skin (summer) for 10-15min/day), or see guidelines for osteoporosis therapy

Calcium: 1000 mg / day

Iron: Fe (II) 100-200mg/d, until deficit is adjusted; if oral application is not tolerated i.v. application; see guidelines for treatment of Iron deficit and anemia

Thiamin: in case of deficiency oral 30-50mg/d; in case of severe clinical symptoms (Wernike-Korsakow): initially parenteral loading dose

Folic acid: 0.5-1 mg / day, until deficit is adjusted; then 0.4-1mg/d (see RDA)

Recommended diagnostic (► Chapter 4.3 ▣ Table 12.5):

Month 1, 3, 6, 12 and afterwards yearly:

- weight control, evaluation of nutrition habits, psychological and physical problems: comorbidity and therapy associated
- laboratory control standards have to be found, our recommendations see Chapter 4.3 ▣ Table 12.5; attention for folic acid, iron; vitamin B12.
- in case of vomiting: special attention for potassium, vitamin B1, blood glucose, blood cell count, renal and liver function
- in case of very fast loss of weight (>10 kg) between the controls: shorten the intervals to monthly visits, magnesium and phosphor should be measured additionally.

12.5.3 Gastric Bypass (RYGB)

In the beginning the filling volume of the stomach is about 15 - 30 cm³, later it may increase. To avoid deficiencies the patients should be advised to eat fresh fruit and vegetables. These are well tolerated compared red meat with the consequence, that the patients will become vegetarian. In the first months some patients have reduced tolerance to high amounts of lactose and fructose.

Modified eating behaviors, dumping symptoms, reduced of biliary acids and pancreas-enzymes, reduced absorption of minerals and B-vitamins in the upper intestine lead to a variety of deficits, lead mainly anemia and begin of osteoporosis. After gastric bypass in Y-Roux technique regularly deficiency of calcium occurs [40] with the development of osteopenia and metabolic bone disease [41]. This is further enhanced by the patient's immobility and if the patient develops a secondary hyperparathyroidism [42]. Further Wernicke encephalopathy due to thiamin deficiency has been reported [43] especially in case of persisting vomiting. The blood levels of vitamin B 12 and the fat-soluble vitamins should be monitored and regularly supplemented [44]. Iron deficiency is one of the most common nutrient deficiencies that occurs (in 20%–49% of bariatric surgery patients), depending on the type of surgery performed [32]. Nutritional deficiencies are very common after RYGB and occur despite supplementation with a multivitamin preparation 45].

The following nutritional deficiencies are common [2]: calcium, iron, vitamin B12, folic acid, fat-soluble vitamins, mainly vitamin D and thiamin, increased in case of vomiting.

Substitution / supplementation recommended (international guidelines for supplementation are lacking):

Multivitamin: one tablet per day including all vitamins (B, C, fat-soluble) and trace-minerals (see table

RDA). In case of intolerance of tablets liquid preparations should be introduced. If deficiencies according blood levels are apparent following substitution should be performed:

Vit B 12: 1-2 mg / day orally or i.m. /s.c. 1 mg / month (=1000µg) in case of malabsorption; according blood level life long [46]; every 3 months may be enough

Vitamin D: up to 800-1000 IE (= 20-25µg) /day [26], (sun exposition to the skin (summer) for 10-15min/day) or see guidelines for osteoporosis therapy; oral intake may not lead to sufficient blood levels, therefore i.m. substitution should be given in case of permanent low levels every 3-6 months (25-45UI/ml aimed level, normal PTH)

Calcium: 1000-2000 mg / day (better absorption of calcium-citrate compared to calcium-carbonate)

If deficiencies according blood levels are apparent following substitution should be performed:

Iron: 64 mg / d should be given in case of menstruating women or deficiency [47], if oral application is not tolerated: i.v. application (daily or weekly) until deficit is adjusted; see treatment anemia.

Thiamin: in case of deficiency oral 50mg/d; in case of severe clinical symptoms (Wernike-Korsakow): initially parenteral loading dose

Folic acid: 5 mg / day until deficit is adjusted; then 0.4-1md/d

Recommended diagnostic (▶ Chapter 4.3 ◻ Table 12.5):

Month 1, 3, 6, 12 and afterwards yearly:

- ▬ weight control, evaluation of nutrition habits, psychological and physical problems: comorbidity and therapy associated
- ▬ laboratory control standards have to be found, our recommendations see ◻ Table 12.3; longterm controls of micronutrients and parathyroid hormone recommended
- ▬ in case of vomiting: special attention for potassium, vitamin B1, blood glucose, blood cell count, renal and liver function
- ▬ in case of very fast loss of weight (>10 kg) between the controls: shorten the intervals to monthly visits, magnesium and phosphor should be measured additionally; attention for cholestasis.
- ▬ if applicable measurement of the bone density

12.5.4 Biliopancreatic Diversion (BPD) with or without Duodenal switch (DS)

These preferred malabsorptive techniques lead to more than 10 to 40% more weight reduction than the restric-

tive techniques, but they result in many more metabolic changes [44]. Despite iron supplementation, 5% of patients are anemic after BPD and with lack of supplementation 40% after BPD [48] and 32% after BPD-DS [49]. Further, in both malabsorptive techniques, despite supplementation, hypocalcaemia is a major problem. After BPD, in 63% elevated parathyroid hormone levels were seen [25] and mainly after 3-5 years, postoperative patients develop extensive bone demineralization [50]. After BPD-DS, 25% of patients develop hypocalcaemia and more than 50% develop deficiencies in fat-soluble vitamins, despite substitution [49]. Four years after BPD, 69% of patients suffer from vitamin A - , 68% from vitamin K - and 49% from vitamin E deficiencies [51]. This is associated with the lack of fat absorption, which mainly cause the desired weight loss. In addition to the reduced fat absorption, the patients after BPD +/- DS suffer from protein deficiency in up to 17% and need a re-operation in 3.2 % after BPD [48] and in 3% after BPD-DS [49]. As in patients with short bowel syndrome, the intestine left for absorption needs time (6-24 months) to adapt to the situation; it will be able to absorb more and more macronutrients, whereas deficits in vitamins and essential lipid acids will slowly become more evident. Observing patients for nutritional deficiencies after malabsorptive operation is a particular challenge and requires regular monitoring of all vitamins, all trace minerals, electrolytes, and because of the risk of severe malnutrition or liver dysfunction.

Substitution / supplementation recommended (international guidelines for supplementation are lacking):

Multivitamin: one to two tablets per day including all vitamins (B, C, fat-soluble) and trace-minerals (see table RDA). In case of intolerance of tablets liquid preparations should be introduced.

Vit B 12: i.m. 1 mg / month life long [46] or oral 1-2 mg / day ; reduction in case of high blood levels

Vitamin D: up to 800-1000 IE (= 20-25µg) /day [26], (sun exposition to the skin (summer) for 10-15min/day); (25-45UI/ml aimed level, normal PTH)

Calcium: 1000-2000mg / day (better absorption of calcium-cit rate compared to calcium-carbonate)

Iron: 64 mg / d should be given in case of menstruating women or deficiency [Love AL 2008]

Thiamin: in case of deficiency: 50 mg / d

Folic acid: 5 mg / day, or according blood level

Magnesium: 300mg / day or according symptoms or blood level

Zinc: 10mg / day

In case of low levels with oral application for Iron, vitamin B12, and the vitamins A,D,E,K these should be given parenteral monthly or every two to three months, according to blood level. Additionally, proteinpowder and MCT-enriched energiedrinks may be needed to prevent malnutriton. Long-term routine controls once a year may not be enough to assure adequate dosage of supplements.

Recommended diagnostic (▶ Chapter 4.3 ◘ Table 12.5):

Month 1, 3, 6, 12 and afterwards yearly:
- weight control, evaluation of nutrition habits, psychological and physical problems: co morbidity and therapy associated
- laboratory control standards have to be found, our recommendations see ◘ Table 12.3; long-term controls of micronutrients and parathyroid hormone recommended.
- in case of vomiting: special attention to potassium, vitamin B1, blood glucose, blood cell count, renal and liver function
- in case of very fast loss of weight (>10 kg) between the controls: shorten the intervals to monthly visits, magnesium and phosphor should be measured additionally; attention for cholestasis
- if applicable, measurement of bone density

Special attention should be paid to
- mineral disturbances, blood glucose, blood cell count
- renal function , formation of kidney stones; hyperoxaluria [Patel BN et al 2009]

- impaired liver function (NASH- improving or worsening)

Surveillance of the patient's food intake and ingestion of macro- and micronutritients after bariatric surgery is very important [45]. Complications caused by deficiencies can be avoided by regular follow up consultations, diagnostic, evaluation and if necessary, medical substitution. The patient should be seen on a regular basis by a dietician experienced in caring for obese patients after restrictive and malabsorptive surgery.

◘ **Table 12.1** Vitamin body-resources [adapted from Leitzmann, 52]

Vit A	1 - 2 years
Vit B 12	2 - 5 years
Vit D	2 - 6 weeks
Vit E	2 - 6 weeks
Vit K	2 - 6 weeks
Vit B1	4 - 10 days
Vit B2	2 - 6 weeks
Vit B6	2 - 6 weeks
Folic acid	3 - 4 months
Vit C	2 - 6 weeks
Biotin	4 - 10 days
Pantothen acid	4 - 10 days
Niacin	few days - weeks
Beta carotene	no resources

◘ **Table 12.2** Secretion of enzymes and absorption of vitamins and trace minerals according the gastro intestinal site after Suter [11]

Secretion of	Organ	Absorbtion of
gastric acid pepsinogen intrinsic factor (B12)	stomach	alcohol
pancreatic enzymes bile acid	duodenum	iron calcium magnesium, zinc H2O
	proximal small	carbohydrates, aminoacids
		Vit C
intestine enzymes	intestine (jejunum)	Vit B1 Vit B2 Vit B5 Vit B6 folic acid calcium
	distal small intestine (ileum)	amino acids peptides Vit A Vit D Vit E Vit K Vit C Vit B 1 fatty acids
	terminal ileum	Vit B 12
		biliary acids
	colon	Vit K
		short chain fatty acids
		Na, K, H2O

◼ Table 12.3 Vitamins - daily recommended doses

Vitamins	Food an nutrition board Institute of Medicine, USA 1998, 2001 RDA >19y; m f (pregnant)			Upper Level UL	D-A-CH (Europe) 2008 RDA >19y; m f (pregnant)		
Vit B1(mg) Thiamin	1.2	1.1	(1.4)	ND	1.3	1.0	(1.2)
Vit B2(mg) Riboflavin	1.3	1.1	(1.4)	ND	1.0-1.5	1.2	(1.5)
Niacin (mg, Equivalent)	16	14	(18)	30	13-17	13	(15)
Vit B6 (mg) Pyridoxine	1.3 <70y 1.7	1.3 >70	(1.9) 1.5	100	1.4-1.5	1.2	(1.9)
Folic acid (μg DFE)	400	400	(600)	1000	400	400	(600)
Pantothen Acid (mg)	5	5	(6)	ND	6	6	(6)
Biotin (μg)	30	30	(30)	ND	30-60	30-60	
Vit B12 (μg)	2.4	2.4	(2.6)	ND	3	3	(3.5)
Vit. C (mg)	90	75	(85)	2000	100	100	(110)
Vit A (RAE) Carotinoides	700	900		3000 ND	1.0mgRAE	0.8	(1.1)
Vit D (ug)	5 >50y: 10	5 >70y: 15		50	5	5 > 65y: 10	
Vit E (mg TAE)	15	15		1,000	12-15	11-12 (13)	
Vit K (μg)	120	90	(90)	ND	70-80min.	60-65 (60)	
Coments	Recommended daily oral intake, (normal function of GI tract)			UL: likely to pose risk of adverse side effects ND= not determined	daily oral intake; more than double or three times portion not recommended		

◼ Table 12.4 Microelements - daily recommended doses

Trace elements Minerals	Food an nutrition board Institute of Medicine, USA 1998, 2000,2001 RDA >19y, m f (pregnant)			Upper Level UL	D-A-CH (Europa) 2008 RDA >19y, m f (pregnant)	
Chromium(μg /d)	35	25	(30)	ND	30-100	
Copper (μg/d)	900	900 (1,000)		10,000	1-1.5 mg/d	
Fluoride (mg/d)	4	3	(3)	10	3.8	3.1 (3.1)
Iodine (μg/d)	150	150 (220)		1,100	200	
Iron (mg/d)	8	18 <50y 8	(27)	45	10	15 (30)
Manganese (mg/d)	2.3	1.8		11	2 - 5	
Molybdenum(μg/d)	45	45 (50)		2,000	50-100	
Nickel (mg/d)	ND			1.0	ND	
Selenium (μg/d)	55	55 (60)		400	30-70	
Zinc (mg/dl)	11	8 (11)		40	10	
Sodium (mg/d) Chloride (mg/d) Potassium (mg/d) Calcium (mg/d)	1,500 2300 4,700 1,000	1000 (1,000) >70y	1200	2,500	550 (minimum) 830 (min.) 2,000 (min.) 1,000	
Magnesium (mg/d) Phosphorus (mg/dl)	400 700	320 (350) 700		350 3,500	350-400 700	310(310)

◻ **Table 12.5** Recommendation for liquid and pureed diet according 1100 kcal – recomandation University of Freiburg, Medical Center, Department of nutrition and dietetics S. Schmitting-Ulrich, 2009]

breakfast - soup consisting of:		
200	ml	milk low-fat
10	gram	Instant oat-flour or semolina
		crème consisting of:
100	gram	yoghurt low-fat
150	gram	Fresh fruits
lunch - soup consisting of:		
100	gram	mince meat (Beef)
100	gram	Vegetables
100	gram	potatoes
50	ml	vegetable – or meat stock
1	teaspoon	Oil
Curd of fruits:		
100	gram	curd low-fat
150	gram	Fresh fruits
supper - soup consisting of:		
1	piece	Egg
100	gram	Vegetable
100	gram	potatoes
50	ml	vegetable – or meat stock
2	teaspoon	Oil
250	ml	buttermilk

Purée everything; flavour optional

The composition is low caloric (1100 kcal/d) and rich in protein (70g/d)); because of deficits in micronutrients 1tablet of vitamins and trace minerals should be added

Literature

1. Folope V, M-F Hellot, J-M Kuhn, P Ténière, M Scotté and PO Déchelotte. Weight loss and quality of life after bariatric surgery: a study of 200 patients after vertical gastroplasty or adjustable gastric banding. European Journal of Clinical Nutrition (2008) 62, 1022-1030
2. Bloomsberg RD, Fleishman A, Nalle JE, et al. Nutritional deficiencies following bariatric surgery: what have we learned ?. Obes Surg 2005; 15:145.
3. Tomé D. Protéines alimentaires. In: Basdevant A, Laville M, Lerebours E, editors. Traité de nutrition clinique de l'adulte. 2001. p. 121-30 (Paris).
4. Poitou-Bernert C, Ciangura C, Coupaye M et al. Nutritional deficiency after gastric bypass: diagnosis, prevention and treatment. Diabetes & Metabolism 33 (2007) 13-24
5. Sundbom M, Mardh E, Mardh S, Ohrvall M, Gustavsson S. Reduction in serum pepsinogen I after Roux-en Y gastric bypass. J Gastrointest Surg 2003; 7:529-35
6. Kushner R. Managing the obese patient after bariatric surgery: a case report of severe malnutrition and reciew of the literature. JPEN J Parenter Enteral Nutr 2000; 24:126-32
7. Skroubis G, Sakellaropoulos G, Pouggouras K, Mead N, Nikiforidis G, Kalfarentzos F. Comparison of nutritional deficiencies after Roux-en-Y gastric bypass and after biliopancreatic diversion with Roux-en Y gastric bypass. Obes Surg 2002; 12:551-8
8. Lerebours E, Savoye G, Ducrotte T. Physiologie du tube digestif. In: Physiologie du tube digestif. 2001. p. 35-44.
9. Cummings S Case study: A patient with diabetes and weight-loss surgery. 2007 spectrum.diabetes journals.org
10. Ponsky TA, Brody F, Pucci E. Alterations in gastrointestinal physiology after Roux-en-Y gastric bypass. J Am Coll Surg 2005; 201:125-31.
11. Suter PM, Checkliste Ernährung; Georg Thieme Verlag 3. Edition 2008
12. Deutsche Gesellschaft für Ernährung, Österreichische gesellschaft für Ernährung, Schweizerische Gesellschaft für Ernährungsforschung, Schweizerische Vereinigung für Ernährung (D-A-CH). Referenzwerte für die Nährstoffzufuhr. 3. Auflage Frankfurt, Umschau Braus GmbH 2008
13. Gubler, CJ. Thiamin. In: Handbook of vitamins: Nutritional, biochemical, and clinical aspects, Machlin, LJ (Ed), Marcel Dekker, New York 1984. p.245.
14. Chaves LC, Faintuch J, Kahwage,S, Alencar Fde A. A cluster of polyneuropathy and Wernicke-Korsakoff syndrome in a bariatric unit. Obes Surg 2002; 12:328–334
15. Sales-Salvado J, Garcia-Lorda P, Cuatrecasas G, et al. Wernicke's syndrome after bariatric surgery. Clin Nutr 2000; 19:371-3.
16. Towbin A, Inge TH, Garcia VF, et al. Beriberi after gastric bypass surgery in adolescence. J Pediatr 2004; 145:263–267
17. Food and Nutrition Board-Institute of Medicine. Dietary reference intakes. National Academy Press, Washington DC 1997,1998, 2000, 2001.
18. Wilson, JA. Vitamin deficiency and excess. In: Harrison's principlesof internal medicine Harrison's Principles of Internal Medicine, 14th edition, Fauci, AS, Braunwald, E, Isselbacher, K, (Eds) et al, McGraw-Hill, New York 1998.p. 481.
19. Prousky, JE. Pellagra may bea rare secondary complication of anorexia nervosa: a systematic review of the literature. Altern Med Rev 2003; 8:180–185
20. Brolin RE, Gorman JH, Gorman RC, et al. Are vitamin B12 and folate deficiency clinically important after Roux-en-Y gastric bypass? J Gastrointest Surg 1998; 436-42
21. Brolin RE. Gastric bypass. Surg Clin North Am 2001; 81:1077-95
22. Jacob, R. Vitamin C. In: Modern nutrition in health and disease, Shils, M, Olson, J, Shike, M, Ross, AC (Eds), Lippincott, Philadelphia 2000. p. 467.
23. Janczewska, I, Ericzon, BG, Eriksson, LS. Influence of orthotopic liver transplantation on serum vitamin A levels in patients with chronic liver disease. Scand J Gastroenterol 1995; 30:68–71
24. Ginde AA, Mansbach JM, Camargo CA Jr. Association between serum 25-hydroxyvitamin D level and upper respiratory tract infection in the Third National Health and Nutrition Examination Survey. Arch Intern Med. 2009 23;169:384-90.

25. Newbury L, Dolan K, Hatzifotis M et al. Calcium and vitamin D depletion and elevated parathyroid hormone following bilio-pancreatic diversion. Obes Surg 2003; 13:893-5.

26. Goode LR, Brolin RE, Chowdhury HA, Shapses SA. Bone and gastric bypass surgery: effects of dietary calcium and vitamin D. Obes Res 2004; 12:40-7.

27. Kumar, N. Nutritional neuropathies. Neurol Clin 2007; 25:209.

28. Still, CD. Management of morbid obesity: before and after surgery: the team approach to management. J Fam Pract 2005; Suppl: S18.

29. Ludwig K, Schneider-Koriath S, Prinz C, Bernhardt J. Nachsorge und Supplementation nach Adipositaschirurgie. Adipositas 2008;2:26-30

30. Presutti, RJ, Gorman, RS, Swain, JM. Primary care perspective on bariatric surgery. Mayo ClinProc 2004; 79: 1158.

31. Von Drygalksi A and Andris DA. Anemia after bariatric surgery: more than just iron deficiency. Nutr Clin Pract 2009; 24:217-226

32. Kumpf VJ, Slocum K, Binkley J and Jensen G. Nutrition in clinical practice 2007; 22: 673-678

33. Malone M. Recommended nutritional support supplements for bariatric surgery The annals of pharmacotherapy 2008; 42: 1851-1858

34. Kalfarentzos F, Kechagias I, Soulikia K et al. Weight loss following vertical banded gastroplasty: intermediate results of a prospective study. Obes Surg 11, 2001, 265-270.

35. MacLean LD, Rhode BM, Shizgal HM. Nutrition following gastric operations for morbid obesity. Ann Surg. 1983, 347-355.

36. Seehra H, MacDermott N, Lascelles RG, Taylor TV. Wernicke's encephalopathy after vertical banded gastroplasty for morbid obesity. BMJ. 1996 17;312:434

37. Houdent C, Verger N, Courtois H et al. Wernick's encephalopathy after vertical banded gastroplasty for morbid obestity. Rev Med Interne 2003, 24; 476-477.

38. Quar Bozbora A, Coskun H, Ozarmagan S, Erbil Y, Ozbey N, Orham Y (2000). A rare complication of adjustable gastric banding: Wernicke's encephalopathy. Obes Surg 10, 274-275.

39. Lannelli A, Dainese R, Piche T et al. Laparascopic gastrectomy for morbid obesity. World j Gastroenterol 2008; 14:821-827

40. Johnson JM, Maher JW, DeMaria EJ et al. The Long-term Effects of Gastric Bypass on Vitamin D Metabolism. Ann Surg. 2006;243:701-705.

41. De Prisco C & Levine SN. Metabolic bone disease after gastric bypass surgery for obesity. Am J Med Sci 2005; 329:57–61

42. Coates PS, Fernstrom JD, Fernstrom MH, et al. Gastric bypass surgery for morbid obesity leads to an aincrease in bone turnover and a decrease in bone mass. J Clin Endocrinol Metab 2004; 89:1061–1065

43. Singh S, Kumar A. Wernicke encephalopathy after obesity surgery: a systematic review. Neurology 2007; 68:615–616

44. Prager G, Langer F. Chirurgische Therapie der Adipositas. Möglichkeiten und Grenzen. Der Diabetologe 2006; 3: 243-249

45. Gasteyger C, Suter M, Gaillard RC, et al. Nutritional deficiencies after Roux-en-Y gastric bypass for morbid obesity often cannot be prevented by standard multivitamin supplementation. Am J Clin Nutr 2008; 87: 1128-33

46. Ledoux, S, Msika, S, Moussa, F, et al. Comparison of nutritional consequences of conventional therapy of obesity, adjustable gastric banding, and gastric bypass. Obes Surg 2006; 16:1041–1049

47. Love AL, Billett HH. Obesity, bariatric surgery, and iron deficiency: true, true, ture and related. Am J Hematol 2008; 83:403–409

48. Scopinaro N, Gianetta E, Adami GF et al. Biliopancreatic diversion for obesity at eighteen years. Surgery. 1996; 119:261-8.

49. Dolan K, Hatzifotis M, Newbury L et al. A clinical and nutritional comparison of biliopancreatic diversion with and without duodenal switch. Ann Surg. 2004;240:51-6

50. Scopinaro N, Adami GF, Marinari GM et al. Biliopancreatic diversion.World J Surg. 1998; 22:936-46.

51. Slater GH, Ren CJ, Siegel N et al. Serum fat-soluble vitamin deficiency and abnormal calcium metabolism after malabsorptive bariatric surgery. J Gastrointest Surg 2004; 8:48-55

52. Leitzmann C in Huth K, Kluthe R Lehrbuch der Ernährungstherapie Georg Thieme Verlah Stuttgart New York 1995, 1-49

53. Decker GA, Swain JM, Crowell MD Gastrointestinal and Nutritional Complications after Bariatric Surgery. Am J Gastroenterol 2007; 102:2571-2580

II Preoperative Evaluation and Indications for Surgery

Psychological and Psychiatric Contraindications

Claus Michael Gross, MD, Ludger Tebartz van Elst, MD

13

Challenges of Anesthesia

Heike Kaltofen, MD

The anesthesiologist will care for an increasing number of obese patients undergoing bariatric surgery. However, anesthesia for bariatric surgery is challenging and must take into account the specific pathophysiology, co-morbidities, and related complications of obesity, as morbid obesity is an independent determinant of death among surgical critically ill patients. Progress in anesthesia knowledge and techniques contributes essentially to a safe perioperative management of the patient presenting for bariatric surgery [1-6].

14.1 Risk Assessment

Data regarding the safety and risk of bariatric surgery are limited. The reported in-hospital mortality for bariatric surgery is 0.1–0.2%; pulmonary complications occur in 4–7%, cardiac complications in 1.0–1.4% of patients [7]. Obese patients have a greater prevalence of co-morbidities such as coronary artery disease, hypertension, type-2 diabetes, steatohepatitis, sleep apnea, and pulmonary hypertension elevating their perioperative risk [8]. Bariatric surgery should thus be considered intermediate- to high-risk noncardiac surgery [9]. However, obesity alone does not seem to be a risk factor for postoperative complications [10]. Childhood obesity as well is associated with a number of medical co-morbidities including type-2 diabetes, asthma, sleep apnea, and heart disease. A recent study revealed a greater incidence of difficult mask ventilation, airway obstruction, bronchospasm, major oxygen desaturation, and overall critical respiratory events in these patients compared with non-obese children, but there were no serious sequelae [11]. Pulmonary embolism is a leading cause of perioperative mortality in bariatric surgery. Risk factors for thromboembolism include history of a prior thromboembolic event, central fat distribution, smoking, female gender, age, venous insufficiency, sleep apnea, hypercoagulable state, and use of oral contraceptives [12]. Patients at highest risk may profit from preoperative placement of inferior cava filters [13].

14.2 Pathophysiological Changes

14.2.1 Pulmonary Function

Oxygen consumption and carbon dioxide production are increased in the obese, owing to the metabolic activity of the excess fat and the increased workload on supportive tissues. In consequence, the minute ventilation rate is increased [14]. The work of breathing is increased, because more energy must be expended to carry the body mass, while the respiratory muscle function is impaired. Mor-

bid obesity is associated with an exponentially decreasing functional residual capacity (FRC), expiratory reserve volume, and total lung capacity [15]. The residual volume usually is not affected. In the supine position, the expiratory reserve volume can fall below the closing volume, resulting in gas trapping with ventilation- perfusion mismatch, shunting, and hypoxemia. Anesthesia is a further aggravation, such that a 50% reduction in observed FRC occurs in the anesthetized obese patient compared with a 20% fall in the non-obese subject [16]. The addition of positive end-expiratory pressure (PEEP) to the ventilation achieves an improvement in both FRC and arterial oxygen tension, but only at the expense of cardiac output and oxygen delivery [17, 18]. Increased pulmonary blood volume and increased chest wall mass from adipose tissue lead to a reduced compliance of the respiratory system. Abnormal diaphragm position and upper airway resistance increase the work of breathing [19].

14.2.2 Obstructive Sleep Apnea

Undiagnosed obstructive sleep apnea (OSA) is very common in severely obese patients. More than 70% of persons presenting for bariatric surgery were found by polysomnography to have sleep apnea [20, 21]. Risk factors for OSA and clinical signs are male gender, increased neck circumference (men >44 cm / women >41 cm), visceral obesity, snoring, and daytime fatigue. The final diagnosis can be obtained by polysomnography, but to date no study has confirmed a reduced perioperative risk when polysomnography is performed prior to surgery. The major pathophysiological consequences of severe sleep apnea include arterial hypoxemia, recurrent arousals from sleep, increased sympathetic tone, pulmonary and systemic hypertension, and cardiac arrhythmias. Possible mechanisms include hyperleptinemia, insulin resistance, elevated angiotensin II and aldosterone levels, oxidative and inflammatory stress, impaired baroreflex function, and endothelial dysfunction [22]. Magnetic resonance imaging shows that obesity causes OSA by deposition of adipose tissue into pharyngeal tissues, predominantly the lateral pharyngeal walls [23]. In addition, the extraluminal pressure is increased by superficially located fat masses, leading to external compression of the upper airway [24]. Several studies confirm an increased risk of difficult tracheal intubation [25, 26]. Failed intubation occurs in as many as 5% of attempted cases [24]. Patients with OSA may be very sensitive to sedative medications. Such commonly used anesthetic drugs as propofol, thiopental, opioids, benzodiazepines, and even small doses of neuromuscular blocking agents are proven to cause pharyngeal collapse [27]. Even minimal sedation may cause respiratory arrest. Premedication agents should be avoided. Immediate postoperative complications may be attributed to the negative effects of sedative, analgesic, and anesthetic drugs on pharyngeal tone and on the arousal responses to hypoxia, hypercarbia, and upper airway obstruction.

14.2.3 Obesity Hypoventilation Syndrome

The obesity hypoventilation syndrome is defined as an elevated arterial carbon dioxide tension (>45 mmHg) while awake and daytime hypoxemia (<65 mmHg) in association with a BMI >30 kg/m2. The absence of another pulmonary or neuromuscular disease should be confirmed [28]. The syndrome is characterized by somnolence, cardiac enlargement, hypoxemia, hypercarbia, and polycythemia; 85% of cases are associated with OSA. Hypoventilation is caused by central desensitization of the respiratory center to hypercarbia. These patients rely on hypoxic drive for ventilation and are at increased perioperative risk for respiratory failure and pulmonary embolism [14, 29, 30]. Pulmonary hypertension and right heart failure are typical cardiovascular complications. The exact underlying pathophysiological conditions of the obesity hypoventilation syndrome are still unclear.

14.2.4 Pulmonary Hypertension

Data concerning the association of obesity per se and pulmonary hypertension are conflicting [31–33]. Many morbidly obese patients, however, have concomitant cardiopulmonary risk including OSA, increased risk of thromboembolic disease, and use of anorexic drugs. Thus, they are prone to develop pulmonary hypertension [34, 35]. Common symptoms of pulmonary hypertension include exertional dyspnea, fatigue, and syncope. These clinical signs reflect an inability to increase cardiac output during activity [36]. The most useful confirmation of the diagnosis is made by echocardiography showing tricuspid regurgitation and right ventricular impairment [37].

14.2.5 Airway Assessment

Difficult tracheal intubation seems to be more frequent in obese than in lean patients [38]. Increased BMI per se, however, is not a valid predictor of difficult intubation [39]. Predictors of difficult laryngoscopy in obese patients are neck circumference >43 cm at the level of the thyroid cartilage, Mallampati score ≥3, short thyromental distance (<6 cm), and the presence of obstructive sleep apnea [38, 40]. Magnetic resonance imaging measurements and ultrasonographic investigations demonstrated fat deposits in the anterior neck and in areas surrounding the collapsible segments of the pharynx as risk factors for difficult airway management [41, 42].

14.2.6 Cardiovascular System

Endocrine and metabolic abnormalities contribute to the development of arterial hypertension, cardiovascular disease, and heart failure. Common features include activation of the renin-angiotensin system, stimulation of the sympathetic nervous system, increased blood volume and raised cardiac output, proinflammatory and prothrombotic properties. Since the heart rate is normal in obesity, an increase in stroke volume is responsible for the change in cardiac output [43]. Increased stroke volume will result in increased end-diastolic volume and pressure, leading primarily to eccentric hypertrophy in the absence of hypertension. Thus, left ventricular hypertrophy and diastolic dysfunction of the left ventricle are commonly present [44]. Left atrial dilatation may mediate the excess risk of atrial fibrillation associated with obesity [45]. The risk of developing heart failure correlates with the BMI [46]. Associated OSA may cause pulmonary hypertension and resulting right ventricular impairment [23].

14.2.7 Gastrointestinal Changes

Particularly in patients with an android fat distribution, there is an increase of intraperitoneal and omental fat masses. The result may be an elevated intra-abdominal pressure leading to reduced perfusion of the intra-abdominal tissues, especially in the perioperative setting. Renal impairment is not uncommon in the patient undergoing bariatric surgery. The prevalence of fatty liver is up to 90%. The liver may be enlarged, thus making bariatric surgery more difficult. Inflammatory processes may lead to significant liver cirrhosis. Obesity is an important risk factor for type-2 diabetes, often associated with severe insulin resistance and the metabolic syndrome [47].

14.3 Preoperative Evaluation

All admitted patients should have their height and weight recorded and their BMI calculated. Preoperative assessment should be obtained according to the American Society of Anesthesiologists (ASA) routine advisory on preanesthesia evaluation [48]. Extensive routine preoperative testing is not necessary for every obese patient undergoing bariatric surgery [49]. Assessment of the airway should include head and neck flexion, jaw mobility and mouth opening, measure of thyromental distance and neck circumference, inspection of oropharynx and dentition, inspection of previous anesthesia records, and a systematic enquiry concerning OSA [14]. Patients with suspicion of obesity hypoventilation syndrome should be screened by room air pulse oximetry. If the O_2 saturation is below 96%, an arterial blood gas analysis should be obtained in order to look at possible CO_2 retention. Echocardiography seems prudent in patients with a history of thromboembolic disease, exertional dyspnea, anorectic drug use, or OSA. Despite expected known pathological findings, spirometry is of no added value in these patients, unless COPD is suspected [34]. In these patients, a reagibility of the bronchial system to β_2-sympathicomimetics should be tested. If appropriate, a bronchodilator therapy should be started for several weeks in order to reduce the rate of perioperative pulmonary complications. Patients suspicious for OSA should be evaluated by polysomnography and may benefit preoperatively from nocturnal continuous positive airway pressure (CPAP). Pre-anesthesia cardiac evaluation should be focused on signs of right and left ventricular dysfunction, ischemic heart disease, and arterial hypertension. According to the guidelines of the American College of Cardiology and the American Heart Association, patients presenting for bariatric surgery should have an ECG based upon age and the presence of concomitant medical illnesses rather than on obesity per se [48, 50]. A history of chest pain and shortness of breath should be evaluated by further preoperative cardiologic testing (i.e., echocardiography, radionucleotide imaging, stress testing, coronary artery angiography) [9]. However, cardiologic investigations may be limited by the body mass of the obese patient. Morbidly obese patients have a high incidence of type-2 diabetes. They should be assessed for the adequacy of glucose control and also for the presence of co-morbidities due to diabetes. Dietary advice and careful glucose control perioperatively may reduce complications such as infection or ketoacidosis [51]. Preoperative minimum laboratory testing of hematocrit, glucose, creatinine, and urea is recommended [52]. Further testing of liver function parameters and evaluation of the thyroid function may be useful if dysfunction is suspected clinically.

14.4   Premedication

The patient's usual medication should be continued until surgery, with the exception of (a) oral antidiabetics, because of the risk of hypoglycemia, and (b)

ACEinhibitors/ AT2-receptor-antagonists, which should be stopped, since their presence can lead to profound hypotension during anesthesia. Blood sugar must be monitored closely. Because of the high prevalence of OSA in these patients, the risk of upper airway obstruction should be avoided by omitting a sedative agent in the preoperative setting. If anxiolysis is essential, oral benzodiazepines should be administered carefully while oxygen saturation is monitored by pulse oximetry. Pharmacologic intervention with H2-receptor antagonists, nonparticulate antacids, or proton pump inhibitors will reduce gastric volume and acidity, thereby reducing the risk of aspiration of gastric contents [53]. Prophylaxis with antibiotics is recommended because of the increased incidence of wound infection. The choice of antibiotic should be discussed with the surgeon and a microbiologist, if appropriate [14]. Morbidly obese patients are at increased risk of thromboembolism and should receive prophylactic low-molecular-weight heparin until they are fully mobile in the postoperative phase. Antithrombotic stockings or pneumatic leggings should be used, if possible. Vagolytic medication may be useful to reduce saliva secretions if fiberoptic bronchoscopic intubation is considered.

14.5   Monitoring/Vascular Access

Most bariatric operations are performed via laparoscopic access. Basic monitoring includes electrocardiography, pulse oximetry, measurement of noninvasive blood pressure, capnography, and monitoring of neuromuscular function. In many morbidly obese patients, accurate noninvasive measurement of blood pressure is impossible due to the conical shape of the upper arm. Falsely high blood pressure values can be measured by cuffs too small for the arm. Alternative sites are the wrist or ankle, if special cuffs are available [54]. Cannulation of the radial artery should be considered and is generally easy to achieve, as the artery normally is palpable even in morbidly obese patients. An arterial line is useful not only for accurate blood pressure monitoring but also for perioperative arterial blood gas sampling. A large-bore peripheral venous cannula should be inserted. Obtaining adequate venous access can be difficult; the dorsum of the hand and the flexor side of the forearm are the best options. In case of limited venous access, a central line may be required for surgery and postoperative needs. Central lines are useful in cardiopulmonary compromised patients and for major laparotomy. It can be difficult to gain access to the central veins due to obscured landmarks and increased depth of insertion. Ultrasound guidance seems to reduce the risk of failed catheter placement and complications [55, 56]. A second person can help by retracting the adipose tissues of the breast away from the neck in order to gain better anatomical conditions.

14.6   Anesthetic Drugs in Obese Patients

Drug dosing is generally based on the volume of distribution for the loading dose and on the clearance for maintenance. The volume of distribution is increased in the obese patient if the drug is distributed in both lean and fat tissues, whereas the renal drug clearance is usually normal or increased. Distribution volume is influenced by composition of tissues, regional blood flow, and protein binding capacity. Obesity leads to increased lean body mass and a greater fat body mass. Several formulas exist to estimate the ideal body weight, which is valuable for dosing weak lipophilic drugs. A practicable method of calculation could be the formula from Lemmens et al. [57]: ideal body weight (IBW) = 22 x H2 (height in meters). Adding 20% to the calculated IBW dose of a hydrophilic drug includes the amount necessary to be applied for the increased lean mass of obese patients [53]. Thiopental and benzodiazepines are lipophilic drugs and should be administered according to the total body mass because of the increased volume of distribution, but prolonged action time is to be expected [58, 59]. Propofol is a highly lipophilic drug with rapid onset and a short, predictable duration of action. Following continuous administration for sedation, there is no delay in emergence compared with non-obese patients [60]. The induction and maintenance-dose regimen of propofol should be estimated based on total body weight [61]. Succinylcholine is recommended for rapid sequence induction in the obese patient, if there are no contraindications. A dose of 1 mg/kg total body weight provides adequate neuromuscular blockade for acceptable laryngoscopy conditions within 1 min [62]. Non-depolarizing relaxants are hydrophilic drugs and should be administered based on IBW + 20% of the estimated dose (i.e., lean body mass). Rocuronium, administered in a dose estimated on the basis of total body weight, results in prolonged action time [63]. If non-depolarizing muscle relaxants are dosed based upon IBW, there are no significant differences in pharmacokinetics and pharmacodynamics compared with non-obese persons [64, 65]. The new volatile anesthetics desflurane and sevoflurane have low lipid solubility and have been suggested to be the volatile agents of choice for obese patients because of their rapid recovery profile [66, 67]. Desflurane would appear to be the first choice,

because recovery time in unpremedicated obese patients is significantly faster than in patients treated with sevoflurane, and the oxygen saturation seems to be higher at the time of entry to the post-anesthesia care unit. This advantage of desflurane persists for up to 2 h after surgery and is associated with earlier mobilization of the patient [66, 68, 69]. Another advantage of desflurane concerns the very low metabolism rate, as higher fluoride serum concentrations are reported following sevoflurane anesthesia in obese patients. However, no renal dysfunction has been described [61]. Synthetic opioids, such as fentanyl, alfentanil, sufentanil, and remifentanil, are widely used for anesthesia of the obese patient. They all are very lipophilic drugs, theoretically suggesting that the loading dose should be estimated based on total body weight. However, significantly slower elimination rates require careful dosing according to lean body mass [61, 70]. In any case, the risk of postoperative respiratory depression and hypoxemia should be kept in mind. The volume of distribution of remifentanil is less than expected, probably because of rapid metabolism by blood and tissue esterases [71]. Remifentanil should be dosed based upon ideal body weight.

14.7   Patient Positioning

Specially designed operating tables may be required for very obese patients. Once the patient has moved himself onto the table, particular attention should be paid to protecting pressure areas, as the risk of neural injuries is greater in the obese [72]. Compression of the inferior vena cava should be avoided with a left lateral tilt of the operating table. Pre-oxygenation should be performed in a reversed Trendelenburg position at 25–30°, as this prolongs the time to desaturation during apnea [73, 74]. The morbidly obese patient should be placed with her head, upper body, and shoulders significantly elevated above the chest; this can be achieved by placing folded blankets under the upper body, neck, and head of the patient. This position provides better conditions for mask ventilation and laryngoscopy [75].

14.8   Induction of Anesthesia

The obese patient presents with an increased intrapulmonary shunt and a reduced functional residual capacity. Apnea results in a much more rapid arterial desaturation than would be the case in non-obese patients. Pre-oxygenation time should be at least 5 min [47]. Application of consequent continuous positive airway pressure (10 cm

H_2O) until the trachea is intubated increases nonhypoxic apnea tolerance by 50% [76]. Obesity is one of many factors contributing to the risk of gastric aspiration during anesthesia [77]. There are conflicting data concerning the risk of gastroesophageal reflux in obese patients [78, 79]. On the other hand, obese patients are at risk of difficult airway management. A rapid sequence technique remains important in obese patients with symptomatic reflux, diabetes mellitus, or gastrointestinal disorders but is debatable in fasted patients without additional risk [80]. Adequate depth of anesthesia and muscle relaxation during induction are essential, because coughing or straining are major factors contributing to the risk of pulmonary aspiration. The use of cricoid pressure has been questioned recently [81, 82]; its efficiency in preventing pulmonary aspiration has not yet been proven in a randomized controlled study. In case of worsened intubation conditions, cricoid pressure should be released to facilitate tracheal intubation. If rapid sequence induction is required, succinylcholine remains the neuromuscular blocking agent of choice because of its short duration of action in the presence of suspected difficult airway management [80].

14.9 Airway Management

Airway management of the obese patient can be challenging. A BMI >26 kg/m² is a strong predictor of higher risk of difficult mask ventilation [83]. Upper airway obstruction and reduced compliance of the respiratory system are reasons for difficult mask ventilation. In addition, morbidly obese patients are at increased risk of difficult tracheal intubation [84], although tracheal intubation and positive pressure ventilation are mandatory. The choice between awake fiberoptic intubation and conventional asleep intubation depends upon the experience of the anesthesiologist, who should take into account the previously described predictors of difficult airway management. Alternative difficult airway devices – for example video-laryngoscope, Bullard laryngoscope, intubating laryngeal mask, ProSeal laryngeal mask, tracheal esophageal combitube, and the laryngeal tube – should be available for temporary ventilation [85]. Cricothyrotomy and tracheostomy are often difficult to carry out because of the subcutaneous adipose tissues of the neck and anatomical distortion of the trachea.

14.10 Mechanical Ventilation during Anesthesia

Hypoxemia during mechanical ventilation in obese patients is mediated, at least in part, through unopposed increases in intra-abdominal pressure that reduce lung volumes, resulting in ventilation-perfusion mismatch [86]. Beach chair position and the application of PEEP 10 cm H_2O seem to improve lung volume, oxygenation, and respiratory mechanics [87]. Recruitment maneuvers followed by PEEP improve intraoperative oxygenation in morbidly obese patients, but the effect disappears immediately after extubation of the trachea [88, 89]. Delivered tidal volumes should be calculated based on ideal body weight to avoid high airway pressures, alveolar overdistention, and barotrauma. End-tidal CO_2 monitors are less reliable in predicting arterial PCO_2 because of the widened alveolo-arterial gradients present in most obese patients [90].

14.11 Laparoscopic Procedures in the Obese Patient

Most bariatric operations are carried out via the laparoscopic approach, as it is less invasive, with a reduced risk of both postoperative complications and postoperative pain. A recent study [91] compared the laparoscopic versus the open technique for Roux-en-Y and found a shorter duration of surgery, fewer wound infections, and shorter hospital stay with the laparoscopic approach. Bariatric surgery usually is performed with the patient in the reverse Trendelenburg position. Lifting the patient into the head-up position reduces venous return and cardiac output as a consequence of venous pooling in the lower limbs. The degree of intra-abdominal pressure caused by insufflation of carbon dioxide into the abdomen determines the further effect on venous return [92]. At an intra-abdominal pressure <10 mmHg, there is an increase in venous return, probably sequestered from the splanchnic region. Compression of the inferior vena cava seems to occur at a pressure >20 mmHg [92]. Possible results are splanchnic ischemia, renal impairment, and venous blood flow reduction in the lower limbs with an increased thromboembolic risk. Resorption of the insufflated carbon dioxide can lead to respiratory acidosis and activation of the sympathetic tone. Pneumoperitoneum markedly affects gas exchange and lung/chest compliance in morbidly obese patients, while positioning of the patient in a 25° reverse Trendelenburg position has no beneficial effect [93]. A recent study showed that the beach chair position and PEEP may both be used to counteract the major derangements produced by anesthesia and paralysis in morbidly obese patients. They similarly improved lung volume, oxygenation, and respiratory mechanics. During pneumoperitoneum, only the combination of the two was able to improve oxygenation [87]. Despite the known pathophysiological changes in the cardiopulmonary system, obese patients tolerate laparoscopic procedures well if appropriate cardiovascular and respiratory monitoring is used.

14.12 Regional Anesthesia

The use of combined general and epidural anesthesia is recommended for open bariatric surgery. The advantages of thoracic epidural anesthesia include improved analgesia, less respiratory depression, prevention of deep venous thrombosis, and earlier recovery of intestinal motility, but reduced mortality is not yet proven [94]. Oxygen consumption and left ventricular stroke work can be reduced [95]. Postoperative spirometry is less impaired in obese patients receiving epidural analgesia, and pulmonary recovery may be faster [96]. However, administration of epidural anesthesia for obese patients may be challenging because of difficulties in positioning of the patient and identification of anatomical landmarks. Needles must be of adequate length. An analysis of 9340 different regional blocks (including neuroaxial blocks) revealed a slightly higher rate of block failure, multiple attempts at the same block, and overdose in obese patients. Obesity was associated with a statistically significant higher rate of complications, but the overall complication rate was very low at 0.3% [97, 98]. The few data concerning regional anesthesia and obesity are gained mostly from obstetrical patients. Obese parturients experienced higher levels of epidural blockade than normal-weight obstetrical patients with identical local anesthetic doses [99]. Neuroaxial anesthesia causes significant decreases in lung volumes of spontaneously breathing obese patients [100, 101]. Further studies are warranted to evaluate the benefit and risk of regional anesthesia for bariatric surgery in particular.

14.13 Recovery and Pain Therapy

During emergence from anesthesia, there is an increased risk of hypoxia due to formation of atelectasis and upper airway obstruction [24, 102]. Another great risk of spontaneous ventilation against an obstructed airway is the rapid development of severe negative pressure pulmonary edema. Full recovery from neuromuscular blockade should be proven by a neuromuscular blockade monitor. The trachea should be extubated with the patient in a semi-upright position and fully awake. If upper airway obstruction is suspected, an oropharyngeal or nasopharyngeal airway should be kept in situ. The patient should have an adequate blood level of narcotics, as indicated by a respiratory rate of 12–14 breaths/min [24]. Obstructive sleep apnea is considered to be an indication for continuous respiratory monitoring as long as opioid analgesia is needed [103]. Continuous positive airway pressure (CPAP) devices can be used safely without increasing the risk of postoperative anastomotic leak [104]. Conversely, using bilevel positive airway pressure (BIPAP) may lead to anastomotic insufficiency [105]. An opioid-based PCA (patient-controlled intravenous analgesia) combined with local anesthetic wound infiltration and adjunct nonsteroidal anti-inflammatory analgesics in a multimodal approach is recommended as standard pain therapy for laparoscopic bariatric surgery [52]. The initial PCA dose setting should be based on estimated lean body mass. A routine use of continuous opoid background infusion should be avoided [106]. In case of open bariatric surgery, pain therapy by thoracic epidural analgesia including local anesthetics and opioids is favorable. The amount of analgesics to be administered should be calculated on the basis of estimated lean body mass. More profound analgesia and faster recovery of the bowel function are provided. In any case, the patient presenting for bariatric surgery should have access to the acute pain service of the department

References

1. Bjorntop P (1997) Obesity. Lancet 350:423–426
2. Consensus Development Conference Panel (1991) NIH conference: Gastrointestinal surgery for severe obesity. Ann Intern Med 115:956–961
3. Buchwald H, Avidor Y, Braunwald E et al (2004) Bariatric surgery: a systematic review and meta-analysis. JAMA 292:1724–1737
4. Sjöström L, Lindroos AK, Peltonen M et al (2004) Lifestyle, diabetes, and cardiovascular risk factors 10 years after bariatric surgery. N Engl J Med 351:2683–2693
5. Adams T, Gress R, Smith S et al (2007) Long-term mortality after gastric bypass surgery. N Engl J Med 357:753–761
6. Stanley A, Nasraway J; Matthew A et al (2006) Morbid obesity is an independent determinant of death among surgical critically ill patients. Crit Care Med 34:964 –970
7. Santry HP, Gillen DL, Lauderdale DS (2005) Trends in bariatric surgical procedures. JAMA 294:1909–1917
8. Mun EC, Blackburn GL, Matthews JB (2001) Current status of medical and surgical therapy for obesity. Gastroenterology 120:669–681
9. Guliotti D, Grant P, Jaber W et al (2008) Challenges in cardiac risk assessment in bariatric surgery patients. Obes Surg 18:129–133
10. Dindo D, Muller M, Weber M, Clavien P (2003) Obesity in general elective surgery. Lancet 361:2032–2035
11. Tait A, Voepel-Lewis T, Burke C, Kostrzewa A, Lewis I (2008) Incidence and risk factors for perioperative adverse respiratory events in children who are obese. Anesthesiology 108:375–380
12. Saltzman E, Anderson W, Apovian C, Boulton H, Chamberlain A, Cullum-Dugan D et al (2005) Criteria for patient selection and multidisciplinary evaluation and treatment of the weight loss surgery patient. Obes Res 13:234–243

13. Sapala JA, Wood MH, Schuhknecht MP, Sapala MA (2003) Fatal pulmonary embolism after bariatric operations for morbid obesity. A 24-year retrospective analysis. Obes Surg 13:819–825

14. Adams JP, Murphy PG (2000) Obesity in anaesthesia and intensive care. Br J Anaesth 85:91–108

15. Pelosi P, Croci M, Ravagnan I et al (1998) The effects of body mass on lung volumes, respiratory mechanics, and gas exchange during general anesthesia. Anesth Analg 87:654–660

16. Damia G, Mascheroni D, Croci M, Tarenzi L (1988) Perioperative changes in functional residual capacity in morbidly obese patients. Br J Anaesth 60:574–578

17. Pelosi P, Ravagnan I, Giurati G, Panigada M, Buttoni N, Tredici S (1999) Positive end-expiratory pressure improves respiratory function in obese but not in normal subjects during anesthesia and paralysis. Anesthesiology 91:1221–1231

18. Santesson J (1977) Oxygen transport and venous admixture in the extremely obese. Influence of anesthesia and artificial ventilation with and without positive end-expiratory pressure. Acta Anaesthesiol Scand 21:56–61

19. Pelosi P, Croci M, Ravagnan I, Vicardi P, Gattinoni L (1996) Total respiratory system,lung, and chest wall mechanics in sedated-paralyzed postoperative morbidly obese patients. Chest 109:144–151

20. Frey WC, Pilcher J (2003) Obstructive sleep-related disorders in patients evaluated for bariatric surgery. Obes Surg 13:676–683

21. Keeffe T, Patterson EJ (2004) Evidence supporting routine polysomnography before bariatric surgery. Obes Surg 14:23–26

22. Wolk R, Shamsuzzaman A, Somers VK (2003) Obesity, sleep apnoe and hypertension. Hypertension 42:1067–1074

23. Strollo PJ,Rogers RM (1996) Obstructive sleep apnoe. N Engl J Med 334:99–104

24. Benumof J (2004) Obesity, sleep apnoe, the airway and anesthesia. Curr Opin Anaesthesiol 17:21–30

25. Siyam MA, Benhamou D (2002) Difficult endotracheal intubation in patients with sleep apnoe syndrome. Anesth Analg 95:1098–1102

26. Kim JA, Lee JJ (2006) Preoperative predictors of difficult intubation in patients with obstructive sleep apnoe syndrome. Can J Anaesth 53:393–397

27. Nanddi PR, Charlesworth CH, Taylor SJ, Nunn JF, Dore CJ (1991) Effect of general anaesthesia on the pharynx. Br J Anaesth 66:157–162

28. Olson AL, Zwillich C (2005) The obesity hypoventilation syndrome. Am J Med 118:948–956

29. Teichtahl H (2001) The obesity-hypoventilation syndrome revisited. Chest 120:336–339

30. DeMaria EJ, Portenier D, Wolfe L (2007) Obesity surgery mortality risk score to predict mortality risk in patients undergoing gastric bypass. Surg Obes Relat Dis 3:134–140

31. Sajkov D, Wang T, Saunders NA et al Daytime pulmonary hemodynamics in patients with obstructive sleep apnea without lung disease. Am J Respir Crit Care Med 1999 159:1518–1526

32. Sanner BM, Doberauer C, Konermann M et al (1997) Pulmonary hypertension in patients with obstructive sleep apnoea syndrome. Arch Intern Med 157:2483–2487

33. Bady E, Achkar A, Pascal S et al (2000) Pulmonary arterial hypertension in patients with sleep apnoea syndrome. Thorax 55:934–939

34. Michelakis ED, Weir FK (2001) Anorectic drugs and pulmonary hypertension from the bedside to the bench. Am J Med Sci 21:292–299

35. Kaw R, Aboussouan L, Auckley D et al (2008) Challenges in pulmonary risk assessment and perioperative management in bariatric surgery patients. Obes Surg 18:134–138

36. Nauser TD, Stites SW (2001) Diagnosis and treatment of pulmonary hypertension. Am Fam Physician 63:1789–1798

37. Schiller NB (1990) Pulmonary artery pressure estimation by Doppler and two-dimensional echocardiography. Cardiol Clin 8:277–287

38. Gonzalez H, Minnville V, Delanoue K, Mazerolles M, Concina D,Fourcade O (2008) The importance of increased neck circumference to intubation difficulties in obese patients. Anesth Analg 106:1132–1136

39. Ezri T, Medalion B, Weisenberg M et al (2003) Increased body mass index per se is not a predictor of difficult laryngoscopy. Can J Anaesth 50:179–183

40. Brodsky J, Lemmens H, Brock-Utne J, Vierra M, Saidman L (2002) Morbid obesity and tracheal intubation. Anesth Analg 94:732–736

41. Horner DD, Mohiaddin RH, Lowell DG et al (1989) Sites and sizes of fat deposits around the pharynx in obese patients with obstructive sleep apnoea and weight-matched controls. Eur Resp J 2:613–622

42. Ezri T, Gewürtz G, Sessler DI et al (2003) Prediction of difficult laryngoscopy in obese patients by ultrasound quantification of anterior neck soft tissue. Anaesthesia 58:1111–1114

43. De Divitiis O, Fazio S, Petitto M, Maddalena G, Contaldo F, Mancini M (1981) Obesity and cardiac function. Circulation 64:477–482

44. Govindarajan G, Alpert M, Tejwani L (2008) Endocrine and metabolic effects of fat: cardiovascular implications. Am J Med 121:366–370

45. Wang TJ, Parise H, Levy D et al (2004) Obesity and the risk of new-onset atrial fibrillation. JAMA 292:2471–2477

46. Kenchaiah S, Evans J, Levy D et al (2002) Obesity and the risk of heart failure. N Engl J Med 347:305–313

47. Bellamy M, Struys M (eds) (2007) Anesthesia for the overweight and obese patient. Oxford University Press, Oxford, pp 25–28

48. Task Force on Preanesthesia Evaluation (2002) Practice advisory for preanesthesia evaluation. Anesthesiology 96:485–496

49. Ramaswamy A, Gonzales R, Smith CD (2004) Extensive preoperative testing is not necessary in morbidly obese patients undergoing gastric bypass. J Gastrointest Surg 89:159–164

50. Eagle KA, Berger PB, Calkins H et al (2002) ACC/AHA guideline update for perioperative cardiovascular evaluation for noncardiac surgery. Circulation 105:1257–1267

51. The Association of Anaesthesists of Great Britain and Ireland (2007) Peri-operative management of the morbidly obese patient. AAGBI, London

52. Schumann R, Jones S, Ortiz V et al (2005) Best practice recommendations for anesthetic perioperative care and pain management in weight loss surgery. Obes Res 13:254–266

53. Ogunnaike B, Jones S, Jones D, Provost D, Whitten C (2002) Anesthetic considerations for bariatric surgery. Anesth Analg 95:1793–1805

54. Emerick DR (2002) An evaluation of non-invasive blood pressure (NIBP) monitoring on the wrist: comparison with upper arm NIBP measurement. Anaesth Intensive Care 30:43–47

55. Hind D, Calvert N, McWilliams R et al (2003) Ultrasonic locating devices for central venous canulation: meta-analysis. BMJ 327:361

56. Jefferson P, Ball DR (2002) Central venous access in morbidly obese patients. Anesth Analg 95:782

57. Lemmens,HJ,Bernstein DP, Brodsky JB (2005) Estimating ideal body weight – new formula. Obes Surg 15:1082–1083

58. Jung D, Mayersohn M,Perrier D et al (1982) Thiopental disposition in lean and obese patients undergoing surgery. Anesthesiology 56:269–274

14

59. Greenblatt DJ, Abernethy DR, Locniskar A et al (1984) Effect of age, gender, and obesity on midazolam kinetics. Anesthesiology 62:27–35

60. Servin F, Farinotti R, Haberer JP, Desmonts JM (1993) Propofol infusion for maintenance of anesthesia in morbidly obese patients receiving nitrous oxide. A clinical and pharmacokinetic study. Anesthesiology 78:657–665

61. Casati A, Putzu M (2005) Anesthesia in the obese patient: pharmacokinetic considerations. J Clin Anesth 17:134–145

62. Lemmens HJ, Brodsky JB (2006) The dose of succinylcholine in morbid obesity. Anesth Analg 102:438–442

63. Leykin Y, PellisT, Lucca M, Lomangino G, Marzano B, Gullo A (2004) The pharmacodynamic effects of rocuronium when dosed according to real body weight or total body weight in morbidly obese patients. Anesth Analg 99:1086–1089

64. Varin F, Ducharme J, Theoret Y, Besner JG, Bevan DR, Donati F (1990) Influence of extreme obesity on the body disposition and neuromuscular blocking effect of atracurium. Clin Pharmacol Ther 48:18–25

65. Schwartz AE, Matteo RS, Ornstein E, Halevy JD, Diaz J (1992) Pharmacokinetics and pharmacodynamics of vecuronium in the obese surgical patient. Anesth Analg 74:515–518

66. Juvin P, Vadam C, Malek L, Dupont H,Marmuse JP,Desmonts JM (2000) Postoperative recovery after desflurane,propofol, or isoflurane anesthesia among morbidly obese patients. A prospective randomized study. Anesth Analg 91:714–719

67. Torri G, Casati A, Albertin A et al (2001) Randomized comparison of isoflurane and sevoflurane for laparoscopic gastric banding in morbidly obese patients. J Clin Anesth 13:565–570

68. La Colla L, Albertin A, La Colla G, Mangano A (2007) Faster wash-out and recovery for desflurane vs sevoflurane in morbidly obese patients when no premedication is used. Br J Anesth 99:353–358

69. Strum EM, Szenohradszki J, Kaufman WA, Anthone GJ, Manz IL, Lumb PD (2004) Emergence and recovery characteristics of desflurane versus sevoflurane in morbidly obese adult surgical patients: a prospective, randomized study. Anesth Analg 99:1848–1853

70. Schwartz AE, Matteo RS, Ornstein E, Young WL, Myers KJ (1991) Pharmacokinetics of sufentanil in obese patients. Anesth Analg 73:790–793

71. Egan TD, Huizinga B, Gupta SK et al (1998) Remifentanil pharmacokinetics in obese versus lean patients. Anesthesiology 89:562–573

72. Warner MA, Warner ME, Martin JT (1994) Ulnar neuropathy: incidence, outcome, and risk factors in sedated or anesthetized patients. Anesthesiology 81:1332–1340

73. Altermatt FR, Munoz HR, Delfino AE, Cortinez LI (2005) Pre-oxygenation in the obese patient: effects of position on tolerance to apnoea. B J Anaesth 95:706–709

74. Dixon BJ, Dixon JB, Carden R et al (2005) Preoxygenation is more effective in the 25 degrees head-up position. Anesthesiology 102:1110–1115

75. Collins J, Lemmens H, Brodsky J, Brock-Utne J, Levitan R (2004) Laryngoscopy and morbid obesity: a comparison of the "sniff" and "ramped" positions. Obes Surg 14:1171–1175

76. Gander S, Frascarolo P, Suter M, Spahn D, Magnusson L (2005) Positive end-expiratory pressure during induction of general anesthesia increases duration of nonhypoxic apnea in morbidly obese patients. Anesth Analg 100:580–584

77. Kluger MT, Short TG (1999) Aspiration during anesthesia: a review of 133 cases from the anaesthetic incident monitoring Study (AIMS). Anaesthesia 54:19–26

78. Warner MA, Warner ME, Webber JG (1993) Clinical significance of pulmonary aspiration during the perioperative period. Anesthesiology 78:56–62

79. Fisher BL, Pennathur A, Mutnick JL et al (1999) Obesity correlates with gastroesophageal reflux. Dig Dis Sci 44:2290–2294

80. Freid E (2005) The rapid sequence technique revisited: obesity and sleep apnea syndrome. Anesthesiol Clin North Am 23:551–564

81. Smith KJ, Dobranowski J, Yip G et al (2003) Cricoid pressure displaces the esophagus: an observational study using magnetic resonance imaging. Anesthesiology 99:60–64

82. Meek T, Gittins N, Duggan JE (1999) Cricoid pressure: knowledge and performance amongst anaesthetic assistants. Anaesthesia 54:59–62

83. Langeron O, Masso E, Huraux C et al (2000) Prediction of difficult mask ventilation. Anesthesiology 92:1229–1236

84. Juvin P, Lavaut E, Dupont H et al (2003) Difficult tracheal intubation is more common in obese than in lean patients. Anesth Analg 97:595–600

85. Gaszynski T (2004) Anesthetic complications of gross obesity. Curr Opin Anaesthesiol 17: 271–276

86. Pelosi P, Croci M, Ravagnan I (1997) Respiratory system mechanics in sedated, paralyzed, morbidly obese patients. J Appl Physiol 82:811–818

87. Valenza F, Vagginelli F, Tiby A et al (2007) Effects of the beach chair position, positive end-expiratory pressure, and pneumoperitoneum on respiratory function in morbidly obese patients during anesthesia and paralysis. Anesthesiology 107:725–732

88. Whalen F, Gajic O, Thompson G et al (2006) The effects of the alveolar recruitment maneuver and positive end-expiratory pressure on arterial oxygenation during laparoscopic bariatric surgery. Anesth Analg 102:298–305

89. Chalhoub V, Yazigi A, Sleilaty G et al (2007) Effect of vital capacity manoeuvres on arterial oxygenation in morbidly obese patients undergoing open bariatric surgery. Eur J Anaesthesiol 24:283–288

90. El-Solh AA (2004) Clinical approach to the critically ill, morbidly obese patient. Am J Respir Crit Care Med 169:557–561

91. Sekhar N, Torquati A, Youssef Y et al (2007) A comparison of 399 open and 568 laparoscopic gastric bypasses performed during a 4-year period. Surg Endosc 11:377–397

92. Chui PT, Gin T, Oh TE (1993) Anaesthesia for laparoscopic surgery. Anaesth Intensive Care 21:163–171

93. Casati A, Comotti C, Tommasino C et al (2000) Effects of pneumoperitoneum and reverse Trendelenburg position on cardio-pulmonary function in morbidly obese patients receiving laparoscopic gastric banding. Eur J Anaesthesiol 17:300–305

94. Rigg JR, Jamrozik K, Myles PS et al (2002) MASTER Anaesthesia Trial Study Group. Epidural anaesthesia and analgesia and outcome of major surgery: a randomised trial. Lancet 13:276–282

95. Gelman S, Laws HL, Potzick J et al (1980) Thoracic epidural vs. balanced anesthesia in morbid obesity: an intraoperative and postoperative hemodynamic study. Anesth Analg 59:902–908

96. von Ungern-Sternberg BS, Regli A, Reber A, Schneider MC (2004) Effect of obesity and thoracic epidural analgesia on perioperative spirometry. Br J Anaesth 94:121–127

97. Cotter JT, Nielsen KC, Guller U et al (2004) Increased body mass index and ASA physical status IV are risk factors for block failure in ambulatory surgery- an analysis of 9,342 blocks. Can J Anaesth 51:810–816

98. Nielsen KC, Guller U, Steele SM et al (2005) Influence of obesity on regional anesthesia in the ambulatory setting: an analysis of 9,038 blocks. Anesthesiology 102:181–187

99. Hodgkinson R, Husain FJ (1980) Obesity and the cephalad spread of analgesia following epidural administration of bupivacaine for cesarean section. Anesth Analg 59:89–92

100. von Ungern-Sternberg BS, Regli A, Bucher E et al (2004) Impact of spinal anaesthesia and obesity on maternal respiratory function during elective cesarean section. Anaesthesia 59:743–749

101. Regli A, Ungern-Sternberg BS, Reber A et al (2006) Impact of spinal anaesthesia on peri-operative lung volumes in obese and morbidly obese female patients. Anaesthesia 61:215–221

102. Eichenberger AS, Proietti S, Wicky S et al (2002) Morbid obesity and postoperative pulmonary atelectasis: an underestimated problem. Anesth Analg 95:1788–1792

103. Bryson GL, Chung F, Finegan BA et al (2004) Patient selection in ambulatory anesthesia- an evidence-based review: Part I. Can J Anaesth 51:768–781

104. Huerta S, DeShields S, Shpiner R et al (2002) Safety and efficacy of postoperative continuous positive airway pressure to prevent pulmonary complications after Roux-en-Y gastric bypass. J Gastrointest Surg 6:354–358

105. Vasquez TL, Hoddinott K (2004) A potential complication of bi-level positive airway pressure after gastric bypass surgery. Obes Surg 14:282–284

106. Schug SA, Torri JJ (1993) Safety assessment of postoperative pain management by an acute pain service. Pain 55:387–391

Patient Selection and Choice of the Procedure

Robert E. Brolin, MD

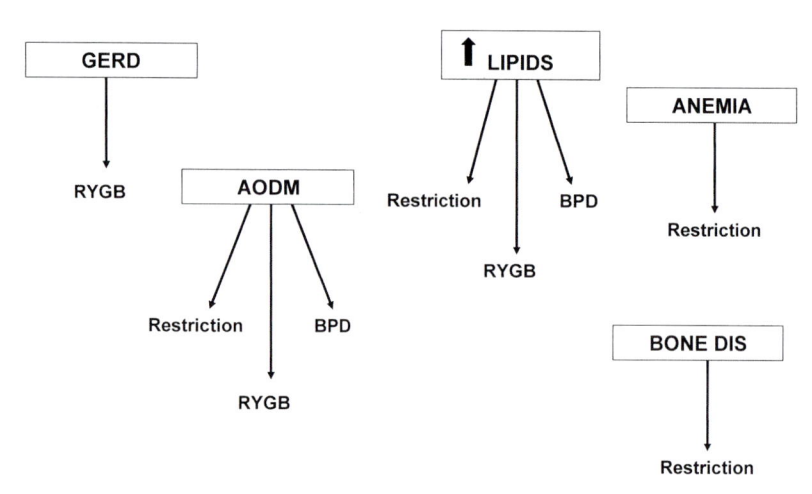

Fig. 15.2. This algorithm is based upon a number of cohort studies which have shown superior results in amelioration of type-2 diabetes (*AODM*) and hypercholesterolemia after operations that incorporate either duodenal or intestinal exclusion. Conversely, pre-existing bone disease (osteoporosis) or anemia might be exacerbated by intestinal exclusion operations, thus making a purely restrictive procedure a better choice. RYGB is an excellent operation for GERD, since more than 95% of the stomach is excluded and the small stomach pouch produces very little acid

[26, 38]. Although isolated cases of hepatic failure have been reported after biliopancreatic diversion, other investigators, including our group, have shown that RYGB and BPD-DS have salutary effects in patients with NASH [38, 39]. A complex algorithm that is focused on the relationship between various preoperative diseases and specific bariatric operations is shown in ▫ Fig. 15.2.

15.7 Algorithm Based on Preoperative Eating Behavior

Sugerman et al. were the first to suggest that weight loss outcome after bariatric surgery could be affected by preoperative eating behavior [23]. After demonstrating in a prospective randomized study that RYGB provided significantly greater weight loss than VBG, Sugerman's group subsequently showed that selective assignment of "sweets eaters" to RYGB rather than VBG resulted in significantly improved weight loss among the VBG patients [40]. Our group attempted to replicate these results using a similar approach for assignment of patients to have VBG or RYGB (▫ Fig. 15.3). We utilized more objective nutritional information than Sugerman et al., in that dietary intake of protein, carbohydrate, and fat was quantified, along with intake of high-calorie liquids and ice cream. In addition, we attempted to identify "gorgers" vs "snackers" and assigned the gorgers to the VBG group. Our findings were somewhat surprising, in that VBG resulted in significantly increased postoperative intake of ice cream and solid sweets in comparison with preoperative intake [41]. Moreover, weight loss after RYGB was significantly greater than after VBG, despite assignment of the snackers and sweets eaters to the RYGB group. Sugerman et al. also identified "high starch nibblers" as patients who were

prone to weight loss failure after RYGB and suggested that BPD might be the procedure of choice for this incorrigible group [40]. The Monash group has subsequently refuted the sweets-eater gastric restrictive contraindication theory with Lap Band patients [21]. In that study there was no difference in weight loss between sweets eaters and non-sweets eaters. These investigators subsequently identified "grazing" and "uncontrolled eating" as two behaviors that work against successful weight loss after LAGB [42].

15.8 Algorithm for Revisional Surgery

Because some patients either will not achieve satisfactory weight loss or will regain a substantial amount following the primary bariatric operation, revisional surgery may be considered in some cases. In the early era of bariatric surgery, attempts at revising a failed restrictive operation to another pure restrictive procedure almost invariably failed to result in satisfactory weight loss [43, 44]. Conversely, revision of a failed restrictive operation to RYGB was frequently successful [44, 45]. This dictum was rarely violated until recently, when Bessler et al. reported successful weight loss in eight patients who had laparoscopic adjustable gastric banding after failing to achieve satisfactory weight loss following conventional RYGB [46]. Prior to Bessler's publication, patients who failed RYGB were revised by adding malabsorption, via lengthening of the measurements of either the Roux or biliopancreatic limbs. Sugerman et al., Fobi, and our group have independently shown satisfactory outcomes in the majority of patients who were treated using this approach [47–49]. The Cornell group recently reported excellent results after failed RYGB by revision to a BPD-DS [50]. The drawback of this approach is the frequent need for

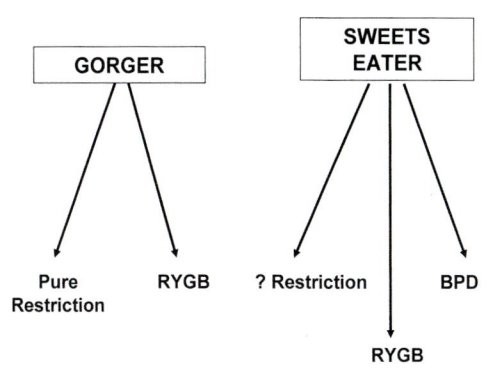
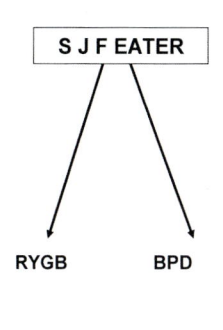

Fig. 15.3. This algorithm is based upon the limited and controversial data which suggest that eating sweets may be curtailed by the dumping symptoms associated with RYGB. Conversely, operations that produce the most effective and permanent restriction of intake would be well-suited for "gorgers" or high-volume eaters. Since salty junk food (*SJF*) is easy to consume after restrictive procedures, operations that incorporate malabsorption of ingested fat would seem best-suited for these problematic patients

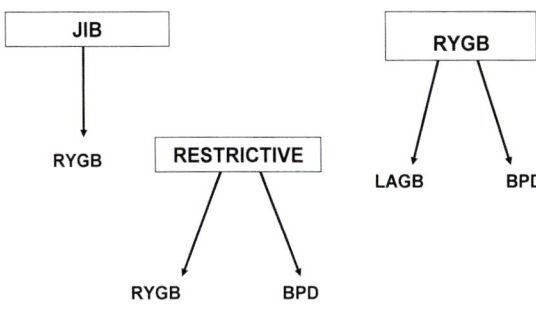
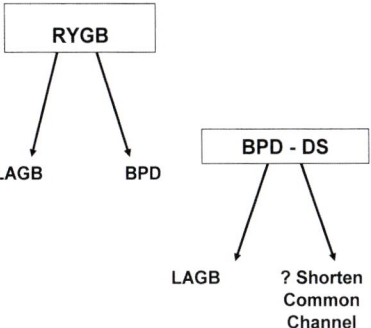

Fig. 15.4. This algorithm is based upon the limited information on weight loss outcome after revisional surgery for weight loss failure. The preponderance of data suggest that failed restrictive operations can be successfully converted to either RYGB or BPD, and that JIB failures can sometimes achieve success after revision to RYGB. There are conflicting data regarding the best approach for revision of failed RYGB – either better restriction (*LAGB*), more malabsorption (*BPD*), or both. Only anecdotal information is available regarding management of patients who fail to lose enough weight after BPD

two separate staged operations in order to complete the procedure. Revision of jejunoileal bypass is occasionally required for unsatisfactory weight loss. Although there is a paucity of published weight loss results in this group of patients, our group reported successful weight loss after conversion to conventional RYGB [49]. Likewise, there is a paucity of information regarding revision of BPD-DS for unsatisfactory weight loss. There are anecdotal reports that resecting or banding the gastric sleeve have resulted in less than impressive weight loss. Likewise, extending the length of excluded intestine has produced inconsistent results. Overall, the results of revisional operations for unsatisfactory weight loss are more problematic than those of primary bariatric procedures in terms of both weight loss and postoperative complications [43, 47]. A hypothetical algorithm of revisional operations for weight loss failure is shown in Fig. 15.4.

References

1. National Institutes of Health Consensus Development Panel (1992) Gastrointestinal surgery for severe obesity. Am J Clin Nutr 55 [Suppl]:615–619
2. Wadden TA, Foster GD (1992) Behavioral assessment and treatment of markedly obese patients. In: Wadden TA, VanItallie TB (eds) Treatment of the seriously obese patient. Guilford Press, New York, pp 290–330
3. National Institutes of Health (2000) Clinical guidelines on the identification, evaluation and treatment of overweight and obesity in adults. The evidence report. NHBL), Bethesda, MD
4. Livingston EH, Huerta H, Arthur D et al (2002) Male gender is a predictor of morbidity and age a predictor of mortality for patients undergoing gastric bypass surgery. Ann Surg 236:576–582
5. Flum DR, Salem L, Broechel et al (2005) Early mortality among Medicare beneficiaries undergoing bariatric surgical procedures. JAMA 294:1903–1908
6. DeMaria EJ, Portenier D, Wolfe L (2007) Obesity surgery mortality risk score: proposal for a clinically useful score to predict mortality risk in patients undergoing gastric bypass. Surg Obes Rel Dis 3:134–140
7. Bloomston M, Zervos EE, Camps MA et al (1997) Outcome following bariatric surgery in super versus morbidly obese patients: Does weight matter? Obes Surg 7:414–419
8. Sugerman HJ, Sugerman EL, Wolfe L et al (2001) Risks/benefits of gastric bypass in morbidly obese patients with severe venous stasis disease. Ann Surg 234:41–46
9. Podnos YD, Jimenez JC, Wilson SF et al (2003) Complications after laparoscopic gastric bypass. A review of 3464 cases. Arch Surg 138:957–961
10. Suggs WJ, Kouli W, Lupovici M, Chau WY, Brolin RE (2007) Complications at gastrojejunostomy after laparoscopic Roux-en-Y gastric bypass: comparison between 21- and 25-mm circular staplers. Surg Obes Rel Dis 3:508–514
11. Brolin RE (1996) Surgery for morbid obesity. In: Current practice of surgery, vol 3, chap 8. Churchill-Livingstone, New York, pp 417–424

12. Balsiger BM, Poggio JL, Mai J et al (2000) Ten and more years after vertical banded gastroplasty as primary operation for morbid obesity. J Gastrointest Surg 4:598–605

13. Scopinaro N, Gianetta E, Adami GF et al (1996) Biliopancreatic diversion for obesity at eighteen years. Surgery 119:261-8

14. MacDonald KG, Long SD, Swanson MS et al (1997) The gastric bypass operation reduces the progression and mortality of non-insulin dependent diabetes mellitus. J Gastrointest Surg 1:213–320

15. Position Statement (2007) Sleeve gastrectomy as a bariatric procedure. Surg Obes Rel Dis 3:573–576

16. Himpens J, Dapri G, Cadiere CB (2006) A prospective randomized study between laparoscopic gastric banding and laparoscopic isolated sleeve gastrectomy: results after 1–3 years. Obes Surg 16:1450–1456

17. Karamanakos SN, Konstantinos V, Kalfarentzos F, Alexandrides TK (2008) Weight loss, appetite suppression and changes in fasting and postprandial ghrelin and peptide-YY levels after Roux-en-Y gastric bypass and sleeve gastrectomy. Ann Surg 247:401–407

18. Mason EE, Doherty C, Maher JW et al (1987) Super obesity and gastric reduction procedures. Gastroenterol Clin North Am 16:495–502

19. Shikora SA, Kim JJ, Tarnoff ME et al (2005) Laparoscopic Roux-en-Y gastric bypass. Results and learning curve of a high-volume academic program. Arch Surg 140:362–367

20. Brolin RE, Kenler HA, Gorman JH, Cody RP (1992) Long-limb gastric bypass in the superobese. A prospective randomized study. Ann Surg 215:387–392

21. Hudson SM, Dixon JB, O'Brien PE (2002) Sweet eating is not a predictor of outcome after Lap Band placement. Can we finally bury the myth? Obes Surg 12:789–794

22. Browne WB, Kelly J, Castro AE et al (2006) Laparoscopic gastric bypass in superior to adjustable gastric band in super morbidly obese patients. Arch Surg 141:683–689

23. Sugerman HJ, Starkey JV, Birkenhauer R (1987) A randomized prospective trial of gastric bypass versus vertical banded gastroplasty for morbid obesity and their effects on sweets versus non-sweets eaters. Ann Surg 205:613–624

24. Lechner GW, Callender K (1981) Subtotal gastric exclusion and gastric partitioning: a randomized prospective comparison of one hundred patients. Surgery 90:637–644

25. Pories WJ, Flickinger EG, Meelheim D et al (1982) The effectiveness of gastric bypass over gastric partition in morbid obesity. Consequence of distal gastric and duodenal exclusion. Ann Surg 196:389–399

26. Brolin RE, LaMarca LB, Kenler HA, Cody RP (2002) Malabsorptive gastric bypass in patients with super obesity. J Gastrointest Surg 6:195–205

27. Lagace M, Marceau P, Marceau S et al (1995) Biliopancreatic diversion with a new type of gastrectomy: some previous conclusions revisited. Obes Surg 5:411–416

28. Prachand VN, DaVee RT, Alverdy JC (2006) Duodenal switch provides superior weight loss in the superobese (BMI >50 kg/m^2) compared with gastric bypass. Ann Surg 244:611–619

29. Murr MM, Balsiger BM, Kennedy FP et al (1996) Malabsorptive procedures for severe obesity: Comparison of pancreaticobiliary bypass and very, very long Roux-en-Y gastric bypass. J Gastrointest Surg 3:607–612

30. DeMaria EJ, Sugerman HJ, Meador JG et al (2001) High failure rate after laparoscopic adjustable silicone gastric banding for treatment of morbid obesity. Ann Surg 233:809-18

31. Schauer PR, Barguera B, Ikramuddin S et al (2003) Effect of laparoscopic Roux-en-Y gastric bypass on type 2 diabetes mellitus. Ann Surg 238:467–484

32. Gleysteen JJ, Barboriak JJ, Sasse EA (1990) Sustained coronary-risk factor reduction after gastric bypass for morbid obesity. Am J Clin Nutr 51:774–778

33. Brolin RE, Bradley LJ, Wilson AC, Cody RP (2000) Lipid risk profile and weight stability after gastric restrictive operations. J Gastrointest Surg 4:464–469

34. Buchwald H, Stoller DK, Campos CT et al (1990) Partial ileal bypass for hypercholesterolemia: 20- to 26-year follow up of the first 57 consecutive cases. Ann Surg 212:318–331

35. Buchwald H, Campos CT, Matts JP et al (1992) Women in the POSCH Trial: effects of aggressive cholesterol modification in women with coronary heart disease. Ann Surg 216:389-400

36. Compston JE, Vedi S, Gianetta E et al (1984) Bone histomorphometry and Vitamin D status in patients with biliopancreatic bypass. Gastrointerol 87:350–356

37. Marceau P, Biron S, Lebel S et al (2002) Does bone change after biliopancreatic diversion? J Gastrointest Surg 6:690–698

38. Marceau P, Biron S, Hould FS et al (1997) The metabolic syndrome as a risk for liver disease. Hepatology 26:556A

39. Brolin RE, Bradley LJ, Taliwal R (1998) Unsuspected cirrhosis discovered during elective obesity operations. Arch Surg 133:84–88

40. Sugerman HJ, Londrey GL, Kellum JM et al (1989) Weight loss with vertical banded gastroplasty and Roux-en-Y gastric bypass for morbid obesity with selective vs random assignment. Am J Surg 157:93–102

41. Brolin RE, Robertson LB, Kenler HA, Cody RP (1994) Weight loss and dietary intake after vertical banded gastroplasty and Roux-en-Y gastric bypass. Ann Surg 220:782–790

42. Colles SL, Dixon JB, O'Brien PE Grazing and loss of control related to eating: two high-risk factors following bariatric surgery. Obesity 2008 16:615-22

43. Yale CE Conversion surgery for morbid obesity: complications and long term weight control. Surgery 1989 106:474-80

44. Linner JH, Drew RD Reoperative surgery – indications, efficacy and long-term follow-up. Am J Clin Nutri 1992 55:606S-10S

45. Weber M, Muller MK, Michel JM et al (2003) Laparoscopic Roux-en-Y gastric bypass, but not rebanding, should be proposed as rescue procedure for patients with failed laparoscopic gastric banding. Ann Surg 238:827–834

46. Bessler M, Doud A, DiGiorgi MF et al (2005) Adjustable gastric banding as a revisional bariatric procedure after failed gastric bypass. Obes Surg 15:1443–1448

47. Sugerman HJ, Kellum JM, DeMaria EJ (1997) Conversion of proximal to distal gastric bypass for failed gastric bypass for superobesity. J Gastrointest Surg 1:517–525

48. Fobi Mal, Lee H, Igwe D et al (1984) Revision of failed gastric bypass to distal Roux-en-Y gastric bypass. A review of 65 cases. Am J Surg 148:331–336

49. Brolin RE, Cody RP (2008) Weight loss outcome of revisional bariatric operations varies according to the primary procedure. Ann Surg 248:227–32

50. Parikh M, Pomp A, Gagner M (2007) Laparoscopic conversion of failed gastric bypass to duodenal switch: technical considerations and preliminary outcomes. Surg Obes Rel Dis 3:611–618

III Surgical Procedures

Pathophysiology of Restrictive Procedures

Giovanni Dapri, MD, G.B.Cadière, MD, Jaqules Himpens, MD

There are three different types of restrictive surgical procedures for morbid obesity: vertical banded gastroplasty (VBG), adjustable gastric banding (AGB), and sleeve gastrectomy (SG). These procedures are currently realized via laparoscopy. The mechanism of VBG is related to the size of the gastric pouch and to the calibrated outlet. After a solid meal, patients describe a sensation of fullness and satiety or even epigastric or low-retrosternal discomfort, indicating pouch fullness; at this point the patient must stop eating. If eating continues, discomfort increases until voluntary or spontaneous regurgitation of the excess food occurs. Satiety is dependent on the thickness and consistency of the food eaten; hence patients who consume mainly liquids usually have less weight loss. Gastric motility may play a part in the rate of drainage of the gastric pouch, and excessive motility may be responsible for poor weight loss in some cases. The variability in weight loss after gastroplasty and other restrictive procedures highlights the fact that the final amount of weight loss depends on patient-controlled factors as well as on the surgical procedure. Following placement of laparoscopic AGB (LAGB), as soon as the patient ingests two spoonfuls the small gastric compartment above the band is filled and he or she experiences a feeling of fullness. Since it takes a long time for this compartment to empty because of the narrowed stoma, more food can be ingested only after substantial time has elapsed. The patient must therefore eat at a much slower pace, and this slower pace allows the satiety center to be stimulated. As the hunger sensation is no longer present, overall food intake is reduced. The major advantage of LAGB is the possibility to adjust the size of the outlet. Another hypothesis not confirmed as the mode of action of gastric banding was gut hormone modulation. The mechanism of action of laparoscopic SG (LSG) is not only the restriction obtained by resecting part of the body and the entire fundus of the stomach, leaving a small gastric tube of 100–150 ml. Hormonal changes following this procedure must also be considered. Ghrelin is a 28-amino-acid orexigenic peptide, secreted essentially by the fundus of the stomach, which stimulates feeding behavior and hunger. In LSG, the gastric fundus is resected and plasma ghrelin levels are expected to decrease following surgery. Another mechanism explaining weight loss after LSG could be the relationship between appetite and gastric emptying, as the gastric clearance seems to be improved.

16.1 Basics

A traditional classification of the different procedures for the treatment of morbid obesity is based on their mode of action. Three groups can be identified: restrictive, mixed, and malabsorptive procedures. Restrictive procedures for morbid obesity are represented by three different types:
- Vertical banded gastroplasty (VBG)
- Adjustable gastric banding (AGB)
- Sleeve gastrectomy (SG)

The most common restrictive and malabsorptive procedure is Roux-en-Y gastric bypass (RYGBP).

16.1.1 Vertical Banded Gastroplasty

In 1966 Mason and Ito performed the first gastric bypass for morbid obesity [1]. In 1971, Mason reasoned that if the mechanism of weight loss in this procedure was food intake reduction, a small gastric pouch emptying directly into the distal stomach should be equally effective in promoting weight loss. Hence some complications of the gastric bypass, such as micronutrient deficiency, could be avoided, making surgery easier and safer. The first gastroplasty performed by Mason divided the stomach into a smaller upper section and a larger distal part connected by a channel on the greater curve. This procedure was unsuccessful in maintaining weight loss [2, 3]. Mason and Gomez performed various modifications of the gastroplasty procedure. The last variation was realized in 1980, the so-called vertical banded gastroplasty (VBG) (◘ Fig. 16.1) [4]. This procedure employed a lesser-curve stoma supported by a Marlex band (1.5 cm wide and 5.5 cm long) passed through a window created by a circular

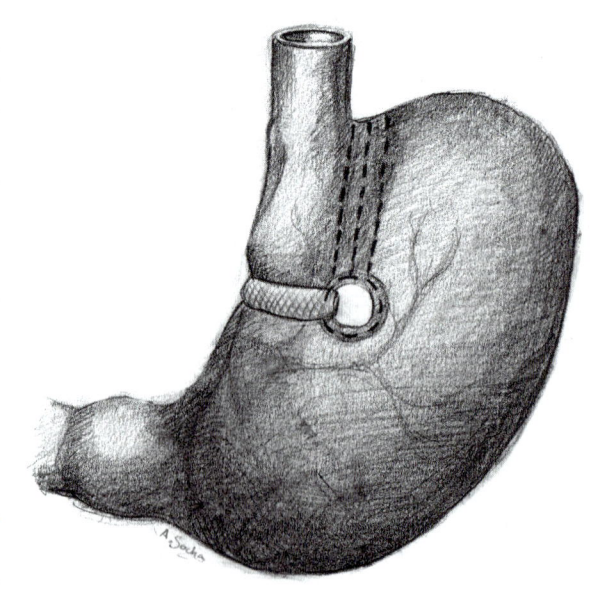

◘ **Fig. 16.1.** Mason's vertical banded gastroplasty

stapler [5]. One year later, Laws and Piatadosi replaced the Marlex band with a silastic ring as a permanent non-expandable support for the VBG [6]. The procedure was called silastic ring vertical banded gastroplasty (SRVBG). At the time, VBG became the most popular procedure for the treatment of morbid obesity. Technical principles of the mechanism of this procedure are related to the size of the gastric pouch, which measures 50 ml or less, and to the calibrated outlet, which measures between 10 and 12 mm in diameter. In the era of minimally invasive surgery, VBG was first performed via laparoscopy in 1993 by Chua and Mendiola [7]. This new approach boosted its popularity [8, 9]. Gastroplasty and its many variants rely on the physical restriction of food intake in order to achieve weight loss by radical reduction of energy intake over the first year. After the first year a moderate restriction remains, which allows weight stabilization and prevents future weight regain. The advantage of this restrictive approach is that micronutrient deficiencies (iron, calcium, vitamin B12) are less likely to occur. It has been demonstrated that a pouch volume of about 20 ml or less is important for good weight loss. Liquids pass easily and rapidly through the empty pouch according to their viscosity and the rate at which they enter the pouch. Solids pass through much more slowly, depending on the particle size of the swallowed food and on its consistency and the degree of resistance at the stoma. After a solid meal, patients describe a sensation of fullness and satiety or even epigastric or low-retrosternal discomfort, indicating pouch fullness. At this point the patient must stop eating. If eating continues, discomfort increases until voluntary or spontaneous regurgitation of the excess food occurs. There is no nausea, despite a definite feeling of relief after regurgitation. Patients should be advised not to eat until the next meal. The feeling of satiety induced by filling the gastric pouch is a very important factor in weight loss. Satiety is dependent on the thickness and consistency of the food eaten; hence patients who ingest mainly liquids usually have poor weight loss, whereas those who can cope with solid food do much better. If the gastric stoma is made too large, weight loss is poor. Similarly, if there is breakdown of the partition of the stoma, patients report an increase in hunger and an earlier loss of postprandial satiety as well as an increased volume of intake accompanying their weight regain. Patients must be advised to avoid eating and drinking at the same time. If a small amount of solid food is followed by a mouthful of liquid, the food will be washed through into the distal stomach. Satiety will not be achieved, and the sequence can be repeated over and over, resulting in excessive intake of food. Some patients use this strategy to appear to be eating more normally when coping with socially difficult situations, but if it is used at all meals, weight loss will be inadequate. Gastric motility may play a part in the rate of drainage of the gastric pouch, and excessive motility may be responsible for poor weight loss in some cases. The variability in weight loss after gastroplasty and other restrictive procedures highlights the fact that the final amount of weight loss depends on patient-controlled factors as well. Lack of dietary counseling may result in poor weight loss, since surgery cannot control the following four aspects:

- The type or caloric content of food: fats, oils, sweet foods are easy to chew
- The frequency of eating: small amounts taken frequently add up to a large amount
- The amount or quality of liquids: liquids can be drunk almost without limit
- The consumption of food and drink beyond what is needed for adequate nutrition

16.1.2 Adjustable Gastric Banding

Wilkinson and Peloso in 1981 [10], Kolle in 1982 [11], and Molina and Oria in 1983 [12] have been credited with initiating the nonadjustable gastric banding approach to restrictive bariatric surgery [13]. An adjustable technique, based on a liquid-filled silastic cuff, was introduced because of a high number of reoperations [14]. After the first adjustable gastric banding (AGB) was realized by Kuzmak [15] in 1986, further successful developments in human subjects were the adjustable silicone gastric band (ASGB) and the Swedish adjustable gastric band (Swedish band) [16], both initially placed by open surgery. The laparoscopic technique was introduced in 1992 by Cadiere et al. [17]. Thanks to laparoscopy, LAGB gained in popularity, owing to less invasiveness and to the option of adjustment of the stoma offered to the patient. The adjustable gastric band is implanted to reduce the stomach's volume by dividing it into two compartments through an adjustable restricted opening (stoma): a small gastric pouch of 25 cc and the rest of the stomach (◉ Fig. 16.2). As soon as two spoonfuls are ingested, the first compartment is filled and one experiences a feeling of fullness. Since it takes a long time for the first compartment to empty because of the narrowed stoma, more food can be ingested only after substantial time has elapsed. One must therefore eat at a much slower pace, and this allows the satiety center to be stimulated. As the hunger sensation is no longer present, overall food intake is reduced [18]. Finally, weight loss achieved with this procedure is determined mainly by changes in eating behavior [19]. The major advantage of LAGB is the possibility to adjust the

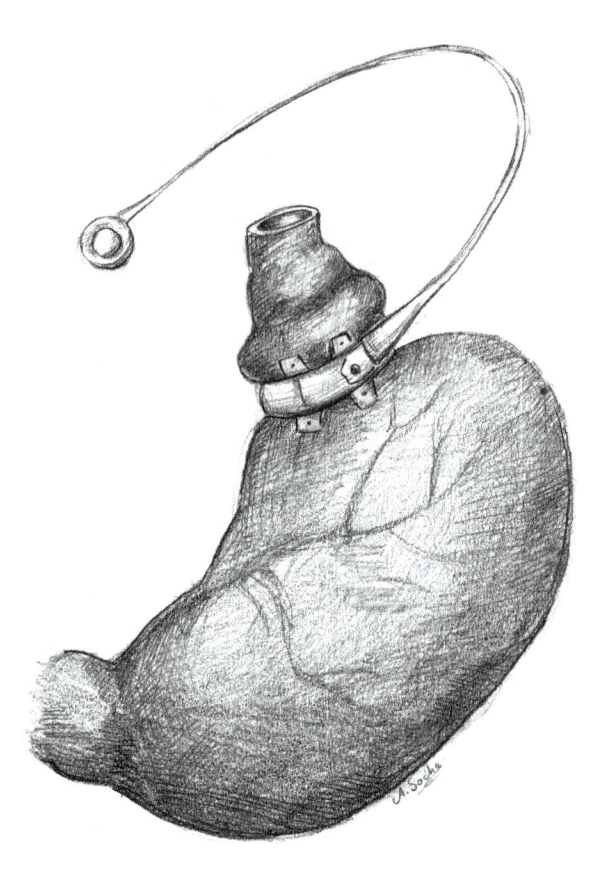

◘ **Fig. 16.2.** Adjustable gastric banding

subjected to LAGB [21, 22]. The role played by other hormones such as glucagon-like-peptide-1 (GLP-1) and peptide-YY (PYY) in weight loss after LAGB was also studied [24], but no known hormonal changes can demonstrate a relation with weight loss after the procedure of gastric banding. There may be still another mechanism, in addition to mechanical restriction, which explains satiety: the presence of a foreign body in contact with the gastric wall, which contains afferent as well as efferent vagus nerve fibers. This assumption needs to be confirmed by research on the electrophysiology of the banded stomach. The possible link between pressure, volume, the physical behavior of implanted bands, and the physiology of the banded patient constitutes the "pressure-volume theory". Hopefully, the ongoing laboratory and clinical investigation of the pressure-volume theory will come up with data to provide clear guidelines for further band engineering and band adjustment policies [25].

16.1.3 Sleeve Gastrectomy

Sleeve gastrectomy (SG) is an essentially restrictive procedure for morbid obesity (◘ Fig. 16.3). It was first described in 1988 as part of the procedure of biliopancreatic diversion with duodenal switch by Hess and Hess [26], and Marceau et al. [27]. In 1993 the SG was reported in isolated form by Johnston et al. [28]. This procedure targets the same patient group as LAGB. It is more invasive, however, and not reversible, and it carries a longer learning curve. In the literature it has been reported mostly as the first step in another bariatric procedure, such as biliopancreatic diversion with duodenal switch [29–33] or gastric bypass [34–37]. SG is justified as a first step, owing to decreased postoperative morbidity in super-obese (BMI >50 kg/m^2) or super super-obese patients (BMI >60 kg/m^2). This first step allows the surgeon to perform the second bariatric procedure under better and safer conditions. The mechanism of action of this procedure is not only the restriction obtained by resecting part of the body and the entire fundus of the stomach, leaving a small gastric tube of 100–150 ml. The Banded Sleeve Gastrectomy (LBGS) is developing even more restriction (◘ Fig. 16.4). Many surgeons are convinced that 90% reduction of the gastric volume and thus decreasing caloric intake early postoperatively may explain the resolution of diabetes after the operation [38]. However, the hormonal changes following this procedure have to be considered as well. The gastric fundus, known as the main source of ghrelin-producing cells, is resected by SG, and plasma ghrelin levels are expected to decrease following surgery. Fruhbeck et al. [39] described reduction of the circulating

size of the outlet (stoma) without anesthesia by injecting or withdrawing saline via the percutaneous access port, thereby inflating or deflating the inflatable portion of the silicone band. The adjustments should be based on objective criteria, including documented dietary inquiry, postoperative weight loss curves, and radiological studies. Another hypothesis regarding the mode of action of AGB is gut hormone modulation. Numerous studies on the relationship between the ghrelin hormone and appetite suppression with LAGB have been reported [19–22]. Ghrelin, a 28-amino-acid orexigenic peptide, is secreted essentially by the fundus of the stomach [23] and acts on the hypothalamic arcuate nucleus, which stimulates feeding behavior and hunger. Serum ghrelin levels increase during fasting and decrease after a meal. Uzzan et al. [20] found a significant increase of ghrelin expression 1 year after gastric banding, which seems to exclude the role of ghrelin in weight loss following laparoscopic AGB. Decrease of hunger with increasing fasting plasma ghrelin following gastric banding was demonstrated by Schindler et al. [19]. Together with other reports, these data seem to confirm the absence of a relationship between ghrelin fluctuations and appetite modifications in patients

4

4

4

4

4

4

4

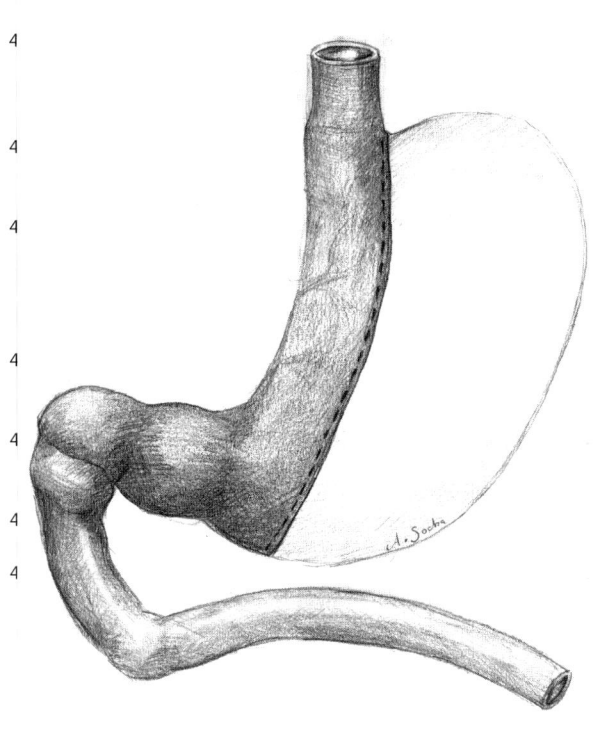

Fig. 16.3. Sleeve gastrectomy

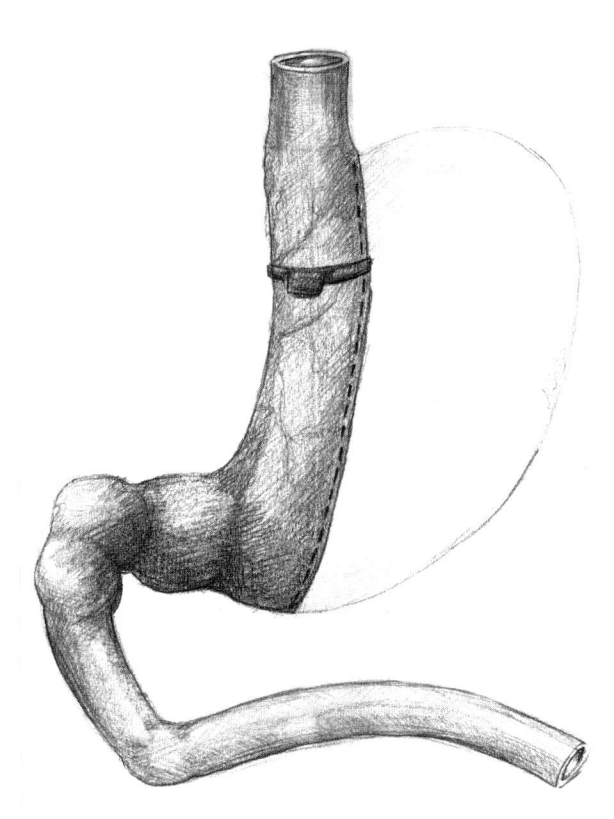

Fig. 16.4. Banded Sleeve Gastrectomy

ghrelin concentrations after bariatric operations depending on the degree of fundus exclusion and subsequent isolation of ghrelin-producing cells from direct contact with ingested nutrients. In a study comparing the effects on plasma ghrelin levels after laparoscopic SG and LAGB, Langer et al. [40] showed a significant decrease of plasma ghrelin levels at day 1 after laparoscopic SG compared with the preoperative levels. Moreover, plasma ghrelin remained stable at 1 month and 6 months postoperatively. In contrast, patients who underwent LAGB showed no change of plasma ghrelin levels at day 1, while a significant increase was found at 1 month and 6 months of follow-up. Thus, the reduction of ghrelin production after SG, unlike after LAGB [21], could explain the superior weight loss achieved after laparoscopic SG [41]. Another study [42] compared the modifications of ghrelin levels in super super-obese patients submitted to laparoscopic SG. The authors confirmed the reduction of ghrelin levels after laparoscopic SG but found a significant increase of this hormone after LAGB. An interesting study by Karamanakos et al. [43], comparing the weight loss and the fasting ghrelin levels between laparoscopic SG and laparoscopic RYGBP at 6 and 12 months, showed a significant difference in favor of laparoscopic SG. After laparoscopic RYGBP, fasting ghrelin levels did not change significantly compared with baseline and did not decrease significantly following meals, unlike laparoscopic SG, where a marked reduction in fasting ghrelin levels and significant suppression after meals was observed. Another mechanism to explain weight loss after SG could be the relationship between appetite and gastric emptying. A randomized and double-blind trial reported by Bergmann et al. [44] showed an association between gastric emptying as evaluated by echography and appetite. The more the antrum is expanded, the less the feeling of hunger seems to be. This mechanism can be linked to the new anatomy of the stomach after SG. The gastric emptying mechanisms were studied and compared in three different groups: control patients, obese patients, and patients submitted to a procedure similar to SG called the Magenstrasse and Mill technique [45]. This study showed no statistically significant differences in the emptying times between the three groups and concluded that a procedure similar to SG achieved acceptable weight loss while preserving gastric emptying mechanisms and minimizing possible side effects such as vomiting. Melissas et al. [46] confirmed improved gastric clearance after laparoscopic SG, which also explains less vomiting than after VBG. Almost all patients have the feeling of satiety after LSG. Strong restriction alone could partly explain the situation; on the other hand, the early vagal stimulation due to postprandial increased tensile pressure on the

The Gastric Banding

Tomasz Szewczyk MD, Bogdan Modzelewski MD

One of the treatments for pathological obesity is adjustable gastric banding. An adjustable gastric band is applied to the stomach via laparoscopy (laparoscopic adjustable gastric banding – LAGB). This is one of the so-called restrictive surgical methods for treating obesity and, in comparison with other techniques of bariatric surgery, is the least invasive for the anatomy of the gastrointestinal tract. The gastric band is used worldwide. It is most popular in Australia, Europe, and South America and is less used in the USA and Mexico. The procedure is based on the idea of dividing the stomach into two parts, the upper part of which has a capacity of 20–50 ml. The width of the passage between these two parts is regulated by filling the gastric band with fluid, making it possible to control the rate of passage of the gastric content from the upper to the lower part of the stomach. Filling of the "upper" stomach produces the feeling of satiety, perceived by the patient as a signal to stop eating. In this way, the volume of food intake and, consequently, the amount of energy supplied to the organism is reduced. Advantages of the gastric band include the small extent of injury associated with the surgical procedure, short duration of the surgery and anesthesia, preservation of the natural anatomy of the gastrointestinal tract, no anastomoses, and preservation of the natural route of the food. Additionally, the possibility of regulating the width of the passage between two parts of the stomach makes it possible to control the rate of weight loss. The disadvantages of the method include the presence of foreign bodies (the gastric band and port), inconvenience for the patient associated with the necessity of periodic regulation of the band volume, complications resulting from compression of the gastric wall by the band (migration), possibility of band displacement (slippage), the presence of the port (causing problems with plastic surgery of the abdominal wall – if it is located on the abdomen, it interferes with physiotherapy and NMR imaging). Moreover, many authors claim that weight loss with this method is insufficient, and it should therefore not be used in patients with a BMI exceeding 50 kg/m^2.

17.1 Pathophysiology

The adjustable gastric band (AGB) was first applied in 1986 by Lubomyr Kuzmak. The Ukrainian, born in Baligrod on August 2, 1929, graduated in 1953 from the Medical Faculty of the Medical University of Lodz (Poland), and then worked in Bytom, in the Silesian Medical University. In 1965 he emigrated to the USA, where he performed the first gastric banding surgery in Irvington Hospital in 1983. He published a report of his achievements in 1986 [1]. Initially, the band was applied by open surgery, and it was not until 1993 that Belachev, first used laparoscopy for this purpose. The adjustable gastric band (AGB) is a typical restrictive method; it limits the amount of food ingested at a single meal. On the other hand, it neither alters the route of food nor influences digestion and absorption of nutrients in the gastrointestinal tract (❑ Fig. 17.1). The effect of the band involves mechanical restriction of passage of the gastric content from the upper, small portion of the stomach to the distal part of the stomach below the band. When the band is properly adjusted, i.e., with the internal diameter optimal for the patient, the passage of gastric content between the "upper" and the "lower" stomach is limited. During meals, the patient should heed the signals coming from his stomach. When the ingested food fills the "upper" stomach, the patient's brain receives the information: "You are full". The patient can, of course, overcome the resistance of esophageal structures and of the upper part of the stomach and eat more, causing the "upper" stomach to distend and the esophagus to widen and to serve as a reservoir of food. Often, such a situation ends with rapid voiding of the esophagus and

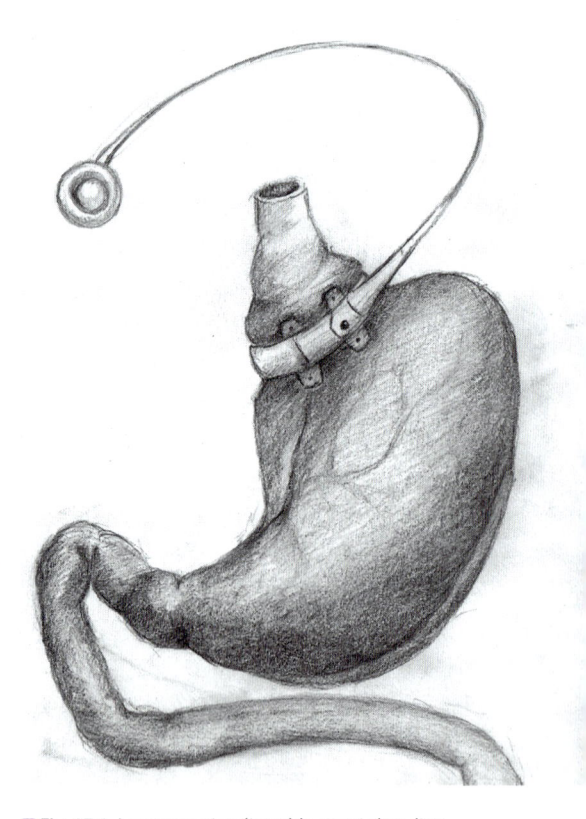

❑ **Fig. 17.1.** Laparoscopic adjustable gastric banding

the "upper" stomach by vomiting. If this happens occasionally, it has practically no significance, but if it is repeated more frequently, the esophageal widening may become permanent, and the volume of the food reservoir above the band may be increased, which will result in no weight loss, as well as in irritation of the esophageal wall and esophagitis, eventually leading to a condition identical to achalasia.

17.2 The Various Bands

The products of a few companies are currently the most common and available on the market:

1. AMI (Austria): A low-pressure band, manufactured in two sizes (cuff length 100 and 115 mm), and as a model with a "basket", applicable in case of coincidental hiatus hernia. The band is passed behind the stomach and equipped with a safe fastening system. Two types of ports, with heights of 13.3 and 9.8 mm, are available.
2. Helioscopie (France), *Heliogast*: A high-pressure band, manufactured in three sizes (31, 27.5, and 25.5 mm in diameter). The band is passed behind the stomach from the side of a drain connecting it to the port. It has a safe fastening system. One port type is used.
3. Bariatric Solutions (Switzerland), *MiniMizer Regular:* A high-pressure band with a two-stage fastening system. The first stage yields an inner diameter of 31 mm; band length 10.5 cm. The second, closing stage yields an inner diameter of 26 mm with a band length of 9.75 cm. The band is passed behind the stomach from the side of a drain connecting it to the port, but fastening requires the use of a special closing instrument (10 mm). Two port types of 13 and 18 mm diameters are used.
MiniMizer Extra: The band has loops on the upper and lower edge, allowing it to be sutured to the gastric wall without plication.
4. Inamed/Allergan (USA), *Lapband*: A high-pressure band, manufactured in three sizes (cuff length 97.5 mm; 100 mm – *Vanguard* – and 110 mm). The band is passed behind the stomach from the side of a drain connecting it to the port and has a safe fastening system. Two port types are used.
5. Obtech/Johnson &Johnson (USA): A low-pressure band available in one size. The currently manufactured model has a double safeguard fastening system and a port prepared for implantation onto the fascia with a quick-fix device (Velocity) (included in the kit).

6. Medical Innovation Developpement (France), *MID-BAND*: A low-pressure band, passed behind the stomach from the side of a drain connecting it to the port, with a safe, double-fastening system. The direction of passage through the band is marked on the drain.

17.3 The Operative Techniques

Initially, the band was placed during an open surgical procedure. When laparoscopy was introduced in 1993, this open surgical method was replaced by the so-called perigastric technique (■ Fig. 17.2). The technique was abandoned after some time because of the high complication rate with slippage, especially posterior, and gastric wall injuries occurring frequently. Currently, the pars flaccida technique is commonly used (■ Fig. 17.3).

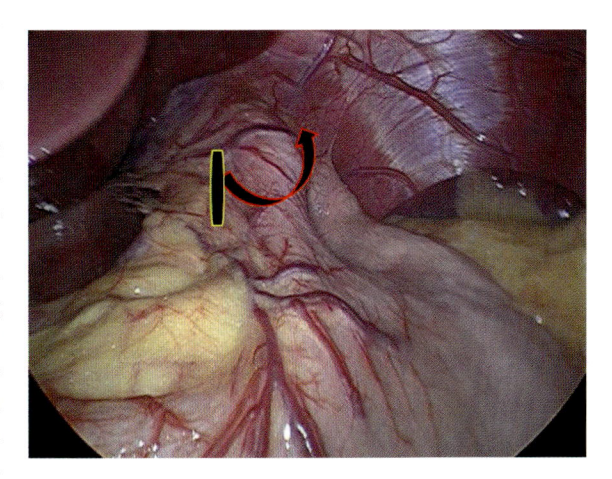

■ **Fig. 17.2.** Perigastric technique

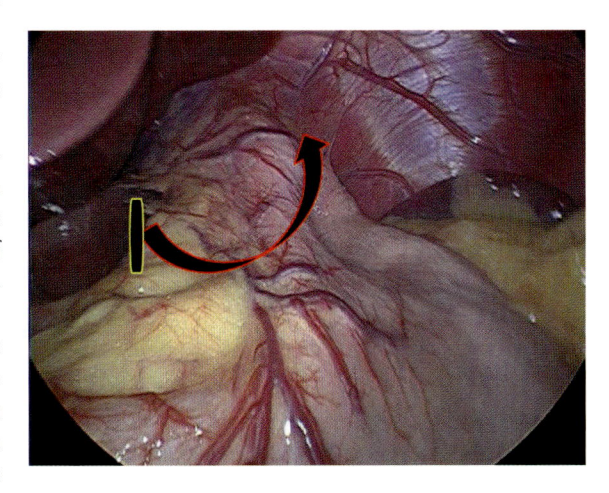

■ **Fig. 17.3.** Pars flaccida technique

Trocar positions are presented in ◘ Fig. 17.4. Most center-related variations concern the position of the hepatic retractor trocar. The retractor is applied most frequently below the xyphoid process, left of the medial line, or in the right epigastrium. Trocars of 5 and 10 mm are used; because of the enlarged, brittle liver, very often seen in obese patients, the 10-mm size is recommended. The typical set of trocars includes:
- 10 mm – optic path
- 10/5 mm – working; the operator's left hand
- 10/5 mm – hepatic retractor
- 12/15/18/20 mm – working, used for band insertion (size dependent on the band type); the operator's right hand

Instrumentarium required (◘ Fig. 17.5):
- Oblique optics 30°
- Veres needle
- Coagulation
- Two atraumatic graspers

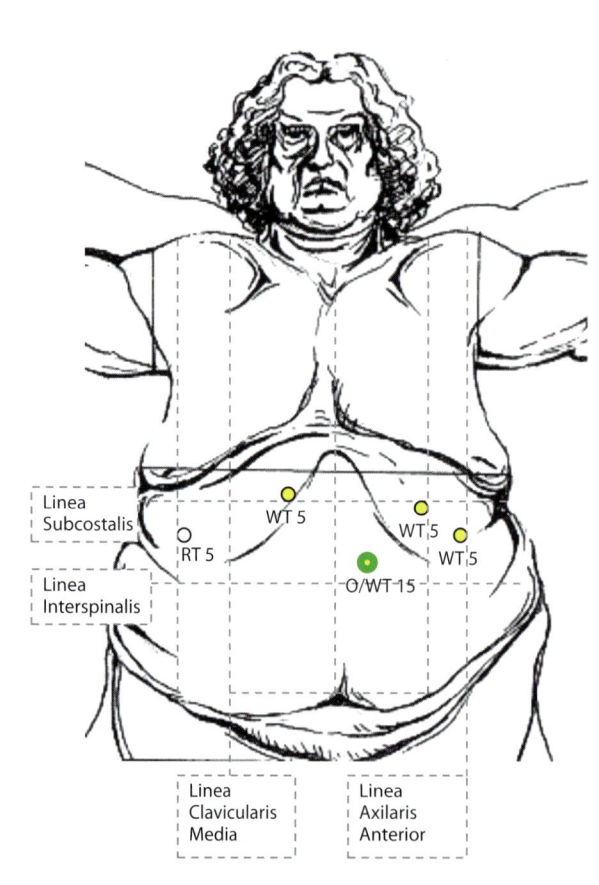

- A tool for retrogastric tunnel formation (e.g. Goldfinger)
- Hepatic retractor

The patient is positioned on the operating table with his legs apart, in a semi-reclining position, protected from slipping. The operator stands between the patient's legs. After pneumoperitoneum is obtained, the trocars are inserted in a horizontal position and the liver is retracted; the peritoneum is incised in the region of the angle of Hiss, and the pars flaccida is dissected. From the side of the pars flaccida, the left crux of the diaphragm is visualized. The next stage involves making a small incision between the diaphragm and the gastric wall, situated on the right (from the operator's point of view). (NOTE: the inferior vena cava is situated to the left of the crux of the diaphragm, which poses a risk). The instrument is introduced into the incision site to form the tunnel behind the stomach in right cruss/ His angle direction. After it has been passed behind the stomach, the instrument is aimed at the incision in the region of the angle of Hiss. Various instruments are used for this purpose, from a simple grasper to special tools that change their shape gradually, offered by band manufacturers, e.g. the Goldfinger. (NOTE: it is possible to push the instrument too far, beyond the left diaphragmatic crux and into the pleural cavity). At this point, it is advisable to control the position of the instrument in relation to the stomach, because in very obese patients the band may be inadvertently passed between the anterior gastric wall and the thick adipose tissue layer in front of the stomach. This check can be accomplished with a gastric probe; some operators also use an endoscope. The right trocar is used for insertion of the band. After being connected to the instrument previously inserted retrogastrically, the band

◘ **Fig. 17.4.** Schedule of Port's placement by Laparoscopical Adjustable Gastric Banding (LAGB); WT- working trockar, retractor trockar, optic trockar, 5 or 15mm.

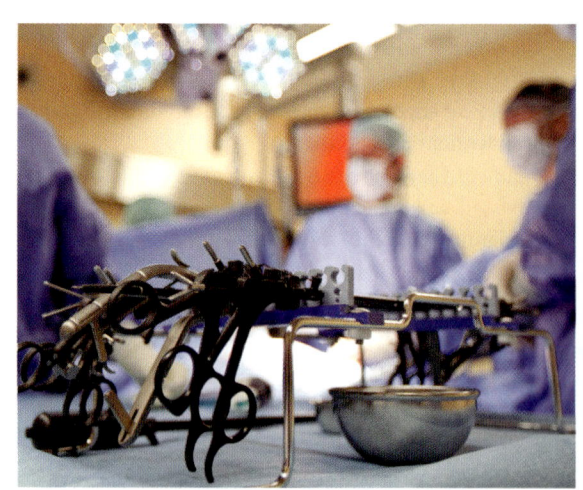

◘ **Fig. 17.5.** LAGB instrumentarium

is passed through the formed tunnel (from the side of the band or the drain connecting it to the port, depending on the manufacturer's instructions) and fastened (in case of some models with a special tool). If several internal band diameters are available, the operator should decide which of them is to be used. The MiniMizer bands have a two-stage fastening system, so the diameter can be adjusted the anatomical conditions after the band has been introduced into the abdominal cavity.

If there is too much fat anterior to the stomach, making it difficult to fasten the band, the fat should be dissected, or a canal between the gastric wall and the adipose tissue layer should be formed for passage of the band. The anesthesiologist inserts a calibration probe and fills the balloon with a specified volume of fluid (15–25 ml). Many experienced surgeons do not use band calibration, but determine the placement site on the basis of their experience. Following the fastening and positioning of the band, plication is performed; i.e., the gastric wall above the band is attached with two to three sutures to the wall below to prevent displacement of the band. At many centers, this stage is omitted as unnecessary (◘ Fig. 17.6). The MiniMizer Extra has special loops which allow for direct fixation of the band with sutures to the gastric wall instead of plication (◘ Fig. 17.7).

Then the drain connecting the band to the port is passed outside (usually through a working puncture on the patient's left side) and connected to the port implanted in the abdominal layer. Obtech offers a special device (Velocity) for fixation of the port on a muscle fascia. All ports have openings allowing them to be sutured to the surrounding tissues. They are usually placed on the sternum, left costal arch, in the subcutaneous tissue. If the location of the port is distant from the point of drain origin, the drain is conducted through a tunnel formed in the subcutaneous tissue. Each port location has its supporters, although no location has been demonstrated to be superior (◘ Fig. 17.8) [2–5]. In the evening of the day of surgery, the patient can

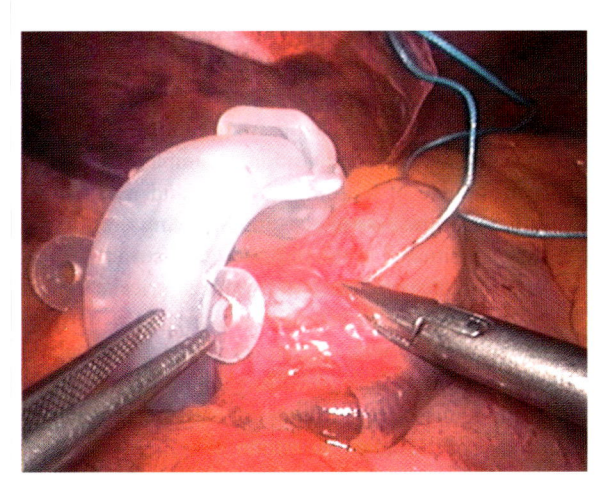

◘ Fig. 17.6. Band plication

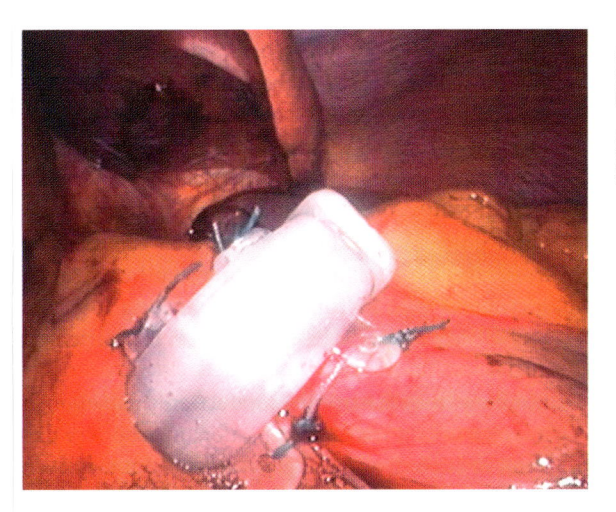

◘ Fig. 17.7. Suturing of a MiniMizer Extra band

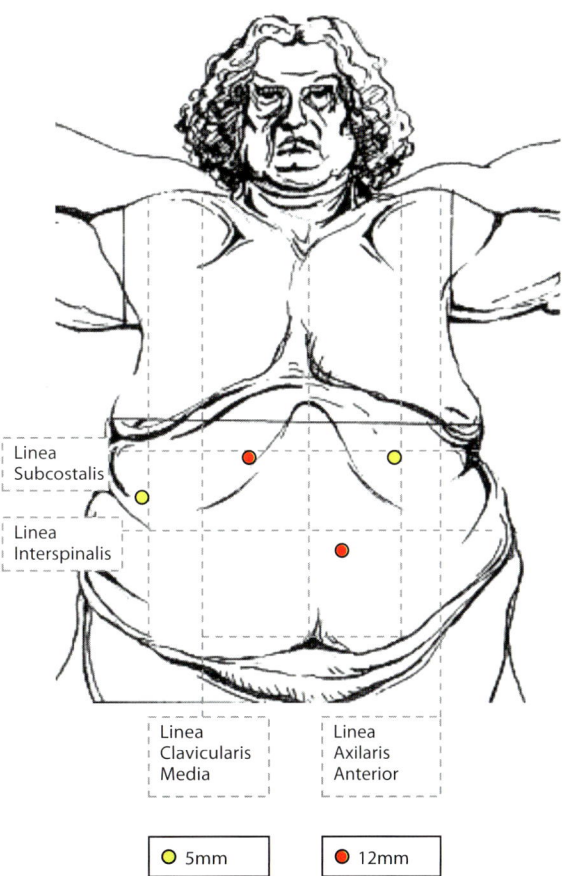

Linea Subcostalis

Linea Interspinalis

Linea Clavicularis Media

Linea Axilaris Anterior

○ 5mm   ● 12mm

◘ Fig. 17.8. Typical ports locations (implantation sites)

often with obstruction at the band site associated with too large "volume" of the gastric wall inside the band lumen. Conservative management (loosening of the band, liquid diet) can be attempted, but most cases require surgical correction (restoration of the previous band placement with fixation, sometimes replacement of the band with another one, another bariatric procedure) [25, 29–34].

— Port infection, due to the lack of aseptic conditions during adjustments, with persistent inflammatory reaction in the region of the port, resistant to antibiotics.

— Ascending infection along the drain with subsequent bacterial colonization of the band, manifested as internal infection with high fever and chills and requiring surgical removal of the band followed by antibiotic therapy. Antibiotic therapy alone is ineffective [14].

— Mechanical wear of the band or its elements, including damage to the port membrane, e.g., through use of an inappropriate needle; mechanical drain damage (puncture in an attempt to puncture the port); band rupture, e.g., due to too much fluid used, or mechanical damage due to manufacturing defects (e.g. lock failure with opening of the band) require replacing the band with a new one [14].

— Rotation of the port, especially if it is placed in loose adipose tissue, which can be prevented by port fixation. If the port is placed subcutaneously, in case of body weight reduction and consequent flabbiness of the skin, it can be grasped with the hand and positioned correctly; this is impossible in a patient before body weight reduction because of tense skin and a thick layer of subcutaneous fat [10, 12, 14, 34–37].

— Reversible widening of the esophagus, due to excessive food ingestion despite signals of stomach filling. It is largely dependent on psychological factors, is often manifested by large amounts of frothy saliva secreted at night, is easily recognizable by X-ray control,

◻ **Table 17.4** Late complications

Reference	Complication (%)			
	Migration	**Slippage**	**Problems with port and band**	**Psychical intolerance**
Montgomery et al. [10]	0.6	0.3	2.2	
te Riele et al. [17]		1.9		
Taylor and Layani [35]		2.5	5	
Bucter et al. [23]	1			
Favretti et al. [36]	0.9	3.9	11.2	0.7
Naef et al. [14]	1.55		5.45	
Arvind et al. [37]		13.8		
Korenkov et al. [11]		1.38		
Lee et al. [12]			3.7	0.94
Schouten et al. [39]	2.8	9.6	1.1	1.7
Suter et al. [13]	9.5	6.3	7.6	
Lattuoda et al. [24]	0.8	2.5	2.0	0.8
Boschi et al. [21]	0.25	4.0	4.5	
Himpens et al. [25]	2.5	7.5	7.5	
Belachev et al. [15]	0.9		2.5	
Holeczy et al. [34]		8.33	13.9	
Doldi et al. [16]	0.6	5.8		
Chevalier et al. [40]	0.3	7.8		

and requires loosening of the band for a period of ca. 4 weeks [13, 38].

— Persistent vomiting due to dietary mistakes (too-large food bolus obstructing the passage to the lower stomach); sometimes voiding the band is sufficient, but if this method fails, endoscopic intervention is necessary. Sometimes vomiting can be caused by mucous membrane edema (often seasonal – in the spring or autumn, or associated with stress); this requires band voiding, proton pump blockers, and local anti-inflammatory agents (lavage with hydrocortisone, chamomile solution). Vomiting can be also caused by an allergic reaction to the band, which is very rare but may result in cicatrization, narrowing the stomach at the band placement site. Such a complication often requires removal of the band, surgical widening of the stenosis site, e.g., with an endoscope, and application of another bariatric procedure. The incidence of these complications is presented in Gastric banding is not mortality-free. The mortality associated with this procedure has been estimated at 0.0– 0.44% and is most frequently due to disturbances associated with anesthesia, cardiac and pulmonary issues, and frequently, despite correct anticoagulant prophylaxis with low-molecular-weight heparins, to thromboembolic complications [13, 14, 17, 45]. The weight reduction effect (%EWL) after gastric banding is assessed in different ways in the literature. Some reports are enthusiastic, valuing the method highly, but there are also some reports emphasizing that because of an inadequate weight reduction effect (%EWL <40) the band should be used in subjects with BMI not exceeding 45–50 kg/m^2. The assessment of long-term effects of gastric banding is presented in ◘ Table 17.6 [25, 46, 47].

◘ **Table 17.5** Rare complications

Complication	Reference
Venous thrombosis of the upper extremity	Montgomery et al. [10]
Aspiration pneumonia	Montgomery et al. [10]
Bezoars	Parameswaran et al. [41]
Obstruction of small intestine due to drain	Zappa et al.[42]
Recurrent pneumonia	Hofer et al. [43]
Arrhythmia	Reijnen and Janssen [44]

◘ **Table 17.6** Long-term effects of gastric banding

Reference	Percent per period of time					
	12 months	24 months (2 years)	36 months (3 years)	60 months (5 years)	288 months (12 years)	Not available
Montgomery et al. [10]	44.0	51.1				
te Riele et al. [17]	34.4	43.4				
Taylor and Layani [35]		54.0				
Favretti et al. [36]	40.3	43.7			49.2	
Naef et al. [14]	33.3	45.5		57.4		
Korenkov et al. [11]						61.9
Lee et al. [12]	44.7	44.8				
Himpens et al. [25]	41.4		48.0			
Doldi et al. [16]						62.5
Chevallier et al. [47]						52.7
Fielding and Duncombe [49]						51.2
Ponce et al. [61]		63.3				
O'Brien et al. [48]						53.0

17.5   Discussion: Gastric Banding – Aspects of Metabolic Surgery

Initially, the "perigastric" banding technique was used (▶ Fig. 17.4). However, the literature contains numerous reports concerning high rates of complications in the form of slippage (especially posterior) associated with the use of this technique. The introduction of the pars flaccida technique (▶ Fig. 17.5) reduced the occurrence of this complication [17, 33, 36, 39, 48, 49]. The operation could be associated with technical problems due to the individual anatomical variations encountered. One of them is an enlarged, edematous left hepatic lobe, often with lesions of the hepar moschatum type. Raising it with a retractor can be helpful, so as to cause minimal injury to the delicate liver tissue. Thus, the instrument should be 10 mm rather than 5 mm in diameter. Nevertheless, small subcapsular hematomas may be observed on the lower surface at the end of the procedure. Such complications subside after a short time and do not affect the patient's general condition. In order to improve visibility in the angle of Hiss region, the left lobe can be released by dissection of the left triangular ligament. Such a maneuver considerably improves visibility in the operating area. The term "sea of fat" is often used in cases of a large amount of visceral fat. Surgery is more difficult in such situations because of the lack of a distinct pars flaccida, usually seen as a thin, transparent membrane. In such a case, the surgeon reaches the region of the right diaphragmatic crux. There are currently no satisfactory explanations concerning the mechanism of the two most serious complications of gastric banding – migration and slippage. Abnormal reaction of the stomach to the band material is most frequently mentioned as a cause of migration, observed in less than 1% of the patients. Reports associating this complication with the use of high-pressure bands have not been confirmed in the literature. It is commonly believed that avoidance of maximal band inflation can prevent this complication. Microscopic investigations of the gastric wall tissues at the interface with the gastric band revealed the presence of fibrosis, or a chronic inflammatory process, but failed to contribute to the solution of the migration problem [14, 24]. Slippage, which may occur anterior or posterior - the latter considerably less frequent after introduction of the pars flaccida technique – is observed in 0.3–9.5% of patients. It is very often preceded by vomiting. In the authors' experience, slippage occurred in 3.2% of cases.

Detailed anamnesis established that vomiting was most often caused by dietary mistakes (too large food bolus) or a systemic infection (e.g. viral). The literature fails to confirm the thesis that slippage is caused by no plication (tunnelization) of the band, i.e., application of sero-serous sutures connecting the gastric wall above and below the band (▶ Fig. 17.6), or, conversely, that the complication can be prevented by such suturing. The MiniMizer Extra band, equipped on the upper and lower edge with special loops allowing it to be sutured to the gastric wall, is an interesting solution intended to prevent both slippage and migration [14, 17, 21, 29, 30, 39, 40, 50]. Esophageal distention, subsiding after periodic "loosening" of the band, and requiring its removal in extreme cases, depends on the effect of the band on the LES mechanism. According to Marconi, the occurrence of this complication is dependent on preoperative disturbances in esophageal motor function. The author suggests routine manometry before the surgery; however, he considers it striking that this complication became manifest in his patients so late – 19 months after surgery [38, 43, 51, 52].

The surgical techniques of LAGB demonstrate the most variety in the location and method of implantation of the port. It is most frequently implanted in the left epigastric region, on the left costal arch, or on the sternum. Fixing the port to a bony structure (the sternum or a rib) ensures its immobility and good access for regulation. In patients who have lost a considerable amount of adipose tissue, the port becomes very visible and the skin covering it very tense, which may lead to injuries exposing the port. Implantation of the port into a muscle fascia may cause problems associated with accessibility – especially during the initial period of weight loss (thick subcutaneous fat layer) – involving the necessity of using a long needle, which may be troublesome in view of the hard, resistant port membrane. The authors prefer subcutaneous implantations of the port, a few centimeters medial to the location of the right working trocar (20 mm). This allows easy identification of the port and, in case of its rotation, access even to the membrane which has turned upside down. The height-to-diameter ratio is considered to be important for the rotation potential. The lower it is, the lower the risk of port rotation [37]. As after any bariatric operation, the success of the procedure, assessed in terms of body weight reduction, is dependent in the majority of cases on good patient compliance. It is recommended that the patient eat frequently, in small quantities, masticate the food thoroughly, and not drink during the meal. Fizzy drinks (mineral water, sweetened beverages, beer, champagne) are absolutely contraindicated, because in a warm environment (such as the gastrointestinal tract) they release large volumes of gas, which may cause distention of the "upper" stomach or the esophagus. Soups, puree, ice-cream, honey, and sweetened beverages are contraindicated because they pass through even a very tightly closed band and supply an enormous amount of calories. We advise our patients to sit at the table with their families and eat the same foods, but using plates "for dolls". However, it is important to take the same amount of time for such small amounts of food as for a normal portion, according to the principle: "if you chew long, you live long." It is difficult to devise an ideal and obligatory diet, because patients have individual dietary likes and dislikes. Unlike slimming diets, dietary "offenses" do not disturb the process of body weight reduction, if they occur only occasionally. The patient can be informed that once a week, or to celebrate some slimming achievements (body weight reduction to the next 10 kg or below the "magic" threshold of 100 kg, BMI change from obese to overweight) he or she can eat "as a reward" a small (!!!) amount of some favorite food. Coffee, tea, and alcohol are not contraindicated, but without sugar or with only a small amount. As it is impossible for the patient to drink a large amount of fluid at a time, the patients should drink low volumes of fluids between meals, but practically on a continuous basis. This is particularly vital in case of considerable fluid loss – in subjects doing manual jobs, living in low-humidity, air-conditioned premises, in tropical climates, or in moderate zones in the summer. Reduced fluid supply leads in many patients to defecation disturbances, such as chronic constipation, due to excessive resorption of water from the large intestine. Particular problems may arise for Muslims during Ramadan – i.e., ritual fasting from sunrise to sunset; unlike other patients, they cannot compensate fluid deficiency quickly. Gastric banding, like other bariatric operations, has been observed to result in regression of type-2 diabetes, manifested by dose reduction or withdrawal of anti-diabetic medications, normalization of arterial blood pressure, and regression of articular symptoms caused by overload. Numerous studies comparing various types of bariatric procedures demonstrated no changes in ghrelin and leptin activity in patients with gastric bands; the regression of coincidental conditions was associated only with body weight reduction, with no changes in endocrine function [54–62]. Despite 25 years of use, LAGB is still a dynamic and developing method. As with other procedures, the indications for gastric banding are being extended gradually, with respect to BMI lower than 35 and the patient's age (reports concerning gastric banding in adolescents and children are becoming more and more frequent). As far as the development of the band itself is concerned, the manufacturers compete in improving and modernizing their product, introducing simpler, safer fastening systems, solutions aimed at homogeneous compression along the whole circumference of the stomach by the band balloon, and use of materials minimizing tissue reactions, which could reduce the complication rates. The introduction of bands allowing remote control of compression parameters, so-called telemetric bands, is important for the patients. They make it possible to avoid port punctures, which will eliminate a wide spectrum of complications associated with this procedure [54].

References

1. Oria HE, Doherty C (2007) Farewell to a pioneer: Lubomyr Kuzmak. Obes Surg 17:141-142
2. Kuzmak LI (1991) A review of seven years' experience with silicone gastric banding. Obes Surg 1:403–408
3. Ren CJ, Fielding GA (2003) Laparoscopic adjustable gastric banding: surgical technique. J Laparoendoscopic Adv Surg Techniques 13:257–263
4. Weiner RA (2005) Gastric banding: chirurgisch–technische Aspekte. Chirurg 76:678–688
5. Arata JE, Perry AJ (1991) Adjustable gastric banding. Obes Surg 1:103–104
6. Fried M, Hainer V, Basdevant A et al (2007) Interdisciplinary European guidelines for surgery for severe (morbid) obesity. Obes Surg 17:260–270
7. Cottam DR, Atkinson J, Anderson, Grace AB, Fisher B (2006) A case-controlled matched-pair cohort study of laparoscopic Rouxen- Y gastric bypass and Lap-Band patients in a single US center with three-year follow-up. Obes Surg 16:534–540
8. Colles SL, Dixon JB, O'Brian PE (2008) Hunger control and regular physical activity facilitate weight loss after laparoscopic adjustable gastric banding. Obes Surg 18:833–840
9. Kirchmayr W, Klaus A, Muhlmann G, Mittermair R, Bonatti H, Aigner F, Weiss H (2004) Adjustable gastric banding: assessment of safety and efficacy of bolus-filling during follow-up. Obes Surg 14:387–391
10. Montgomery KF, Watkins BM, Ahroni JH et al (2007) Outpatient laparoscopic adjustable gastric banding in super-obese patients. Clin Anesth 17:711–716
11. Korenkov M, Shah S, Sauerland S, Duenschede F, Junginger T (2007) Impact of laparoscopic adjustable gastric banding on obesity co-morbidities in the medium and long term. Obes Surg 17:679–683
12. Lee WJ, Wang W, Yu PJ, Wie PL, Huang MT (2006) Gastrointestinal quality of life following laparoscopic adjustable gastric banding in Asia. Obes Surg 16:586–591
13. Suter M, Calmes JM, Paroz A, Giusti V (2006) A 10-year experience with laparoscopic gastric banding for morbid obesity: high longterm complication and failure rates. Obes Surg 16:829–835
14. Naef M, Naef U, Mouton WG, Wagner E (2007) Outcome and complications after laparoscopic Swedish adjustable gastric banding: 5-year results of a prospective clinical trial. Obes Surg 17:195–201
15. Belachew M, Belva PH, Desaive C (2002) Long-term results of laparoscopic adjustable gastric banding for the treatment of morbid obesity. Obes Surg 12:564–568
16. Doldi SB, Micheletto G, Lattuada E, Zappa MA, Bona D, Sonvico U (2000) Adjustable gastric banding: 5-year experience. Obes Surg 10:171–173
17. te Riele WW, Vogten JM, Boerma D, Wiezer MJ, van Ramshorst B (2008) Comparison of weight loss and morbidity after gastric bypass and gastric banding. A single-center European experience. Obes Surg 18:11–16

18. Boschi S, Fogli L, Berta RD et al (2006) Avoiding complications after laparoscopic esophago-gastric banding: experience with 400 consecutive patients. Obes Surg 16:1166–1170

19. Lagandre S, Arnalsteen L, Vallet B et al (2006) Predictive factors for rhabdomyolysis after bariatric surgery. Obes Surg 16:1365–1370

20. Ettinger JEMTM, de Souza CAM, Santos-Filho PV et al (2007) Rhabdomyolysis: diagnosis and treatment in bariatric surgery. Obes.Surg 17:525–5327

21. Boschi S, Fogli L, Berta RD et al A (2006) Voiding complications after laparoscopic esophago-gastric banding: experience with 400 consecutive patients. Obes Surg 16:1166–1170

22. Rao AD, Ramalingam G (2006) Exsanguinating hemorrhage following gastric erosion after laparoscopic adjustable gastric banding. Obes Surg 16:1675–1678

23. Bueter M, Thalheimer A, Meyer D, Fein M (2006) Band erosion and passage, causing small bowel obstruction. Obes Surg 16:1679–1682

24. Lattuada E, Zappa MA, Mozzi E et al (2006) Histologic study of tissue reaction to the gastric band: does it contribute to the problem of band erosion? Obes Surg 16:1155–1159

25. Himpens J, Dapri G, Cadiere GB (2006) A prospective randomized study between laparoscopic gastric banding and laparoscopic isolated sleeve gastrectomy: results after 1 and 3 years. Obes Surg 16:1450–1456

26. Campos J, Ramos A, Galvao NM et al (2007) Hypovolemic shock due to intragastric migration of an adjustable gastric band. Obes Surg 17:562–564

27. Vertruyen M, Paul G (2003) 11-cm Lap-band system placement after history of intragastric migration. Obes Surg 13:435–438

28. Meir E, Van Baden M (1999) Adjustable silicone gastric banding and band erosion: personal experience and hypotheses. Obes Surg 9:191–193

29. Sherwinter DA, Powers CJ, Geiss AC, Howard M, Warman J (2006) Posterior prolapse: an important entity even in the modern age of the pars flaccida approach to lap-band placement. Obes Surg 16:1312–1317

30. Yitzhak A, Mizrahi S, Avinoach E (2006) Laparoscopic gastric banding in adolescents. Obes Surg 16:1318–1322

31. Abuzeid AW, Banerjea A, Timmis B, Hashemi M (2007) Gastric slippage as an emergency: diagnosis and management. Obes Surg 17:559–561

32. Lanthaler M, Mittermair R, Erne B, Weiss H, Aigner F, Nehoda H (2006) Laparoscopic gastric re-banding versus laparoscopic gastric bypass as a rescue operation for patients with pouch dilatation. Obes Surg 16:484–487

33. Zappa MA, Micheletto G, Lattuada E et al (2006) Prevention of pouch dilatation after laparoscopic adjustable gastric banding. Obes Surg 16:132–136

34. Holeczy P, Novak P, Kralova A (2001) 30% complications with adjustable gastric banding: what did we do wrong? Obes Surg 11:748–751

35. Taylor CJ, Layani L (2006) Laparoscopic adjustable gastric banding in patients ≥60 years old: is it worthwhile? Obes Surg 16:1579–1583

36. Favretti F, Segato G, Ashton D et al (2007) Laparoscopic adjustable gastric banding in 1791 consecutive obese patients: 12-year results. Obes Surg 17:168–175

37. Arvind N, Bates SE, Morgan JD, Hewin DF, Frering VM, Norton SA (2007) Fixation of the access-port is not required in gastric banding. Obes Surg 17:577–580

38. Facchiano E, Scaringi S, Sabate JM et al (2007) Is esophageal dysmotility after laparoscopic adjustable gastric banding reversible? Obes Surg 17:832–835

39. Schouten R, van Dielen FM, Greve JW (2006) Re-operation after laparoscopic adjustable gastric banding leads to a further decrease in BMI and obesity-related co-morbidities: results in 33 patients. Obes Surg 16:821–828

40. Chevallier JM, Zinzindohoue F, Douard R et al (2004) Complications after laparoscopic adjustable gastric banding for morbid obesity: experience with 1000 patients over 7 years. Obes Surg 14:407–414

41. Parameswaran R, Ferrando J, Sigurdsson A (2006) Gastric bezoar complicating laparoscopic adjustable gastric banding with band slippage. Obes Surg 16:1683–1684

42. Zappa MA, Lattuada E, Mozzi E et al (2006) An unusual complication of gastric banding: recurrent small bowel obstruction caused by the connecting tube. Obes Surg 16:939–941

43. Hofer M, Stollberger C, Finsterer J, Kriwanek S (2007) Recurrent aspiration pneumonia after laparoscopic adjustable gastric banding. Obes Surg 17:565–567

44. Reijnen MM, Janssen IM (2004) Cardiac arrhythmias after laparoscopic banding. Obes Surg 14:139–141

45. Chapman AE, Kiroff G, Game P et al (2004) Laparoscopic adjustable gastric banding in the treatment of obesity – a systematic literature preview. Surgery 135:326–351

46. Schweitzer DH, Dubois EF, van den Doel-Tanis N, Oei HI (2007) Successful weight loss surgery improves eating control and energy metabolism: a review of the evidence. Obes Surg 17:533–539

47. Chevallier JM, Zinzindohoue F, Elian N et al (2002) Adjustable gastric banding in a public university hospital: prospective analysis of 400 patients. Obes Surg 12:93–99

48. O'Brien PE, Dixon JB, Laurie C, Anderson M (2005) A prospective randomized trial of placement of the laparoscopic adjustable gastric band: comparison of the perigastric and pars flaccida pathways. Obes Surg 15:820–826

49. Fielding GA, Duncombe JE (2005) Clinical and radiological follow- up of laparoscopic adjustable gastric bands, 1998 and 2000: a comparison of two techniques. Obes Surg 15:634–640

50. Szewczyk T, Modzelewski B (2006) Perioperative comparison of the MiniMizer extra band with the other laparoscopic gastric bands. Obes Surg 16:646–650

51. Tolonen P, Victorzon M, Niemi R, Makela J (2006) Does gastric banding for morbid obesity reduce or increase gastroesophageal reflux? Obes Surg 16:1469–1474

52. Dargent J (2005) Esophageal dilatation after laparoscopic adjustable gastric banding: definition and strategy. Obes Surg 15:843–848

53. Rocha AT, de Vasconcellos AG, da Luz Neto ER, Araujo DMA, Alves ES, Lopes AA (2006) Risk of venous thromboembolism and efficacy of thromboprophylaxis in hospitalized obese medical patients and in obese patients undergoing bariatric surgery. Obes Surg 16:1645–1655

54. Weiner RA, Korenkov M, Matzig E, Weiner S, Karcz WK, Junginger T (2007) Early results with a new telemetrically adjustable gastric banding. Obes Surg 17:717–721

55. Uzzan B, Catheline JM, Lagorce C et al (2007) Expression of ghrelin in fundus is increased after gastric banding in morbidly obese patients. Obes Surg 17:1159–1164

56. Baranova A, Gowder SJ, Schlauch K et al (2006) Gene expression of leptin, resistin, and adiponectin in the white adipose tissue of obese patients with non-alcoholic fatty liver disease and insulin resistance. Obes Surg 16:1118–1125

57. Ballantyne GH, Farkas D, Laker S, Wasielewski A (2006) Short-term changes in insulin resistance following weight loss surgery for morbid obesity: laparoscopic adjustable gastric banding versus laparoscopic Roux-en-Y gastric bypass. Obes Surg 16:1189–1197

58. Coupaye M, Bouillot JL, Poitou C, Schutz Y, Basdevant A, Oppert JM (2007) Is lean body mass decreased after obesity treatment by adjustable gastric banding? Obes Surg 17:427–433

59. Hernandez-Morante JJ, Milagro FI, Larque E et al (2007) Relationship among adiponectin, adiponectin gene expression and fatty acid composition in morbidly obese patients. Obes Surg 17:516–524

60. Ram E, Vishne T, Maayan R et al (2005) The relationship between BMI, plasma leptin, insulin and proinsulin before and after laparoscopic adjustable gastric banding. Obes Surg 15:1456–1462

61. Ponce J, Haynes B, Paynter S et al (2004) Effect of lap-band-induced weight loss on type 2 diabetes mellitus and hypertension. Obes Surg 14:1335–1342

62. Weiss H, Labeck B, Klocker J et al (2001) Effects of adjustable gastric banding on altered gut neuropeptide levels in morbidly obese patients. Obes Surg 11:735–739

The Sleeve Gastrectomy

Daniel Krawczykowski, MD

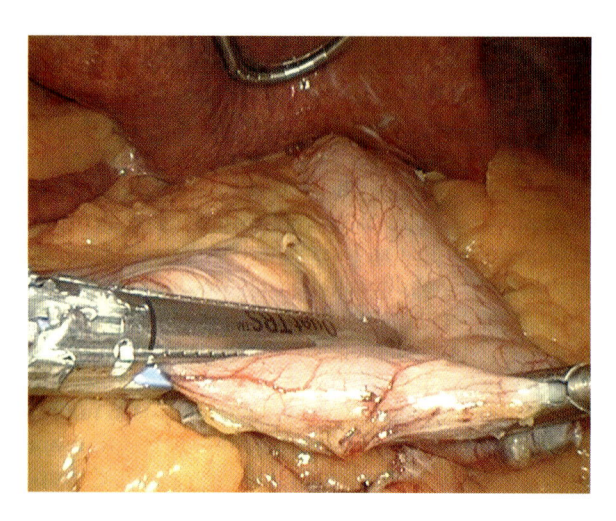

■ **Fig. 18.4.** The transomental approach for SG: section of the stomach prior to mobilization of the greater curvature

5 years. Even if the size of the meal is small, the volume of the remaining stomach is larger by far than after purely restrictive procedures (gastric banding, vertical banded gastroplasty). Melissas et al. demonstrated an accelerated gastric emptying of solid food into the duodenum and the intestine at 6 and 24 months, and this could explain some enterohormonal changes [36, 37]. In addition to these mechanical effects, SG has hormonal effects. This operation is "anorexigenic"; the patients feel little hunger and have only a mild interest in eating. Most of them could skip a meal each day for at least 1 year after surgery. The fundus is known to be the major source of ghrelin, an orexigenic hormone. It has been proved that the level of ghrelin is dramatically reduced after the currently performed SG with the entire fundus resected, and to a higher degree than with gastric banding [38] or gastric bypass [39]. Other hormonal changes have been noted, such as a rise in the level of fasting PYY or GLP1, a hormone that induces also a feeling of satiety [39]. This latter point has yet to be assessed in human beings [40, 41]. These incretin modifications could play a role in the remarkable short-term effects observed on diabetes [41, 42]. Thus it appears that LSG is a multifactorial procedure with a mild restrictive aspect and a complex neurohormonal aspect [37].

18.3 Indications for LSG

As mentioned above, ISG has been performed as the first stage several months prior to DS or gastric bypass in staged surgery to reduce the mortality of laparoscopic BPD/DS and bypass surgery in high-risk patients: i.e.,

either super-super-obese patients (BMI >55) or patients with cardiac, respiratory, or hepatic conditions [9, 12, 15, 24, 43]. SG has been also described as revision surgery for gastric banding failure with inadequate weight loss, slippage, erosion, or a port problem [7, 44–47]. Currently, ISG is proposed as a single surgical procedure by some authors instead of gastric banding or a bypass for low BMI (35–45) patients, for adolescents, for the elderly, for high-risk patients, for transplant candidates, for those who require periodical monitoring of their stomach (gastritis, *Helicobacter pylori* infection, ulcers), and for those patients for whom a malabsorptive procedure would be dangerous because of concomitant anti-inflammatory treatment, chronic anemia, an inflammatory bowel disease, or AIDS [14, 16, 18, 48, 49]. Other indications found in the literature are poor intraoperative exposure [50] and following a malabsorptive procedure such as jejuno-ileal bypass [51]. A hiatal hernia of 5 cm or less should not be a contraindication; however, for larger hernias or for severe gastric reflux, patients would be better treated with a gastric bypass [35, 46]. The advantages of this procedure are limited surgical intervention and no foreign body. It is a "low-maintenance" procedure: no adjustment is required; there are neither port- nor band-related complications; the dietary restrictions are fewer than after other restrictive procedures, and consequently, the quality of life is better; there is no dumping syndrome, there are no ulcers, and no major nutritional deficiencies are to be expected. Vomiting is seldom encountered after 6 months [37]. However, a case of Wernicke's syndrome has been reported by Makarewicz et al. [52], so even though it is rare (fewer than 2.5% [48]), patients who are vomiting must be checked for thiamine deficiency. Baltasar has argued that LSG could be a multi-purpose bariatric operation [12]. However, we think that this enthusiasm should be tempered: If the patients are in a very poor condition and cannot tolerate a complication, they should either not be operated on or they would be better served by a gastric banding procedure because there is no stapling, the operating time is shorter, and the rate of major complications remains lower. A contraindication could be ulcers in the lesser curvature of the stomach and Barret's esophagus, should the greater curvature be needed in reconstructive surgery after esophagectomy [30].

18.4 Results (■ Table 18.1)

At 1 year, the % EWL achieved with an ISG is in the range of 33–83.3% [5, 53]. In the short term, the % EWL is greater with SG than with an intragastric balloon [54], comparable to that of a bypass [55], and in a randomized study, greater at 3 years, than that obtained with gastric banding [48]. However, we do not yet have any long-term results, and patients should be informed that an additional malabsorptive procedure may be necessary in case of inadequate weight loss or weight regain. A particular case is super and super-super-obese patients, who often require combined surgery to achieve weight reduction and almost normal BMI. Improvement in the co-morbid conditions is obvious, as for other bariatric procedures. For hypertension, the resolution/improvement rates are (62.5–93%) / (25–7%); for

hyperlipidemia: (45–73%) / (30–5%); for sleep apnea: (56.2–80%) / (31.2–7%) [10, 15, 43, 53]. SG improves the candidacy for transplantation of patients with cirrhosis and end-stage lung disease [56]; it reduces the ASA score in super-obese patients undergoing two-stage BPD/DS [10]. Special mention must be made of type-2 diabetes mellitus (T2DM): In a Korean study, Moon Han et al. reported that all (100%) cases of T2DM were improved by SG at 6 months [16]. In a matched study for T2DM duration and type of treatment, Vidal et al. showed that at 4 months SG was as effective as gastric

Table 18.1 Sleeve gastrectomy: technical aspects and results

Ref.	Patients (n)	Initial BMI	Bougie calibration in F	Starting from pylorus (in cm)	Size of residual stomach	% IEWL	Morbidity, major complications (%)	Leaks (%)	Mortality (%)
[23]	230	40–64	36 34 32	5–6		62 60 58 at 3 yr	4	2.5	0
[24]	21[1]	57.7 (53–71.5)			100	47 at 1 yr	20		0 late 14
[12]	31	three series	32	2	<60	42–100	3.2	0	3.2
[44]	8[3]	50.5 (37–74)	34			57 at 1 year	0	0	0
[13]	50[2]	37.9 (32.9–46.8)	32	2–3	75 ±22		2	?	0
[43]	126[2]	65.4 ±9 (45–91)	46–50	5		45 ±17 at 1 yr	14	1.6	0 late 0.75
[14]	126[2,3]	48.1±8.7	48	Crow's foot		At 20 months: 64% of patients loss >50% 6.8% loss <25%	3.17	2.4	0
[15]	118[1,2]	55 (37–108)				49.4 (26.8–79.6) at 1 yr 47.3 at 2 yr	15.3	1.7	0.85
[48]	40[2]	39 (30–53)	34	Crow's foot		57.7 (0–125.5) at 1 yr 66 (-3.1–152.4) at 3 yr	5	1 gastric ischemia	0
§	206[2]	45 ±7.2 (33.8–82.2)	36	Crow's foot	±120	83.0 ± 26.1 at 1 yr 80.1 ± 26.7 at 2 yr 66.8 ±23.4 at 3 yr	5.8	3.4	0
▼	83[3]	45.2 ±6.4 (35.9–65.4)	36			71.6 ±24.8 at 1 yr 74.4 ±27.1 at 2 yr 77.7 ±26.5 at 3 yr	16.7	13.3	Late 1.2

◻ **Table 18.1** *Continued*

Ref.	Patients (n)	Initial BMI	Bougie calibration in F	Starting from pylorus (in cm)	Size of residual stomach	% IEWL	Morbidity, major complications (%)	Leaks (%)		Mortality (%)
[59]	148[2] 16[3]	44 (35–64)	52-42				2.9	0.7		0
[38]	23[2]	48.5 ±6.9 (40–73)	48	Crow's foot		56 at 1 yr				
[18]	216[2]	49 ±11	32	6–8	60–80	59 ±17 at 1 yr	4.6	1.4		0
[53]	130[2]	30–56	48		50–60	83.3 at 1 yr	2.9	0.7		0.7
[75]	135[2]	60±10.6	40	4–6		47.3±16 at 1 yr	7	1.5		Late 0.7
[19]	140[2] 22[3]	45.9	36	Crow's foot		59.45 at 1 yr 61.52 at 2 yr	15	3.66	1.22 2.44	0
[41]	68[2] 47[2]	63.1±8.1 55.1±11.5	60 40	Crow's foot Crow's foot		45.4±14.9 51.9±20.9 at 1 yr				
[5]	14[2]	58-71	60	Crow's foot		33 at 11 months	21.4	0		0
[68]	120 (100[2], 20[3])	43±5 (30–60)	48	6–7		53±24 at 11.7 months		0		0
[10]	41[2]	57.3±	48	7–8	120–150		12.1	2.4		0
[33]	93 (90[2], 3[3])	46.9±6.5 (37–66)	36	3–4	<100	67.2 at 12 months	8.6	4.3		0

[1] Open surgery
[2] Primary
[3] Secondary, after gastric banding
[5] Krawczykowski, not published; IEWL initial excess weight loss

bypass in inducing T2DM remission, and their data suggest that mechanisms beyond weight loss may be implicated [41].

18.5 Drawbacks of the Operation

The two major drawbacks of the SG are the long staple line that carries the risk of morbidity and mortality and the irreversible nature of gastric resection. Indeed, SG is so far the only definitively non-reversible bariatric surgery. In the position statement on SG as a bariatric procedure endorsed by the ASMBS, the complication rate is in the range of 0–24% and the perioperative mortality is 0.39% [21]. – Bleeding at the staple line was reported by

Silecchia et al. in 7.3% of patients in a series of super-obese patients, but only one of the three patients needed a laparoscopic reoperation for extraluminal bleeding [10]. Endoluminal bleeding was ruled out by intraoperative gastroscopy [31]. The risk of hemorrhage from the line of section is usually around 0.7%, and it can be reduced by reinforcing the stapling with a running suture, with fibrin glue [43], or by using Gore Seamguard® bioresorbable staple line reinforcement [57]. Bovine pericardium reinforcement has been used but seems to migrate [58]. At present, we make separate Vicryl 2/0 stitches if occasional hemostasis is needed. Bleeding may also occur from spleen or liver laceration, as well as from the trocar site [12, 59]. Leakages are the main concern with this surgical procedure. They may occur in the range of

0–4.3% [33, 53, 59], with extremes as high as 10% when the surgery is performed in super-obese patients [42] or when it is a revision after gastric banding, especially after gastric erosion [14, 60] Leaks usually occur at the esophageal-gastric junction. Tests should be carried out with methylene blue and/or by insufflation of air, but they do not always reveal a leak which will show up during oral re-feeding on the 2nd or even up to the 5th day. Nevertheless, some have been described that appear late, after 3 weeks: four cases in our series, one in Weiner's series [29], and one in Silecchia's [10]. Leaks are either slight and well-tolerated (usually the late leaks, which may resolve with i.v. antibiotics and parenteral nutrition) [10], or dramatic, with hyperthermia, tachycardia (>120/min) not explained by dehydration or pain, tachypnea (>20/min), a decrease in left basal breath sounds, left lumbar pain, or pain in the left hypochondrium. If not well-drained, these leaks may lead to a cascade of complications: subphrenic collection/abscess, reactional pleural effusion, fistulation to the pleural cavity and to the left lung, and pseudoaneurysm (infectious) of the splenic artery with the possibility of cataclysmic hemorrhage and eventually sepsis that will progress rapidly to multiple organ failure. There may also be a progressive leukocytosis and rise in CRP, often with a fall in serum albumin requiring diagnostic and appropriate treatment, i.e., repeat laparoscopy. Paraclinical examinations, particularly to exclude a pulmonary embolism, must not delay this revision, even if the gastrographin swallow that we normally carry out on day 1 or day 2 is considered fine and does not show a leak. The goals are the safety of the patient and healing of the leak. The former is achieved by creating a gastrocutaneous fistula that prevents collection by directing the juices out of the body; the latter is obtained by reducing the output, keeping the patient well-nourished, and treating problems that might compromise the healing (strictures). Whenever possible, suturing the leak and apposition of an omental patch should be attempted; these are often ineffective for upper fistulas but usually effective for lower fistulas. Usually we debride the false membranes, perform thorough lavage, place a drain in contact with the leak, and, given time for improvement, we perform an alimentary jejunostomy. When leak drainage has been inadequate or protracted (more than 3 weeks), coated self-expanding stents have been fitted with success [35, 61, 62], but a Roux en Y limb draining the leak [63, 64] and total gastrectomies have been also described [65]. Stomaphyx® could be another option [66]. The mechanism of these leaks and factors favoring them are still not clear. Ischemia, thickness of the stomach, and technical problems concerning the staples and stapling are prime concerns. A long gastric sleeve and, even more a distal stenosis, do not create leaks but do contribute to their delayed healing. Leaks may be prevented by observing the principles for use of viscerosynthesis material: (a) using stapling equipment and staples according to the standards laid down by the manufacturers (60-mm Ethicon Endo-Surgery Echelon Endopath® Stapler with green or gold cartridges or green Covidien Endo GIA® staples); (b) keeping to a tissue compression time before stapling, avoiding crossing staples, dissecting to preserve good vascularization [67]. The ischemic risk is real [48]. It is possible that the calibration of the sleeve on a small-diameter Faucher tube (36 F and below) may encourage leaks. The final stapling must be made towards the greater curvature to avoid encroachment on the esophagus. Even though some authors advocate oversewing [68] or buttressing material [57], there is no evidence that staple-line reinforcement is of any use in reducing the rate of leaks [69]. Unstapling may occur during the operation, particularly in the antral part of the stomach, which is sometimes thick. This is dealt with by using a running suture, as restapling could narrow the sleeve.

The frequency of gastric strictures is between 0.7 and 4% [43, 59]. They are sometimes related to stapling too close to the incisura angularis, but oversewing of the staple-line has been also implicated [43]. They can delay the healing of a proximal fistula and, in theory, contribute to dilatation upstream. When induced by hematoma or edema, they are transient. Endoscopic dilation has been advocated for non-resolving strictures and when there is a proximal non-healing leak [43, 59]. Seromyotomy is also an option [35]. Regaining weight is not a complication but is the natural history of all types of bariatric surgery. The rate of gastric sleeve dilatation is still not established, but it will probably be more frequent with wide calibration [29]. To prevent gastric enlargement, wrapping the SG using polytetrafluoroethylene mesh has been assessed in a porcine model and has shown a lesser weight gain at 8 weeks [70]. Banded SG has been described with a view to improving and maintaining the weight loss for SG calibrated with a 50-F bougie; the bands were located over a 38-F bougie and 6 cm below the esogastric junction. The initial results were comparable to those of gastric bypass [71]. Unlike other, we do not consider the progressive dilatation of the stomach to be the main aspect: such dilatation is rare, and significant weight loss is obtained with relatively wide (48-F) calibrations [55]. Weight regain is related more to the ingestion of calorific foods with a soft or liquid consistency [33, 72] and, in our experience, to the lack of physical activity adjusted to weight loss. That being the case, if there is a lack of cooperation by the patient, or if it is impossible for him to make radical changes in the quality of his diet and in his physical activity, he can be offered an additional malabsorptive procedure, as long as he accepts the risks of a new operation, metabolic monitoring, and taking vitamin and trace-element supplements daily. Re-sleeve gastrectomy has been described with good results in patients regaining weight, particularly after BPD/DS when the stomach was calibrated with a 60-F tube [73], but also for failure after ISG [28]. High-BMI patients should be enrolled in a program of sequential or two-stage BPD/DS [10, 30, 74, 75]. A wide proximal gastric pouch with a funnel-like appearance or the appearance of a proximal gastric diverticulum is the result of incomplete dissection and resection of the fundus. These aspects are most often encountered in revision procedures after gastric banding [44]. Low initial weight loss could result from an incomplete resection of the fundus. Langer et al. [55] described such a case where the ghrelin level did not fall postoperatively, and the patient returned to his original weight after moderate weight reduction. A re-sleeve gastrectomy or the addition of malabsorptive surgery should be taken into consideration if the pouch poses a problem or if the patient regains weight. The Stomaphyx® device could be an option to reduce the size of the enlarged pouch.

Gastroesophageal reflux: The SG procedure has the reputation of encouraging gastroesophageal reflux disease (GERD) by removing the anti-reflux system. It is true that early on, 11.8–21.8% of patients complain of reflux occurrence, which usually responds to proton pump inhibitors (PPI) [48, 19]. Nevertheless, this problem, which appears shortly after the operation, may sometimes correct itself after the phase of weight loss. Some patients with reflux treated during the operative period, on the other hand, experience improvement, or the reflux disappears and they stop all PPI treatment after the SG [48, 37]. A gastric bypass can be performed if GERD is severe [55]. A repeat SG was performed by Gagner for a patient complaining of GERD and who regained weight after a BPD/DS [76].

Rhabdomyolysis has been reported but is related to the operating time and not specific to this procedure [33, 77]. Mucocele of the gastric tube has been described after conversion of a vertical banded gastroplasty to duodenal switch [78, 79].

Metabolic sequelae: We presented our results at the 6th International Obesity Surgery Expert Meeting in Saalfelden in 2008: Two years after primary ISG, there was no low albumin, no vitamin B12 deficiency, and no anemia, but the rate of patients with low ferritin rose from 4.2% before surgery to 19.5% at 2 years, probably because of a low desire on the part of the patients to eat red meat. A transient iron deficiency has been observed by Skrekas et al. [33].

18.6 Our Experience

We have been performing ISGs in a two-stage BPD/DS program since December 2001 in patients with a complication or failure of gastric banding, and since December 2002 in patients who do not wish to have a gastric band (LASGB) [7].

The Patients. Up to March 2009, 84 patients underwent SG as a second-line treatment after gastric banding. The indications were: 33 slippage, 21 inadequate weight loss, 21 intolerance, five esophageal dilatation, three erosion, one G-G fistula. The demographics for secondary SG after gastric banding were age: 43.2 years (25–67); sex ratio: 6 M/78 F; mean BMI before LASGB: 44.2 (35.9–61.7); before SG: 39.3 (27.9–59.4); mean time between LASGB and SG: 51.9 months (6–120); 32 SG were delayed and in 52 cases the SG was performed simultaneously with band withdrawal. Up to March 2009, 207 patients underwent ISG as a first-line treatment. The demographics for the primary isolated SG were age: 40 years (18–67); sex ratio: 28 M/179 F; mean BMI: 45 (33.8–82.2); seven had an intragastric balloon to initiate weight loss (four have decreased their weight by about 10 kg and three have gained weight).

The Technique. At the beginning of our experience, we were using 45-mm staplers with either green or blue cartridges, depending on the thickness of the gastric wall. The rate of leaks was 3.1% in primary surgery (one of 32 patients). Then we started a trial of oversewing the entire staple line with a continuous running suture using Vicryl 2/0, Mersuture 2/0, or Prolene 1. The rate of leaks was 6.1% (two of 33 patients). Next we used Gore *Seamguard®* Bioabsorbable Staple Line Reinforcement, and the rate of leaks was 6.9% (two of 29 patients). Eventually, in October 2006, we switched to the transomental approach and introduced the 60-mm stapling device (EndoGIA, Covidien, USA). Since February 2007, we have changed the stapler device and the technique for secondary SG after gastric banding. The current technique and results were presented at the First International Consensus Summit for Sleeve Gastrectomy in New York City, October 25–27, 2007 [22], and they are described below. We usually do not drain the patients but we have a very low threshold for re-laparoscopy whenever there is unexplained tachycardia, tachypnea, pain, fever, high white cell count, or high CRP.

The Results. The operative problems encountered with primary ISG were: seven reopening at the antrum, five bleeding: four at the splenic hilum, one at the posterior gastric artery, and one section of the calibrating tube at the last firing that led us to convert to an open bypass procedure. Following secondary SG after gastric banding, the operative complications were mainly difficulties in dissecting the angle of Hiss, one section of the calibrating tube resulting in conversion to an open gastric bypass (the patient is excluded from the series); two cases of re-opening of the staple line at the site of the previous band – these were sutured by laparoscopy; and two cases of bleeding – one from the spleen, one from the posterior gastric artery – that were managed by laparoscopy. We had no mortality within 30 days, but three patients died later (one patient died at 6 weeks of a pulmonary embolism, one committed suicide at 9 months, and one suffered a myocardial infarction at 33 months). New developments with the stapling device and the technique have dramatically reduced the rate of leaks to 1.8 % (two of the most recent 112 patients) for primary ISG and 6.5% (two of 31 patients) for secondary SG after LASGB. Our results in terms of weight loss and morbidity are compared to those in the literature in ◘ Table 18.1 and detailed in ◘ Table 18.2. Additional DS was performed at patients' request for inadequate weight loss (BMI >30) and curable co-morbid conditions (diabetes mellitus, high cholesterol). At 3 and 4 years, respectively, additional DS was performed in 11.3% and 20% of patients for primary SG, and the rates were 26% and 39%, respectively, for SG after gastric banding. For those who underwent an additional DS, the initial BMI was 50 for primary SG and 43.5 for secondary SG. This leads us to think that even with a BMI lower than 50, certain patients would benefit from malabsorptive surgery, but for some patients, ISG alone could be sufficient. Eventually we found that there are several advantages to the two-stage strategic approach:

- It gives restrictive surgery a chance and avoids patients' having to undergo complex surgery as a first-line procedure.

- A malabsorptive procedure (bypass or DS) can be added without re-operating on the esophageal-gastric junction.
- Sometimes patients who are fragile are in a better condition to face a second procedure which, in addition, will be easier.
- The cumulative rate of complications is lower when the two components of the BPD/DS are performed separately [5, 8].
- The result in terms of EWL is the same for the two-stage surgery as for the one-stage BPD/DS [8].

18.7 The Technique of SG after Gastric Banding

We use eight trocars and a 0°optic, and no long instruments. We work on two arcs of a circle (◘ Fig. 18.5). The first (superior) arc provides a perfect view of the esophageal-gastric junction, while the second (inferior) arc provides a view of the greater curvature of the stomach. The patient is positioned supine. The surgeon stands between the patient's legs. Since May 2008, the camera (0° optical system) is no longer held by an assistant but rather by an optic-holding device fixed to the right of the patient. The scrub nurse assists from the left side of the patient. Insufflation is undertaken using a Palmer needle into the left hypochondrial area until a pneumoperitoneum of 15 mmHg is obtained. We introduce the first 10-mm trocar (T1) on the median line 10 cm from the xiphoid process, then, under visual control, a 5-mm trocar (T2) below the xiphoid for the retractor, which pushes aside the left lobe of the liver and usually gives a perfect view of the esophageal-gastric junction. Between these two trocars, a right paramedian 5-mm trocar (T3) is placed 10 cm from the median line for the forceps held by the surgeon, which allows exposure by

◘ Table 18.2 Early reoperations for complications after sleeve gastrectomy

Reoperation for postoperative complications		Leaks				Hemor-rhage	Re-look laparoscopy
		Staple 45 mm	Staple 45 mm + running suture	Staple 45 mm + Seamguard	Staple 60 mm		
206 primary ISG		1/32, 3.1%	2/33, 6%	2/29, 6.9%	2/112, 1.8%	0	5
83 secondary ISG	simultaneous	0/10	2/16	2/4	2/21	0	0
	delayed	0/2	1/3	4/17	0/10	1	2

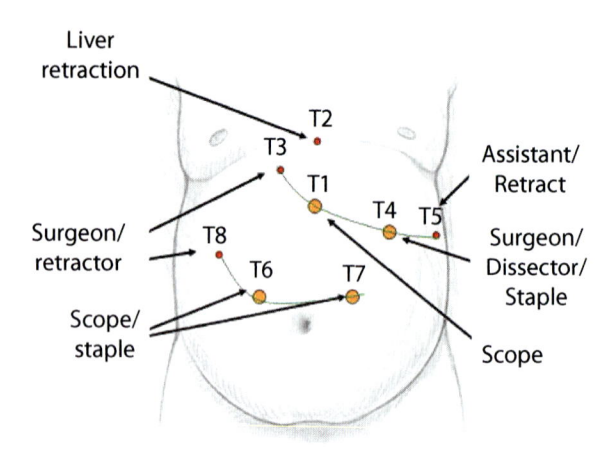

□ Fig. 18.5. Placement of ports

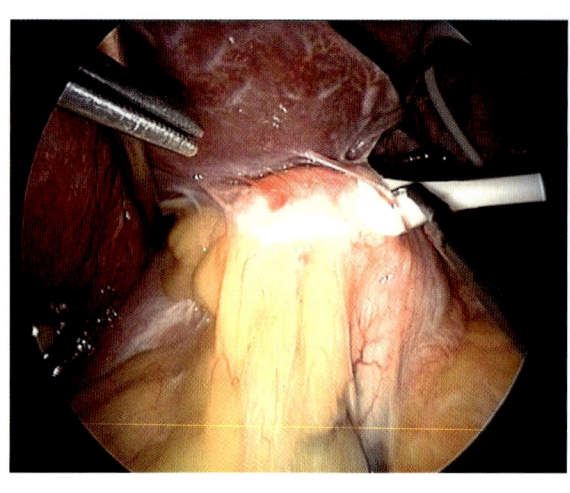

□ Fig. 18.6.

traction on the stomach. A 12-mm trocar with a reducer (T4) is inserted on the left side, on the medioclavicular line and in line with trocars T1 and T3, thus slightly offset downwards. In the first instance, this allows the introduction of scissors or the ultrasonic dissector, then at the end of the operation, of the stapler. On this same T1 and T3 line, where it crosses the anterior axillary line, a 5-mm trocar (T5) is inserted, which allows traction to be put on the omentum during the dissection of the angle of Hiss, then during freeing of the stomach from the omentum, and also holds the stomach during stapling. On the inferior arc, 5 cm on either side of the umbilicus, two 12-mm trocars (T6 and T7) are inserted which will alternatively admit the optic and the stapler. Finally, in the prolongation of the medioclavicular line, a 5-mm trocar (T8) is placed which exposes the greater curvature during its dissection and after its stapling. We always start with dissection of the angle of Hiss. This is easier if the band is still in place. After tracing the connecting tube to the buckle, we re-open the wrapping covering the band (□ Fig. 18.6 and 18.7). The adhesions between the left lobe of the liver and the esophageal-gastric junction (EJ) have to be severed (□ Fig. 18.8). For SG after gastric banding, we move to the greater curvature of the stomach and opposite to Latarjet's nerve; between 6 and 8 cm upstream of the pylorus, which may be palpated, we begin to free the stomach from the greater omentum using an ultrasonic dissector (□ Fig. 18.9). The stomach is freed as far as the band, with great care taken near the short vessels, moving the optic from trocar T7 to trocar T1. All the posterior attachments of the stomach, including the ramifications of the posterior gastric artery, are freed where they contact the stomach. Gentle pulling on the band helps to dissect the fibrotic tissue

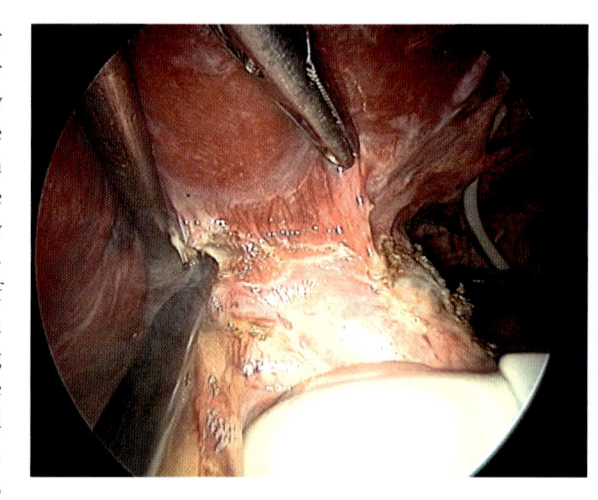

□ Fig. 18.7.

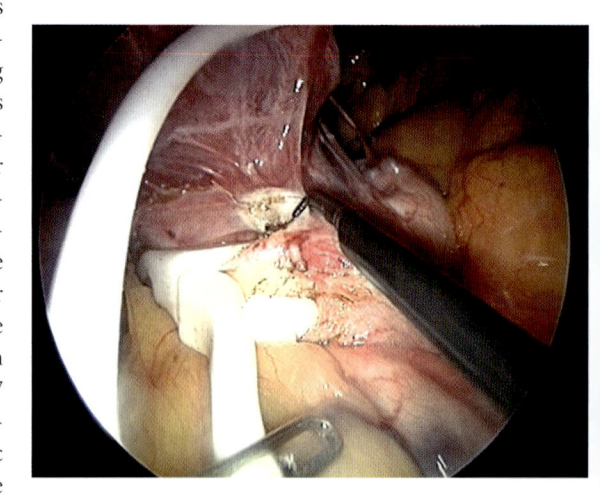

□ Fig. 18.8.

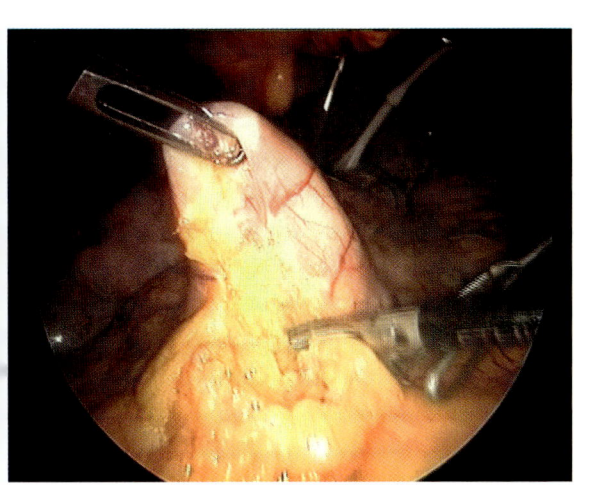

Fig. 18.9.

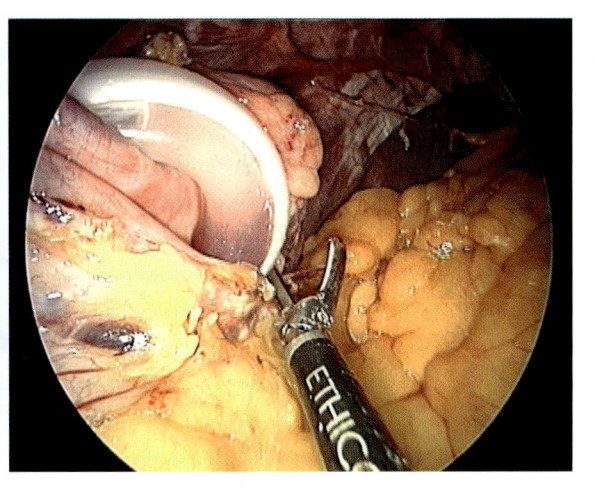

Fig. 18.10.

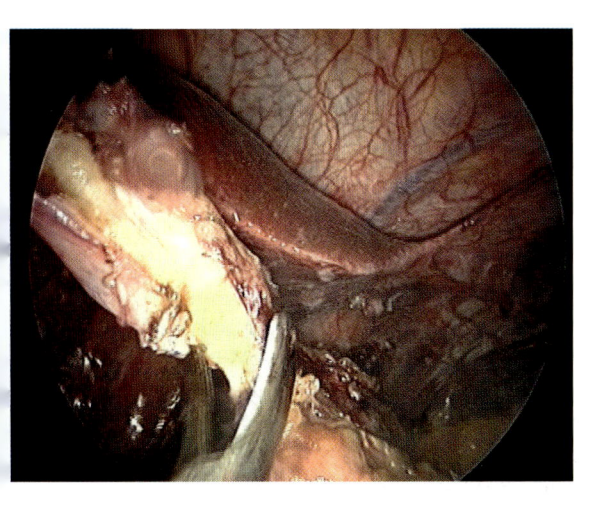

Fig. 18.11.

that fixes the posterior aspect of the stomach to the left crus (**Fig. 18.10**).

The fatty roll covering the EJ is dissected and excised, particularly if it is voluminous (**Fig. 18.11**). The band is then severed (**Fig. 18.12**), and the fibrotic tissue underneath is at least partially removed to allow this part of the stomach to be released (**Fig. 18.13**). The fundus often has a posterior development which must be completely dissected. The left pillar must be completely in view. The anesthetist passes a 36-F Faucher tube under the control and with the assistance of the surgeon, who directs the tube towards the pylorus.

The tube is held in contact with the lesser curvature. The stomach is moderately stretched out, and stapling begins with green or gold 60-mm Ethicon Endo-Surgery Endopath® Echelon Stapler cartridges, depending on the thickness of the antrum, with the optic in T6 and the stapler in T7 (**Fig. 18.14–18.16**). Stricture at the angulus must be avoided and the calibrating tube mobilized to be sure that it is not taken in the stapler. Final stapling is done with the stomach stretched out by gentle traction on the posterior wall of the fundus in the direction of the patient's left shoulder, to avoid not only encroachment on the esophagus but also taking in too much tissue and risking unstapling or leaving too wide a residual stomach (**Fig. 18.16 and 18.17**). We no longer reinforce our staple line with a running suture. In our experience, this running suture generally takes nearly half an hour, the appearance of the sleeve is sometimes irregular, and the rate of fistula is equivalent to that with 45-mm staples. We think that a running suture on a narrow sleeve is a factor encouraging complications: The start of the running suture may be the origin of tension on the bottom of the esophagus and may cause shearing of the gastric serous membrane. We carry out a test with methylene blue, clamping the stomach at the pylorus, which gives us an idea of the residual gastric volume (usually between 100 and 120 ml), then an immersed air insufflation test. The stomach is extracted in a surgical glove via the orifice of trocar T4, which is enlarged and closed with Vicryl at the end of the procedure. We systematically carry out a hepatic biopsy; cholecystectomy is performed only if gall stones are present. We drain only occasionally. The nasogastric catheter remains in place for 24 h to prevent vomiting and to check on the absence of bleeding. The patients are given prophylactic antibiotic treatment (second-generation cephalosporin) before the incision is made. Thrombosis prophylaxis is started the day before the operation and continued for a month, and patients wear support stockings. They are asked to walk about once they have come around. They are allowed to begin a liquid diet following a water-soluble swallow check on

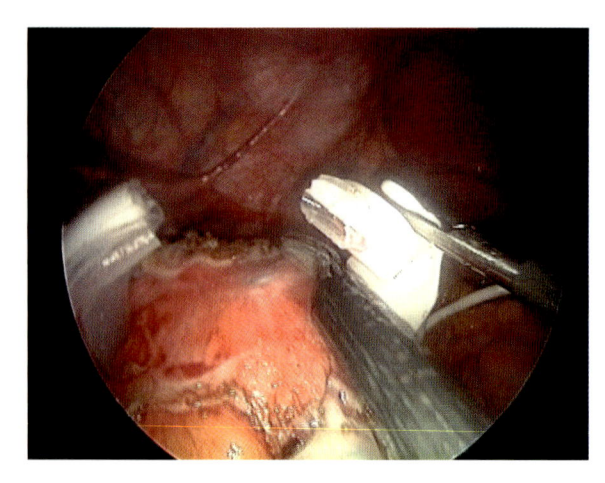

Fig. 18.12.

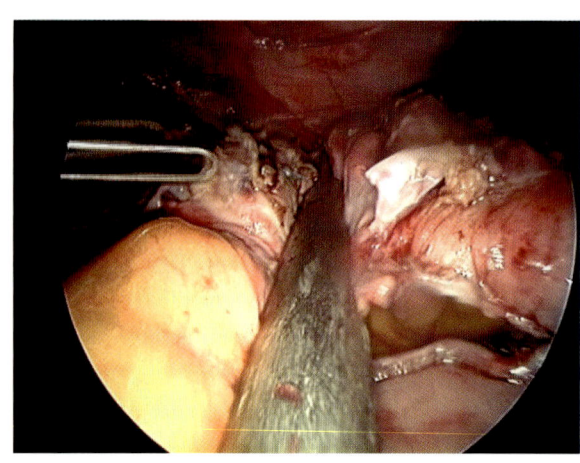

Fig. 18.15.

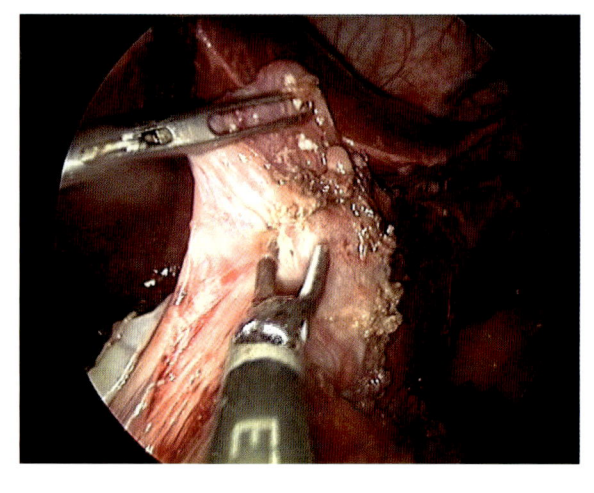

Fig. 18.13.

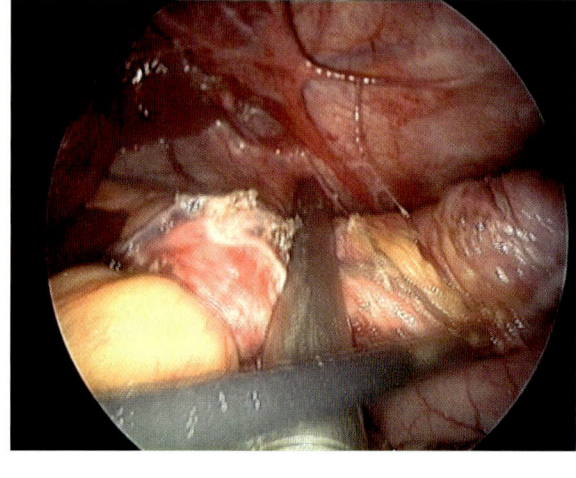

Fig. 18.16.

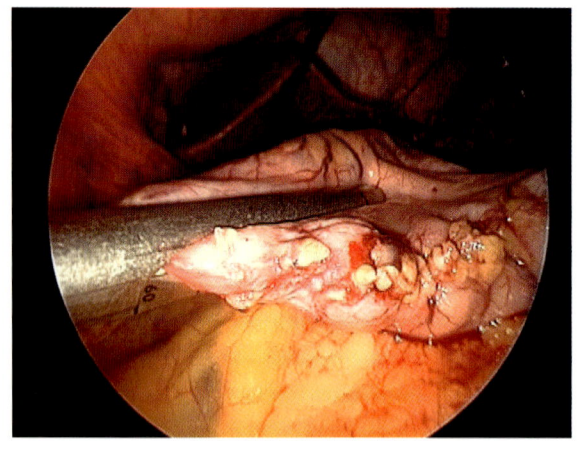

Fig. 18.14.

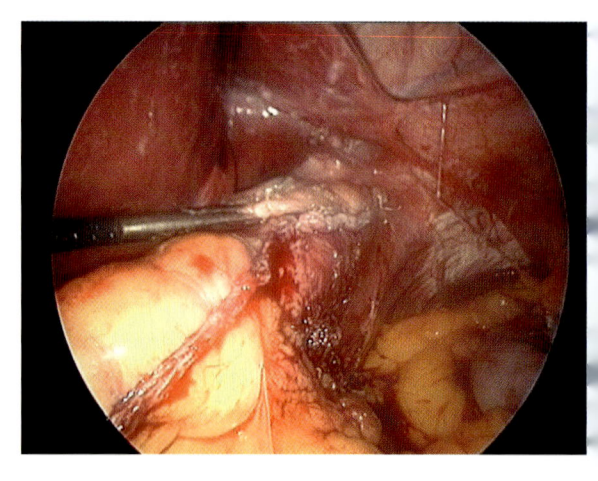

Fig. 18.17.

day 2, and are discharged on the 5th day with a blended soft diet and purees up to the 3rd week.

18.8   Conclusion

SG is not a new operation, but carrying it out as an isolated procedure is a new surgical approach to obesity. Initially, SG was reserved for high-BMI/ high-risk patients, but since the morbidity and mortality are lower than for bypasses, the technique is less demanding, and the early results are as good and there has even been an increase in the number of indications with regard to comorbidities. The anatomical landmarks for performing a proper SG are becoming more precise. It appears that SG is more than a restrictive procedure: enterohormonal effects are being investigated. Short-term results are very promising, but it is still too early to define the real position of ISG in the armamentarium of bariatric surgery as an isolated procedure as long as long-term results are lacking. Even if the stomach resection is definitive, no major metabolic deficiencies are expected and this operation does not burn bridges to other options. Therefore, SG fits perfectly in a strategic approach to obesity, which is currently an incurable disease. Patients should be informed that second-stage surgery might be necessary.

References

1. Hess DS, Hess DW (1998) Biliopancreatic diversion with duodenal switch. Obes Surg 8:267–282
2. Lagace M, Marceau P, Marceau S, Hould F-S, Potvin M, Bourque R-A Biron S (1995) Biliopancreatic diversion with a new type of gastrectomy: some previous conclusions revisited. Obes Surg 5:411–418
3. Marceau P, Biron S, Bourque RA (1993) Biliopancreatic diversion with a new type of gastrectomy. Obes Surg 3:29–36
4. Marceau P, Hould F, Lebel S, Marceau S, Biron S (2001) Malabsorptive obesity surgery. Surg Clin North Am 81:1113–1127
5. Regan JP, Inabnet WB, Gagner M, Pomp A (2003) Early experience with two stage laparoscopic Roux-en-Y gastric bypass as an alternative in the super-super obese patient. Obes Surg 13:861–864
6. Ren C, Patterson E, Gagner M (2000) Early results of laparoscopic biliopancreatic diversion with duodenal switch: a case series of 40 consecutive patients. Obes Surg 10:514–523
7. Krawczykowski D, Lecko M, Nore O (2005) Preliminary results with laparoscopic sleeve gastrectomy. Chir Gastroenterol 21[Suppl 1]:26–30
8. Krawczykowski D One or two stages BPD/DS. (abstract) Surg Obes Relat Dis 2008 4:334
9. Nguyen NT, Longoria M, Gelfand DV, Sabio A, Wilson S (2005) Staged laparoscopic Roux-en-Y: a novel two-stage bariatric operation as an alternative in the super-obese with massively enlarged liver. Obes Surg 15:1077–1081
10. Silecchia G, Boru C, Pecchia A, Rizzello M, Casella G, Leonetti F, Basso N (2006) Effectiveness of laparoscopic sleeve gastrectomy (first stage of biliopancreatic diversion with duodenal switch) on co-morbidities in super-obese high-risk patients. Obes Surg 16:1138–1144
11. Scopinaro N, Marinari GM, Prestolesi F, Papadia F, Murelli F, Marini P, Adami GF (2000) Energy and nitrogen absorption after biliopancreatic diversion. Obes Surg 10:436–441
12. Baltasar A, Serra C, Pérez N, Bou R, Bengochea M, Ferri L (2005) Laparoscopic sleeve gastrectomy : a multi-purpose bariatric operation. Obes Surg 15:1124–1128
13. Braghetto I, Korn O, Valladares H, Gutiérrez L, Csendes A, Debandi A, Castillo J, Rodriguez A, Burgos AM, Brunet L (2007) Laparoscopic sleeve gastrectomy: surgical technique, indications and clinical results. Obes Surg 17:1442–1450
14. Felberbauer FX, Langer F, Shakeri-Manesch S, Schmaldienst E, Kees M, Kriwanek S, Prager M, Prager G (2008) Laparoscopic sleeve gastrectomy as an isolated bariatric procedure: intermediate-term results from a large series in three Austrian centers. Obes Surg 18:814–818
15. Hamoui N, Anthone GJ, Kaufman HS, Crookes PF (2006) Sleeve gastrectomy in the high-risk patient. Obes Surg 16:1445–1449
16. Moon Han SM, Kim WW, Oh JH (2005) Results of laparoscopic sleeve gastrectomy at 1 year in morbidly obese Korean patients. Obes Surg 15:1469–1475
17. Krawczykowski D, Lecko M (2006) Is isolated laparoscopic sleeve gastrectomy an option in bariatric surgery? (abstract) Surg Obes Relat Dis 2:339
18. Lee C, Cirangle PT, Jossart G (2007) Vertical gastrectomy for morbid obesity in 216 patients: report of two-year results. Surg Endosc 21:1810–1816
19. Nocca D, Krawczykowski D, Bomans B, Noël P, Picot MC, Blanc PM, de Seguin de Hons C, Millat B, Gagner M, Monnier L, Fabre JM (2008) A prospective multicenter study of 163 sleeve gastrectomies: results at 1 and 2 years. Obes Surg 18:560–565
20. Roa PE, Kaidar-Person O, Pinto D, Cho M, Szomstein S, Rosenthal RJ (2006) Laparoscopic sleeve gastrectomy as treatment for morbid obesity: technique and short-term outcome. Obes Surg 16:1323–1326
21. ASMBS position statement on sleeve gastrectomy as a bariatric procedure
22. Deitel M, Crosby RD, Gagner M (2008) First international consensus summit for sleeve gastrectomy, New York City, October 25-27, 2007. Obes Surg 18:487–496
23. Johnston D, Dachter J, Sue-Ling H, King R, Martin L (2003) The Magenstrasse and Mill operation for morbid obesity. Obes Surg 13:10–16
24. Almongy G, Crookes PF, Anthone G (2004) Longitudinal gastrectomy as a treatment for the high-risk super-obese patient. Obes Surg 14:492–497
25. Saber AA, Elgamal MH, Itawi EA, Rao AJ (2008) Single incision laparoscopic sleeve gastrectomy: a novel technique. Obes Surg 18:1338–1342
26. Marchesini JC, Cardoso AR, Nora M, Neto MG, Mottin CC, Baretta G, Padoin AV, Moretto M, Maggioni L, Alves LB, Kupski C (2008) Laparoscopic sleeve gastrectomy with NOTES visualization a step toward NOTES procedures. Surg Obes Relat Dis 4:773–776
27. Ramos AC, Zundel N, Neto MG, Maalouf M (2008) Human hybrid NOTES transvaginal sleeve gastrectomy: initial experience. Surg Obes Relat Dis 4:660–663
28. Baltasar A, Serra C, Pérez N, Bou R, Bengochea M (2006) Re-sleeve gastrectomy. Obes Surg 16:1535–1538

29. Weiner RA, Weiner S, Pomhoff I, Jacobi C, Makarewicz W, Weigand G (2007) Laparoscopic sleeve gastrectomy- Influence of sleeve size and resected gastric volume. Obes Surg 17:1297–1305
30. Parikh M, Gagner M, Heacock L, Strain G, Dakin G, Pomp A (2008) Laparoscopic sleeve gastrectomy: does bougie size affect mean % EWL? Short-term outcomes. Surg Obes Relat Dis 4:528–533
31. Frezza EE, Barton A, Herbert H, Wachtel MS (2008) Laparoscopic sleeve gastrectomy with endoscopic guidance in morbid obesity. Surg Obes Relat Dis 4:575–580
32. Sanchez-Pernaute A, Rodriguez R, Rubio MA, Pérez-Aguirre E, Cardenas Crespo S, Cano Valderrama O, Talavera P, Méndez R, Diez-Valladares L, Torres A (2007) Gastric tube volume after duodenal switch and its correlation to short-term weight loss. Obes Surg 17:1178–1182
33. Skrekas G, Lapatsanis D, Stafyla V, Papalambros A (2008) One year after laparoscopic "tight" sleeve gastrectomy: technique and outcome. Obes Surg 18:810–813
34. Yehoshua RT, Eidelman LA, Stein M, Fichman S, Mazor A, Chen J, Berstine H, Singer P, Dickman R, Shikora SA, Rosenthal RJ, Rubin M (2008) Laparoscopic sleeve gastrectomy Volume and pressure assessment. Obes Surg 18:1083–1088
35. Dapri G, Vaz C, Cadière GB, Himpens J (2007) A prospective randomized study comparing two different techniques for laparoscopic sleeve gastrectomy. Obes Surg 17:1435–1441
36. Melissas J, Koukouraki S, Askoxylakis J, Stathaki M, Daskalakis M, Perisinakis K, Karkavitsas N (2007) Sleeve gastrectomy – a restrictive procedure? Obes Surg 17:57–62
37. Melissas J, Daskalakis M, Koukouraki S, Askoxylakis J, Metaxari M, Dimitriadis E, Stathaki M, Papadakis JA (2008) Sleeve gastrectomy – a "food-limiting" operation. Obes Surg 18:1251–1256
38. Langer FB, Hoda R, Bohdjalian A, Felberbauer FX, Zacherl J, Schindler K, Luger A, Ludvik B, Prager G (2005) Sleeve gastrectomy and gastric banding: effects on plasma ghrelin levels. Obes Surg 15:1024–1029
39. Karamanakos SN, Vagenas K, Kalfarentzos F, Alexandrides TK (2008) Weight loss, appetite suppression, and changes in fasting and postprandial ghrelin and peptide-YY levels after Roux-en-Y gastric bypass and sleeve gastrectomy: a prospective, double blind study. Ann Surg 247:408–410
40. Sabench Perreferrer F., Hernandez Gonzalez M., Blanco Blasco S., Morandeira Rivas A, del Castillo Dejardin D (2008) Influence of sleeve gastrectomy on several experimental models of obesity: metabolic and hormonal implications. Obes Surg 18:97–108
41. Vidal J, Ibarzabal A, Nicolau J, Vidov M, Delgado S, Martinez G, Balust J, Morinigo R, Lacy A (2007) Short-term effects of sleeve gastrectomy on type 2 diabetes mellitus in severely obese subjects. Obes Surg 17:1069–1074
42. Wheeler A, Morales M, Fearing NScott J, de la Torre R, Ramaswamy A (2008) Laparoscopic sleeve gastrectomy in the super morbidly obese is effective treatment for diabetes mellitus and obstructive sleep apnea (abstract). Surg Obes Relat Dis 4:351–352
43. Cottam D, Qureshi FG, Mattar SG, Sharma S, Holover S, Bonanomi G, Ramanathan R, Schauer P (2006) Laparoscopic sleeve gastrectomy as an initial weight-loss procedure for high-risk patients with morbid obesity. Surg Endosc 20:859–863
44. Bernante P, Foletto M, Busetto L, Pomerri F, Pesenti F, Pelizzo MR, Nitti D (2006) Feasibility of laparoscopic sleeve gastrectomy as a revision procedure for prior laparoscopic gastric banding. Obes Surg 16:1327–1330
45. Dapri G, Cadière GB, Himpens J (2009) Feasibility and technique of laparoscopic conversion of adjustable gastric banding to sleeve gastrectomy. Surg Obes Relat Dis 5:72–76
46. Gagner M, Gumbs A (2007) Gastric banding: conversion to sleeve, bypass, or DS. Surg Endosc 21:1931–1935
47. Krawczykowski D, Lecko M, Nore O (2006) A comparative study between primary and secondary isolated laparoscopic sleeve gastrectomy: preliminary results (abstract). Obes Surg 16:1009
48. Himpens J, Dapri G, Cadiere GB (2006) A prospective randomized study between laparoscopic gastric banding and laparoscopic isolated sleeve gastrectomy: results after 1 and 3 years. Obes Surg 16:1450–1456
49. Till H, Blüher S, Hirsch W, Kiess W (2008) Efficacy of laparoscopic sleeve gastrectomy as a stand-alone technique for children with morbid obesity. Obes Surg 18:1047–1049
50. Quesada BM, Roff HE, Kohan G, Oria AS, Porras LTC (2008) Laparoscopic sleeve gastrectomy as an alternative to gastric bypass in patients with multiple intra abdominal adhesions. Obes Surg 18:566–568
51. Lutrzykowski M (2007) Vertical gastric resection (sleeve gastrectomy) in a morbidly obese patient with past jejunoileal bypass. Obes Surg 17:423–425
52. Makarewicz W, Kaska L, Kobiela J, Stankiewicz M, Wujtewicz MA, Lachinski AJ, Sledzinski Z (2007) Wernicke's syndrome after sleeve gastrectomy. Obes Surg 5:704–706
53. Moon Han S, Kim WW, Oh JH (2005) Results of laparoscopic sleeve gastrectomy at 1 year in morbidly obese Korean patients. Obes Surg 15:1469–1475
54. Milone L, Strong V, Gagner M (2005) Laparoscopic sleeve gastrectomy is superior to endoscopic intragastric balloon as a first-stage procedure for super-obese patients (BMI >50). Obes Surg 15:612–617
55. Langer FB, Bohdjalian A, Felberbauer FX, Fleischmann E, Reza Hoda MA, Ludvik B, Zacherl J, Jakesz R, Prager G (2006) Does gastric dilation limit the success of sleeve gastrectomy as a sole operation for morbid obesity? Obes Surg 16:166–171
56. Takata MC, Campos GM, Ciovica R, Rabl C, Rogers SJ, Cello JP, Ascher NL, Posselt AM (2008) Laparoscopic bariatric surgery improves candidacy in morbidly obese patients awaiting transplantation. Surg Obes Relat Dis 4:159–165
57. Consten ECJ, Gagner M, Pomp A, Inabmet WB (2004) Decreased bleeding after laparoscopic sleeve gastrectomy with or without duodenal switch for morbid obesity using a stapled buttressed absorbable polymer membrane. Obes Surg 14:1360–1366
58. Consten EC, Dakin GF, Gagner M (2004) Intraluminal migration of bovine pericardial strips used to reinforce the gastric staple-line in laparoscopic bariatric surgery. Obes Surg 14:549–554
59. Lalor PF, Tucker ON, Szomstein S, Rosenthal RJ (2008) Complications after laparoscopic sleeve gastrectomy. Surg Obes Relat Dis 4:33–38
60. McBean E, Szomstein S, Rosenthal R (2008) Laparoscopic sleeve gastrectomy: an alternative approach for failed laparoscopic adjustable gastric banding in the treatment of morbid obesity. (abstract) Surg Obes Relat Dis 4:353–354
61. Eisendrath P, Cremer M, Himpens J, Cadière G-B, Le Moine O, Devière J (2007) Endotherapy including temporary stenting of fistulas of the upper gastrointestinal tract after laparoscopic bariatric surgery. Endoscopy 39:625–630
62. Serra C, Baltasar A, Andreo L, Perez N, Bengochea M, Chisbert JJ (2007) Treatment of gastric leaks with coated self-expanding stents after sleeve gastrectomy. Obes Surg 17:866–872
63. Baltasar A, Bou R, Bengochea M, Serra C, Cipagauta L (2007) Use of a Roux limb to correct esophagogastric junction fistulas after sleeve gastrectomy. Obes Surg 17:1408–1410

64. Baltasar A, Serra C, Bengochea M, Bou R, Andreo L (2008) Use of Roux limb as remedial surgery for sleeve gastrectomy fistulas. Surg Obes Relat Dis 4:759–763

65. Serra C, Baltasar A, Pérez N (2000) Total gastrectomy for complications of duodenal switch with reversal. Obes Surg 16:1082–1086

66. Overcash WT (2008) Natural orifice surgery (NOS) using StomaphyX™ for repair of gastric leaks after bariatric revisions. Obes Surg 18:882–885

67. Baker RS, Foote J, Kemmeter P, Brady R, Vroegop T, Serveld M (2004) The science of stapling and leaks. Obes Surg 14:1290–1298

68. Rubin M, Tzioni R, Stein M, Lederfein D, Fichman S, Berstine H, Eidelman LA (2008) Laparoscopic sleeve gastrectomy with minimal morbidity. Early results in 120 morbidly obese patients. Obes Surg 18:1567–1570

69. Kasalicky M, Michalsky D, Housova J, Haluzik M, Housa D, Haluzikova D, Fried M (2008) Laparoscopic sleeve gastrectomy without an over-sewing of the staple line. Obes Surg 18:1257–1262

70. Ueda K, Gagner M, Milone L, Bardaro SJ, Gong K (2008) Sleeve gastrectomy with wrapping using polytetrafluoroethylene to prevent gastric enlargement in a porcine model. Surg Obes Relat Dis 4:84–90

71. Alexander JW, Goodman H (2007) Initial experience with banded sleeve gastrectomy. Surg Obes Relat Dis 3:(P 54):317

72. Burgmer R, Grigutsch K, Zipfel S, Wolf A-M, de Zwaan M, Husemann B, Albus C, Senf W, Herpertz S (2005) The influence of eating behavior and eating pathology on weight loss after gastric restriction operations. Obes Surg 15:684–691

73. Gagner M, Rogula T (2003) Laparoscopic reoperative sleeve gastrectomy for poor weight loss after biliopancreatic diversion with duodenal switch. Obes Surg 13:649–654

74. Krawczykowski D, Lecko M (2008) La derivation bilio-pancréatique avec duodenal switch: l'approche en un temps versus l'approche séquentielle. J Coelio-chir 66:40–47

75. Moy J, Pomp A, Dakin G, Parikh M, Gagner M (2008) Laparoscopic sleeve gastrectomy for morbid obesity. Am J Surg 196:e56–e59

76. Parikh M, Gagner M Laparoscopic hiatal hernia repair and repeat sleeve gastrectomy for gastroesophageal reflux disease after duodenal switch. Surg Obes Relat Dis 2008 4:73–75

77. Forestieri P, Formato A, Pilone V, Romano A, Monda A, Tramontano S (2008) Rhabdomyolisis after sleeve gastrectomy: increase in muscle enzymes does not predict fatal outcome. Obes Surg 18:349–351

78. Baltasar A (2006) Mucocele of the gastric tube after conversion of VBG to DS. Obes Surg 16:528

79. Sanchez-Pernaute A, Pérez-Aguirre E, Talavera P, Robin A, Diez-Valladares L, Cabrerizo L, Rubio MA, Méndez R, Santos E, Torres A (2006) Mucocele of the gastric tube after conversion of vertical banded gastroplasty to duodenal switch: not just a radiological image. Obes Surg 16:524–527

The Conventional Gastric Bypass

Oliver Thomusch, MD, W. Konrad Karcz, MD

After the Second World War during the 1950's, subtotal gastrectomy with the Billroth II reconstruction was the surgical treatment of choice for peptic ulcer disease. Post-operative weight loss and early satiety were frequently observed in these patients, and these observations led Mason in 1966 to begin restrictive bariatric surgery by introducing the gastric bypass procedure. The initial technique involved a horizontal proximal gastric division of 10% of the stomach with a gastric pouch of approximately 100–150 ml. Mason reconstructed the alimentary passage with a short afferent biliopancreatic limb and a 12-mm in diameter end-side gastrojejunal anastomosis, and then left the residual distal stomach in place. Later on, Mason improved early satiety and post-operative weight loss by reducing the gastric pouch to 50 ml. Further improvements and modifications were made by Ward Griffen, who introduced the retrocolic Roux-en-Y loop reconstruction. He excluded the biliopancreatic juices and thereby reduced the risk of gastrojejunal fistulas. Griffen and Alden modified this technique with a simple division of the stomach without performing a complete transection. Jose Torres and Clemente Oca introduced the prototype of the modern gastric bypass procedure. They created the gastric pouch on the lesser curvature, 4 cm distal to the cardia, and separated the gastric pouch from the rest of the stomach. They created a gastric pouch with 35 ml volume. The jejunum was dissected 45 cm from the ligament of Treitz, and the gastroentero-anastomosis (GEA) was performed with a 21-mm circular stapler, with the anvil inserted through a gastrostomy in the upper part of the anterior wall of the pouch. The end-loop with the end-side anastomosis was created at 90 cm. The first laparoscopic gastric bypass was performed by Wittgrove in 1994. Later, several technical variations were introduced with sometimes mechanical, sometimes manual, gastroentero-anastomosis. The stomach is always transected, and the gastric pouch is usually vertical and on the lesser gastric curvature. The alimentary, common, and biliopancreatic limbs are of variable length and depend on the intention to enhance either the restrictive or the malabsorptive potency of the procedure.

19.1 Mechanisms of Action

Overall, the complete mechanism of action of the gastric bypass is not yet fully understood. Up to now it is clear that it is a combination of food restriction, modification of eating behavior, endocrine modification of enteropeptides, and at least a component of energy malabsorption in case of a distal enteroentero-anastomosis.

19.1.1 Restrictive Component

First of all, the gastric bypass works by restricting food intake. As demonstrated by the development of the gastric bypass technique, post-operative weight loss and weight loss maintenance are inversely related to the gastric pouch volume. In the beginning, pouch volumes around 100 ml and more were common. Initial weight loss was satisfactory, but long-term weight loss reduction failed because the gastric pouch was too large. Later on, the vertical gastric pouch was reduced to volumes of 20–25 ml with a consequently improved long-term food restriction and therefore long-term weight loss reduction.

19.1.2 Modification of Eating Behavior

Excluded from the function of the pylorus and the duodenal and early jejunal passage, the food arrives early in the upper small intestine and causes a reduction of hunger and the appearance of a postcibal syndrome comparable to the well-known early dumping syndrome after gastric surgery. This modification of the gastrointestinal passage leads to a profound modification of eating behavior. The dumping syndrome occurred in varying degrees in up to 70% of patients questioned but was severe in less than 5% [1]. It is regarded as a beneficial feature of this bariatric operation because patients learn to avoid calorie-dense foods and to eat less at one time to avoid postprandial discomfort such as sweating, flushing, dizziness, weakness, tachycardia, nausea, cramping, bloating, and diarrhea.

Ernst et al. [2] compared the eating behavior of patients after gastric bypass surgery with that of obese control subjects and found significant differences. Patients after gastric bypass surgery more often consumed poultry, fish, cooked vegetables, and eggs, while they consumed less chocolate, cake, biscuits and cookies, and soda. A trend was also noted to less frequent consumption of white bread and toast and whole-grain bread. This pattern of changes in food selection after gastric bypass surgery strongly suggests that patients can, at least in part, follow the advice they receive during dietary counseling. Furthermore, the exclusion of the fundus and the duodenum leads to a depletion of the orexic enterohormone ghrelin and thus to less feeling of hunger. In contrast to other forms of hypocaloric diets accompanied by an increased level of ghrelin and thus an increased feeling of hunger, patients with weight loss after the gastric bypass had lower levels of ghrelin with a disappearance of daytime and meal-related fluctuation of serum levels

[3]. This effect reduced the feeling of hunger and resulted in much better post-operative diet compliance, with a reduction in food intake and meal frequency.

19.1.3   Endocrine Metabolic Component

Several reviews have addressed changes in gut hormones after bariatric surgery. The two major gut hormones that have been identified as incretins are gastric inhibitory peptide (GIP) and glucagon-like peptide-1 (GLP-1). GIP is secreted from the K cells located mainly in the duodenum, while GLP-1 is secreted from L cells found mainly in the ileum [4, 5]. The main function of incretins is to stimulate glucose-dependent insulin secretion. Both in vivo and in vitro studies showed that GLP-1 in pancreatic β-cells stimulates insulin biosynthesis [6, 7]. In addition to its insulinotropic effects, GLP-1 exerts its glucose-lowering effects through inhibition of gastric emptying [8], restoration of insulin sensitivity [8], and inhibition of glucagon secretion [9], which may result in the decrease of hepatic glucose production [10]. The changes in GLP-1 levels after bariatric surgery have been extensively studied in the past 10 years. The postprandial GLP-1 response increases during an oral glucose tolerance test (OGTT) or a mixed test meal after gastric bypass in obese patients [11, 12] as well as in patients with type-2 diabetes [13]. The GLP-1 increase occurs as early as 2 days after GBP [14] and persists at 6 months and 1 year [15]. Purely restrictive procedures do not result in an increase of GLP-1. Furthermore, the incretin GIP levels also increased during an OGTT 1 month after GBP [16].

In addition to the increase of meal- or glucose-stimulated GLP-1 and GIP levels occurring after GBP, studies have also demonstrated that insulin secretion, impaired in patients with type-2 diabetes, returns to the level of controls 1 month after the surgery [16]. The normalization of the incretin effect in patients with recently diagnosed type-2 diabetes (less than 5 years) persists at 1 year after surgery [15]. Moreover, GBP surgery interferes with the hepatic glucose production and reduces the endogenous glucose production. This effect also seems to be long-lasting, for at least 1–4 years [17]. One major characteristic of type-2 diabetes is insulin resistance, normally manifesting as a reduced insulin-mediated glucose uptake. After gastric bypass, GLP-1 may improve insulin sensitivity [8, 9], but its role and that of other gut peptides such as peptide YY (PYY) [18] and ghrelin [19] in increasing insulin sensitivity, above and beyond caloric restriction and weight loss, is not totally clear [20]. The above-described effects seem to occur soon after gastric bypass surgery and often prior to substantial weight loss [21, 22].

Several mechanisms have been proposed for the increase in incretin levels after GBP, although to date none have been clearly established, and the results of many studies often conflict with one another [20]. Existing data suggest that weight loss contributes to increased incretin levels, because the surgical nature of GBP appears to play a much greater role in the increase than weight loss per se [13]. The "rapid hindgut delivery hypothesis" states that the rapid exposure of the lower small intestine to nutrients leads to an increased level of incretins after GBP. Another hypothesis, that of the "foregut exclusion", proposes that the exclusion of the foregut from nutrient exposure is responsible for the increased incretin levels after GBP. Overall, gut motility and gastric emptying may also play an important role in postprandial glucose control [23].

A recent study demonstrated accelerated gastric emptying and shortened intestinal transit time in morbidly obese subjects 6 weeks after GBP. This phenomemon was accompanied by an increased postprandial GLP-1 response, which was significantly correlated with the gastric-emptying response after surgery [24]. In addition to incretins, a number of other hormones are altered after GBP that may be integral to the maintenance of glucose homeostasis [20]. Ghrelin is a hormone produced by the stomach and may play a role in short- and long-term energy balance. Administration of ghrelin or its analogs stimulates food intake. Obese individuals have lower circulating ghrelin levels. Weight loss by diet increases ghrelin levels, and consequently leads to increased food intake [3]. In contrast, ghrelin levels do not rise after GBP in spite of considerable weight loss [3, 25]. PYY is co-secreted with GLP-1 from intestinal L cells in response to food intake. PYY has been shown to decrease food intake in human subjects [26]. Several working groups [17, 27] reported increased PYY levels after GBP, which may partially explain the reduced caloric intake after surgery. Leptin, which is secreted from adipose tissue, is also involved with food intake and long-term energy regulation [28]. However, in contrast to ghrelin, leptin levels are generally higher in obese individuals. Several studies showed a reduction of leptin levels after GBP [29, 30] which was partly correlated with weight or BMI.

19.2   Indications for the Gastric Bypass Procedure

Severe obesity is a biological, psychological, and social disaster. The co-morbid conditions associated with obesity are chronic and ultimately life-threatening. Diabetes, hypertension, dyslipidemia, heart disease, respiratory failure, joint degeneration, and cancer have all been

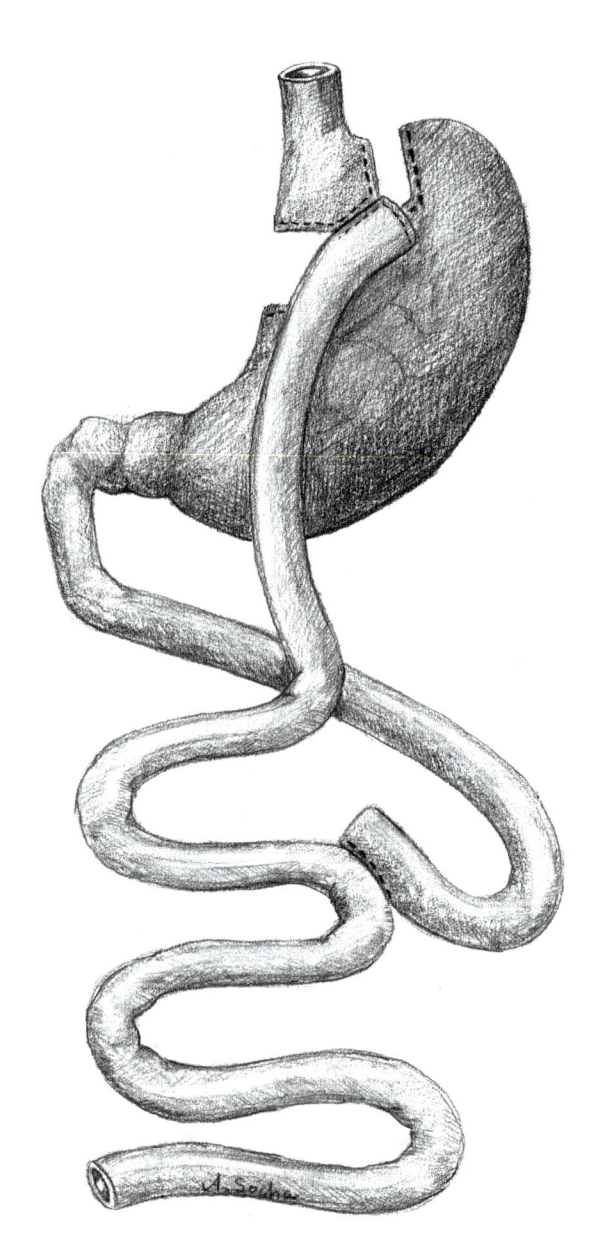

▫ Fig. 19.1.

and experienced in this work. A proper operating table and equipment, anesthesia, monitoring, and support staff are required. The surgeon or the institution and the patient must be committed to lifelong follow-up. Proper patient selection is mandatory, and the surgeon should refuse the belligerent, non-cooperative, or uncontrolled psychotic patient [39]. The criteria for gastric bypass surgery are:

- Presence of serious sequelae of massive obesity
- Exclusion of endocrine diseases causing obesity (hypothyroidism, Cushing's disease)
- Exclusion of psychotic diseases (depression, schizophrenia)
- Exclusion of eating disorders (binge eating, anorexia)
- BMI ≥40 kg/m^2 or >35 kg/m^2 with extenuating circumstances
- Failure of sustained weight loss on extensive supervised dietary and conservative regimens over the years
- Patient cooperation with long-term follow-up
- Acceptable operative risk

However, patients with a BMI >40 kg/m^2 or with a BMI >35 kg/m^2 with serious co-morbidities (e.g., debilitating arthritis of weight-bearing joints, severe reflux esophagitis, diabetes, hypertension, obesity-hypoventilation syndrome, infertility, or psychosocial or economic problems) related to obesity are generally candidates for surgery [39, 40].

19.3 Surgical Technique

Patient Preparation. The patient is placed in the reverse Trendelenburg position, nearly sitting (beach chair position) with legs wide apart, and wearing antithrombosis stockings and intermittent pneumatic compression boots. Both arms are positioned in abduction, accessible to the anesthesiologist. The operating field is prepared with iodopolividone solution. The patient is covered with a special drape securing the operating field and covering the rest of the body including both arms and legs.

Surgical Team Position. The laparoscopic gastric bypass procedure is performed by two surgeons. The first surgeon (operator) stands between the patient's legs, the second surgeon to the patient's right. The scrub nurse stands on the first surgeon's left side next to the patient's right foot.

Trocar Placement. The capnoperitoneum is insufflated with a 12-mm separator trocar (Applied Medical). When an intra-abdominal pressure of 14 mmHg is reached, four

connected with excessive weight. Life expectancy and quality of life are also reduced in the obese (Consensus 1991). Gastric bypass surgery is the bariatric procedure performed most often worldwide and is still the gold standard operation for both weight loss and reduction of co-morbidities. There is now abundant published literature supporting the short-, medium-, and long-term efficacy of gastric bypass surgery [31–38].

Gastric bypass surgery is a specialized field requiring extensive knowledge in laparoscopic surgery, and GBP (▫ Fig. 19.1) must be performed by a surgeon interested

19

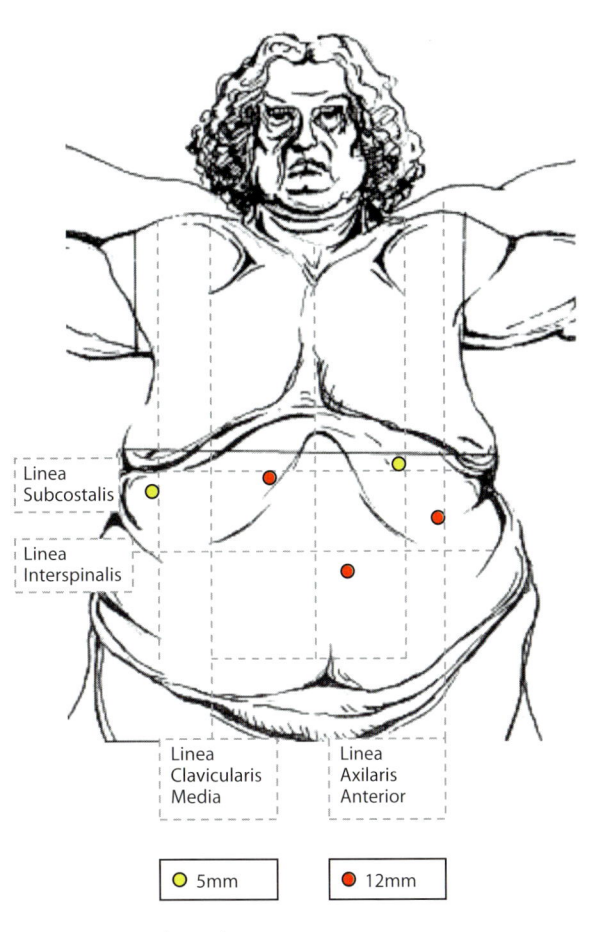

Linea
Subcostalis

Linea
Interspinalis

Linea
Clavicularis
Media

Linea
Axilaris
Anterior

○ 5mm   ● 12mm

Fig. 19.2. Typical ports locations

more work trocars are placed similarly to the fundoplication position under direct vision (■ Fig. 19.2). The first step of the procedure is a meticulous inspection of the complete abdominal cavity to exclude serious diagnoses of importance such as bulky ovarian tumors or complex adhesions.

Preparation of the Gastric Pouch. The subcardiac area is exposed by lifting the left hepatic lobe and pulling down the fundus of the stomach. Using a 30° optic (HDTV, STORZ), the operator commences exploration of the region of interest. Perigastric dissection is started in the region of the angle of Hiss with Ligasure Advanced (Covidien Valley Lab) just above the first short gastric artery and towards the left crus of the diaphragm. Using an endograsper, the second surgeon fixes the gastric wall near the operator's dissection point, pulling the stomach ventrally and laterally towards the patient's left. Having entered the retrocavity, the surgeons ensure that there are no posterior adhesions, and the anesthesiologist removes

the nasogastric tube. Then the surgeons begin the dissection in the region of the small curvature of the stomach and continues until the retrogastric space is reached. At times, dense adhesions to the pancreas are encountered. Visualization is enhanced by opening a gastrocolic window and approaching this area from behind the stomach. The surgeons take care to avoid thermal injury to the adjacent viscera and vagal nerves. The inferior aspect of the gastric pouch is determined with the first horizontal stapler. All subsequent firings are vertically oriented. Three to four linear Endo-GIA® (Covidien, Auto Suture) 60-mm staplers with blue cartridges are used to completely transect the stomach after the removal of the calibration tube (32-F). The dissection thus continues up to the angle of Hiss for a complete partition of the stomach. This technique enables adequate direct visualization and thus objective evaluation of the anterior and posterior aspects of the pouch and distal stomach for tears, leaks, bleeding, and visual estimation of the pouch size. Sometimes the cut edge of the proximal and the distal stomach are reinforced with Hemoclips (Apply Medical). The pouch size is usually estimated at 10–25 ml.

Preparation of the Alimentary Limb. An alimentary limb of Roux-en-Y is created by dividing the jejunum 50 cm below the ligament of Treitz with a 45-mm Endo-GIA® stapler with a white vascular cartridge. The transposition of the jejunal alimentary limb is performed in an antecolic and antegastric position. In patients with an extremely thick and fat greater omentum, additional omentum division is performed with a LigaSure® dissector.

The Gastrojejunal Anastomosis. The formation of the gastrojejunostomy begins with single stitches at the posterior, exterior layer using 3-0 polyglactin (Vicryl®) sutures to create a double-lined posterior wall anastomosis. Beginning distally and sewing proximally, the surgeon approximates the antimesenteric side of the alimentary Roux limb to the inferior staple line of the gastric pouch, incorporating the staples in the suture line. Enterotomies are performed on the gastric pouch and Roux limb adjacent to the suture line. Afterwards, a 45-mm Endo-GIA stapler (blue cartridge) is inserted and the second line of the gastrojejunostomy is created. The anterior suture lines are run from the distal anterior aspect of the enterotomy, the first being full thickness and the second line seromuscular. Prior to completion of the anastomosis, a 12-mm obturator is used to calibrate the stomal opening as well as to provide assurance of patency. The anterior sutures are tied with their respective posterior counterparts. Afterwards, the anastomosis is tested for leakage by insufflating methylene-blue through the gastric tube and placing the bowel clamp on the intestinal limb distal to the anastomosis.

The Jejunojejunostomy. The omentum is displaced cephalad to expose the ligament of Treitz. The alimentary limb is then measured and a side-to-side stapled jejunojejunostomy is created, typically 150 cm below the GEA. After determining the length of the alimentary limb, the operator passes the measured alimentary limb to the second surgeon to hold in the left lower part of the abdomen. By retrieving the end of the biliopancreatic limb, the surgeon fixes both ends to secure the latter to the end loop of the alimentary limb. Using LigaSure® (Covidien, Valley Lab) an incision is performed in the biliopancreatic and alimentary limb to insert the 45-mm Endo-GIA stapler (white cartridge), and to create the jejunojejunostomy on the antimesenteric border. The anastomosis is checked for possible bleeding and the opening is closed with running absorbable suture. The mesenteric defect must be closed with non-absorbable suture to limit the possibility of internal herniation.

Prevention of Internal Hernias. Internal hernias are prevented by closing the gap between the alimentary jejunal limb and the transverse mesocolon with interrupted non-absorbable sutures. The area of the GEA is drained with a Blake drain if needed, and the operation is finished without closure of any abdominal fascial openings. The port sites are inspected for bleeding when the trocars are withdrawn, and the skin is closed with simple absorbable monofilament sutures.

19.4 Perioperative Complications

Excluding pulmonary embolism, anastomotic leakage is the major cause of death (Table 19.1). The fistula is located mostly at the gastrojejunal anastomosis and very rarely in the excluded stomach remnant or at the distal enteroentero-anastomosis. Accidental perforations of the colon or the small intestine are also described in the literature but are even rarer. Clinical signs after leakages are often sub-clinical, and even results of diagnostic tests such as endoscopy or CT scans are negative. Any clinical suspicion of leakage – e.g., the persistence of tachycardia above 120 b/min; a pain in the hypochondrium, sometimes radiating to the left shoulder, with hyperthermia, dyspnea, an increase in white blood cells, an increased CRP, or procalcitonin level – should lead to an intensified diagnostic workup of the patient with at least emergency exploratory laparoscopy. However, if the fistula is discovered with instrumental tests, conservative treatment can be applied, using CT-guided percutaneous drainage combined with specific antibiotic therapy, possibly combined with the application of intraluminal stents [48].

Pulmonary embolism is the second most life-threatening complication and should be treated by thromboembolic prophylaxis with low-molecular-weight heparin, antithrombosis stockings, intermittent pneumatic compression in the perioperative phase, and early mobilization during the first several hours after the procedure. In any case, the onset of respiratory symptoms or pain in the thorax combined with a worsening of the hemodynamic parameters should lead to a prompt clinical workup and/or to the prompt start of thromboembolism treatment. The incidence of digestive hemorrhage from anastomotic bleeding of the stapler lines is reported to be between 0 and 3%. All bleeding episodes can be easily detected by a regular check of hemoglobin and can be effectively treated by interventional endoscopy.

The most frequent late postoperative complications after gastric bypass surgery are stenosis of the gastrojejunal anastomosis, anastomotic ulcer, and intestinal obstructions caused mainly by internal hernias (Table 19.2). The incidence of anastomotic stenosis varies extremely, from 0.8% to 34.5%, and is related to the surgical technique. Some surgeons try to increase the restrictive character of gastric bypass surgery by creating a very small gastrojejunal anastomosis. In case of a symptomatic stenosis, dilation by endoscopy is the treatment of choice. Anastomotic ulcer development occurs in about 4–12% of patients, and there are probably two different behaviors regarding the appearance of marginal ulcer after gas-

Table 19.1 Early postoperative complications

Complication	Range (%)	Reference
Anastomotic dehiscence	4.4	Shauer et al. [41]
	0	White et al. [38]
	4	Lujan et al. [42]
	1.3	Nguyen et al. [43]
Pulmonary embolism	0	Higa et al. [44]
	1.1	DeMaria et al. [45]
	0.6	Nguyen et al. [43]
Hemorrhage	2.4	Smith et al. [34]
	3.2	Nguyen et al. [46]
	6	Lujan et al. [42]
	3.2	Bakhos et al. [47]

◘ Table 19.2 Late postoperative complications

Complication	Range (%)	Reference
Anastomotic stenosis	4	White et al. [38]
	6	Lujan et al. [42]
	7.1	Nguyen et al. [43]
Anastomotic ulcer	6	White et al. [38]
	6 early, 0.6 late	Csendes et al. [49]

tric bypass: there is a relatively high incidence (4–12%) 1 month after surgery and a very low incidence 1 or 2 years after surgery. These findings suggest that there are probably different etiological factors in the pathogenesis of marginal ulcer. Three to four weeks after the initial gastric bypass with a small gastric pouch and very few parietal cells, it is hard to believe that the ulcer is caused by excessive production of acid. This early onset is probably due more to a combination of such factors as the use of electrocautery, some degree of ischemia, or an inflammatory reaction to the surgical suture [49]. Later, after 1 or 2 years, marginal ulcers are probably due to a higher acid output in a dilated gastric pouch with increased parietal cell mass. If an early or late marginal ulcer is found on endoscopy, acid suppression therapy should be employed. This treatment should be administered for at least 3–6 months. Overall, after Roux-en-Y gastric bypass GERD symptoms and esophageal acid exposure are generally reduced in morbidly obese patients [50].

19.5 Follow-up Examinations

Due to the bypassing of the duodenum and the upper jejunum, vitamin-iron-calcium-zinc supplements are mandatory, with surveillance for anemia due to a deficiency of iron (especially in menstruating women), vitamin B12, and calcium. After a Roux-en-Y gastric bypass, the patients require life-long multivitamin supplementation [51]. There are no objective data regarding the exact dose of any nutrients that should be administered to these patients, and there is no standardized recommendation for vitamin supplementation [52]. Many studies have found that iron deficiency is the main cause of anemia following GBP surgery. The amount of elemental iron in commercial multivitamins is usually small (10–20 mg per tablet), and it is clearly insufficient to prevent iron deficiency in GBP patients. Current recommendations for iron deficiency prophylaxis include the administration of

40–65 mg of elemental iron per day (200–400 mg ferrous sulfate). In women of reproductive age, recommendations for iron supplementation increase to 100 mg elemental iron per day (400–800 mg ferrous sulfate) [52]. Additional vitamin C may improve absorption. Iron measurements should be followed closely in these patients, and if they fail to respond adequately despite escalated doses, or if patients cannot tolerate an adequate dose of oral iron, a course of intravenous iron therapy is indicated [53, 54]. Post-operative supplementation with calcium and vitamin D partially corrects osteoporosis. Following gastric bypass surgery, patients need periodic follow-ups for bone mineral density, parathormone, calcium, serum vitamin D, and markers of bone resorption and formation, especially postmenopausal women [55]. The incidence of cobolamin deficiency after Roux-en-Y gastric bypass has been reported as 26–70% [56, 57]. Nevertheless, multivitamin supplements with low amounts of vitamin B12 (6–25 μg per tablet) are not sufficient to prevent the deficiency. Published reports recommend B12 prophylaxis in a range of 350–500 μg oral cobalamin per day, or the intramuscular administration of 1000–3000 μg every month for up to 6 months [51].

Folate deficiency is rare and is present in only 1% of all patients after GBP surgery [58]. This situation may be because folate absorption is adequate in the distal segment of the small intestine. Multivitamin prophylaxis with 400- 500 μg folate per tablet seems to be sufficient to prevent the deficiency. Most authors recommend 1 mg oral folic acid per day [54]. Nevertheless, during pregnancy, folate requirements increase five- to tenfold because of the transfer of folate to the growing fetus. Lactation also aggravates folate deficiency.

19.6 Results

Weight Loss. Gastric bypass is generally regarded as the gold-standard operation. Most reports of gastric bypass document a mean %EWL of 65–75% after 2–5 years [31–38].

Metabolic Syndrome. That improvement in co-morbidities is accomplished by bariatric surgery is now well documented [35, 37, 38, 59]. Adams et al. demonstrated in their study that long-term mortality from any cause in the surgery group decreased by 40%, as compared with that in the control group. The cause-specific mortality in the surgery group decreased by 56% for coronary artery disease, by 92% for diabetes, and by 60% for cancer. Overall, the estimated number of lives saved after a mean follow-up of 7.1 years was 136 per 10,000 gastric bypass

59. Simard B, Turcette H, Marceau P et al (2004) Asthma and sleep apnea in patients with morbid obesity: outcome of bariatric surgery. Obes Surg 14:1381–1388
60. Arterburn D, Schauer DP, Wise RE, Gersin KS, Fischer DR, Selwyn CA, Risman A, Tsevat J (2009) Change in predicted 10-year cardiovascular risk following laparoscopic Roux-en-Y gastric bypass surgery. Obes Surg 19:184–189
61. Carson L, Ruddy ME, Duff AE, Holmes NJ, Cody RP, Brolin RE (1994) The effect of gastric bypass surgery on hypertension in morbidly obese patients. Arch Intern Med 154:193–200
62. Jones KB (1992) The effect of gastric bypass on cholesterol, HDL, and the risk of coronary heart disease. Obes Surg 2:83–85
63. Buchwald H, Avidor Y, Braunwald E et al (2004) Bariatric surgery: a systemic review and meta-analysis. JAMA 292:1724–1737
64. Mottin CC, Padoin AV, Schroer CE, Barancelli FT, Glock L, Repetto G (2008) Behavior of type 2 diabetes mellitus in morbid obese patients submitted to gastric bypass. Obes Surg 18:179–181
65. Alexandrides TK, Skroubis G, Kalfarentzos F (2007) Resolution of diabetes mellitus and metabolic syndrome following Roux-en-Y gastric bypass and variant of biliopancreatic diversion in patients with morbid obesity. Obes Surg 17:176–184
66. Scheen AJ, Luyckx FH, Lefebvre PJ (1998) The place of bariatric surgery in the management of the obese type 2 diabetic patient. Int Diab Monitor 10:1–7
67. Foley EF, Benotti PN, Borlase BC et al (1992) Impact of gastricrestrictive surgery on hypertension in the morbidly obese. Am J Surg 163:294–297
68. Cowan GS jr, Buffington CK (1998) Significant changes in blood pressure, glucose, and lipids with gastric bypass surgery. World J Surg 22:987–992
69. Gleysteen JJ (1992) Results of surgery: long-term effects on hyperlipidemia. Am J Clin Nutr 55:591S–593S
70. Reaven GM, Lithell H, Landsberg L (1996) Hypertension and associated metabolic abnormalities – the role of insulin resistance and the sympathoadrenal system. N Engl J Med 334:374–381
71. Ferrannini E, Buzzigoli G, Bonadonna R et al (1987) Insulin resistance in essential hypertension N Engl J Med 317:350–357
72. DeFronzo RA, Ferrannini E (1991) Insulin resistance. A multifaceted syndrome responsible for NIDDM, obesity, hypertension, dyslipidemia, and atherosclerotic cardiovascular disease. Diabetes Care 14:173–194
73. Stubbs RS, Wickremesekera SK (2001) Insulin resistance and type 2 diabetes: time for a new hypothesis. NZ Med J 114:239–240

The Banded Gastric Bypass

Mal Fobi, MD, Malgorzata V. Stanczyk, MD, Joseph Naim, MD, Kekah Che-Senge, MD

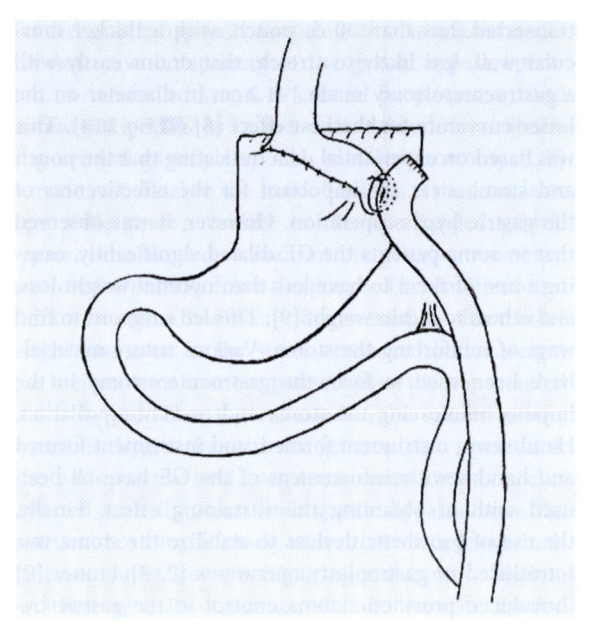

☐ **Fig. 20.5.** Linner's banded RYGB

☐ **Fig. 20.6.** The banded stoma transaction

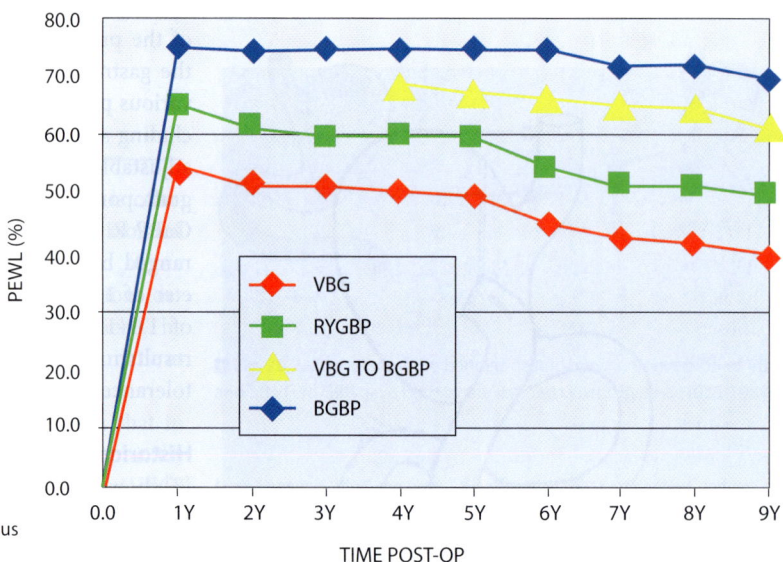

☐ **Fig. 20.7.** Long-term weight loss with various procedures evolving to the BGBP

the band resulted in better weight loss and longer weight loss maintenance than was observed in the gastric bypass or gastroplasty operations (☐ Fig. 20.7). Published series [14–22] with 6–14 years follow-up substantiate more weight loss and more weight loss maintenance in more patients, even in super-obese patients, with a banded gastric bypass.

Prospective Randomized Data. Three classic prospective evaluations of the vertical banded gastroplasty ver-

sus the gastric bypass have been published. The results with the gastroplasty were identical in all three studies, whereas the results with the gastric bypass were identical in two of the studies while in one of the studies where the banded gastric bypass was used the weight loss and weight loss maintenance were superior [21–23].

Fobi et al. [24] published a prospective randomized study comparing a transected versus a non-transected banded gastric bypass, and the weight loss and maintenance in both groups were identical to those reported by

Howard et al. [23] in his prospective study and better than had been reported for the non-banded gastric bypass.

Comparative studies of gastric bypass with or without the ring in the treatment of morbid obesity show that the banded gastric bypass effects more weight loss in more patients maintained for a longer period than the non-banded gastric bypass [25, 26].

A European multicenter prospective evaluation is currently underway using the GaBP Ring device, a pre-fabricated, standardized, sterilized, and auto-locking ring in varying sizes that will replace "the surgeon-fashioned rings and bands" currently used. This study will compare the banded vs. the non-banded gastric bypass. Hopefully, this will deliver the ultimate verdict on whether the band in the gastric bypass makes a difference.

Experimental Data. Gastric isotope emptying studies in banded versus non-banded gastric bypass showed significantly slower emptying in the banded than in the non-banded gastric bypass [27, 28].

Anecdotal Data. Published reports with band placement in failed gastric bypass documented increased weight loss and weight loss maintenance [29–31].

More and more surgeons are placing a band as a revision operation of failed gastric bypass (J. Himpens, personal communication) [32].

CSTO Experience. At our Center for Surgical Treatment of Obesity (CSTO), we have made the following observations: Patients who have had the band removed after a banded gastric bypass, because of either band migration or intolerance, have shown weight regain significantly more than banded patients.

Standard gastric bypasses have been revised by placing a band proximal to the gastroenterostomy with successful weight loss and weight loss maintenance.

A review of CSTO patients with perioperative leaks identified patients in whom the band was removed because of the leak and contamination and patients whose bands were left in place either because the treatment was nonoperative or the contamination was minimal. The weight loss in the de-banded patients was significantly less than in the patients with the band in place.

20.3 Surgical Technique of the Banded Gastric Bypass

The open approach to performing the BRYGB has been published previously [33] and will not be presented here because the laparoscopic approach has replaced it.

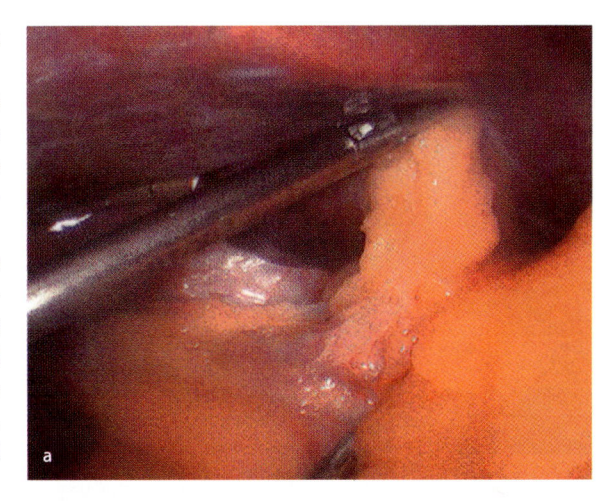

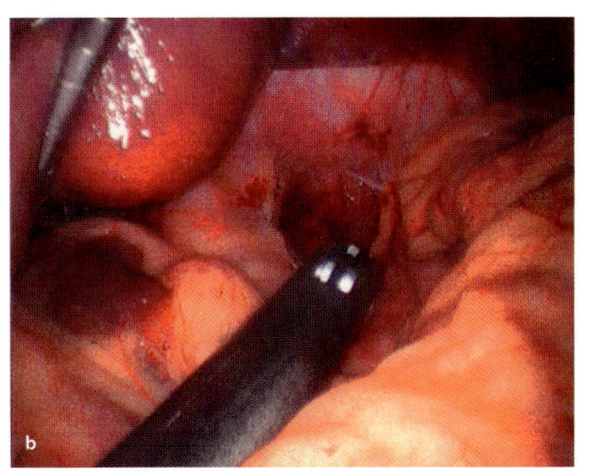

◘ **Fig. 20.8.** Mobilization of the GE junction

Creation of the Pouch. Five to six trocars are used to perform the BRYGB. Once the peritoneum is insufflated and the liver is retracted to expose the gastroesophageal junction, a size-34 lavacuator tube is inserted into the stomach by the anesthesiologist and the stomach is decompressed of air and any other contents. Using a harmonic scalpel the fat pad on the left of the gastroesophageal junction, part of the gastrophrenic ligament, is taken down and an esophageal retractor is used to bluntly mobilize the stomach caudally (◘ Fig. 20.8). A defect 1 cm wide is made at a point 4–5 cm from the GE junction on the lesser curvature, between the stomach serosa and the neurovascular bundle. The stapler is passed through this defect and the stomach is transected horizontally. The lavacuator tube should be mobilized to make sure it is not stapled. The next application of the stapler is placed to cut the stomach vertically. The lavacuator tube should be mobilized so that the vertical pouch formed by the vertical transaction is tubular, small, and barely

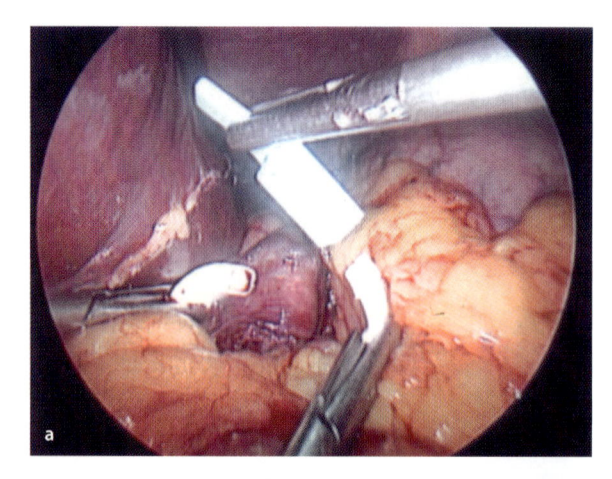

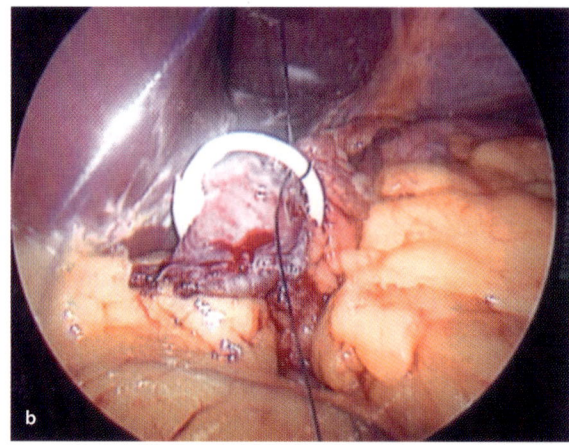

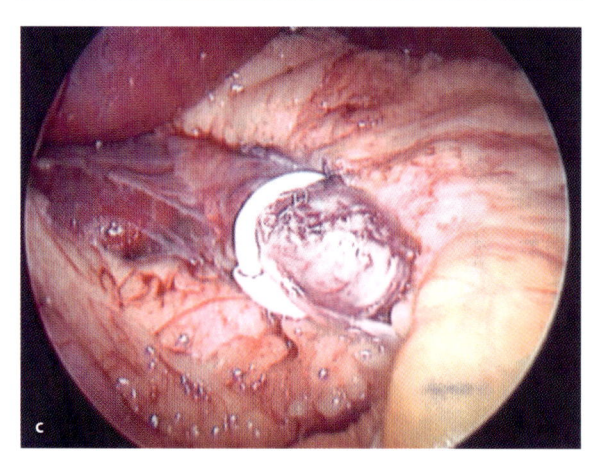

Fig. 20.9a–c. Band placement: a placement and closure of the ring; b suturing of the ring in place; c proper placement of the ring

sure it is not entrapped in the stapler. The proposed pouch is examined visually to make sure it is not more than 25 cc in size. The stapler should be kept closed for at least 20 s to squeeze the fluid out of the tissue within the stapler blade; then the stapler is fired to staple and transect the pouch. It may take two to three or more applications of the stapler to complete the transection of the pouch. Most surgeons use a staple-line-reinforcing prosthesis such as Seamguard™, Surgisis™, Peri-strip™, or Duet TRS™. The tube should be withdrawn and reinserted into the proximal pouch to ensure that the tube is not stapled and that there is a patent pouch attached to the esophagus. The pouch is again examined on both the anterior and the posterior surface to make sure a small pouch has been formed. If the pouch is deemed to be too large, another application of the stapler is required to reduce the pouch to the desirable size. The diaphragm, esophagus, stomach, and pancreas are carefully examined to make sure there are no tears or avulsed vessels that may bleed later. The cut edges of both the pouch and the bypassed stomach are examined for bleeding and for the integrity of the staples. It should be noted that the staplers are designed to transect and seal the tissues but to permit vascular supply and flow.

A band is passed through a window made on the lesser curvature 2–2.5 cm from the caudal tip of the pouch and placed around the pouch and sutured to hold it in place until a capsule is formed around it (Fig. 20.9a–c). This band provides a reinforced stoma that does not dilate. This leaves a pouch between the esophagus and the band about 15–20 cc in size. The retrogastric space of the bypassed stomach is mobilized to make sure there is a clear space through which the Roux limb can be brought once it is formed. This may not be necessary if an antecolic ante-gastric Roux limb is used.

Creation of the Roux-en-Y Limb. The omentum is mobilized at this point to expose the small bowel and the ligament of Treitz. The small bowel is transected with a white cartridge stapler at a point 30–40 cm from the ligament of Treitz. The small bowel mesentery is taken down 2–3 cm using a Seamguard™-reinforced white cartridge stapler or a harmonic scalpel. In transecting the jejunum a good blood supply, both arterial and venous, should be ensured for an adequate Roux limb that will be brought up to establish the gastrointestinal continuity. The biliopancreatic limb is then anastomosed side to side about 60–100 cm from the cut edge of the Roux limb (Figs. 20.10a,b and 20.11). The mesenteric space between the Roux limb and the biliopancreatic limb is closed using non-absorbable 2-0 sutures to minimize the occurrence of internal hernias (Fig. 20.12). Once the Roux limb is created and the mesenteric space is closed, a window is made in the meso-

larger than the tube. This is done by pulling the stomach through the aperture of the stapler to leave as small a pouch as possible. (We have never yet made a pouch too small.) The tube assures the presence of a pouch. The stapling device is closed and the tube is moved in and out to make

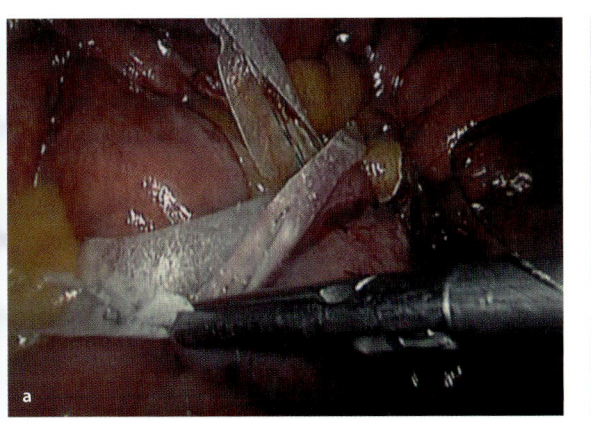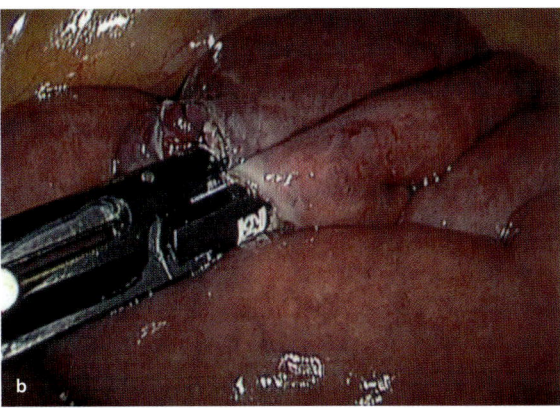

Fig. 20.10a,b. Creation of Roux-en Y limb: a the small bowel mesentery is taken down 2–3 cm; b the biliopancreatic limb is anastomosed side-to-side about 60–100 cm from the cut edge of the Roux limb

colon into the retrocolic and retrogastric space, just above the ligament of Treitz. Fifteen to 20 cm of the Roux limb is then delivered into the retrogastric space (■ Fig. 20.13). The Roux limb is sutured to the mesocolon to prevent prolapse into the retrogastric space. The space between this Roux limb and the retroperitonium (Peterson's defect) is closed with 2-0 silk sutures to minimize internal herniation and volvulus formation (■ Fig. 20.14a–c). The previously made entero-enterostomy (EE) is re-examined for bleeding, patency, and kinking. The omentum is then replaced over the small bowel and the patient is placed in a reverse Trendelelberg position.

The Gastrojejunal Anastomosis. At this point, attention is directed to the pouch and the transected bypassed stomach. The Roux limb in the retrogastric space is retrieved, brought up and out, and placed between the pouch and the bypassed stomach (■ Fig. 20.15a–c). The proximal segment of this limb is used to plicate the edge of the pouch from just above the band to just below the band. This takes away any tension on the anastomosis.

A gastrojejunostomy is formed between the pouch and the jejunal limb. This is an end-to-side anastomosis using 3-0 Vicryl for both the serosa and the mucosal layer. The staple line of the pouch is incorporated in the posterior suture line of the gastrojejunostomy. The lavacuator tube should be advanced through the banded stoma and through the gastrojejunostomy into the Roux limb without any assistance.

20.4   Variations in the Surgical Technique

The BRYGB has been performed with various "surgeon-fashioned" bands, using Marlex, Gortex graft, silastic reinforced tubing, Dacron graft and linear alba grafts, but there is currently the GaBP Ring Device™ (■ Fig. 20.16). The Roux and biliopancreatic limbs can be of varying lengths. The Roux limb can be brought up retro-colic, ante-gastric, or ante-colic ante-gastric. The anastomosis can be hand sewn as described or made with a circular or linear stapler.

We routinely place a gastrostomy (■ Fig. 20.15) but most other surgeons do not. We rarely use a drain in primary cases but do so routinely in revision or conversion cases.

20.5   Concurrent Operations

Patients with other surgical pathologies can have them addressed at the time of the RYGB operation. Concurrent operations include but are not limited to lysis of adhesions, cholecystectomy, herniorraphy, ovarian cystectomy, bilateral tubal ligation, hysterectomy, and oophorectomy.

20.6   Secondary Operations

Banded gastric bypass operations are secondary in patients who have undergone previous bariatric surgery such as jejunoileal bypass, gastric banding, various gastroplasties, biliopancreatic diversion, and other gastric bypass operations. These account for about 7% of all the BRYGB operations we perform. A banded bypass following a previous bariatric operation should be undertaken only if a vertical pouch on the lesser curvature can be formed safely. Secondary operations carry a higher incidence of complications than primary operations [34].

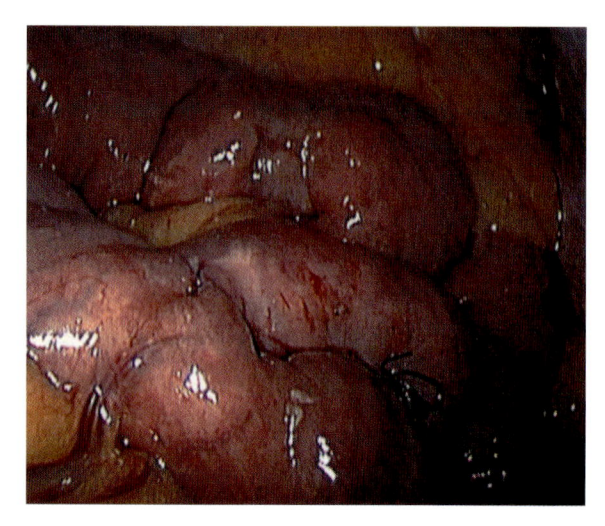

▪ **Fig. 20.11.** Entero-enterostomy is created

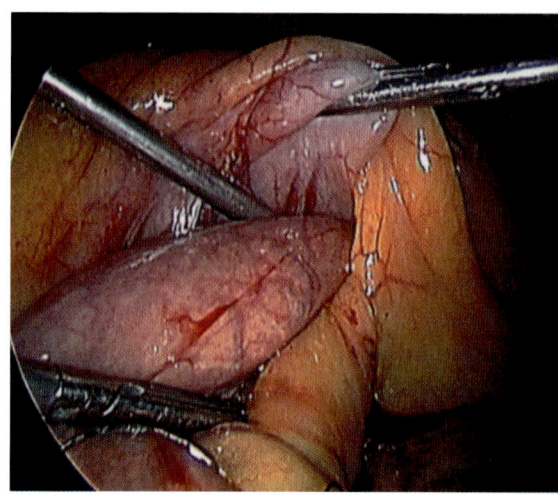

▪ **Fig. 20.13.** The Roux limb is delivered into the retrogastric space

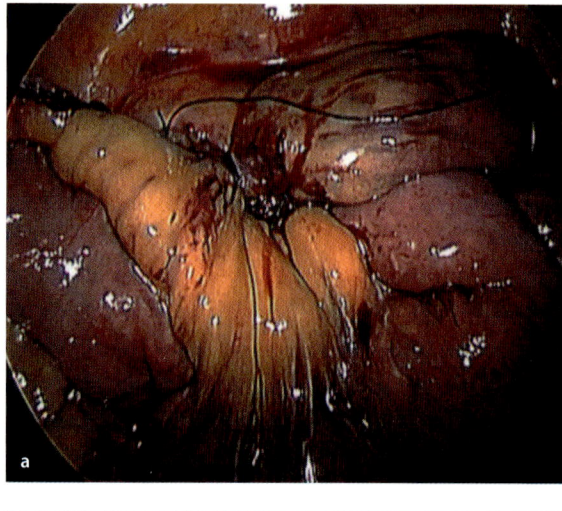

a

b

▪ **Fig. 20.12a,b.** Closure of the mesenteric space between the Roux limb and the biliopancreatic limb

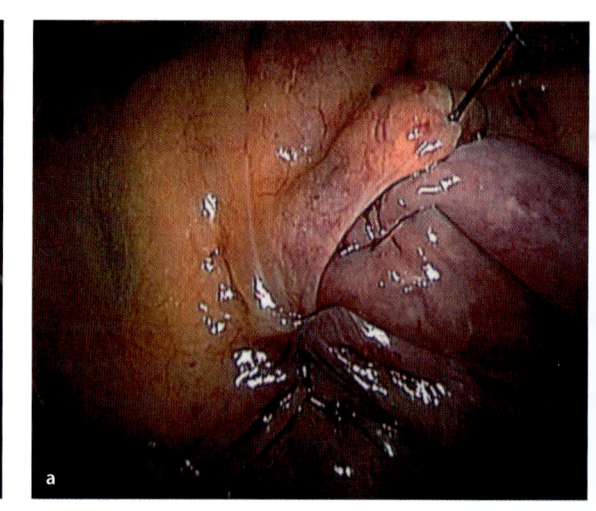

a

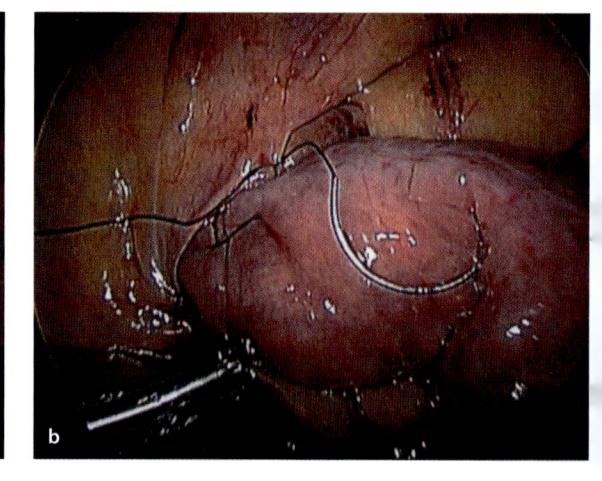

b

▪ **Fig. 20.14a,b.** Space between the Roux limb and the retroperitonium (Peterson's defect) is closed

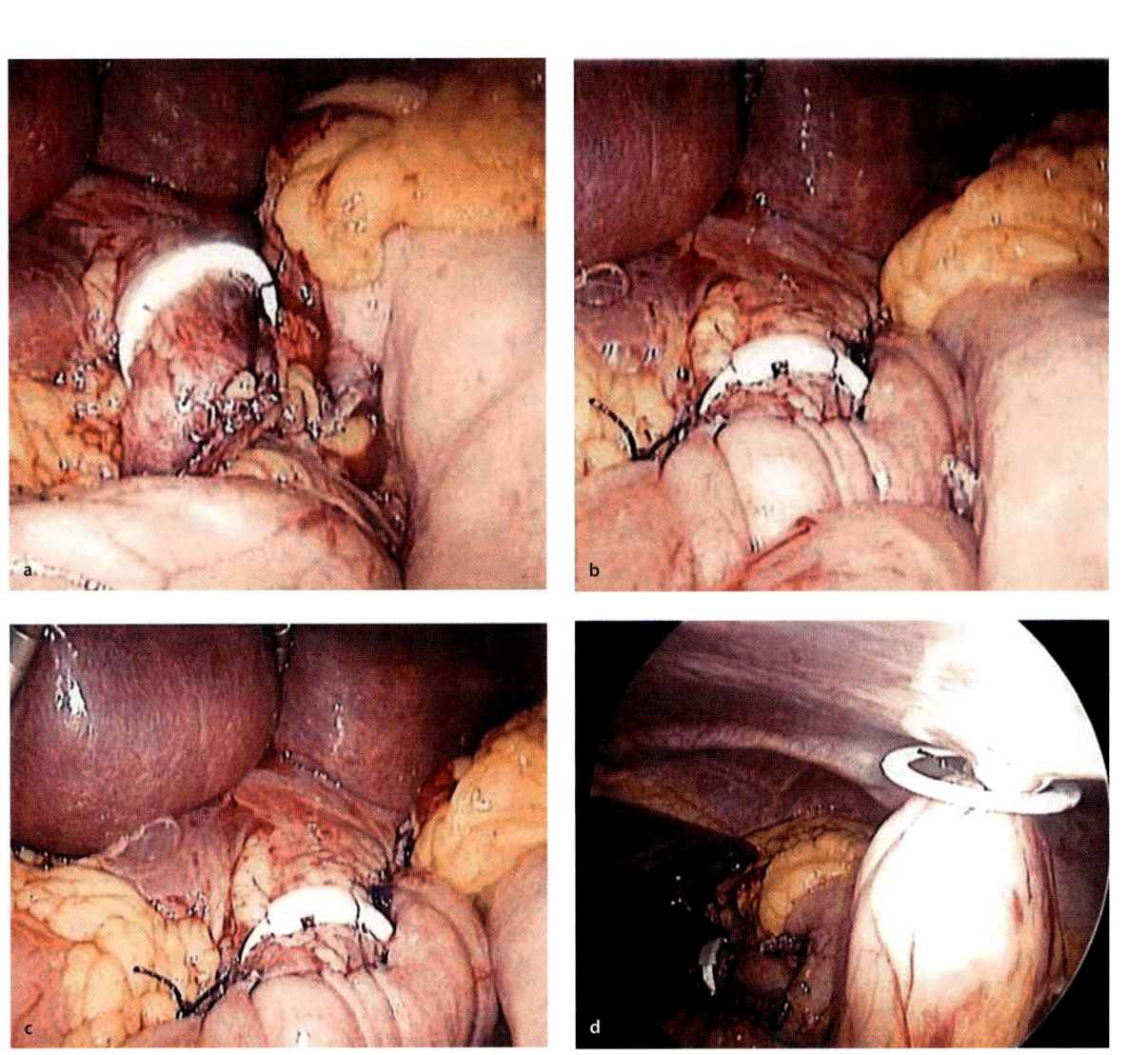

Fig. 20.15a–d. Gastro-jejunostomy is created and the gastrostomy and gastrostomy site marker completes the operation

20.7 Perioperative Care

With a few exceptions, patient selection follows the guidelines of the 1991 NIH consensus statement on gastrointestinal surgery for obesity. Preoperative evaluation entails a complete history and physical exam, including a detailed dietary history and listing of various efforts to lose weight. All patients are seen by a multidisciplinary team including the surgeon, cardiologist, pulmonologist, psychologist/psychiatrist, patient counselor, and nutritionist. Other consultants are used as necessary. All patients get basic laboratory evaluation including *H. pylori* titers, AM cortisol levels, and T3 and T4 levels.

Perioperative antibiotics, sub-Q heparin, TED stockings, sequential compression devices, incentive spirometers, and, when indicated, C-PAP or Bi-PAP machines are used routinely. Early ambulation is routine. Drains are removed as indicated. The gastrostomy tube which is connected to gravity drainage is plugged after 24 h. This tube is removed between 7 and 10 days postoperatively, usually in the office. Patients are started on ice chips 12 h after returning from the operating room. A prescribed diet is started on day 1 after surgery and the patient is followed up with increases in the diet on an outpatient basis. Contrast studies of the pouch and outlet prior to discharge from the hospital are routine.

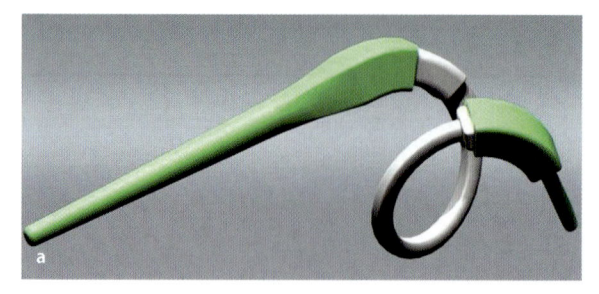

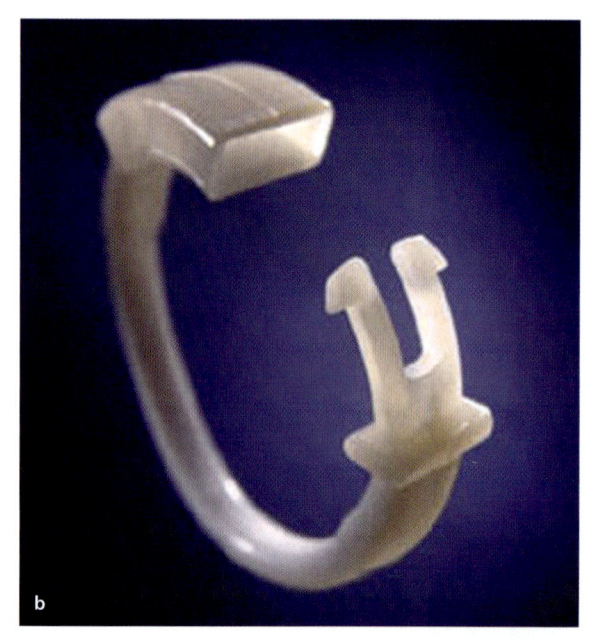

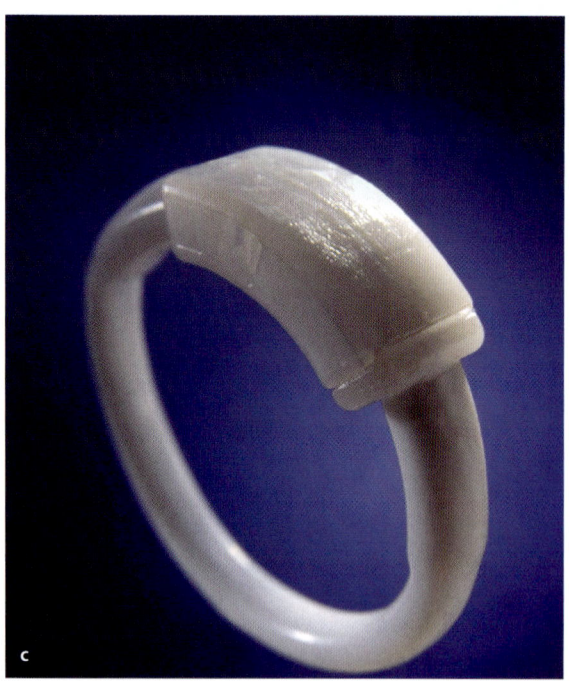

Fig. 20.16. GaBP Ring

20.8   Perioperative Complications

The perioperative complications after the BRYGB are the same as with other short-limb RYGB operations. They include:

- Wound problems/infection/seroma
- Severe nausea, vomiting
- Respiratory problems/atelectasis
- Leaks – pouch/anastomotic
- Pulmonary embolus
- Deep venous thrombosis
- Gastric ileus
- Depression/mood swings
- Death

It should be noted that the band markedly reduces the incidence of outlet stenosis requiring endoscopic dilation.

20.9   Long-term Complications

Long-term complications after the BRYGB are similar to those of short-limb RYGB except that a lower incidence of inadequate weight loss and a lower incidence and magnitude of weight regain are observed. Late complications include:

- Vitamin and mineral deficiencies (vitamins A, D, E, calcium, and iron)
- Weight loss failure, weight regain
- Excessive weight loss
- Transient hair loss
- Anorexia
- Dehydration
- Malnutrition
- Anemia
- Protein malnutrition
- Hypoglycemia
- Dumping syndrome
- Osteoporosis
- Constipation, diarrhea
- Nausea, vomiting
- Marginal ulcers
- Incisional hernias
- Small bowel obstruction

Band complications are seen in just less than 2% of the patients [35]. These include band slippage and erosion with gastrojejunal or gastro-gastric fistula.

20

20.10 Revision/Conversion/Reversal Operations

The common indications for revision of the BRYGB are inadequate weight loss, weight regain, excessive weight loss, mechanical failure of the operation such as outlet stenosis or obstruction, band erosion, and gastro-gastric fistula with marginal ulceration and pain. Other rare indications include patient requests, intractable diarrhea, intractable nausea, recurrent marginal ulcers, intractable anemia, intolerance by the patient, and old age.

The most common revision operation after the BRYGB is shortening of the common limb to effect more weight loss [36]. When weight regain or inadequate weight loss is not due to any mechanical or anatomical dysfunction of the operation, the BRYGB is revised to effect more weight loss by shortening the common limb to increase the malabsorptive component of the operation. Shortening of the common limb is also indicated in patients who experience significant weight regain after band removal. Occasionally, this is also done at the patient's request concurrent with another planned procedure to maximize weight loss. How short the common limb is made depends on how much weight the patient needs to lose and also on his or her current bowel habits. Most commonly, the enteroenteric anastomosis that forms the Roux limb is taken down and a new one is made so that the biliopancreatic limb, the bypassed small bowel, is equal in length to the functional alimentary segment, the efferent limb plus the common limb. Since this revision will result in increased stool frequency with watery consistency, it should not be done in a patient who already has more than six watery stools a day. Patients with increased malabsorption have been documented to lose an average of 7 BMI points or 60 lbs. This is at the cost of increased incidence of protein malnutrition, foul body odor, flatus, and stool odor, and the need for more frequent biochemical monitoring.

There have been a few revision operations to take down a gastro-gastric or gastrojejunal fistula. There have also been conversion operations to a vertical banded gastroplasty because of excessive weight loss, intractable nausea, intractable diarrhea, and intractable marginal ulceration not responsive to medications. Two cases were converted to a banded gastroplasty because of a short-bowel syndrome. Anatomical reversal of the operation has been done at the request of the patients because of recurrent marginal ulcers, patient intolerance, anorexia, old age, and in one patient with Lou Gehrig's disease. All reversal operations have resulted in a rapid regain of the lost weight except in the patient with Lou Gehrig's disease.

20.11 Weight Loss Outcome after Banded Gastric Bypass

Weight loss after the BRYGB is rapid during the first 6 months and continues at a slower pace for up to 18 months after the operation. The percentage excess weight loss in the first year is 77% and this is maintained for 3–5 years. By the 9th year post-op this is around 69.8%. Similarly, the average BMI is maintained below 29.3 kg/m^2 even after 9 years. The success rate after the BRYGB is 90% at 9 years. This means that 90% of those followed had lost and maintained more than 50 %EWL 9 years after the operation.

20.12 Conclusion

The banded gastric bypass operation enhances the restrictive component of the non-banded short limb gastric bypass. The increased benefit of a lesser incidence of outlet stenosis requiring endoscopic dilatation, the increased percentage weight loss in the obese, the morbidly obese, and the super obese, and the increased weight loss maintenance observed with the BRYGB outweigh the 3% incidence of band-related complications which usually have no serious consequences. Fisher and Barber [36] summed up the effectiveness of the banded gastric bypass when they wrote: "… adding the band to the gastric bypass results in more weight loss in more patients that is maintained over a longer period of time." Revision of a failed gastric bypass to a shorter common-limb BRYGB is a simple and effective procedure.

References

1. Fobi MAL, Lee H, Fleming A (1989) Surgical technique of the banded R-Y gastric bypass. JOBWR 8:99–103
2. Mason EE (1982) Vertical banded gastroplasty for morbid obesity. Arch Surg 117:701
3. Laws H, Piantadosi S (1981) Superior gastric reduction procedure for morbid obesity. Am Surg 193:334
4. Crampton NA, Izvomikov V, Stubbs RS (1997) Silastic ring gastric bypass: a comparison of two ring sizes: a preliminary report. Obes Surg 7:495–499
5. Fobi MAL (1991) Marginal ulcer after gastric bypass. Probl General Surg 9: 455–459
6. Capella JF, Capella RF (1996) Staple line disruption and marginal ulceration in gastric bypass procedures for weight reduction. Obes Surg 6:44–49
7. Mason EE, Ito C (1967) Gastric bypass in obesity. Surg Clin 47:1345–1350
8. Torres JC, Oca CF, Garrison RN (1983) Gastric bypass Roux-en-Y gastro-jejunostomy from the lesser curvature. South Med J 76:1217–1220
9. Linner JH, Drew RL (1986) New modifications of Roux-en-Y gastric bypass procedures. Clin Nutr 5:33–37

10. Fobi M, Lee H, Igwe D et al (2001) Band erosion: etiology, management and outcome after banded vertical gastric bypass. Obes Surg 11:699–707
11. Fobi MAL et al (2005) Placement of the GaBP ring system in the banded gastric bypass operation. Obes Surg 15:1196–1201
12. Charuzi I, et al (1989) Presentation at the ASBS Annual Meeting, Toronto Canada June
13. Fobi M (1989) Exhibit, ASBS Annual Meeting, Toronto Canada. June
14. Capella JF, Capella RF (1996) The weight reduction operation of choice: vertical banded gastroplasty of gastric bypass. Am J Surg 17:74–79
15. White S et al (2005) Long-term outcomes after gastric bypass. Obes Surg 15:155–163
16. Zorilla PG, Salinas RJ, Salinas-Martinez AN (1999) Vertical banded gastroplasty – gastric bypass with and without the interposition of jejunum: preliminary report. Obes Surg 9:29–32
17. Fobi MAL, Lee H, Holness R, Cabinda D (1998) Gastric bypass operation for obesity. World J Surg 22:925–935
18. Cruz-Vigo F, Cruz-Vigo J et al Laparoscopic banded gastric bypass, immediate and mid-to long-term results. Obes Surg 2006, 16:232
19. Marema RT (2005) Laparoscopic Roux-en-Y Gastric Bypass: a step-by-step approach. J Am Coll Surg 6:979–982
20. Salinas A, Santiago E, Yeguez J et al (2005) Silastic ring vertical gastric bypass: evolution of an open surgical technique, and review of 1588 cases. Obes Surg 15:1403–1417
21. Sugerman HJ, Starky JV, Birkenhaur R (1987) A randomized prospective trial of gastric bypass versus vertical banded gastroplasty for morbid obesity and their effects on sweets versus non sweets eaters. Ann Surg 205:613–624
22. Fobi M, Fleming AW (1984) Vertical banded gastroplasty vs. gastric bypass in treatment of obesity, J Natl Med Assoc 78:1092
23. Howard L, Malone M, Michalek A et al (1995) Gastric bypass and vertical banded gastroplasty – a prospective randomized comparison and 5-year follow-up. Obes Surg 5:55–60
24. Fobi MA, Lee H, Igwe D jr, Stanczyk M, Tambi JN (2001) Prospective comparative evaluation of stapled versus transected silastic ring gastric bypass: 6-year follow-up. Obes Surg 11:18–24
25. Carvajal JJB et al (2006) Comparative study between gastric bypass with or without ring in the treatment of morbid obesity. Obes Surg 16:225
26. Awad W, Garay A et al (2005) Gastric bypass with and without a ring: the effect on weight reduction and the quality of life. Obes Surg 15:724
27. Luis Vincenti, Jose Pareja et al (2004) Presentation, Brazilian Congress on Obesity Surgery. Rio de Janero
28. Membrives O, Gallardo V et al (2006) Vertical ring gastroplasty and gastric bypass: assessment by gammagraphy with labeled food. Obes Surg 16:233
29. Charuzi I, et al (2001) Use of adjustable silicone gastric banding for revision of failed gastric operations. Obes Surg 11:66–69
30. Bressler M et al (2005) Adjustable gastric banding as a revisional bariatric procrdure after failed gastric bypass. Obes Surg 15:1443–1448
31. Avinoah E, Lantsberg L, Solly M (2006) Proximal gastric banding after failed gastric restrictive operations Obes Surg 16:213
32. Higa K (2004) Revisional Bariatric surgery Course, San Francisco, April
33. Fobi M et al (2007) Banded gastric bypass. In: Buchwald H et al (eds) Surgical management of obesity, chap 27. Saunders Elsevier, Amsterdam, pp 223–230
34. Fobi M et al (2001) Revision of failed gastric bypass to distal Roux-Y gastric bypass: review of 65 cases. Obes Surg 11:195
35. Fobi M, Lee, H, Igwe et al (2000) Transected silastic ring vertical gastric bypass with jejunal interposition a gastrostomy and a gastrostomy site marker (Fobi pouch operation for obesity). In: Deitel M, Cowan GSM (eds) Update: surgery for the morbidly obese patient. FD Communications, Toronto, pp 203–226
36. Fisher BL, Barber AE (1999) Gastric bypass procedures. Eur J Gastroenterol Hepatol 11:93–97

21

Pathophysiology of Malabsorptive Bariatric Procedures

Nicola Scopinaro, MD

protein intake to be sufficient in all cases for nutritional needs. The problem was initially addressed by adopting a 100-cm BPL with the usual 50-cm CL, with almost all of the small bowel remaining in the AL. Later, in order to make sure that sufficient food reached the ileum, an AL of 350 cm was used instead of the usual 250 cm, resulting in 400 cm from the gastroenterostomy to the ICV. This has minimized the risk of protein malnutrition, while also reducing the unpleasant side effects of BPD.

21.6 Conclusion

A good knowledge of the principles of malabsorption helps to avoid or reduce its negative effects to a minimum, while best exploiting its mechanisms of action, which may be adapted to the patient's individual characteristics. The results are excellent weight reduction maintained indefinitely, disappearance or marked reduction of the co-morbidities related to excess weight, and near disappearance of nearly all components of the metabolic syndrome. If the necessary dietary supplements are taken, which represents the only collaboration required from the patient, all the results can be obtained at the negligible cost of only a 1% reoperation rate for late specific complications.

The Biliopancreatic Diversion

W. Konrad Karcz, MD, Luc Lemmens, MD, Waleed Bukhari, MD, Cheng Zhou, MD, Marc Daoud, MD, Simon Küsters, MD

The still increasing number of metabolic operations has led to the creation of many Obesity or Metabolic Surgery Centers. Laparoscopic metabolic surgery has recently become the fastest-growing surgical specialty in many countries. The chapter presents the indications, technique and complications of the biliopancreatic diversion (BPD). The BPD operation is considered as the technique with the best long term weight loss and the highest resolution rate of the co-morbidities. On the other hand there are late complications, even life threatening.

Is the 95% remission rate of T2DM, a complete remission of hypercholesterolemia, a high remission rate of arterial hypertension (AH) and other good results concerning co-morbidities after BPD a factor which can influence the number of BPD-operations and is worth the price of late complications?

22.1 Introduction

It is well accepted now that bariatric surgery is the only treatment with acceptable or even good long term results for the treatment of morbid obesity and metabolic disease. Different conservative therapies do not stabilize weight in the long run [1-5]. Since the first operations in the early fifties, many procedures were developed to treat morbid obesity. Many of them disappeared because of too many complications or insufficient success rate. For a long time the vertical-banded gastroplasty (Mason procedure) was considered the gold standard but completely abandoned since the beginning of the 21st century. Nowadays, gastric bypass is the gold standard in bariatric surgery worldwide [6-8]. The excess body weight loss ranges between 50% and 60% after a gastric bypass procedure in the first postoperative year [8-11]. Unfortunately, long-term follow-up studies have showed that the patients can regain weight later [6;9;12-15].

Malabsorptive procedures – biliopancreatic diversion in its two main forms: traditional BPD by Scopinaro and BPD with Duodenal Switch – have shown better long term weight loss and better remission of the co-morbidities. The 30- year follow-up of the BPD shows a stable weight loss, but life-long medical control is required [16]. The biliopancreatic diversion was developed in 1976 by Nicola Scopinaro as an alternative procedure to jejuno-ileal bypass (JIB) [17]. In 1998 Hess modified this procedure into the BPD-Duodenal Switch (BPD-DS). Later this modification was popularized by Picard Marceau. The idea of this modification was that preserving of the pylorus and the atrum would make the BPD-DS more physiological and could reduce the side effects and com-

plications. Both operations will be described in detail in this chapter.

Michel Gagner performed the first laparoscopic BPD-DS in 1999 [18]. These developments led to an increased number of BPD operations and the development of the "2-step strategy". Because of an increased number of complications and even increased mortality in the super-obese patients, some authors did promote the performance of this operation in two steps. In the first step, a sleeve resection (vertical resection of the stomach) was performed. After a significant weight loss the duodenal switch was then performed as a second step. Since the sleeve resection resulted in a very good weight loss in many patients more and more surgeons started to perform this procedure as a definitive procedure. To improve the weight loss and prevent the weight regain the sleeve became smaller and smaller. This resulted in the narrow sleeve gastrectomy around a 32-34F gastric tube.

This new procedure can be considered as a modification of the vertical banded gastroplasty and Magenstrase procedure [19] but with better metabolic results. The two-step procedure also allows us to discern two groups of patients, those with good weight control after the sleeve gastrectomy who do not need the second step and those with insufficient weight loss or even weight regain who need the second malabsorptive step.

The complementary operation to the sleeve gastrectomy seems to be the duodenal switch [20;21]. In our experience, patients lose significantly more weight after a duodenal switch as a second step than patients undergoing RYGB as a secondary operation. The aim of this chapter is to convince the metabolic surgical community not to be afraid of malabsorption in carefully-selected patients. The surgical complications of a laparoscopic Scopinaro operation or a duodenal switch are not as high as expected, and the benefits can rarely be reached with any other surgical method.

22.2 Indications for malabsorptive surgery

What is the correct place for Biliopancreatic Diversion in Metabolic Surgery? The general indication of a BMI over 40 kg/m^2 does not answer the question. It is difficult to identify the patient who will respond best to the therapy. All patients must fulfill the criteria for bariatric and metabolic surgery as described by the National Institutes of Health Consensus Development Panel in 1991 [22]. There are different indication algorithms, and in our opinion they can serve as a basis for choosing the optimal operation. There are some points which strongly restrict the application of malabsorption. In our opinion, biliopancreatic diversion should not be performed in any form in non-compliant patients, patients needing permanent oral medication, whose absorption is influenced, patients who cannot participate in regular follow-up, patients with chronic bowel disease, patients with severe pychiatric and psychological disorders, patients who are vegetarians or patients who suffer from chronic diarrhea.

In our opinion, the main focus should be placed on obese patients with related metabolic disorders. Both currently performed malabsorptive operations, BPD Scopinaro and BPD with Duodenal Switch lead to good weight reduction and improvement of related metabolic disorders. The laparoscopic BPD operations require relatively high operative skills, especially in patients with a BMI over 60 kg/m². Here the two-step procedure proposed by Gagner allows evaluation of the patient's compliance and helps to avoid high-risk surgery. We found that weight regain, a common problem after restrictive procedures, is much less frequent after malapsorptive operations. In the last few years we observed a beneficial effect on type-2 diabetes after all types of bariatric/metabolic operations. Some scientific evidence exists to show that insulin resistance also improves. More than 95% of prevalent type-2 diabetes is attributable to being overweight or obese. In a recent meta-analysis of 136 controlled trials and case series, Buchwald et al. found that type-2 diabetes showed remission - defined as the ability to discontinue all diabetes medications - in 76.8% of operated patients. The rates differed by operation type: a rate of 98.9% was seen for biliopancreatic diversion, 83.7% for gastric bypass, 71.6% for gastroplasty, and 47.9% for gastric banding. Also, more than 50% of those patients who did not experience complete resolution showed significant improvement for diabetes. In addition, an improvement in diabetic neuropathy after obesity surgery has been noted [6;23].

What has surprised us for years is that the remission of diabetes comes almost directly after surgery, with an improvement in insulin resistance occurring prior to significant weight loss. This observation and the more pronounced changes observed after combined restrictive and malabsorptive procedures (gastric bypass, biliopancreatic diversion) have sparked a great deal of speculation about the role of gut hormones in insulin resistance and the possibility of novel regulatory mechanisms. Accordingly, the impact of various obesity surgery procedures on leptin, ghrelin, resistine, adiponectin, glucagon-like peptide 1, and other satiety mechanisms is receiving increasing attention [24-29]. However, all forms of weight loss surgery lead to weight loss, caloric restriction, decrease in fat mass, and improvement in type-2 diabetes, and the degree of these improvements in the long term seem to be stratified by weight. These observations alternatively suggest that the improvements in glucose metabolism and insulin resistance after obesity surgery may arise primarily from known mechanisms: in the short term due to decreased stimulation of the enteroinsular axis by decreased calorie intake, and in the long term from decreased fat mass and resultant changes in the release of adipocytokines [30]. After over 40 years of bariatric surgery, these findings may mean that time has come to say that Diabetes mellitus therapy should involve bypass surgery.

At the beginning, the indications should be discussed in an interdisciplinary group for all patients with insulin resistance. In the near future, new guidelines for metabolic surgery indications have to consider type-2 Diabetes mellitus. But not only Diabetes mellitus is positively influenced by malabsorptive surgery; positive changes have also been observed in cardiac function leading to improvement of hypertension. Epidemiological studies indicate obesity in up to 50% of patients with prevalent hypertension [31]. The relationship between abdominal obesity and blood pressure is well known [10;12]. It is interesting that weight loss is almost always associated with decreased blood pressure, even in normotensive individuals.

Generally, a 1% decrease in body weight has been associated with decrease of about 1mmHg in systolic blood pressure and about 2 mmHg in diastolic blood pressure. In obese hypertensive patients, a number of randomized controlled trials and prospective cohort studies have shown that intentional weight loss, whether dietary or surgical, leads to reductions of systolic blood pressure, diastolic blood pressure, and decrease of anti-hypertensive medications used [32-34]. Therefore it was not surprising to find that obesity surgery is commonly associated with marked improvements or resolution of clinical hypertension [35].

We can easily find scientific arguments: Sugarman, in a large series of 1000 obese subjects undergoing gastric bypass, found that 75% had a diagnosis of hypertension. One year after bypass surgery, 69 % of patients no longer suffered hypertension, and after 7 years, 66% still had normal blood pressure [36]. In the famous SOS study, a long-term prospective, case-controlled trial, 2-year and 10-year recovery rates from hypertension were greater for patients after obesity surgery than for control subjects [37]. A recent systematic review and meta-analysis by Buchwald et al. found that hypertension was significantly improved in the total population analyzed across all surgical procedures. Specifically, their meta-analysis found the rate of reported hypertension resolution to be 62% and the rate of combined resolution or significant improvement to be 78.5% [6]. Although it is difficult to apply these specific numbers to individual cases due to the nature of meta-analysis, their relative magnitude as well as the diversity of studies from which they were derived emphasizes the profound effect that obesity surgery has on improving or resolving hypertension. Improvement of hypertension seems to be proportional to the amount of weight lost, and not to the final weight. It is important to note that hypertension is often resolved even though patients do not achieve ideal body weight. The improvement of blood pressure positively influences and prevents heart pathology.

The next area of interest directly involved with malabsorptive surgery is lipid disorders. Along with the remission of hypertension, other circulatory diseases can be prevented. Many series have reported a significant improvement in low-density lipoprotein, increased high-density lipoprotein (HDL), and decreased triglycerides [38-40]. Average reductions of as much as 40% of total triglycerides and 25% of total cholesterol have been reported within 6 to 12 months following bypass surgery [40]. The SOS study found significant improvements in triglyccrides and HDL in the surgical group at 2 and 10 years [37]. However, total cholesterol was not significantly different at 2 and 10 years in the entire cohort, while in the bypass subgroup total cholesterol, triglycerides, and HDL were all significantly improved. In general, dyslipidemia, hypercholesterolemia, and hypertriglyceridemia all appear to improve significantly with metabolic surgical procedures.

Disturbances in lipid homeostasis are combined with the liver disorders. The risk of liver diseases in patients who are overweight is higher than in other patients. Fatty liver disorder (FLD) is documented in up to 15 % of the normal population and up to 80 % of obese individuals [41]. Pathophysiology shows hepatocyte triglyceride accumulation because of insulin resistance. The development of FLD following mitochondrial fatty acids oxidation, NF-κB-dependent inflammatory cytokine expression and adipocytokines are all considered to be potential factors causing hepatocyte injury, inflammation and fibrosis. Non-alcohoic FLD was always seen as a benign disorder which may progress to fibrosis in about 30%. But in some cases, hepatocellular carcinoma can result after time. This is the reason not to trivialize NAFLD and to introduce therapy possibly including metabolic surgery [42].

The greatest potential in treatment of these disorders seems to be found in malabsorptive procedures. The lowest lipid levels were registered one year after BPD, an adaptation of the ileum and changes in diet could be responsible for the slight increase after one year [43]. Brizzi et al. showed that the decrease in LDL and trigliceridcs after BPD surgery seems to be independent of recovery of DM as they appeared in patients both with and without diabetes [39;44]. The same technique of BPD is the most effective method for reduction of plasma lipid levels in patients with heterozygous familiar hypercholesterolemia. Here, indications for this procedure should be considered carefully, particularly in view of availability of other dyslipidemia treatments [45].

Another important clinical observation is that abdominal circumference is a risk factor for many diseases. It seems to be important to evaluate the two different fat compartments: visceral and subcutaneous. The visceral fat is reduced much more quickly after metabolic surgery. The improvement of metabolic variables correlates with decrease of BMI and visceral fat. This directly suggests that the visceral fat is mostly responsible for the metabolic disturbances [46]. The effect on hyperlipidemia after ileal bypass was prospectively investigated in the POSCH long-term study. Malabsorptive surgical interventions resulted in normalization of lipid profiles, decreased mortality and increased life expectancy in the long-term observation [45-47]. In 2005 it was seen that only malabsorptivc proccdurcs introduccd sustained and marked reduction of blood LDL cholesterol with increased cholesterol fecal output. Patients who were hypercholesterolemic before surgery showed the highest reduction of serum cholesterol levels. Restrictive bariatric operations alone do not induce similar changes, which leads to the question whether the guidelines should not be modified in terms of favouring malabsorptive procedures in patients with hyperlipidemia. It is well known that lowering LDL cholesterol, a risk factor of arteriosclerosis, can prevent coronary heart disease which is another benefit of malabsorptive procedures [40].

The liver is another organ directly connected with lipid metabolism and diabetes. The status of the liver has to be evaluated before considering malabsorptive surgery. Whereas patients with FLD (caused by alcohol, drugs and toxins), hepatic failure, viral hepatitis or cirrhosis should not be operated on, patients with NAFLD / NASH combined with diabetes, hypertension, obesity and dyslipidemia might be good candidates for biliopancreatic diversion. Thus, the diagnosis of non-alcoholic steatosis hepatis should also be considered as a criteria for the selection of patients for malabsorptive metabolic surgery [38]. The literature shows different examples of the liver as a mirror of metabolic lipid and glucose pathology. Machado et al. investigated a large group of patients in a review article. The severity of obesity and age were not related to liver status, but the metabolic condition with insulin resistance and diabetes mellitus type-2 were related to hepatic pathology. It is also very important to recognize the need to develop criteria for defining NASH to make comparison of different studies much easier [48]. Kral et al. found that not only steatosis hepatis improved after the biliopancreatic diversion but also more advanced pathologies like fibrosis showed recovery after weight reduction. The improvement was directly connected with the protein absorption and diarrhea status [49]. In another large series by Baltasar et al., liver disorders arose in some cases after BPD. On the other hand, all steatosis hepatis problems were resolved by using the same operative technique [50]. It was interesting to find that the fibrosis of the liver slightly increased in a small group of patients after bariatric surgery. The status of the liver has to be evaluated before surgery, possibly including biopsy in carefully-selected cases to avoid progression of liver disease after malabsorptive metabolic surgery. In the biggest series of biliopancreatic diversion, chronic liver damage was not seen, but acute reversible hepatocellular necrosis 2 months after the operation was reported. Scopinaro et al. agree that laboratory examinations and hepatic histology are helpful in identifying patients with increased risk for acute liver damage [51]. With these results came the question: Where does one draw the line when considering a malabsorptive operation? Establishment of a standard BPD-DS operation was also postulated. The enzymatic function of the liver is enhanced in first 12 months and the histological status improves earlier after duodenal switch surgery [52]. Evaluation of hypertension, ALT level and measurement of insulin resistance, diagnostic of dyslipidemia and FLI (Fatty Liver Index) should be performed prior to operations and controlled in the follow-up process. "HAIR" =hypertension, ALT and insulin resistance and "BAAT" = BMI, ALT, age and triglyceride scores can be very useful [53].

The lipid and carbohydrate metabolism homeostasis also have to be monitored before and after biliopancreatic surgery. Soriguer et al. measured a difference in the free fatty acids levels after the intra venous glucose tolerance test between patients with impaired fasting glucose or with diabetes and patients with normal metabolic status. The following relationship was seen: the smaller the glucose metabolism disturbances, the faster the lipid recovery after surgical procedures. This leads us to the conclusion that the greater the lipid pathology indicates that the more potent surgical treatment should be performed [54]. NAFLD is seen as one of the main causes of chronic liver disease, and depicts the hepatic component of the metabolic syndrome. The best regression of metabolic syndrome with improvement of diabetes, hypertension and dyslipidemia with reduction of insulin resistance and improvement of liver histology can be achieved with malabsorptive metabolic surgery. The changes reached with surgery seem to be stable in long-term examinations.

It is obvious that metabolic malabsorptive surgery has to be one of the modern metabolic syndrome therapy options [55]. It is interesting that liver status strongly influences the pathophysiology of circulation, still the most common cause of death, and should thus come in the focus of health care providers as a risk factor [56]. There is no data to scientifically evaluate cardiovascular disease (CVD) as an indication for metabolic surgery. The most important risk factors for CVD, like hypertension, diabetes, high LDL, increased TG, high total cholesterol, metabolic syndrome etc., are very familiar to the metabolic surgeon. Improvement or elimination of these risk factors leads to reduction of myocardial infarction, stroke and cardiovascular death. Only 10% percent reduction of weight in overweight patients leads to 20% decrease of the CVD risk. It was found that congestive heart failure and cardiomyopathy as well as dynamic functions of the heart improve after weight reduction and bariatric surgery. Also the pulmonary manifestations of obesity, including asthma, obstructive sleep apnea, obesity hypoventilation syndrome and pulmonary hypertension, have to be considered as indications for metabolic surgery.

It is already scientifically proven that these diseases improve with weight reduction. Another pathological symptom – increased intra-abdominal pressure – leads to several pathologies like venous stasis, urinary incontinence and pseudotumor cerebri. All the problems can possibly be resolved with the reduction of intra-abdominal fat. They should also be considered as indications for metabolic surgery. Recognizing the pathophysiology of obesity, the indication for metabolic surgery will become even wider in the future and will include areas which today seem to be closed to interventional treatment. But success is only possible with cooperation between all medical disciplines involved.

22.3 Operative technique – the standard BPD as described by Scopinaro

The laparoscopic approach of this technique (LBPD-S) (◘ Fig. 22.1a,b) is used as a standard in bariatric centers. We will describe the method briefly. In the majority of our patients, we perform the operation as a two-surgeon procedure. With the patient in the lithotomic position, and the operating table in a 30 to 40 degree reverse Trendelenburg tilt, the surgeon stands between the patient's legs with one assistant on the left side of the patient at the beginning of the operation. The capnoperitoneum is archieved with a 12 mm separator trocar (Applied Medical, USA). The residual abdominal pressure is much higher in obese patients (12-16 mm Hg) than in patients of normal weight (2-5 mm Hg). When a pressure of 14 mm Hg is reached, four or five more work trocars are

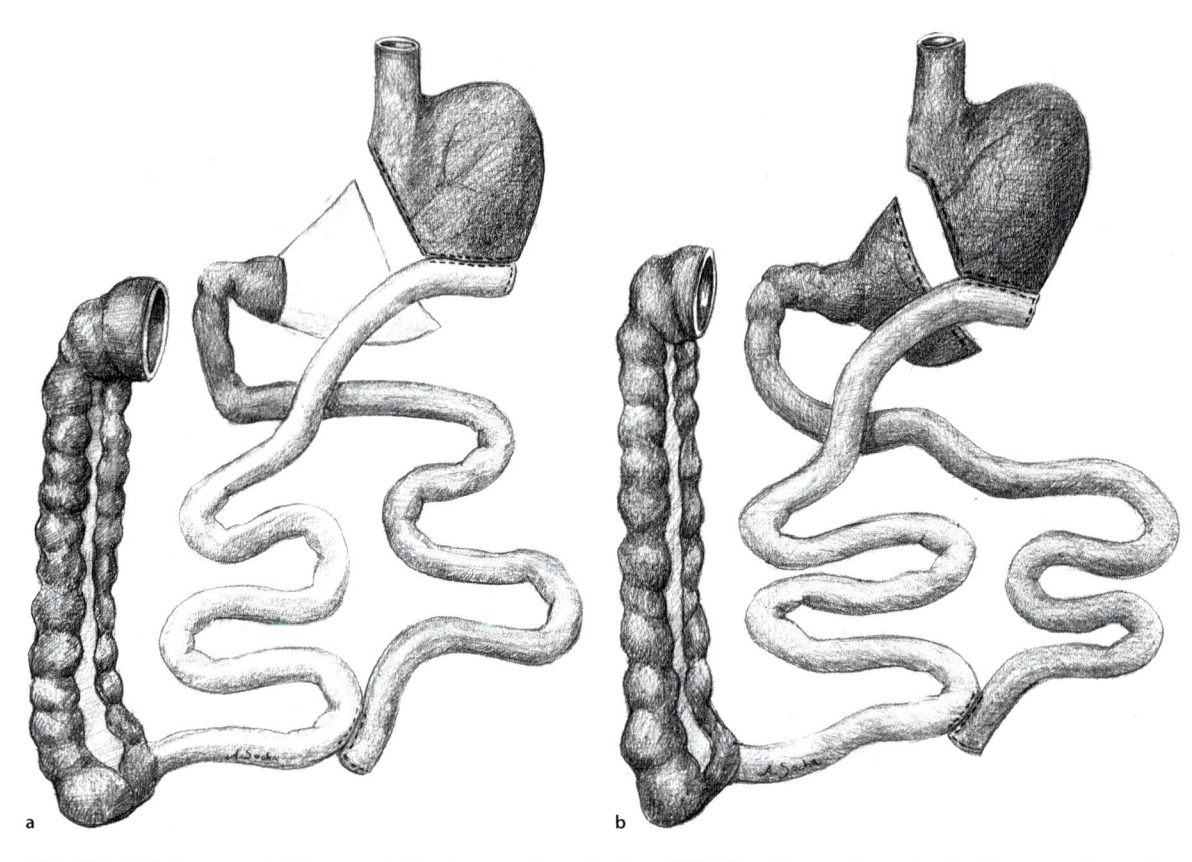

a · b

Fig. 22.1a,b. The Laparoscopic Biliopancreatic Diversion according to Scopinaro (LBPD-S) **a** with stomach resection, **b** without stomach resection.

placed under direct view, as shown (☐ Fig. 22.2). The large curvature is exposed by lifting the anterior stomach wall and dissection is started in the region of the upper stomach with Ligasure®Advanced (Covidien, Valley Lab). As a first step, the bursa omentalis is opened. Then we begin the dissection in the region of the small curvature of the stomach, perigastric 4-6 cm below the cardia, with the aim of also opening the bursa omentalis from the lesser curvature side. Then a gastric pouch with a volume of about 250 to 400 ml is created using 2 linear Endo-GIA® (Covidien, Auto Suture) 60 mm staplers with blue (or green) cartridges to completely transect the stomach. The gastric tube has to be removed from the stomach prior to transection. This technique enables adequate direct visualization and thus objective evaluation of the anterior and posterior aspects of the pouch and distal stomach for leaks or bleeding, and visual estimation of the pouch size. Originally the distal stomach was resected with closing of the duodenum with a GIA stapler. Then the Ileocecal region becomes the area of interest and should be correctly identified.

Standard operation technique includes an appendectomy. The measurement of the common channel has to

be made very precisely starting at the valve of Bauhin. There are two methods which are mostly used: direct measurements using instruments in 5 cm or 10 cm steps or measurement with a band which is 25 cm long. The common channel in the Scopinaro operation always has a length of 50 cm. Then two marks are made with threads, leaving the short mark distal for orientation. After that, the whole intestine should be measured up to the Treiz's band. The diversion should be made with a 45-mm Endo-GIA® stapler with white vascular cartridge at 50% of the total length of the intestine. This is about 250 cm from Bauhin's Valve in the majority of all cases. The mesentery should be divided with GIA 45 Endo-GIA® (Covidien, Auto Suture) white stapler or with the LigaSure®Advanced (Covidien, Valley Lab) for haemostasis. This division is important to reduce tension on the GE anastomosis. The proximal part of the small bowel is positioned in the lower-left part of the abdominal cavity; the distal part is shifted into the right upper part of the abdomen to avoid later distortion. The marker threads show the direction of the ileum. A side-to-side stapled jejunoileostomy connecting the biliopancreatic jejunal limb and the marked side of the terminal ileum is cre-

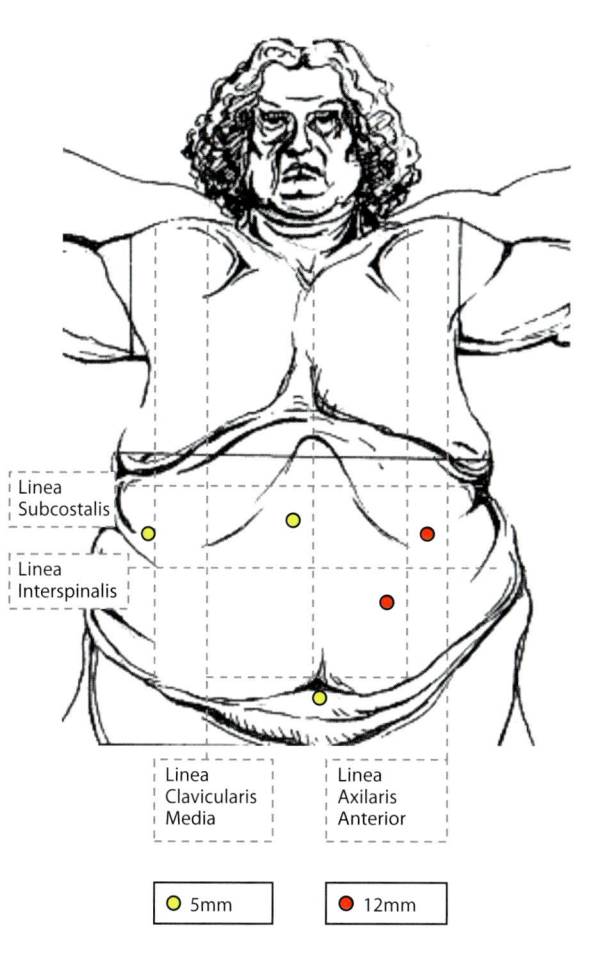

☐ Fig. 22.2. The trocar positions for LBPD-S.

Linea Subcostalis

Linea Interspinalis

Linea Clavicularis Media

Linea Axilaris Anterior

○ 5mm   ● 12mm

GIA® (Covidien, Auto Suture) stapler. Afterwards, the integrity of anastomosis is tested for leakage by using methylene-blue insufflation through the gastric tube and placement of a bowel clamp on the intestinal limb distal to the anastomosis. Prevention of internal hernias is achieved by closing the gap between the alimentary jejunal limb and transverse mesocolon with interrupted non-absorbable sutures. The areas of GEA and IJA are drained with a Blake drain if needed, and the operation is finished without closure of any abdominal fascial openings.

22.4 Operation technique of Standard Laparoscopic Biliopancreatic Diversion with Duodenal Switch

Principally the operation technique is very similar to the classical biliopancreatic diversion. The main difference is the preservation of the pylorus and a vertical, not horizontal stomach resection. As mentioned, it is possible to divide the procedure into two steps with a preliminary sleeve resection to reduce weight and intra-abdominal fat and thus make the second step of intestinal diversion easier. At the beginning, there was no standard to define how the vertical resection should be made. First resections were resections of the larger curvature without calibration of the sleeve. Then 40F gastric tubes were used to calibrate the sleeve. When the two-step procedure was introduced, the sleeve formation was done more restrictively using 32-34F gastric tubes. Later on, the size of the sleeve was measured before the second step operation. The results using the 32F gastric tube showed that the volume of sleeve had approximately doubled one year after the primary operation. In our clinic, all patients with a BMI over 50 are qualified for the two-step operation and for that reason there are no differences between the LSG as a first step operation and the LSG as a sole bariatric operation procedure concerning the size of the gastric tube.

Because in our collective about 30% of the super-obese patients need no second-step operation for sufficient weight reduction after two years, we do rarely perform the one step duodenal switch operation. Instead we perform the isolated duodenal switch operation (without sleeve gastrectomy) in selected patients with severe metabolic disturbances.

The sleeve operation technique was described before; the second-step operation starts with separation of the duodenum with a GIA® (Covidien, Auto Suture) stapler white or blue cartridge. After that, a typical cholecystectomy is performed to avoid the formation of gallstones as

ated using a 45-mm Endo-GIA® (Covidien, Auto Suture) stapler. The opening for the stapler is closed with running absorbable suture. Prevention of internal hernias is achieved by closing the gap between the biliopancreatic jejunal limb and mesoileum with interrupted or continuous non-absorbable sutures. In patients with extremely thick greater omentum, additional omentum division is performed with a LigaSure® (Covidien, Valley Lab) dissector. The distal end of the divided intestine, which is still positioned in the right upper abdominal cavity, is marked with a suture and transported antecolic (the retrocolic laparoscopic approach is technically more difficult in very obese patients) and antegastric (if the distal stomach was preserved).

As a next step, the gastroentero-anastomosis (GEA) is created with a hand running suture end to side, 2 cm long, with a two-layer closure of 2-0/3-0 Vicryl on the side of large curvature. A 12-mm obturator is used to calibrate the stomal opening. The anastomosis can also be made with a CEA® (Covidien, Auto Suture), or with

22

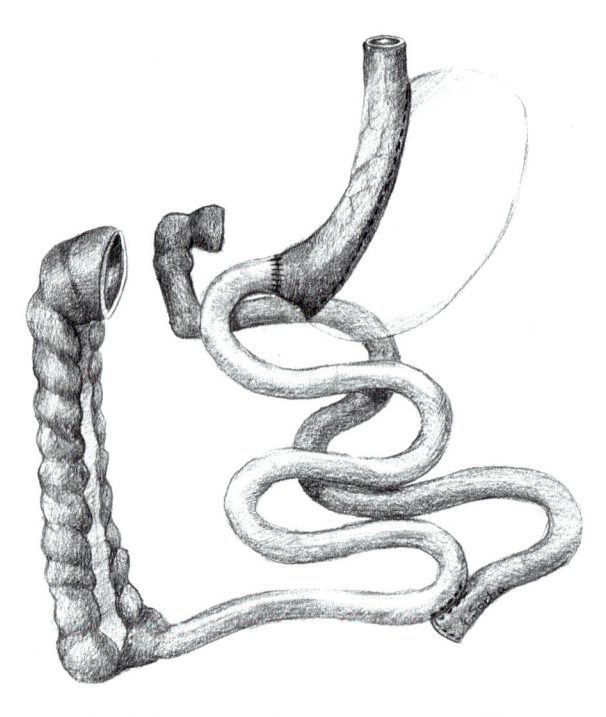

Table 22.1 Early complications after BPD-Scopinaro in a series of 1040 patients (own data, L.Lemmens)

Early complication	Count	[%] of n=1040
Pulmonary embolism	8	076 %
Thrombophlebitis of the lower limb	8	076 %
Abscess	1	0,096 %
Small bowel occlusion	3	0.288 %
Wound problems	2	0.192 %
Wound infection with pus evacuation	4	0.384 %
Mortality Haemorrhage: 1, Pulmonary embolism: 1, Infarction of small intestine: 1	3	0.288 %
Incisional hernia	24	2.31 %

Fig. 22.3. The Laparoscopic Biliopancreatic Diversion with the Duodenal Switch (BPD-DS)

well as adhesions between the duodenal stump and the gallbladder. The next moves are similar to the classical duodenal diversion. The main difference is the length of the common channel which is elongated to 75-100cm in DS. The division of the intestine is done as described above. The second difference is the ileo-duodenostomy which can be performed in different ways. We prefer the end (duodenum) to side (ileum) or end to end manual double line suture. The other options used contain CEA® or GIA (Covidien, Auto Suture) stapler anastomoses which are technically difficult. Of course all the openings of the mesentery are completely closed. (**Fig. 22.3**)

22.5 Early and Late Complications

The introduction of laparoscopy reduced the number of surgical post-operative bariatric complications. The overall complication rate ranges from 20% to 40% [6, 9, 57]. It is proven that among the most influential factors for predicting major complications are: male gender, revisional surgery, age, a BMI >50 kg/m^2, FEV1< 80%, previous abdominal procedures and an abnormal ECG [58]. It is well known that laparoscopic bariatric surgery requires advanced skills. Complication rates of about 9.5% with major and 6.7% minor GI complications are reported after BPD, with a mortality rate of 0.4% (own

data, L.Lemmens) (**Table 22.1**). Suture line leaks occur in 1.2% to 3% and are mostly seen at the beginning of the learning curve, which improves with the surgeon's experience (8). The most common early complications (within 30 days after surgery) include bleeding, followed by gastric leaks and wound infections. Intra-abdominal abscesses, thrombembolisms, subileus, sepsis, thrombophlebitis, pancreatitis, trocar herniation, dysphagia, rhabdomyolysis are rarely found [59].

Anastomotic leakage

The diagnosis of post-operative peritonitis is much more difficult in morbidly-obese patients. Physical manual examination is required, but an additional clinical evaluation is necessary in each case. The canon of symptoms includes tachycardia, incipience of pulmonary insufficiency and worsening of abdominal pain. The diagnostic procedure should be rapidly started with radiological and laboratory examinations. Anastomotic leakage usually occurs within the first 10 days of surgery. The most common site of the leak is the gastroenteric anastomosis. Because sepsis and bowel obstruction are potential manifestations of an anastomotic leak, CT examination is strongly recommended in all patients with unexplained fever, pain and abdominal distension following BPD. If CT examination is not possible, the patient should undergo emergency relaparoscopy. This usually allows improvement of the local status and, depending on the intervention time, makes local surgical intervention or drainage of the infected area possible. For the diagnostic on ICU the LapVision MultiPort system (Pajunk Medizintechnologie) is very useful (◘ Fig. 19.4a,b).

Incisional hernias

It has been shown that the incidence of incisional hernias reaches approximately 13.7% of the rate after open surgery. A port side herniation is reported in 0.5% (8). We have not observed such complications in our series since we started using the separator trocars.

Thromboembolism

An increased risk for venous thromboembolism in obese individuals has been questioned. In prospective studies, neither Hill et al. nor Sue-Ling et al., could demonstrate a correlation between obesity and the incidence of post-operative deep vein thrombosis [61,2]. In a postmortem study of 152 surgical patients by Cullen and Nemeskal, obesity did not seem to be a risk factor for pulmonary embolism, but obesity was not clearly defined [63]. Finally, Flordal et al. evaluated risk factors for thromboembolism in 2,070 patients but failed to prove a correlation between obesity and post-operative thromboembolism. However, all patients had undergone prophylaxis with low-molecular-weight heparin [64]. Gonzalez et al. reported only one popliteal thrombosis in 380 patients with a mean BMI of 48.5 undergoing laparoscopic Roux-en-Y gastric bypass. Intermittent pneumatic calf compression was used in this study, but no pharmacological prophylaxis [65]. In a registry including 3,097 patients undergoing bariatric surgery, 15 patients died within 6 months after surgery. Pulmonary embolism was the cause of death in 13% [66]. But in 10 autopsies of patients who died after bariatric surgery, pulmonary embolism was the cause of death in 30%, and microscopic evidence of pulmonary embolism was found in 8 out of 10 patients, reflecting the difficulties in correctly diagnosing venous thromboembolism in any patient and even more in the very obese [67]. In a review, Rocha et al. found 11 studies supporting the hypothesis that obese patients undergoing bariatric surgery have an increased risk of venous thromboembolism, and only 2 studies disputing this association. They came to the conclusion that the risk of venous thromboembolism exceeds the risk due to the surgical procedure alone in these patients [68]. A 0.21 % rate of fatal pulmonary embolism was detected in a retrospective analysis of 5,554 patients undergoing bariatric surgery in a 24-year period [69].

The co-factors most commonly associated with an increased risk of venous thromboembolism were venous stasis disease, a BMI of more than 60, truncal obesity, and obstructive sleep apnea. To date, eight studies have been published addressing the efficacy of venous thromboembolism prophylaxis, especially in patients undergoing bariatric surgery. In a 5-center retrospective study of 668 obese patients receiving 30 mg or 40 mg enoxaparin once or twice daily, 6 (0.9%) cases of pulmonary embolism were documented by objective testing, and 1 (1%) deep vein thrombosis. This is a low incidence – but virtually all pulmonary emboli derive from deep vein thrombosis, whereas only 25% of deep vein thromboses lead to pulmonary embolism [70]. So a lot of deep vein thrombosis episodes must have been missed in this study, again demonstrating the difficulty in correctly diagnosing deep vein thrombosis in obese patients.

GE anastomosis stenosis

The gastroenteric or duodenoileal anastomosis that drains the stomach pouch or sleeve into the ileum is intentionally small. Larger stomas are not associated with adequate weight loss. As a consequence, stomal stenosis is relatively common. Patients develop dysphagia, vomiting, satiety, upper abdominal pain and gastrooesophageal reflux in an early post-operative period. The incidence of this complication is directly related to the anastomosis technique (round staple, linear staple, hand-anastomosis). The therapy of GE stenosis is based on common endoscopic dilation and there is very seldom need for reanastomosis [59].

◘ **Table 22.2** Incidence of complications between BPD-Scopinaro and BPD-DS including laparoscopic and traditional surgery (87).

[%]	Laparotomy		Laparoscopy	
	BPD-S	BPD-DS	BPD-S	BPD-DS
Anastomosis stenosis	0.7-1.6	0.5-1.9	0.5-1.9	0.4-2.0
Haemorrhage	27-33	17-25	22-28	12-20
Leaks	0.2-1.2	0.5-4.1	1.2	4.1
Pulmonary embolisms	1-3.6	0.7-1.7	1-3.6	0.7-1.7
Wound infections	3-14	3-14	0.8	1.0

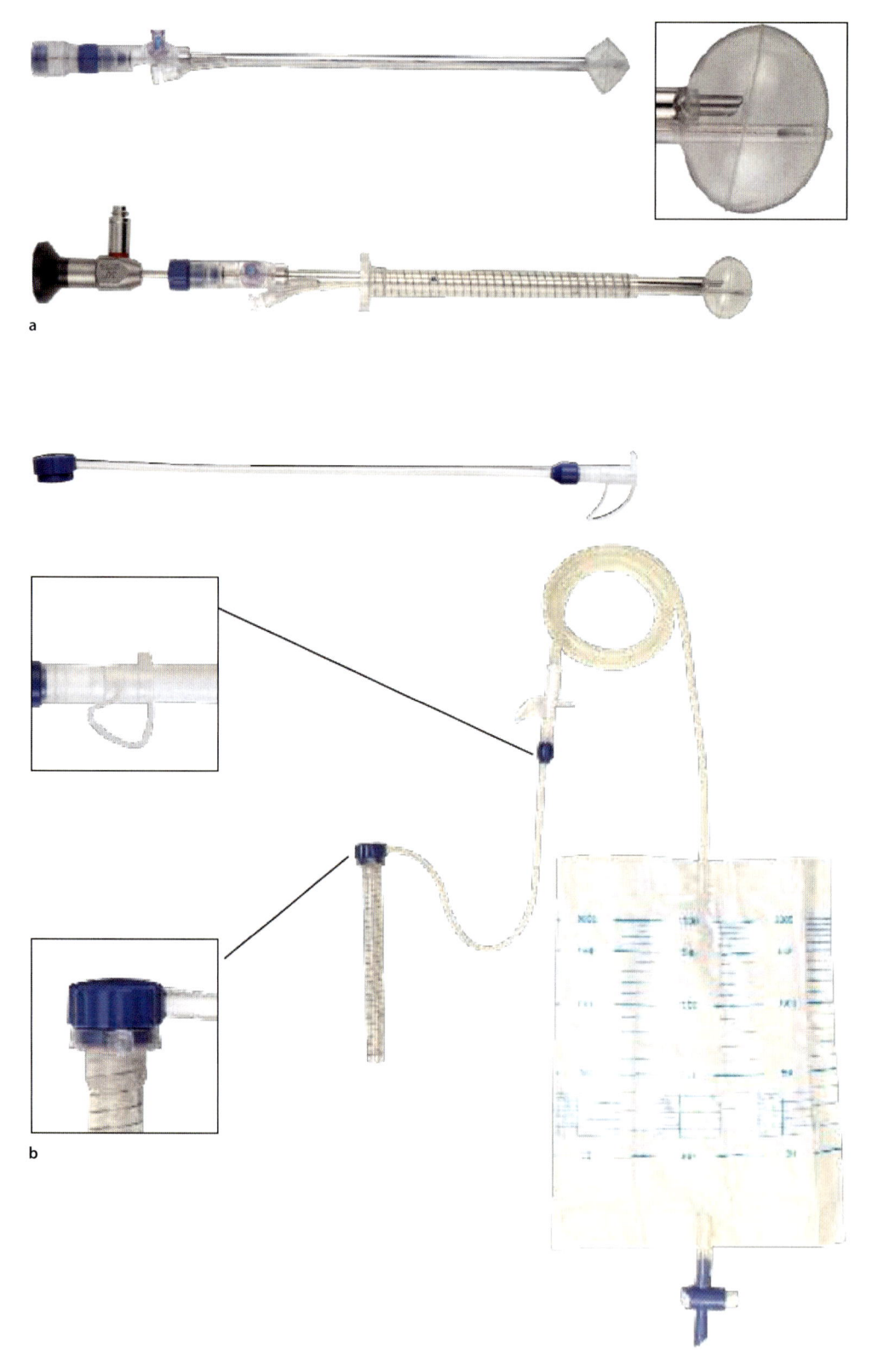

■ **Fig. 22.4a,b. a** The diagnostic balloon system LapVision, a "gas-less" alternative method, permits the organs in the abdomen to be (directly) examined by means of an endoscope introduced via a "two-chambered balloon". **b** The LapVision port can be connected to a drainage system postoperatively.

Regurgitation and oesophagitis

Hypotonia of the lower esophageal sphincter (normal value: 14-34 mmHg) increases the risk of chronic regurgitation. The chance is seven times greater than in patients with normal lower esophagus sphincter pressure. The LES pressure can be measured by oesophageal manometry. In our opinion, this should be done routinely prior to bariatric surgery for the purpose of selecting the operation type. Patients with low LES pressure should undergo conventional RYGB or BPD rather than banded gastric bypass [60, 71, 72]

◼ **Table 22.3** Mortality and Morbidity after BPD-S and BPD-DS in laparoscopic and traditional operative technique (73;74

	Laparotomy		Laparoscopy	
[%]	BPD-S	BPD-DS	BPD-S	BPD-DS
Mortality	0.7-1.6	0.5-1.9	0.5-1.9	0.4-2.0
Morbidity	27-33	17-25	22-28	12-20

Late complications

◼ **Table 22.4** Late complications after conventional BPD operations in a series of 1040 Patients (own data, L.Lemmens)

Late complications	Type	Cases	[%] n=1040
GE ulcerations			
	end to end anastomosis	12 (n=35)	34.28 %
	end to side anastomosis	74 (n=1005)	7.11 %
Anaemia with Fe supplementation			
	Oral	416	40 %
	Intramuscular/or intravenous	31	2.98 %
	Blood transfusion	21	2.01 %
Vitamin D 3 deficiency			
	Intermittent supplementation intramuscular	17	1.63 %
	Osteomalacia	13	1.25 %
Protein manutrition	With hypoalbuminemia	129	12.4%
	With Total Parenteral Nutrition	73	7.02 %
Diarrhoea/ Steatorrhoea			
	< 3 times per day	643	61.28 %
	3 – 5 times per day	312	30 %
	> 5	85	8.17 %
Flatulence and odour problems		104	10%
Polyneuropathy		2	0.19 %
Intestinal occlusion		10	0.96 %
Hepatic failure			
		3	0.288 %
	ethylic	2	0.19 %
Anorexia nervosa		1	0.096 %

22

◼ Table 22.5 Revisionary operations after conventional BPD operations in a series of 1040 Patients (own data, L.Lemmens)

Type of Redo-operation	Cases [12.3% of 1040 patients]	[%] of Revisionary-operation n=128	[%] of all cases in series
Total reversion	17	13.2 %	1.63 %
Elongation of CC	68	53.125 %	6.538 %
Secondary Gastric Bypass	37	28.9 %	3.557 %
Secondary S-Fundus Resection	6	4.68 %	0.577 %

◼ Table 22.6 Revisionary operations after biliopancreatic diversion influence the BMI (own data, L.Lemmens).

	BMI	Before BPD operation	Before Revisionary operation	Year after Revisionary operation
Generally	Mean BMI	41	26	33
Generally	Range	35 – 70.9	18 – 33	26.8 – 54.7
Elongation of CC	Mean BMI	42.5	23.3	27.7
Elongation of CC	Range	37 – 54.7	18 - 33	26.8 – 44.7
Secondary in RYGB	Mean BMI	47.5	28.9	26.6
Secondary in RYGB	Range	35.6 - 70.9	19.1 – 36.6	18.4 – 36.4

◼ Table 22.7 Marginal ulcers and nutritional complications occur at the same frequency independent of laparotomic or laparoscopic technique (75).

	Laparotomy or Laparoscopy	
[%]	BPD-S	BPD-DS
Marginal ulcer	8-15	0
Nutritional complications	40-77	39-77

◼ Table 22.8 The most important specific late complications by Scopinaro (76).

Complication	Cause
Anemia	Chronic bleedings, Compliance
Bone demineralisation	Previously existing bone problems Compliance
Stoma ulceration	Stomach secretion Alcohol and smoking
Neuropathy	Lack of Thiamin Compliance
Protein malnutrition	Compliance Too strong malabsorption

Protein malnutrition

Protein malnutrition mostly appears two or three months after the BPD operation and is directly related to very low patient compliance. It is simple to recognize by the following clinic signs like: alopecia, asthenia, anemia, hypoalbuminemia and oedema. In severe cases, parenteral nutrition has to be conducted for 2 -3 weeks. In case of recurrent hypoproteinemia, elongation of the common channel or transformation into the Roux-en-Y gastric Bypass has to be considered [77,78]. See also the chapter written by Prof. Scopinaro.

Internal hernia

In contrast to open surgery, a small bowel obstruction after laparoscopic surgery is more likely to be caused by an internal hernia than by adhesions. Usually, the small bowel herniates through an abnormal aperture within the peritoneal cavity [79]. The most common internal locations include Petersen's space as the area between the mesentery of the alimentary Roux-limb and the transverse mesocolon, the mesenteric defect at the jejunojejunostomy and in case of a retrocolic Rouxlimb, the transverse mesocolon defect [80]. The incidence of internal hernia after Roux-en-Y gastric bypass has been described as less than 1% and up to 4.5% in large series with the retrocolic approach associated with significantly higher internal hernia rates due to three defects which are created compared to two defects in the currently more-favoured antecolic reconstruction [79-81]. Exact location of internal hernia varies with the surgeon's preference of either retrocolic or antecolic Roux-limb. In their large series of more than 1,000 laparoscopic RYGB procedures, Garza et al. reported as most common clinical symptoms: intermittent, postprandial abdominal pain (88%) and / or nausea and vomiting (65%) with mean duration of symptoms of 16 days. Mean time from first operation to intervention was 225 days.

The location of abdominal pain seems to correlate with the side of internal herniation [80]. Paroz et al. describe very similar symptoms with a mean occurrence at 29 months post-operative and a mean weight loss of over 14 BMI units [82]. We have observed similar results in our patients. In our collective, most patients had atypical abdominal pain, not as a postprandial event. All of our patients were re-operated because of internal hernia more than a year after the primary procedure. Except in the acute setting of a small bowel obstruction, the exact diagnosis is hard to find. CT scan examination of the abdomen and the pelvis should be performed with both oral and intravenous contrast.

Abnormal clusters of bowel loops were shown to be the best predictors of internal hernia. Small bowel loops in the left or right upper quadrant, evidence of small bowel mesentery traversing the transverse colon mesentery and/or location of the jejunojejunostomy above the transverse colon are suggestive of internal hernia. In addition, crowding, stretching and engorgement of the main mesenteric trunk to the right may be seen [80]. But one should not forget the limited diagnostic reliability. Higa et al. presented 20% negative CT scans in patients with proven internal hernia, and furthermore Garza et al. showed only 64 % positive CT scans in patients with internal hernia [80, 81, 83]. This is the reason why it is suggested that a diagnostic laparoscopy

be performed in patients with atypical abdominal pain, if it is not possible to find a cause for the abdominal tenderness, to ensure the diagnosis and to avoid further complications. A negative CT scan examination in case of a present herniation was even higher in our collective and reached 50%. This inaccuracy is likely to have been caused by the inexperience of radiologists diagnosing internal hernias.

Despite the mean time-frames until diagnosis mentioned above, surgeons must be very suspicious of internal hernias post-operatively irrespective of the interval after surgery. To improve the results and reduce surgical reintervention, it is obligatory to carefully close each aperture created in the primary procedure. The surgeon has to control the Petersen space and other apertures and when needed create closure with non-resorbable sutures in all patients who undergo abdominal operations for whatever reason. For re-operations, only very few patients need an open approach, so mostly it remains a less invasive procedure requiring 1 to 4 days of hospital stay [80]. All defects should be repaired with non-absorbable, preferentially running sutures [82]. Other abdominal hernias should be operated with general indications and techniques, giving preference to less invasive procedures. See also the chapter written by Prof. Brolin. Supplementations and nutritional problems after biliopancreatic diversion are discussed in the chapters by Prof. Engelhardt and Prof. Swierczynski.

22.6   Weight loss and Benefits

The influence of malabsorption on the percentage of excess weight loss within the first year is between 81.3 and 73.5. After two years, the percentage ranges around 80%, and at 5-year follow-up, an EWL of about 75% can be found. In comparison to Laparoscopic Conventional Roux-en-Y Gastric Bypass (LCRYGB) the Biliopancreatic Diversion with or without Duodenal Switch shows better EWL. Only a slight weight regain of 3-4% is observed in some series between the second and fifth post-operative year (Lemanns), whereas in LCRYGB, a weight regain rate of over 10% is reported in the same period. The differences in excess weight loss between conventional BPD and BPD with DS are minimal and were between 61-78% and 66-80% in big series (84). The laparoscopic approach shows no difference in effect on EWL in the two operations. The EWL after conventional gastric bypass reaches 58.2% after five years in the best series [9]. Banded gastric bypass leads to almost the same weight control as BPD and BPD-DS, with lower incidence of subsequent biliopancreatic diversion disadvantages like diarrhea, gas

22

■ **Table 22.9** Beneficial effects of BPD on obesity-related diseases.

Problem	Minimal Follow up In Months	Disappeared [%]	Improved [%]	Unchanged [%]	Impaired [%]
Pickwickian Syndrome (2%)	2	100	-	-	-
Somnolence (5%)	2	100	-	-	-
Hypertension (37%)	12	81	13	6	-
Steatosis hepatis (48%)	24	87	9	4	-
Leg oedemas (27%)	12	45	39	16	-
Hypercholesterolemia (53%)	2	100	-	-	-
Hypertriglyceridemia (32%)	12	95	5	-	-
Hyperglycemia (14%)	4	100	-	-	-
Diabetes mellitus Type 2	4	100	-	-	-
Diabetes mellitus requiring insulin (2%)	12	100	-	-	-
Hyperuricemia (18%)	4	94	-	3	3
Gout (2%)	4	100	100	-	-

bloat syndrome, protein malnutrition, foul body odour, stool odour or flatus.

22.7 Conclusions

It is observed that 90% of all operated patients are pleased with the BPD procedure. The weight loss is stable in the long-term observation. Thereby, patients are eating normal portions of food and leading an active life. About 10% of them complain about frequent stools. The re-operation rate is low (8%) in comparison with other bariatric procedures. Certainly, malabsorptive operations need constant and long-term follow-up but the procedures show the best influence on metabolic disorders. We generally welcome the findings of the international consensus conference Diabetes Surgery Summit Consensus 2009 to use und study of gastrointestinal surgery to treat type-2 diabetes. The acceleration of pathological metabolic changes can be stopped or at least slowed after metabolic operation. Even if the metabolic syndrome with all components returns after a number of years, a benefit of the metabolic operation is reached. The patients experienced a period of time without or with reduced symptoms of disease. Such profit should be considered by the providers in our health systems. The BPD has the most potent effect on several pathological disturbances and can be safely used

under the conditions of precise indication, compliance of the patient and regular follow-up.

References

1. Dansinger ML, Gleason JA, Griffith JL, Selker HP, Schaefer EJ. Comparison of the Atkins, Ornish, Weight Watchers, and Zone diets for weight loss and heart disease risk reduction: a randomized trial. JAMA 2005 Jan 5;293(1):43-53.
2. Fried M, Hainer V, Basdevant A, Buchwald H, Deitel M, Finer N, et al. Interdisciplinary European guidelines for surgery for severe (morbid) obesity. Obes Surg 2007 Feb;17(2):260-70.
3. Heshka S, Anderson JW, Atkinson RL, Greenway FL, Hill JO, Phinney SD, et al. Weight loss with self-help compared with a structured commercial program: a randomized trial. JAMA 2003 Apr 9;289(14):1792-8.
4. Martin LF, Tan TL, Horn JR, Bixler EO, Kauffman GL, Becker DA, et al. Comparison of the costs associated with medical and surgical treatment of obesity. Surgery 1995 Oct;118(4):599-606.
5. Peeters A, Barendregt JJ, Willekens F, Mackenbach JP, Al MA, Bonneux L. Obesity in adulthood and its consequences for life expectancy: a life-table analysis. Ann Intern Med 2003 Jan 7;138(1):24-32.
6. Buchwald H, Avidor Y, Braunwald E, Jensen MD, Pories W, Fahrbach K, et al. Bariatric surgery: a systematic review and metaanalysis. JAMA 2004 Oct 13;292(14):1724-37.
7. Tsai AG, Wadden TA. Systematic review: an evaluation of major commercial weight loss programs in the United States. Ann Intern Med 2005 Jan 4;142(1):56-66.

8. Wittgrove AC, Clark GW. Laparoscopic gastric bypass, Roux-en-Y-500 patients: technique and results, with 3-60 month follow-up. Obes Surg 2000 Jun;10(3):233-9.

9. Maggard MA, Shugarman LR, Suttorp M, Maglione M, Sugerman HJ, Livingston EH, et al. Meta-analysis: surgical treatment of obesity. Ann Intern Med 2005 Apr 5;142(7):547-59.

10. Stevens VJ, Obarzanek E, Cook NR, Lee IM, Appel LJ, Smith WD, et al. Long-term weight loss and changes in blood pressure: results of the Trials of Hypertension Prevention, phase II. Ann Intern Med 2001 Jan 2;134(1):1-11.

11. Obesity: preventing and managing the global epidemic. Report of a WHO consultation. World Health Organ Tech Rep Ser 2000;894:i-253.

12. Anderson JW, Konz EC. Obesity and disease management: effects of weight loss on comorbid conditions. Obes Res 2001 Nov;9 Suppl 4:326S-34S.

13. Christou NV, Sampalis JS, Liberman M, Look D, Auger S, McLean AP, et al. Surgery decreases long-term mortality, morbidity, and health care use in morbidly obese patients. Ann Surg 2004 Sep;240(3):416-23.

14. Fobi MA. Placement of the GaBP ring system in the banded gastric bypass operation. Obes Surg 2005 Sep;15(8):1196-201.

15. Martin LF, White S, Lindstrom W, Jr. Cost-benefit analysis for the treatment of severe obesity. World J Surg 1998 Sep;22(9):1008-17.

16. Scopinaro N, Papadia F, Marinari G, Camerini G, Adami G. Long-term control of type 2 diabetes mellitus and the other major components of the metabolic syndrome after biliopancreatic diversion in patients with BMI < 35 kg/m2. Obes Surg 2007 Feb;17(2):185-92.

17. Scopinaro N, Gianetta E, Civalleri D, Bonalumi U, Bachi V. Biliopancreatic bypass for obesity: II. Initial experience in man. Br J Surg 1979 Sep;66(9):618-20.

18. Ren CJ, Patterson E, Gagner M. Early results of laparoscopic biliopancreatic diversion with duodenal switch: a case series of 40 consecutive patients. Obes Surg 2000 Dec;10(6):514-23.

19. Baltasar A, Serra C, Perez N, Bou R, Bengochea M, Ferri L. Laparoscopic sleeve gastrectomy: a multi-purpose bariatric operation. Obes Surg 2005 Sep;15(8):1124-8.

20. Gagner M, Deitel M, Kalberer TL, Erickson AL, Crosby RD. The Second International Consensus Summit for Sleeve Gastrectomy, March 19-21, 2009. Surg Obes Relat Dis 2009 Jul;5(4):476-85.

21. Nocca D, Krawczykowsky D, Bomans B, Noel P, Picot MC, Blanc PM, et al. A Prospective Multicenter Study of 163 Sleeve Gastrectomies: Results at 1 and 2 Years. Obes Surg 2008 Mar 4.

22. Hubbard VS, Hall WH. Gastrointestinal Surgery for Severe Obesity. Obes Surg 1991 Sep;1(3):257-65.

23. Buchwald H, Estok R, Fahrbach K, Banel D, Jensen MD, Pories WJ, et al. Weight and type 2 diabetes after bariatric surgery: systematic review and meta-analysis. Am J Med 2009 Mar;122(3):248-56.

24. Pories WJ, Swanson MS, MacDonald KG, Long SB, Morris PG, Brown BM, et al. Who would have thought it? An operation proves to be the most effective therapy for adult-onset diabetes mellitus. Ann Surg 1995 Sep;222(3):339-50.

25. Rubino F. Bariatric surgery: effects on glucose homeostasis. Curr Opin Clin Nutr Metab Care 2006 Jul;9(4):497-507.

26. Valverde I, Puente J, Martin-Duce A, Molina L, Lozano O, Sancho V, et al. Changes in glucagon-like peptide-1 (GLP-1) secretion after biliopancreatic diversion or vertical banded gastroplasty in obese subjects. Obes Surg 2005 Mar;15(3):387-97.

27. Sancho V, Trigo MV, Martin-Duce A, Gonz LN, Acitores A, Arnes L, et al. Effect of GLP-1 on D-glucose transport, lipolysis and

lipogenesis in adipocytes of obese subjects. Int J Mol Med 2006 Jun;17(6):1133-7.

28. Mingrone G, Nolfe G, Gissey GC, Iaconelli A, Leccesi L, Guidone C, et al. Circadian rhythms of GIP and GLP1 in glucose-tolerant and in type 2 diabetic patients after biliopancreatic diversion. Diabetologia 2009 May;52(5):873-81.

29. Salani B, Briatore L, Andraghetti G, Adami GF, Maggi D, Cordera R. High-molecular weight adiponectin isoforms increase after biliopancreatic diversion in obese subjects. Obesity (Silver Spring) 2006 Sep;14(9):1511-4.

30. Guidone C, Manco M, Valera-Mora E, Iaconelli A, Gniuli D, Mari A, et al. Mechanisms of recovery from type 2 diabetes after malabsorptive bariatric surgery. Diabetes 2006 Jul;55(7):2025-31.

31. Nguyen NT, Magno CP, Lane KT, Hinojosa MW, Lane JS. Association of hypertension, diabetes, dyslipidemia, and metabolic syndrome with obesity: findings from the National Health and Nutrition Examination Survey, 1999 to 2004. J Am Coll Surg 2008 Dec;207(6):928-34.

32. Nguyen NT, Varela JE, Sabio A, Naim J, Stamos M, Wilson SE. Reduction in prescription medication costs after laparoscopic gastric bypass. Am Surg 2006 Oct;72(10):853-6.

33. Bueter M, Ahmed A, Ashrafian H, le Roux CW. Bariatric surgery and hypertension. Surg Obes Relat Dis 2009 Sep;5(5):615-20.

34. Segal JB, Clark JM, Shore AD, Dominici F, Magnuson T, Richards TM, et al. Prompt reduction in use of medications for comorbid conditions after bariatric surgery. Obes Surg 2009 Dec;19(12):1646-56.

35. Pontiroli AE, Laneri M, Veronelli A, Frige F, Micheletto G, Folli F, et al. Biliary pancreatic diversion and laparoscopic adjustable gastric banding in morbid obesity: their long-term effects on metabolic syndrome and on cardiovascular parameters. Cardiovasc Diabetol 2009;8:37.

36. Sugerman HJ, Wolfe LG, Sica DA, Clore JN. Diabetes and hypertension in severe obesity and effects of gastric bypass-induced weight loss. Ann Surg 2003 Jun;237(6):751-6.

37. Karlsson J, Taft C, Ryden A, Sjostrom L, Sullivan M. Ten-year trends in health-related quality of life after surgical and conventional treatment for severe obesity: the SOS intervention study. Int J Obes (Lond) 2007 Aug;31(8):1248-61.

38. Zambon S, Romanato G, Sartore G, Marin R, Busetto L, Zanoni S, et al. Bariatric surgery improves atherogenic LDL profile by triglyceride reduction. Obes Surg 2009 Feb;19(2):190-5.

39. Vila M, Ruiz O, Belmonte M, Riesco M, Barcelo A, Perez G, et al. Changes in lipid profile and insulin resistance in obese patients after Scopinaro biliopancreatic diversion. Obes Surg 2009 Mar;19(3):299-306.

40. Corradini SG, Eramo A, Lubrano C, Spera G, Cornoldi A, Grossi A, et al. Comparison of changes in lipid profile after bilio-intestinal bypass and gastric banding in patients with morbid obesity. Obes Surg 2005 Mar;15(3):367-77.

41. Hodgson M, van Thiel DH, Goodman-Klein B. Obesity and hepatotoxins as risk factors for fatty liver disease. Br J Ind Med 1991 Oct;48(10):690-5.

42. Duvnjak M, Lerotic I, Barsic N, Tomasic V, Virovic JL, Velagic V. Pathogenesis and management issues for non-alcoholic fatty liver disease. World J Gastroenterol 2007 Sep 14;13(34):4539-50.

43. Garcia-Diaz JD, Lozano O, Ramos JC, Gaspar MJ, Keller J, Duce AM. Changes in lipid profile after biliopancreatic diversion. Obes Surg 2003 Oct;13(5):756-60.

44. Brizzi P, Angius MF, Carboni A, Cossu ML, Fais E, Noya G, et al. Plasma lipids and lipoprotein changes after biliopancreatic diversion for morbid obesity. Dig Surg 2003;20(1):18-23.

45. Moghadasian MH, Frohlich JJ, Saleem M, Hong JM, Qayumi K, Scudamore CH. Surgical management of dyslipidemia: clinical and experimental evidence. J Invest Surg 2001 Mar;14(2):71-8.

46. Pontiroli AE, Frige F, Paganelli M, Folli F. In morbid obesity, metabolic abnormalities and adhesion molecules correlate with visceral fat, not with subcutaneous fat: effect of weight loss through surgery. Obes Surg 2009 Jun;19(6):745-50.

47. Buchwald H, Williams SE, Matts JP, Nguyen PA, Boen JR. Overall mortality in the program on the surgical control of the hyper-lipidemias. J Am Coll Surg 2002 Sep;195(3):327-31.

48. Machado M, Marques-Vidal P, Cortez-Pinto H. Hepatic histology in obese patients undergoing bariatric surgery. J Hepatol 2006 Oct;45(4):600-6.

49. Kral JG, Thung SN, Biron S, Hould FS, Lebel S, Marceau S, et al. Effects of surgical treatment of the metabolic syndrome on liver fibrosis and cirrhosis. Surgery 2004 Jan;135(1):48-58.

50. Baltasar A, Serra C, Perez N, Bou R, Bengochea M. Clinical hepatic impairment after the duodenal switch. Obes Surg 2004 Jan;14(1):77-83.

51. Papadia F, Marinari GM, Camerini G, Adami GF, Murelli F, Carlini F, et al. Short-term liver function after biliopancreatic diversion. Obes Surg 2003 Oct;13(5):752-5.

52. Keshishian A, Zahriya K, Willes EB. Duodenal switch has no detrimental effects on hepatic function and improves hepatic steatohepatitis after 6 months. Obes Surg 2005 Nov;15(10):1418-23.

53. de Andrade AR, Cotrim HP, Alves E, Soares D, Rocha R, Almeida A, et al. Nonalcoholic fatty liver disease in severely obese individuals: the influence of bariatric surgery. Ann Hepatol 2008 Oct;7(4):364-8.

54. Soriguer F, Garcia-Serrano S, Garcia-Almeida JM, Garrido-Sanchez L, Garcia-Arnes J, Tinahones FJ, et al. Changes in the serum composition of free-fatty acids during an intra-venous glucose tolerance test. Obesity (Silver Spring) 2009 Jan;17(1):10-5.

55. Mattar SG, Velcu LM, Rabinovitz M, Demetris AJ, Krasinskas AM, Barinas-Mitchell E, et al. Surgically-induced weight loss significantly improves nonalcoholic fatty liver disease and the metabolic syndrome. Ann Surg 2005 Oct;242(4):610-7.

56. Vuppalanchi R, Chalasani N. Nonalcoholic fatty liver disease and nonalcoholic steatohepatitis: Selected practical issues in their evaluation and management. Hepatology 2009 Jan;49(1):306-17.

57. Higa KD, Boone KB, Ho T. Complications of the laparoscopic Roux-en-Y gastric bypass: 1,040 patients--what have we learned? Obes Surg 2000 Dec;10(5):509-13.

58. Yu J, Turner MA, Cho SR, Fulcher AS, DeMaria EJ, Kellum JM, et al. Normal anatomy and complications after gastric bypass surgery: helical CT findings. Radiology 2004 Jun;231(3):753-60.

59. Weiner S, Karcz W, Rosenthal A, Pomhoff I, Weiner R. [Surgical treatment of obesity and its side effects is effective]. MMW Fortschr Med 2006 May 4;148(18):29-32.

60. Fobi MA, Lee H, Felahy B, Che K, Ako P, Fobi N. Choosing an operation for weight control, and the transected banded gastric bypass. Obes Surg 2005 Jan;15(1):114-21.

61. Hills NH, Pflug JJ, Jeyasingh K, Boardman L, Calnan JS. Prevention of deep vein thrombosis by intermittent pneumatic compression of calf. Br Med J 1972 Jan 15;1(5793):131-5.

62. Sue-Ling HM, Johnston D, McMahon MJ, Philips PR, Davies JA. Pre-operative identification of patients at high risk of deep venous thrombosis after elective major abdominal surgery. Lancet 1986 May 24;1(8491):1173-6.

63. Cullen DJ, Nemeskal AR. The autopsy incidence of acute pulmonary embolism in critically ill surgical patients. Intensive Care Med 1986;12(6):399-403.

64. Flordal PA, Berggvist D, Burmark US, Ljungstrom KG, Torngren S. Risk factors for major thromboembolism and bleeding tendency after elective general surgical operations. The Fragmin Multicentre Study Group. Eur J Surg 1996 Oct;162(10):783-9.

65. Gonzalez QH, Tishler DS, Plata-Munoz JJ, Bondora A, Vickers SM, Leath T, et al. Incidence of clinically evident deep venous thrombosis after laparoscopic Roux-en-Y gastric bypass. Surg Endosc 2004 Jul;18(7):1082-4.

66. Omalu BI, Luckasevic T, Shakir AM, Rozin L, Wecht CH, Kuller LH. Postbariatric surgery deaths, which fall under the jurisdiction of the coroner. Am J Forensic Med Pathol 2004 Sep;25(3):237-42.

67. Melinek J, Livingston E, Cortina G, Fishbein MC. Autopsy findings following gastric bypass surgery for morbid obesity. Arch Pathol Lab Med 2002 Sep;126(9):1091-5.

68. Rocha AT, de Vasconcellos AG, da Luz Neto ER, Araujo DM, Alves ES, Lopes AA. Risk of venous thromboembolism and efficacy of thromboprophylaxis in hospitalized obese medical patients and in obese patients undergoing bariatric surgery. Obes Surg 2006 Dec;16(12):1645-55.

69. Sapala JA, Wood MH, Schuhknecht MP, Sapala MA. Fatal pulmonary embolism after bariatric operations for morbid obesity: a 24-year retrospective analysis. Obes Surg 2003 Dec;13(6):819-25.

70. Hamad GG, Choban PS. Enoxaparin for thromboprophylaxis in morbidly obese patients undergoing bariatric surgery: findings of the prophylaxis against VTE outcomes in bariatric surgery patients receiving enoxaparin (PROBE) study. Obes Surg 2005 Nov;15(10):1368-74.

71. Arasaki CH, Del Grande JC, Yanagita ET, Alves AK, Oliveira DR. Incidence of regurgitation after the banded gastric bypass. Obes Surg 2005 Nov;15(10):1408-17.

72. Stubbs RS, O'brien I, Jurikova L. What ring size should be used in association with vertical gastric bypass? Obes Surg 2006 Oct;16(10):1298-303.

73. Schirmer B. Laparoscopic bariatric surgery. Surg Endosc 2006 Apr;20 Suppl 2:S450-S455.

74. Ren CJ, Patterson E, Gagner M. Early results of laparoscopic biliopancreatic diversion with duodenal switch: a case series of 40 consecutive patients. Obes Surg 2000 Dec;10(6):514-23.

75. Schirmer BD. Laparoscopic bariatric surgery. Surg Clin North Am 2000 Aug;80(4):1253-67, vii.

76. Scopinaro N. Biliopancreatic diversion: mechanisms of action and long-term results. Obes Surg 2006 Jun;16(6):683-9.

77. Hamoui N, Chock B, Anthone GJ, Crookes PF. Revision of the duodenal switch: indications, technique, and outcomes. J Am Coll Surg 2007 Apr;204(4):603-8.

78. Kuesters S, Marjanovic G, Karcz WK. [Redo operations after bariatric and metabolic surgery]. Zentralbl Chir 2009 Feb;134(1):50-6.

79. Blachar A, Federle MP, Brancatelli G, Peterson MS, Oliver JH, III, Li W. Radiologist performance in the diagnosis of internal hernia by using specific CT findings with emphasis on trans-mesenteric hernia. Radiology 2001 Nov;221(2):422-8.

80. Garza E Jr, Kuhn J, Arnold D, Nicholson W, Reddy S, McCarty T. Internal hernias after laparoscopic Roux-en-Y gastric bypass. Am J Surg 2004 Dec;188(6):796-800.

81. Higa KD, Ho T, Boone KB. Internal hernias after laparoscopic Roux-en-Y gastric bypass: incidence, treatment and prevention. Obes Surg 2003 Jun;13(3):350-4.

82. Paroz A, Calmes JM, Giusti V, Suter M. Internal hernia after laparoscopic Roux-en-Y gastric bypass for morbid obesity: a continuous challenge in bariatric surgery. Obes Surg 2006 Nov;16(11):1482-7.

83. DeMaria EJ, Sugerman HJ, Kellum JM, Meador JG, Wolfe LG. Results of 281 consecutive total laparoscopic Roux-en-Y gastric bypasses to treat morbid obesity. Ann Surg 2002 May;235(5):640-5.

84. Schirmer B, Watts SH. Laparoscopic bariatric surgery. Surg Endosc 2003 Dec;17(12):1875-8.

85. Schirmer B. Laparoscopic bariatric surgery. Surg Endosc 2006 Apr;20 Suppl 2:S450-S455.

86. Schirmer BD. Laparoscopic bariatric surgery. Surg Clin North Am 2000 Aug;80(4):1253-67, vii.

23

Surgical Treatment focused of T2DM: Looking for The Limits

Michael Frenken, MD, Simon Kuesters, MD, W.Konrad Karcz, MD

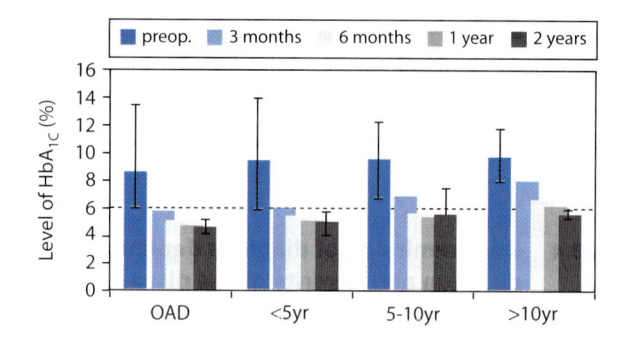

Fig. 23.5. HbA1C levels after BPD-DS dependent on preoperative duration of insulin usage. Group I "OAD" was treated with oral anditiabetics. HbA1c levels were below 6% starting 3 months after the operation. Group II had used insulin for less than 5 years preoperatively and also showed normal levels of HbA1c from 3 months after the operation on. Group III had used insulin for 5 to 10 years. Mean HbA1c had normalized 6 months after the operation. Group IV had used insulin for more than 10 years. Mean HbA1c in this group did not normalize until 2 years after the operation.

this group, the time course of remission is significantly longer and a small percentage of patients will not be completely free of insulin probably due to secondary beta cell failure. Nevertheless, HbA1c of these patients is significantly lower and less insulin is needed.

23.5 Mechanisms of diabetes remission after gastrointestinal surgery

The effect of gastrointestinal surgery on glucose metabolism is not fully understood. For sure, the restrictive effect of bariatric surgery leads to an improvement of glucose homeostasis and T2DM in the long run, equivalent to a diet and accompanied by weight loss. This effect can be seen after gastric banding [15]. Remarkably, the antidiabetic effect after gastric bypass surgery and BPD occurs a few days after surgery, long before a significant loss of excess weight is achieved [16]. Thus other mechanisms beside the "dietary" effect must exist. Those mechanisms are independent of, and additive to weight loss. A crucial point seems to be that the duodenum and proximal jejunum are excluded from the passage of nutrients (foregut hypothesis) [17]. Remarkably, this effect has also been seen in diabetic patients after subtotal gastrectomy due to ulcer or cancer [18, 19]. Insulin secretion and glucose homeostasis are influenced via a so-far unknown neuronal, hormonal or chemical signalling on an entero-pancreatic axis. This weight-independent antidiabetic effect is absent in the solely restrictive bariatric procedures of gastric banding; however, the also restrictive procedure

of sleeve gastrectomy shows an early effect on T2DM, similar to that of gastric bypass [20].

23.6 Morbidity and mortality of anti-diabetic surgery

Bariatric surgery is associated with low postoperative mortality with rates between 0.25% and 0.5% [1, 21] which compares to mortality rates after elective laparoscopic cholecystectomy [22]. Postoperative complications have also declined, since more and more operations are performed laparoscopically. Most common complications are anastomotic leak, hemorrhage, wound infection and pulmonary events [23]. In the long term, nutritional deficiencies can occur, especially after BPD and mostly including protein, vitamin B12, vitamin D3 and iron. Severe problems can be largely avoided with stringent follow up and constant supplementation.

Concerning mortality, it must be considered that diabetes itself has considerable long-term mortality. A retrospective study by MacDonald et al. compared obese patients with type 2 DM after gastric bypass surgery to obese diabetics who were scheduled for bypass surgery but were not operated (due to missing approval of their health insurance, e.g.) [24]. For every year of follow-up, patients in the non-operated group had a 4.5% chance of dying vs. a 1.0% chance for the operated patients. This was primarily due to a decrease in the number of cardiovascular deaths. Adams et al. also recognised an improvement in long-term survival after gastric bypass [25]. An elective operation with low mortality and morbidity can resolve or at least improve diabetes and thus probably prevent severe complications of diabetes like renal failure, coronary and vascular disease, diabetic foot syndrome, other infections and blindness. Furthermore, diabetes-caused operations (e.g. amputations, coronary bypass surgery, vascular surgery) might be prevented – which have higher complication rates because they often are not elective operations in a patient with poorly-controlled diabetes.

Reference

1. Buchwald H, Avidor Y, Braunwald E, Jensen MD, Pories W, Fahrbach K, Schoelles K. Bariatric surgery: a systematic review and meta-analysis. JAMA 2004;292:1724-1737.
2. Rubino F. Is type 2 diabetes an operable intestinal disease? A provocative yet reasonable hypothesis. Diabetes Care 2008;31 Suppl 2:S290-S296.
3. Noya G, Cossu ML, Coppola M, Tonolo G, Angius MF, Fais E, Ruggiu M. Biliopancreatic diversion preserving the stomach and

pylorus in the treatment of hypercholesterolemia and diabetes type II: results in the first 10 cases. Obes Surg 1998;8:67-72.

4. Cohen R, Pinheiro JS, Correa JL, Schiavon CA. Laparoscopic Roux-en-Y gastric bypass for BMI < 35 kg/m(2): a tailored approach. Surg Obes Relat Dis 2006;2:401-4, discussion.

5. Cohen RV, Schiavon CA, Pinheiro JS, Correa JL, Rubino F. Duodenal-jejunal bypass for the treatment of type 2 diabetes in patients with body mass index of 22-34 kg/m2: a report of 2 cases. Surg Obes Relat Dis 2007;3:195-197.

6. Hess DS, Hess DW, Oakley RS. The biliopancreatic diversion with the duodenal switch: results beyond 10 years. Obes Surg 2005;15:408-416.

7. Standards of medical care in diabetes--2009. Diabetes Care 2009;32 Suppl 1:S13-S61.

8. Standards of medical care in diabetes--2010. Diabetes Care 2010;33 Suppl 1:S11-S61.

9. Rubino F, Kaplan LM, Schauer PR, Cummings DE. The Diabetes Surgery Summit consensus conference: recommendations for the evaluation and use of gastrointestinal surgery to treat type 2 diabetes mellitus. Ann Surg 2010;251:399-405.

10. Cho EY, Tunger S, Röhrig I, Frenken M. Duodenal Switch Operation for the Treatment of Insulin-Dependent Type 2 Diabetes Mellitus: 1-Year Results. Obes Surg 2008;18:458.

11. Scopinaro N, Marinari GM, Camerini GB, Papadia FS, Adami GF. Specific effects of biliopancreatic diversion on the major components of metabolic syndrome: a long-term follow-up study. Diabetes Care 2005;28:2406-2411.

12. Frenken M, C, EY. Homa in Obese Patients with Type 2 Diabetes Mellitus Undergoing BPD-DS: Is the Rapid Postoperative Increase in Insulin Sensitivity Dependent on Severity of Diabetes or on BMI? Obes Surg 2009;19:1004.

13. Matthews DR, Hosker JP, Rudenski AS, Naylor BA, Treacher DF, Turner RC. Homeostasis model assessment: insulin resistance and beta-cell function from fasting plasma glucose and insulin concentrations in man. Diabetologia 1985;28:412-419.

14. Cho EY, Tunger S, Röhrig I, Frenken M. Biliopancreatic Diversion with Duodenal Switch in Patients with Type 2 Diabetes Mellitus: is the Chance of Cure Dependent on Severity and Duration of the Disease? Obes Surg 2009;19:927.

15. Dixon JB, O'Brien PE, Playfair J, Chapman L, Schachter LM, Skinner S, Proietto J, Bailey M, Anderson M. Adjustable gastric banding and conventional therapy for type 2 diabetes: a randomized controlled trial. JAMA 2008;299:316-323.

16. Pories WJ, Swanson MS, MacDonald KG, Long SB, Morris PG, Brown BM, Barakat HA, deRamon RA, Israel G, Dolezal JM, . Who would have thought it? An operation proves to be the most effective therapy for adult-onset diabetes mellitus. Ann Surg 1995;222:339-350.

17. Rubino F, Forgione A, Cummings DE, Vix M, Gnuli D, Mingrone G, Castagneto M, Marescaux J. The mechanism of diabetes control after gastrointestinal bypass surgery reveals a role of the proximal small intestine in the pathophysiology of type 2 diabetes. Ann Surg 2006;244:741-749.

18. FRIEDMAN MN, SANCETTA AJ, MAGOVERN GJ. The amelioration of diabetes mellitus following subtotal gastrectomy. Surg Gynecol Obstet 1955;100:201-204.

19. NGERVALL L, DOTEVALL G, TILLANDER H. Amelioration of diabetes mellitus following gastric resection. Acta Med Scand 1961;169:743-748.

20. Rizzello M, Abbatini F, Casella G, Alessandri G, Fantini A, Leonetti F, Basso N. Early postoperative insulin-resistance changes after sleeve gastrectomy. Obes Surg 2010;20:50-55.

21. Buchwald H, Estok R, Fahrbach K, Banel D, Sledge I. Trends in mortality in bariatric surgery: a systematic review and meta-analysis. Surgery 2007;142:621-632.

22. Shea JA, Healey MJ, Berlin JA, Clarke JR, Malet PF, Staroscik RN, Schwartz JS, Williams SV. Mortality and complications associated with laparoscopic cholecystectomy. A meta-analysis. Ann Surg 1996;224:609-620.

23. Wittgrove AC, Clark GW. Laparoscopic gastric bypass, Roux-en-Y-500 patients: technique and results, with 3-60 month follow-up. Obes Surg 2000;10:233-239.

24. MacDonald KG, Jr., Long SD, Swanson MS, Brown BM, Morris P, Dohm GL, Pories WJ. The gastric bypass operation reduces the progression and mortality of non-insulin-dependent diabetes mellitus. J Gastrointest Surg 1997;1:213-220.

25. Adams TD, Gress RE, Smith SC, Halverson RC, Simper SC, Rosamond WD, Lamonte MJ, Stroup AM, Hunt SC. Long-term mortality after gastric bypass surgery. N Engl J Med 2007;357:753-761.

IV Accessory Medical Problems after Metabolic Surgery

Postoperative Management

Magnus Kaffarnik, MD, Carolin Kayser, MD, Stefan Utzolino, MD

Most bariatric surgery patients return directly to the surgical ward postoperatively. Although the overall mortality and morbidity of bariatric surgery is less than 1% and 15%, respectively, certain groups require intermediate-level care (IMC) or the intensive care unit (ICU). The reasons for this are a higher risk for complications because of co-morbidities, failed postoperative extubation, or intraoperative complications.

Bariatric surgery, especially in the morbidly obese, can be associated with serious postoperative complications. Besides surgical complications requiring reoperation, pre-existing diseases can worsen during the postoperative period. Common causes include acute respiratory failure and pulmonary embolism. One of the most challenging issues is the early identification and management of postoperative intra-abdominal sepsis (IAS) prior to the onset of organ dysfunction. IAS is usually due to perforation after gastric restrictive procedures or to anastomotic leakage.

Traditional approaches to nursing care must be reconsidered in dealing with morbidly obese patients. Early and frequent ambulation is thought to reduce the risk of decubitus ulcers, deep vein thrombosis, re-sedation, pain, pneumonia, and atelectasis. To prevent back problems in employees it is necessary to provide appropriate support with special beds and lifting and transfer devices. This chapter reviews postoperative IMC/ICU care management with a detailed focus on the special needs of morbidly obese patients.

24.1 Introduction

Following bariatric surgery, the majority of patients are directly triaged to the surgical ward. For patients at high risk due to co-morbidities such as sleep apnea, intermediate level care (IMC) is used. Others who have suffered intraoperative complications or failed extubation require intensive level care (ICU). Special needs for these patients include pain and fluid management, management of sleep apnea, mobilization, and prevention of decubitus ulcers. The presence of co-morbidities such as diabetes and cardiovascular and chronic obstructive lung diseases poses significant challenges that may affect ICU survival. For patients who need IMC/ICU care for a longer period, enteral or parenteral nutrition has to be mentioned. Assessment of patients with early signs of complications is an important part of IMC/ICU care. One of the most difficult issues is the early recognition and management of severe intra-abdominal sepsis due to postoperative perforation or anastomotic leakage. To optimize treatment and to keep a quality-controlled high standard of postoperative care it is recommended that standardized clinical routines be established.

24.2 Fluid Management

Traditionally, many patients undergoing major gastrointestinal surgery receive large volumes of crystalloids intravenously. It was taught that hypotension is best treated with volume rather than with inotropic agents. Recently, however, several studies have shown that postoperative fluid excess may have negative effects on recovery of the cardiopulmonary and the coagulatory-fibrinolytic systems and is a major cause of postoperative paralytic ileus and delayed gastric emptying [1]. With a "goal-directed fluid therapy" a reduction of morbidity and length of hospital stay was demonstrated in patients undergoing major abdominal surgery [2, 3]. With the restricted fluid management, gastric emptying returned sooner and the patients were capable of tolerating oral intake. Bowel movements were observed several days earlier than in patients receiving liberal fluid administration [4, 5]. The best amount and composition (crystalloid vs. colloid) of fluid replacement is not yet clear, but the target of fluid therapy is a regulated salt and water balance. There is a need to develop optimal techniques for monitoring postoperative normovolemia. Clinical signs (wrinkles, dry tongue, and edema) are generally difficult to interpret in obese patients. Daily measurement shows short-term differences in patients' weight. Be sure to use the same scale under the same conditions every day. A standard procedure on IMC/ICU should be the measurement of daily fluid balance (intake and excretion). Passive leg raising increases venous return, generating a sort of "autotransfusion", and increases the aortic blood flow and cardiac output [6]. Patients with rising blood pressure and lowering heart rate during passive leg rising may have fluid demand. Ultrasonography of the vena cava may be helpful in estimating fluid balance. A high inspiratory collapsibility of the superior vena cava may be another sign of fluid demand. A similar phenomenon may occur in the upper portion of the inferior vena cava and can be detected with abdominal ultrasound [7]. These procedures are non-invasive and easy to perform. Central venous pressure is imprecise, but a reasonable alternative is the measurement of central venous saturation ($ScvO_2$). However, a central intravenous line is required. $ScvO_2$ is a surrogate parameter for tissue hypoxia in septic patients. $ScvO_2$ below 65% is correlated with a worse outcome and increased fluid requirement [8]. The situation in non-septic patients is unclear, but in hemodynamically unstable patients in the absence of other reasons, low $ScvO_2$ may also be a sign of fluid demand. The esophageal Doppler technique has a high sensitivity but is an invasive procedure with logistic problems (expensive equipment and need for a specialist). A common limitation of all procedures is that they can predict fluid responsiveness, but they do not indicate the need for fluid. The decision to give fluid depends on the clinical status.

In order to estimate the optimal postoperative fluid amount for an individual patient it is necessary to know the intraoperative fluid intake and the perioperative excretion and loss of blood. The target volume should be 2000 ml fluid intake per day to avoid both hypovolemia and fluid excess. The intravenous fluid replacement should be decreased based on the amount during the first several days if the patient can ingest orally. Be aware of added fluids such as intravenous chemotherapeutics; they can easily amount to more than 500 ml per day.

24.3 Metabolic Management and Perioperative Nutrition

24.3.1 Metabolic Management

The most important metabolic responses after major elective surgery are hyperglycemia and protein catabolism. Some degree of insulin resistance develops after all types of surgery. The severity is related to the scale of the operation and increases with any complications or in sepsis. The development of insulin resistance is independent of the patient's preoperative state. Studies in the past few years clearly showed that postoperative hyperglycemia is also dangerous for non-diabetic patients. Postoperative normoglycemia maintained by insulin infusion reduced the morbidity and mortality by almost half [9, 10]. With a few relatively simple perioperative interventions, metabolic responses can be almost completely attenuated: (a) Preoperative oral carbohydrate treatment (12 and 2–4 h preoperatively) breaks the overnight fasting state and reduces an anabolic state [11, 12]. (b) Early enteral nutrition and postoperative isocaloric feeding prevents insulin resistance and extensive whole-body nitrogen loss [13]. (c) Pain relief and continuous epidural analgesia using local anesthetics have the additive effect of reducing insulin resistance [14].

These data refer to patients undergoing major abdominal surgery. While there are few sophisticated data available for patients following upper gastrointestinal surgery, it is reasonable to extrapolate from these interventions to bariatric surgery patients.

Bariatric patients with apparent diabetes mellitus may be more difficult to treat. The coincidence of type-2

▫ Table 24.1 Improvement of metabolic response in abdominal surgery

Preoperative
Oral carbohydrate 12 and 2-4 hours before operation
Postoperative
Early enteral nutrition and isocaloric feeding
Enhanced pain relief (continuous epidural analgesia / patient controlled analgesia)
Intensive insulin therapy

diabetes and obesity is accelerating [15, 16]. About one quarter of bariatric patients have diabetes [17]. Diabetes mellitus is a well-described risk factor for postoperative complications. There are only few data focusing on bariatric patients with metabolic or endocrine co-morbidities. Diabetic patients undergoing colorectal surgery seem to develop hyperglycemia and protein catabolism more often than non-diabetic patients [18].

To reduce the risk of postoperative complications, intensive insulin therapy is recommended. To avoid hypoglycemia, the blood glucose level should be monitored frequently; it should be in the range of 80–120 mg/dl [9]. The safety of continuous insulin infusion (CII) was proven in many studies, and recent data demonstrated similar results for bariatric patients [19] (▫ Table 24.1).

24.3.2 Perioperative Nutrition

Surgery triggers a series of reactions, including the release of stress hormones and inflammatory mediators. They cause the catabolism of glycogen, fat, and protein, thus releasing glucose, free fatty acids, and amino acids into the circulation. Beyond other factors, recent studies have shown the impact of pre- and postoperative nutrition in reducing the stress of surgery, minimizing catabolism, and supporting anabolism throughout surgical treatment [5].

In former times, fasting of patients before, during, and after surgery was common. This was due mainly to the fear of aspiration and anastomotic leakage. More recently, data have shown that 12 h of preoperative fasting has been associated with prolonged recovery following uncomplicated surgery [12, 21]. Patients with the oral intake of fluids 2-3 h preoperatively have no higher risk of aspiration or regurgitation, since fluid clears the stomach rapidly. Patients may drink clear fluids until 2 h before receiving anesthesia. Exceptions are patients with known delayed gastric emptying or those undergoing emergency surgery.

Preoperative metabolic preparation using carbohydrates not only reduces insulin resistance but also preserves skeletal muscle mass and may have an effect on postoperative nausea and vomiting (PONV) [11, 23]. Data for patients with upper gastrointestinal surgery are rare. Only one study found no effect of preoperative carbohydrate load on the complication rate and length of hospital stay in this group of patients [11]. With good data for elective abdominal surgery and a lack of data for bariatric patients, it is reasonable to implement preoperative oral carbohydrate treatment in clinical routine. Recommended are 800 ml of a carbohydrate drink the night before and 400 ml the morning before surgery. This regime does not increase the risk of aspiration [24]. (◘ Table 24.2)

Delayed oral intake or esophago-gastric decompression after abdominal surgery failed to show any benefit [25, 26]. Oral nutrition, including clear liquids, can be initiated in most cases immediately after surgery. Early enteral nutrition on the first or second postoperative day after laparoscopic colon resection showed an earlier onset of bowel movement [27]. However, the situation regarding upper gastrointestinal surgery is less clear. It is not reasonable to interrupt oral intake of liquid fluids postoperatively, as

2–3 l of gastric secretions pass through the stomach and bowel per day in any case. Provided that the patient does not suffer from PONV or known delayed gastric emptying, drinking tea in sips 6 h after surgery is allowed. On the first postoperative day drinking is allowed and the patient can have an additional 500 ml liquid in the form of immune-modulating nutritional or standard whole-protein formulae. An adequate diet for the second and third postoperative days is balanced puréed fare in combination with immune-modulating or standard whole-protein nutritional formulae. During the next few days light fare is a reasonable diet for the patient. This nutritional regime is reserved for patients with normal bowel movement and an uncomplicated postoperative period (◘ Table 24.3).

For patients with a supposed inadequate oral intake for more than 7 days, nutritional support is indicated. Also patients who cannot maintain oral intake above 60% of the recommended amount for more than 10 days should receive nutritional support [28]. The influence of undernutrition on postoperative mortality and morbidity is well-described, particularly that of inadequate oral intake for more than 14 days [29, 30]. Undernutrition is an independent risk factor for anastomotic leakage after gastrectomy [31]. Most current data show a better outcome with early enteral nutrition support for mortality, morbidity, and length of hospital stay in undernourished patients and compared with delayed enteral nutrition, administration of crystalloids, and parenteral nutrition [28]. In other studies no benefits or even a higher morbidity for early enteral nutrition were observed [32, 33]. These different findings indicate that the exact amount of initial enteral intake in patients with or without nutritional support should be adapted to the individual's tolerance and the state of his or her gastrointestinal function [34].

Compared with parenteral nutrition, enteral nutrition showed a significantly reduced rate of infections and a shortened length of hospital stay [35, 36]. In elective surgery no data regarding combined enteral and parenteral nutrition exist, but it is reasonable to combine both methods of nutritional support in patients who cannot get <60% of their caloric requirement via the enteral route [24]. For patients with a known disturbance of gastrointestinal passage, but no ileus, minimal enteral feeding (e.g. 200–500 ml/day) in combination with parenteral nutrition should be considered. A small amount of enteral diet prevents atrophy of gut mucosa and reduces the risk of bacterial translocation and abdominal sepsis [37, 38].

The enteral route should always be preferred except for patients with ileus, severe shock, or intestinal ischemia, and oral feeding should be favored. For patients who cannot ingest an adequate amount of fare for any reason, tube feeding should be considered. Nasoenteric

◘ **Table 24.2** Influence of preoperative oral carbohydrates on postoperative metabolism

Catabolism	↓
Insulin resistance	↓
Degradation of skeletal muscle mass	↓
PONV	↓
Anabolism	↑

◘ **Table 24.3** Postoperative enteral feeding in patients with normal gastric emptying, without PONV and with uncomplicated postoperative period

6 hours postop.	Tea in sips
Day 1	Liquid fluids, 500 ml immune modulating or standard whole protein formulae
Day 2-3	Balanced puréed fare Immune modulating or standard whole protein formulae
From day 4	Slight fare

tube placement is a less invasive and safe technique for establishing enteral feeding access. In patients with disturbed gastric emptying, nutritional support via an endoscopically placed nasoenteric-jejunal tube is reasonable. For long-term nutritional support percutaneous endoscopic or surgical tube placement provides a more invasive, but durable alternative [39].

24.4   Postoperative Analgesia

Postoperative pain management is of particular importance. An optimized analgesic therapy reduces stress and circulatory disorders and the patient can be mobilized properly. Mobilization prevents deep vein thrombosis and decubitus ulcers and makes the patients feel better. Baseline analgesia in postoperative patients is central effective analgesic substances in combination with peripheral effective analgesics. For severe pain, epidural analgesic techniques with local anesthetics and opioids or patient-controlled analgesia (PCA) also in combination with non-opioid analgesics are required. The multimodal pain management reduces the dose of any single drug and therefore reduces the side effects of opioids.

24.4.1   Continuous Epidural Analgesia and Patient-controlled Analgesia

Continuous epidural analgesia with local anesthetics and/or opioids is one of the most efficient techniques for providing dynamic perioperative pain relief in major operations [40]. Epidural analgesia also has been shown to be associated with fewer pulmonary complications [41], a lower incidence of deep vein thrombosis [42], decreased cardiac morbidity [43], suppression of metabolic neuroendocrine responses [44], and acceleration of postoperative return of gastrointestinal function [45]. Other studies have been published with negative effects, except for the improved pulmonary outcome [56, 47, 48]. These studies have been predominantly opioid-based, which will not provide the stress-reducing effects that are observed when local anesthetics are included [45, 49]. Nevertheless, there are no clear-cut documented benefits for morbidity and hospital stay. However, pain relief and patients' comfort are improved, and a reduction in pulmonary morbidity has been demonstrated in most studies.

Another established procedure is the patient-controlled analgesia (PCA) pump. It is a computerized machine that is attached to a patient's intravenous line. The machine contains a syringe of pain medicine (typically an opioid analgesic). The patient judges when to take more pain-killing drugs by using the PCA pump. When a patient feels pain, he can press the button on the pump for additional pain medicine. The machines have built-in safety features. The total amount of analgesic that the patient can self-administer is within the safe limit. Patients will not be able to self-administer sufficient dynamic pain relief because of opioid-related side effects, and opioids will not provide sufficient incident-related pain relief. Because of the lack of significant stress-reducing effects, PCA has no positive effect on such outcome parameters as cardiopulmonary or thrombembolic complications or hospital stay. However, PCA provides improved patient satisfaction [40, 50] (■ Table 24.4).

Few clinical trials have evaluated different kinds of analgesic management in bariatric patients. One retrospective study compared PCA with epidural analgesia. No superiority of any one procedure was shown [51]. Because of potential technical difficulties and neurological complications associated with epidural catheter placement, PCA with i.v. opioids is an acceptable strategy for pain management in this group of patients.

■ **Table 24.4** Influence of different analgesic procedures on patients' outcome

	Continuous epidural analgesia	Patient-controlled analgesia
Pulmonary complications	+	O
Incidence of deep vein thrombosis	+	O
Cardiac morbidity	+	O
Suppression of metabolic neuroendocrine responses	+	O
Gastrointestinal function	+	-
Patient satisfaction	+	+

+ positive influence; - negative influence; O no influence

24.4.2 Non-steroidal Anti-inflammatory Drugs (NSAID)

NSAIDS are widely used for light and medium-heavy pain and especially as components of balanced analgesia. The most prominent NSAIDS are acetylsalicylic acid, ibuprofen, and metamizole. Acetylsalicylic acid is not recommended for postoperative pain management because it inhibits thrombocyte aggregation and therefore may cause bleeding complications. NSAIDs have both analgesic and anti-inflammatory actions. Their mechanism of action is predominantly inhibition of prostaglandin synthesis by the enzyme cyclo-oxygenase (COX-1 and COX-2 isoenzymes), which catalyzes the conversion of arachidonic acid into various prostaglandins that are the chief mediators of inflammation. NSAIDS have a ceiling effect, and the recommended highest dosage should not be exceeded [52]. Recent meta-analyses have shown that in PCA the combination with NSAIDS significantly reduced the amount of opioids used, the intensity of pain, and the incidence of nausea, vomiting, sedation, ileus, bladder dysfunction, and pulmonary morbidity [53–55]. The incidence of pruritus, urinary retention, and respiratory depression seems not to be reduced by NSAIDS [56]. Due to insufficient study data for selective NSAIDS (selective COX-2-inhibitors), no advantage with respect to reduction of opioid-related side effects has been demonstrated [55, 57, 58]. Following withdrawal of rofecoxib and valdecoxib due to cardiovascular risks and lumiracoxib due to the risk of liver dysfunction, the benefit of selective NSAIDS is now under discussion. The main side effects of both NSAIDS and selective NSAIDS are the risks of gastrointestinal, renal, and cardiovascular dysfunction (◘ Table 24.5).

Gastrointestinal Complications. The use of NSAIDS increases the risk of gastrointestinal complications three- to fivefold [59], depending on the agent, the dosage, and the length of use. Other risk factors are age >75 years, a history of ulcer, use of oral glucocorticoids or anticoagulants, and severe illness [60, 61]. Most data are based on more than 1 month of use. Data on short-term use are missing. Therefore, also in the short term, NSAIDS should not be applied for patients with risk factors.

Selective COX-2 inhibitors have a better risk profile of gastrointestinal side effects. Because they can lead to wound-healing disorders, however, the use of selective COX-2-inhibitors should be avoided in patients with gastric ulcer [61].

Renal Complications. The short-term use of NSAIDS and selective COX-2 inhibitors (7–10 days) causes acute renal failure in 0.5–1% of patients with myocardial insufficiency and renal or hepatic disorders. Following drug withdrawal the acute renal failure is mostly complete reversible [62]. For healthy adults there is no contraindication to the perioperative use of NSAIDS and selective COX-2 inhibitors.

Cardiovascular Complications. Recent data demonstrated an elevated risk of cardiovascular complications with the use of NSAIDS and selective COX-2 inhibitors over the long term [63, 64]. Only few studies have evaluated the risk of short-term use. The results indicate an elevated risk for patients with pre-existing cardiovascular diseases [65, 66].

With long-term use NSAIDS and selective COX-2 inhibitors may have severe side effects; the risk of complications with short-term use is not yet sufficiently investigated. Therefore, the following general contraindications are recommended (◘ Table 24.6):

— History of gastric ulcer
— Renal insufficiency
— Decompensated myocardial insufficiency
— Cardiovascular diseases

◘ **Table 24.5** Riskfactors for complications by intake of NSAIDS and COX-2 inhibitors

Gastrointestinal complications
Age > 75y
Oral glucocorticoids
Oral anticoagulants
Severe illness
Gastric ulcer in history

Renal complications
Myocardial insufficiency
Hepatic disorders
Renal disorders

Cardiovascular complications
Pre-existing cardiovascular diseases

◘ **Table 24.6** Contraindications for NSAIDS and selective COX-2 inhibitors

Gastric ulcer in history
renal insufficiency
Decompensated myocardial insufficiency
cardiovascular diseases

24.4.3 Paracetamol

Paracetamol is not an NSAID. It has analgesic and anti-pyretic properties but few anti-inflammatory effects. It is well-absorbed orally and is metabolized almost entirely in the liver. It has few side effects in normal dosage and is widely used for the treatment of minor pain. It causes hepatotoxicity in overdosage by overloading the normal metabolic pathways with the formation of a toxic metabolite. The analgesic effect is even higher when it is given intravenously.

24.4.4 Infiltration of the Wound

The infiltration of wounds with a long-lasting local anesthetic (e.g. ropivacaine, bupivacaine) is an effective part of the multimodal analgesic concept [67]. In bariatric patients infiltration of the wound is useful after open techniques [68]. Following laparoscopic surgery, the size of the wound is small and a local anesthetic procedure is usually not necessary.

24.4.5 New Substances

Non-competitive N-methyl-D-aspartate (NMDA) Receptor Antagonist. Amino acids like glutamate and aspartate are important transfer agents in neural activity. They activate pre- and postsynaptic localized NMDA receptors and play a major role in the development of pain. The most prominent of the NMDA receptor antagonists is ketamine. The effect of intravenous ketamine on pain is low, but it reduces the usage of opioids and extends the possible administration period [69–71]. Patients with malignancies or chronic pain or patients who are accustomed to opioids may develop a tolerance against opioids. In these patients continuous administration of ketamine may enhance the therapeutic effect of analgesic concepts [72].

Because there are no existing studies, the optimal dosage and period of time are not known. Due to several side effects such as fatigue, sedation, hallucination, and hypersalivation the routine use of NMDA receptor antagonists in postoperative pain management is limited. A new opportunity is systemic administration as a co-analgesic substance in the setting of multimodal analgesic therapy in patients with chronic pain and tolerance to opioids.

Anticonvulsants (gabapentin, pregabalin). The analgesic effect of gabapentin and pregabalin is based on the inhibition of calcium channels, localized on peripheral afferent nerves and central spinal and supraspinal neurons. The inhibition leads to an increased influx of calcium ions and a subsequent release of neurotransmitters such as glutamate and substance P. Glutamate and substance P are involved in nociception, transmitting information about tissue damage from peripheral receptors to the central nervous system to be converted to the sensation of pain. Recent studies demonstrated that a single administration of gabapentin prior to the operation reduces the pain as well as the amount of opioids needed and opioid-related side effects on the first postoperative day [73–75]. Similar results are found in combination with patient-controlled epidural analgesia [76]. The results for pregabalin are comparable, but only a few randomized controlled trials have been performed to date. Before it is adopted into routine use, a recent meta-analysis recommends defining the optimal dosage and investigating whether the positive analgesic effect differs with the type of operation [77].

Corticosteroids. Corticosteroids inhibit the synthesis of prostaglandins and leukotrienes and are therefore well-established in the therapy of chronic inflammatory diseases. Recent data have shown that a single perioperative dose of dexamethasone and methylprednisolone in patients in different surgical settings results in a significant reduction of pain and opioid-caused side effects [78, 79]. A large trial with 1900 surgical patients demonstrated that a single dose of methylprednisolone has no side effects [80].

Before corticosteroids are adopted into routine use following major abdominal surgery, randomized, controlled trials are needed to prove a positive effect in this setting. Furthermore, the optimal dosage and period of administration have to be defined.

24.5 Postoperative Airway Management and Obstructive Sleep Apnea-Hypopnea-Syndrom (OSAS)

Care of the respiratory system is one of the most important tasks in morbidly obese patients. One third of bariatric patients have obstructive sleep apnea-hypopnea (OSA), others suffer from the Pickwickian syndrome or the obesity hypoventilation syndrome. Even when awake, morbidly obese patients have severe alterations of their respiratory mechanics [81, 82]. Among patients with OSA, 10–15% develop hypoventilation, and there is a relationship between the OSA syndrome and the obesity hypoventilation syndrome [83]. Chronic exposure to hypoxia and sleep fragmentation weakens the central ventilatory drive. In healthy patients chronic exposure to hypoxia leads to a reduced hypoxic and hypercapnic ventilatory response. In morbidly obese patients sleep fragmentation also decreases the hypercapnic ventilatory response [84]. The OSA syndrome results in sleep hypoxemia, hypercapnia, and sleep fragmentation and therefore in a diminished ventilatory drive and resultant hypoventilation [83–85]. Hypoventilation and disturbed lung mechanics may prevent restoration of post-apnea eucapnia, which results in more severe exposure to hypoxemia and hypercapnia. These patients may be caught in a vicious circle [83, 86].

Evidence suggests that leptin, a protein produced by adipose tissue, may have an influence on the obesity hypoventilation syndrome. Leptin acts on receptors in the hypothalamus and suppresses the appetite [87–89]. In central respiratory centers, leptin stimulates the ventilation, while a deficiency of the protein has been associated with hypoventilation [90]. Leptin deficiency or resistance may lead to a reduction in ventilation [90–92].

During the postoperative period, morbidly obese patients are more likely to have significant impairment of pulmonary gas exchange and respiratory mechanics [93]. Particular concerns are a decreased chest wall and lung compliance, an increased airway resistance, lower expiratory reserve volumes, and a decreased functional residual capacity [83, 94]. With changes in position from upright to supine, the negative effect of the chest wall and the abdominal adipose tissue on lung compliance, functional residual capacity, and blood oxygenation is exacerbated [95]. During general anesthesia morbidly obese patients develop more atelectasis than non-obese patients. During the postoperative period, pulmonary atelectasis resolves within hours in non-obese patients, while in morbidly obese patients atelectasis persists or increases 24 h after tracheal extubation [96]. For these patients an at least 25° reverse Trendelenburg position is important for full diaphragmatic excursion.

Postoperative cardiopulmonary-associated deaths may relate to cardiac arrhythmias occurring in the setting of OSA. During apneic episodes, arterial hypoxia can be serious. Awakening in response to apnea is associated with a significantly higher sympathetic tone [97]. This spike in the sympathetic tone in the presence of hypoxemia may induce lethal arrhythmias without coronary artery disease. This effect can be worsened in the direct postoperative period, when the lipophilic intravenous narcotics are released from the adipose tissue.

For bariatric surgery patients with a diagnosis of OSA or the obesity hypoventilation syndrome, nocturnal continuous positive airway pressure (CPAP) is usually effective. Delivered by a nasal mask, this therapy provides continuous positive pressure during the respiratory circle. It maintains upper airway patency, eliminates apnea and hypopnea, and restores daytime eucapnia [98]. An easy system for applying positive pressure is the Boussignac CPAP system. It is cheap and effective, requiring only an oxygen source without a special respirator. Besides many other conditions, it is indicated for use in the OSA syndrome, for prevention of postoperative atelectasis, and for weaning after tracheal extubation [100].

Patients who do not respond to CPAP for any reason may require non-invasive mechanical ventilation (NIV) [99]. NIV is the delivery of positive pressure via a tight-fitting mask that covers the nose or both the nose and the mouth of spontaneously breathing patients. Two different procedures can be performed: Bi-level positive airway pressure (BiPAP) permits independent adjustment of inspiratory and expiratory positive airway pressure. Differences between these pressures assist with lung inflation during each respiratory cycle of support ventilation. On the other hand, volume ventilation ensures adequate alveolar ventilation [99].

Because of an unprotected airway, patients requiring CPAP or NIV must have an adequate level of consciousness and airway protective reflexes. It should be avoided in patients who are not hemodynamically stable or have evidence of impaired gastric emptying. These patients have a high risk of life-threatening aspiration. The pressure for non-invasive mechanical ventilation must be set below the opening pressure of the lower esophageal sphincter (20 cm H_2O) to avoid gastric insufflation [101].

Esophageal and gastric surgery are usually considered to be contraindications to the use of CPAP or NIV. Several studies have shown that NIV is a safe method after bariatric procedures and even after esophageal surgery [102–104]. In particular, the rates of anastomotic leakage and pulmonary complications were not higher than in the reference groups. Gastric distension was successfully avoided by the placement of a nasogastral tube.

Evidence suggests that obstructive sleep apnea-hypopnea and obesity hypoventilation syndrome are underrecognized and undertreated. These syndromes are associated with a significant increase in mortality. CPAP and NIV are effective treatment regimens and should be established in postoperative care.

24.6 Perioperative Morbidity and Mortality

Due to their co-morbidities, obese patients have an increased risk of postoperative complications. Diabetes mellitus, hypertension, and obstructive sleep apnea increase the risk of perioperative pulmonary, cardiovascular, and thromboembolic complications. Bariatric surgical procedures carry additional risks. Also contributing to perioperative morbidity and mortality are the expertise of the surgeon and that of the facility in bariatric procedures.

Two retrospective studies investigated indicators of morbidity and mortality specifically related to both open and laparoscopic bariatric surgery. The factors analyzed were age, sex, BMI, hypertension, diabetes mellitus, obstructive sleep apnea and obesity-hypoventilation syndrome. In both studies only age (>55 years) was an independent patient-related risk factor for increased morbidity and mortality [105, 106].

The expertise of the surgeon as related to the outcome after bariatric surgical procedures was analyzed by three major studies. The authors came to the conclusion that the surgeon's experience with laparoscopic gastric bypass was directly related to the incidence of postoperative complications. Surgeons with high expertise in laparoscopic bariatric operations (>100 cases) had a rate of major complications comparable to that with open procedures. Complications unique to laparoscopic bariatric techniques were highest when the surgeon had performed fewer than 75 laparoscopic bariatric operations [107–109].

Overall mortality is significantly lower in facilities with a high volume of bariatric surgical procedures (>100/year) than in low-volume hospitals (<50/year) (0.3–0.5% vs. 1.2%). This factor becomes more important for patients older than 55 years (0.9% vs. 3.1%). Besides lower mortality, high-volume facilities had significantly lower overall complication rates (10.2% vs. 14.5%) and shorter hospital stays (3.8 vs. 5.1 days) [107, 110, 111].

A recent study showed that death within 30 days after bariatric surgery is less than 1% [108]. The fact that data were collected in all institutions of the United States that perform bariatric surgery does not consider differences between experienced and unexperienced facilities. Another study described a lower incidence at high-volume centers (0.3%) [112]. Some authors reported a fourfold 30-day mortality after gastric bypass procedures performed by surgeons in low-volume bariatric surgery facilities compared with procedures performed by experienced surgeons in high-volume bariatric centers [113].

24.6.1 Surveillance of Surgical Site Infections and Therapeutic Options

Chronic wounds and postoperative wound infections are common findings in the obese patient. Wound infections are significantly less common after laparoscopic surgery than after open procedures (3% vs. 7%). In general, avascularity in excessive fatty tissue decreases the ability to combat infection [114, 115]. The overall decreased tissue oxygen level leads to impaired ability of the neutrophils to phagocytose bacteria. Additionally, other metabolic disorders evoked in the metabolic syndrome also lead to decreased immunosufficiency (diabetes, arterial hypertension, elevated blood cholesterol levels, and dyslipidemia). Pulmonary restriction and already impaired and infected skin, problems of mobilization and general nursing also contribute to the higher risk of wound development and healing impairment.

Morbid obesity is a well-known risk factor where surgical site infections and postoperative wound complications are concerned [116–118]. This is due to lower tissue oxygen levels, as mentioned above, and to the impairment of general wound healing by the metabolic syndrome. A higher level of postoperative wound infections can also be attributed to technical difficulties during the operative procedure, increased operation time and therefore increased time for contamination, and increased operative trauma [119].

Wound infection weakens the surgical incision site and may lead to an incisional hernia. Incisional hernias occur more often after open bariatric surgery than after laparoscopic procedures (9% vs. 0.45%) [107]. Subcutaneous wound infections are associated with a higher morbidity because of the long treatment duration and the higher risk of incisional hernia. Deep wound infection such as fascial dehiscence is rare (<1%) but requires immediate surgical therapy [120].

24.6.2 Postoperative Surveillance

A prospective evaluation showed that bariatric surgery does not carry an additional risk of postoperative wound infection in obese patients compared with elective general surgery, although BMI was higher in the bariatric group [121]. However, because of the overall elevated risk of wound complications, strict and structured surveillance of surgical sites should be the rule following bariatric surgery.

A short overview of recommended postoperative examinations and interventions is given in ▢ Table 24.7. This schedule provides easy and inexpensive methods for identifying wound complications and surgical site infections as soon as possible in order to provide the best medical care without delay. Since most bariatric procedures are now performed via laparoscopic surgery, the rate of surgical site infections has dropped. Nevertheless, surveillance must take place on a regular basis.

24

▪ Table 24.7 Schedule for wound surveillance after bariatric surgery			
Postop day	**Laparoscopic surgery**	**Open surgery**	**Additional procedures**
1	Inspection of wound dressing	Inspection of wound dressing	Blood count and CRP-measurement
2	Inspection of wound dressing	Inspection of wound dressing	Change of wound dressing in case of bloody remnants or other peculiarities
			Removal of intra-abdominal drainages
3	Change of wound dressing and inspection of the wound	Change of wound dressing, inspection and ultrasound examination of the wounds	Blood count and CRP-measurement
Discharge			
4	Inspection, no dressing	Change of wound dressing and inspection of the wound	
5	Inspection, no dressing	Change of wound dressing and inspection of the wound	
6	Inspection, no dressing	Inspection, no dressing	
7–10		Removal of suture material	

24.6.3 Signs of Surgical Site Infections in the Obese

Due to the changes in fatty tissue in the morbidly obese, the appearance of a wound infection may also differ from that in patients with lesser amounts of body fat. In some cases, an infection is not noticeable by simply inspecting the wound. Erythema and edema can appear late during the formation of infection because of the vertical depth of the wound. Also, exudation and dehiscence may appear some time after the onset. This delayed formation of the classical signs of wound infection appears especially after laparoscopic surgery, although the rate of infection is lower than after conventional surgery and the symptoms in the patient are rare at the beginning [122]. In some cases not even pathological wound exudation is noticed after surgical re-opening of the skin, although a wound infection is taking place in the depth of the wound. Further examination and imaging are necessary to verify the diagnosis.

Following conventional open surgery, the complete surgical site should be re-opened, even if the area of secondary wound healing reaches quite large dimensions. After only partial re-opening, the remaining surgical stitches are not able to hold against the tension caused by the pull of the fatty tissue of the enlarged abdominal wall in many cases. Rupture of the remaining stitches or the surrounding skin occurs. Additionally, bacteria enter the former regular surgical wound through the already open and infected skin, and the infection spreads despite ongoing treatment.

Following laparoscopic surgery, the ratio between vertical and horizontal wound diameter is even more adverse; the depth of the wound cannot be reached by the surgeon using scissors and forceps. In these cases, re-opening and enlargement of the wound should be considered; although these procedures partially negate the former positive effects of laparoscopic surgery, the risk of abscess formation in the abdominal wall must be minimized.

24.6.4 Therapeutic Options

The therapeutic options for dealing with postoperative wounds in the obese do not generally differ from those available in other patients. In case of an infection, re-opening of the surgical wound is mandatory and moist wound treatment must follow. Indications for dry wound treatment usually do not exist.

24.6.5 Advancement of Secondary Wound Healing

After the surgical wound is re-opened, large wound areas are subject to secondary wound healing. A long period of medical and nursing treatment follows, with high consequential costs and secondary monetary factors in every single case. Acceleration of wound healing has to be attained to minimize the costs and effects on both the patient and the health-care environment. Conventional moist wound treatment with regular changes of the wound dressing and the use of modern dressings can result in complete closure of the wound but can take up to months to achieve.

Vacuum-assisted closure (VAC®-Therapy) is regarded as a powerful device to accelerate wound healing. In addition to the standard therapeutic application, different methods with higher benefit for wound healing are in common use:

Skin Stretching. A standard vacuum therapy is used in the primary step of this treatment. The vacuum generated in the wound area keeps the fatty tissue of the abdominal wall from exerting great tension on the wound, exudates of the wound itself are transported from it, capillary growth is enhanced, and the amount of oxygen and number of immunocompetitive cells in the wound area are therefore increased. After the first few applications of this dressing system, the walls of the wound are adapted by stitches, and the tension generated in the stitching area is minimized by the vacuum still applied to the wound. Additionally, devices for narrowing the wound through the stitches, without changing the stitches themselves and thus adding new trauma to the surrounding skin, have to be put in place (◘ Figs. 24.1–24.3). The pressure put on the tissue by the stitches and the hoist can be minimized by foam or gauze. With this procedure, the wound can be narrowed at every change of the dressing without additional trauma until a definite secondary stitching can be obtained. Even patients with large amounts of fatty tissue on the abdominal wall can be treated; this can also be performed on an outpatient basis in younger and compliant patients.

Partial Secondary Stitching. Following conventional vacuum therapy or narrowing of the wound via skin stretching, a part of the wound can be closed by secondary stitching while the central parts are still subject to secondary wound healing. The tension on the surrounding tissue can be minimized by ongoing vacuum therapy. By these means, gradual wound closure can be obtained. It is important that the stitches be applied with large gaps to keep exudate from collecting distant from the vacuum system and causing new infection. This can also be performed on an outpatient basis, if the patient is capable of understanding the dressing and of solving minor problems by him- or herself.

Preparation for Skin Grafts. In very severe cases of wound infection and very large wound areas, a skin graft can be considered, although this is not a standard thera-

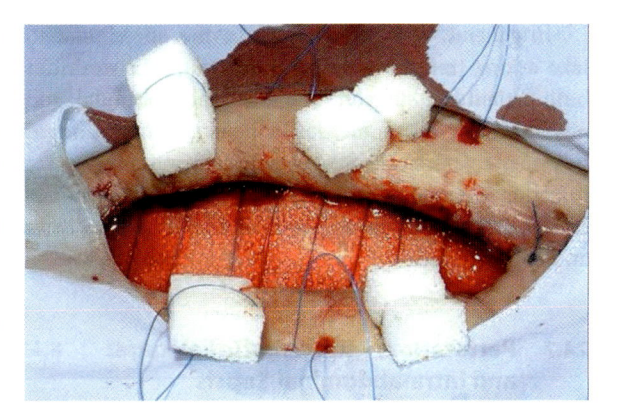

◘ Fig. 24.1. Postoperative wound after conditioning with VAC®-dressing in preparation for skin stretching; parts of the foam are used as cushions to minimize pressure on surrounding skin

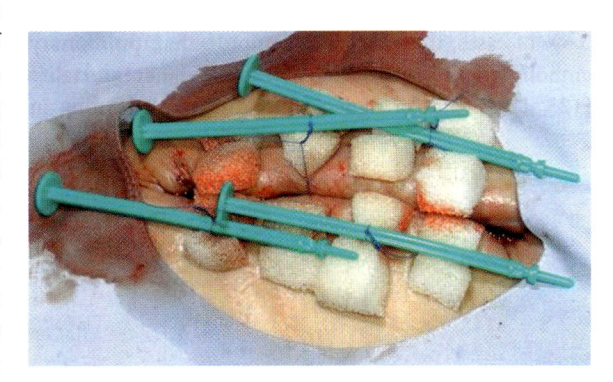

◘ Fig. 24.2. In this example standard stamps of syringes are used as hoists to narrow the wound edges without re-stitching the wound. This additionally minimizes trauma to the surrounding tissue

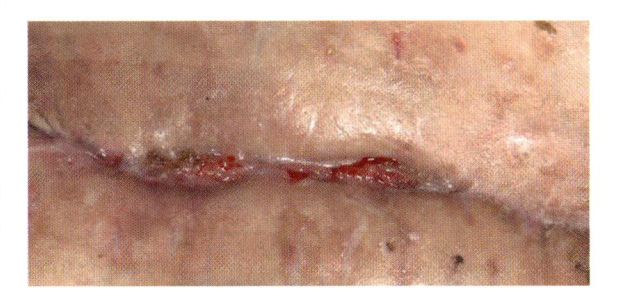

◘ Fig. 24.3. Cosmetic result of a wound closed by skin stretching and secondary stitching

peutic option for surgical site infections. The wound area should also be prepared and conditioned by vacuum application to accelerate the process. It must be mentioned that the cosmetic results of these procedures are limited, and patients face major weight loss following bariatric surgery, which aggravates the results even more.

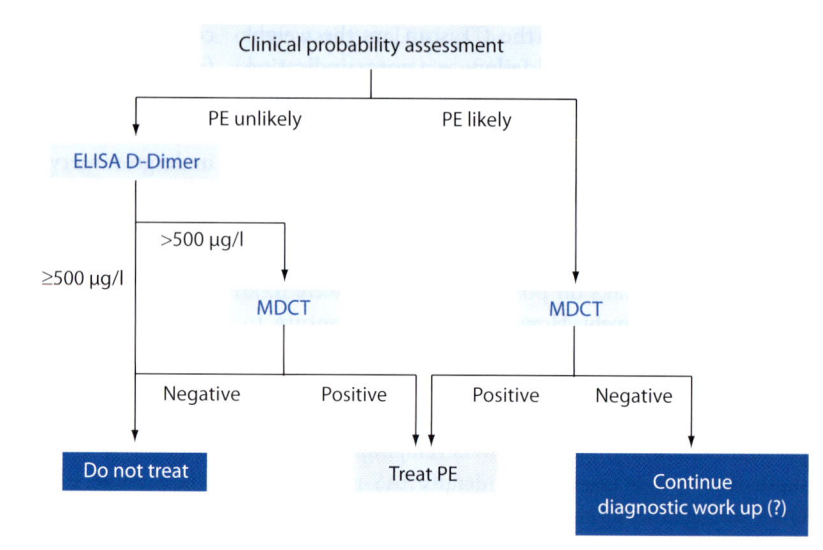

Fig. 24.6. Validated algorithm for diagnosis of pulmonary embolism (PE), based on multidetector row computed tomographic pulmonary angiography (MDCT) [149]

Clinical probability assessment

PE unlikely — ELISA D-Dimer — ≥500 µg/l → Negative → Do not treat; >500 µg/l → MDCT → Positive → Treat PE

PE likely → MDCT → Positive → Treat PE; Negative → Continue diagnostic work up (?)

Table 24.8 Clinical model for predicting pretest probability of DVT [135]

Active cancer (treatment ongoing within previous 6 months or palliative)	1
Paralysis, paresis, or recent plaster immobilization of the legs and feet	1
Recently bedridden >3 days or major surgery within 4 weeks	1
Localized tenderness along the distribution of the deep venous system	1
Entire leg swollen	1
Calf swelling 3 cm greater than asymptomatic leg (measurement 10 cm below tibia tuberosity)	1
Pitting edema (confined to the symptomatic leg)	1
Collateral superficial veins (non-varicose)	1
Alternative diagnosis as likely or greater than that of deep vein thrombosis	1
Pretest probability calculated as follows	-2

		Total points
High	≥3	_____
Moderate	1 or 2	_____
Low	≤0	_____

DVT seldom occurs after bariatric surgery. The incidence does not differ between open and laparoscopic procedures [107]. In addition to several other factors, conditions increasing the likelihood of thrombosis include obesity and surgery [133, 134]. Except for those with contraindications, all surgical bariatric patients should receive prophylaxis for thrombosis. Patients at higher risk of thrombotic disorders (e.g., chronic leg edema, venous insufficiency, stasis dermatitis, oral contraceptives) require special attention.

A clinical probability test based on physical examination and medical history is the first step when DVT is suspected. Patients can be stratified into categories of low, intermediate, or high probability (Table 24.8j) [135].

Typical clinical signs of DVT are swelling of the calf or the entire leg, tenderness along the distribution of the deep venous system, and pitting edema [135].

The only laboratory test which has gained a prominent part in the diagnosis of thrombosis is the measurement of D-dimer. The predictive value of negative

D-dimer together with a low clinical probability safely rules out acute DVT. Positive results are sensitive but not specific. In various situations (e.g., inflammation, cancer, or surgery) D-dimer may be raised [136]. D-dimer is not recommended as a stand-alone test [137].

Venography is still the gold standard, with a high sensitivity and specificity for both proximal and distal DVT, but this diagnostic tool is invasive and has potential contraindications. It should be used in patients with a high clinical probability but suspect or negative non-invasive tests [138].

Compression ultrasonography is the most useful imaging test. For the detection of proximal thrombosis compression ultrasonography has a sensitivity of 97–100% and a specificity of 98–99% [139]. Ultrasonography is less accurate in the detection of calf vein thrombosis, with a sensitivity of 70% and a specificity of 60%. An exclusive calf vein thrombosis rarely results in a pulmonary embolism, and an extension to proximal veins is unusual. Therefore, a combination of clinical assessment, D-dimer measurement, and serial ultrasonography can safely be applied for patients with distal thrombosis [138].

24.8.2 Therapy

Recent data have shown that fixed-dose, weight-adjusted, subcutaneous low-molecular-weight heparin (LMWH) is as effective as intravenous unfractionated heparin [140]. Compared with unfractionated heparin, LMWH has a longer half-life, contains a lower risk of immune-mediated thrombocytopenia or osteoporosis, and has a more predictable dose-response relationship [141, 142]. The monitoring of anti-factor Xa activity 4 h after injection is recommended in patients with impaired renal function and in morbidly obese patients [143]. Unfractionated heparin may be useful in patients with high bleeding risk, because of its shorter half-life and the possibility of quickly antagonizing the effect [138].

Another treatment modality is thrombolytic therapy (systemic or via local catheter-directed infusion). In comparison to standard anticoagulation it carries a higher risk of bleeding, and there is no evidence for a positive effect on preventing the post-thrombotic syndrome [144].

Vena cava filters in patients with proximal vein thrombosis prevent the short-term incidence of pulmonary embolism, but they do not affect mortality [145]. They are used for special indications. In elective bariatric surgery this method does not play any role [146].

The currently preferred mode of long-term therapy following DVT is orally administered vitamin-K antagonist. Several new anticoagulants have been evaluated. An inhibitor of thrombin, ximelagatran, was not inferior to enoxaparin. The advantage of ximelagatran was the oral administration without the need of monitoring [147]. However, because of liver toxicity it was recently phased out. Other agents are not yet used in long-term therapy after DVT. The course and duration of therapy are reviewed in detail in recently published guidelines [148].

24.9 Pulmonary Embolism

24.9.1 Diagnosis

Typical clinical signs of pulmonary embolism (PE) do not exist. Unspecific signs are dyspnea, chest pain, and cardiac arrhythmias. The only factor which clearly determines the diagnostic and therapeutic approach for suspected PE is hemodynamic instability. The sudden pressure overload of the right ventricle leads to acute right ventricle dysfunction and decreased left ventricular preload. The cardiac index is reduced, and the patient is hypotensive and may go into shock. The increased demand for myocardial oxygen may cause myocardial ischemia and infarction.

Massive PE with hemodynamic instability occurs in 5% of all cases and is associated with high in-hospital mortality. The prognosis of non-massive PE in hemodynamically stable patients is favorable if a rapid diagnosis is confirmed and adequate therapy is started immediately [149]. Similar to the diagnostic approach for DVT, patients with suspicion of PE can be stratified into different groups. Validated scores are the revised Geneva and the Wells score (◘ Table 24.9) [150, 151]. The diagnostic procedure depends on the severity of the suspected PE (see ◘ Fig. 24.6).

Massive PE is a life-threatening disorder, and rapid treatment is more important than an accurate diagnosis. Bedside echocardiography is the fastest diagnostic tool and should be performed immediately. It is the most adequate test for confirming acute right heart failure. Additional information obtained from echocardiography includes floating intracardial thrombi, which prompt emergency surgical thrombectomy or thrombolysis, open foramen ovale with a right-to-left shunt or paradoxical thrombembolism, or alternative reasons for cardiac shock (e.g., myocardial infarction, left ventricular failure, valvular disease). If echocardiography is not available or the results are imprecise, spiral computed tomography is the most reliable method. Beyond clinical assessment, performing a D-dimer test is not helpful in patients with cardiac shock. Selective invasive pulmonary angiography is not routinely necessary and is reserved for special situ-

□ Table 24.9 Validated scores for predicting pretest probability of pulmonary embolism [150, 151]

Revised Geneva Score		Wells Score	
Risk factors			
Age >65 years	+1	Previous DVT or PE	+1.5
Previous DVT or PE	+3	Recent surgery or immobilization	+1.5
Surgery or fracture within 1 month	+2	Active cancer	+1
Active cancer	+2		
Symptoms			
Unilateral lower limb pain	+3	Hemoptysis	+1
Hemoptysis	+2		
Clinical signs			
Heart rate 75–94 bpm	+3	Heart rate <100 bpm	+1.5
≥94 beats per minute	+5	Clinical signs of DVT	+3
Pain on lower limb deep vein palpation and unilateral edema	+4		
		Clinical judgement	
		Alternative diagnosis less likely than PE	+3
Clinical probability			
Low	0–3	Low	0–1
Intermediate	4–10	Intermediate	2–6
High	≥11	High	≥7
		Clinical probability (dichotomized)	
		PE unlikely	0–4
		PE likely	>4

ations such as catheter-based aspiration of the pulmonary thrombus [149].

After the clinical probability has been classified, the diagnostic algorithm in normotensive patients with suspected PE depends on the computed tomography scan (CT scan). A single (helical) detector CT scan has a low sensitivity of 60–70%. The combination of negative CT scan, negative lower limb ultrasound, and low or intermediate clinical probability safely rules out PE [149]. Multidetector row CT pulmonary angiography has a high sensitivity and the ability to confirm or rule out PE without the need for venous ultrasound [152]. In some patients, particularly those with severe renal failure or allergy to intravenous contrast agents, CT cannot be used. These patients, as well as those in whom a CT-based strategy is inconclusive, may undergo ventilation-perfusion lung scanning [149]. Negative measurement of D-dimer with a highly sensitive assay is a reliable test to exclude PE in patients with low or intermediate clinical probability [152]. One third of all patients with suspected PE can be managed on the basis of clinical signs and measurement of D-dimer without further imaging techniques [153]. Because of the low reliability, D-dimer as a single test is not recommended for patients with high probability [149]. For patients with an elevated D-dimer level or high clinical probability, lower limb compression ultrasonography is the next step to confirm the diagnosis. It will detect DVT in 10% of all cases. The negative predictive value is low, but it can be used to confirm a positive diagnosis. The Christopher Study investigators showed that combining pretest probability, D-dimer, and CT without ultrasonography effectively rules out

PE [154]. Another study showed that combining clinical probability, D-dimer, and multidetector row CT scan is as safe as the approach of D-dimer, leg ultrasonography, and multidetector row CT scan [152]. In recent years risk stratification has been implemented for normotensive patients with less than massive PE to define certain groups for early thrombolytic therapy. Methods and parameters which have been proposed are the measurement of troponin T or brain natriuretic peptide (BNP) and the severity of right ventricular dysfunction. Firm evidence that these patients will benefit from thrombolysis is lacking [153, 154].

24.9.2 Therapy

For patients with massive PE and cardiogenic shock, immediate recanalization of the occluded pulmonary arteries by thrombolysis or embolectomy should be considered [156, 157]. Currently approved thrombolytic agents are streptokinase, urokinase, and alteplase. Alteplase is generally considered to be the most effective agent. Reteplase and tenecteplase are not yet approved for PE [149]. The systemic intravenous administration of thrombolytic agents is preferred. In special cases, such as in patients with a high bleeding risk (e.g. postoperative), topical administration via a Swan-Ganz catheter is possible. Only small observation studies exist in this regard. In these studies the dosage of thrombolytic agents was as high as in systemic lysis with a comparable mortality and morbidity [158–160]. A thrombolytic effect with lower doses of thrombolytic agents is not yet proven, but there are case reports about successful lysis with a tenth of the recommended dose of alteplase for systemic lysis.

Surgical embolectomy is a rarely performed rescue operation. Recent data show that technical advances may be associated with a better postoperative outcome [161]. For patients with contraindications for thrombolysis, or when thrombolysis has failed, surgical pulmonary embolectomy is a recommended alternative therapeutic approach. Another alternative method is catheter embolectomy or fragmentation. Recommendations or restrictions are the same as for surgical embolectomy. The indication for inferior vena cava filters is reserved for special cases. In elective bariatric surgery this method does not have any impact [146].

Early initiation of anticoagulation therapy is the gold standard for normotensive patients with non-massive PE. A fixed-dose, weight-adjusted, subcutaneous low-molecular-weight heparin (LMWH) is as effective and safe as intravenous unfractionated heparin [148, 162]. In hemodynamically stable patients with non-massive PE,

LMWH is recommended as the initial course of treatment [163]. Currently approved LMWHs include enoxaparin, tinzaparin, and fondaparinux. The administration and monitoring of LMWH are described in the preceding section (DVT). In patients with contraindications for LMWH, such as those with renal failure (creatinine clearance <30 ml/min), intravenous unfractionated heparin is still the preferred mode of anticoagulation. The dosage can be adjusted by measuring the aPTT. In cases of high bleeding risk the effect can be quickly antagonized [149]. Unfractionated heparin and LMWH are associated with the risk of heparin-induced thrombocytopenia. Therefore, monitoring of the platelet count is essential during treatment. Following initial therapy with LMWH or unfractionated heparin, long-term therapy with vitamin-K antagonist is recommended. The course and duration of therapy are reviewed in detail in recently published guidelines [148].

24.10 Peripheral Nerve Injuries

Most peripheral nerve injuries occur in the setting of operative procedures. The most frequent lesions are stretch injuries of the brachial plexus and compression damage to the ulnar nerve due to excessive arm abduction, inadequate support of the outstretched arm, or prolonged flexion of the elbow [164, 165]. Of patients with perioperative ulnar neuropathy, 29% had a body mass index of 38 kg/m^2 and 70% were male [166]. Ulnar nerve lesions also occur in non-surgical departments, suggesting that patient positioning also contributes to this condition. The reasons are the supine position of the patient, the hand resting on the chest or abdomen, or elbows resting on bed rails [167]. Special education of patients, nurses, and physicians is needed regarding arm positions while the patient is in bed. Extended-width beds are essential for critically ill obese patients to prevent their arms from resting on the side rails. Peripheral neuropathies that develop during the postoperative period are more likely to be due to malnutrition (particularly vitamin-B deficiencies) and should be thoroughly investigated [168].

24.11 Nursing Care

24.11.1 Early Ambulation and Mobility

Early and frequent mobilization and ambulation prevents the risk of pulmonary disturbances such as atelectasis and pneumonia, DVT and PE, pain, re-sedation, and decubi-

24

tus ulcers. Non-intubated patients should be ambulated every 2 h while awake, beginning at least 2 h after surgery. The goal of mobilization is not only transfer into a chair, but also walking with the patients on the ward. Special beds are helpful for mobilization (■ Fig. 24.7). With the KCI-BariAir®, morbidly obese patients can get up on their feet without help [169].

Mobilization of intubated patients is also possible. They can be safely moved into a special chair. Some intubated patients cannot be extubated because of pulmonary or laryngeal complications but are awake and spontaneously breathing. The endotracheal tube is well-tolerated, and these patients can be mobilized almost like self-breathing patients (■ Fig. 24.8). Therefore, nurses caring for obese surgical patients require repeated education in this kind of setting [169].

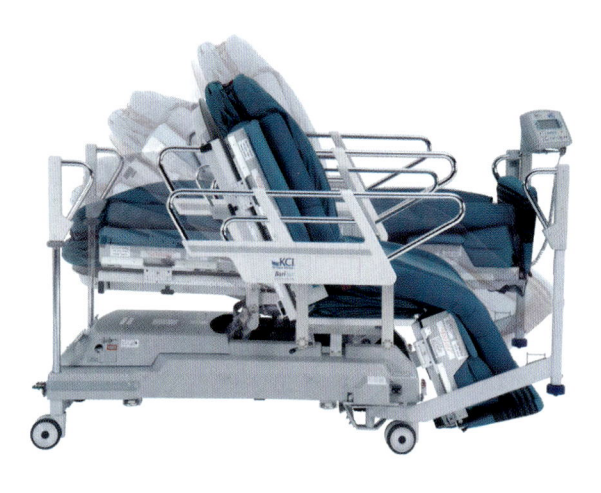

■ **Fig. 24.7.** Special bed for bariatric patients (KCI BariAir©)

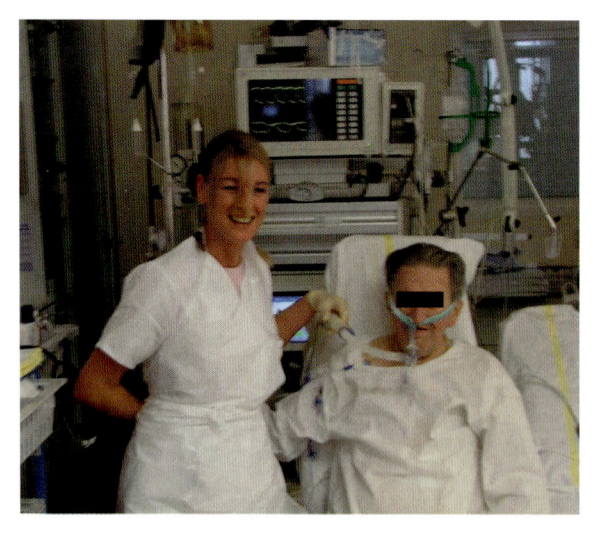

■ **Fig. 24.8.** Mobilization of intubated patient

24.11.2 Prevention of Decubitus Ulcers

Morbidly obese patients have a high risk of developing decubitus ulcers. For critically ill patients, the risk increases dramatically. To decrease the likelihood of decubitus ulcers, critically ill obese patients need special air or rotating mattresses. This special bedding does not relieve the nurse from having to turn the patient manually. Nursing care includes repeated inspection of the of the patient's entire body for cleansing and drying and to ensure that lines and tubes are not caught in skin folds. Arms should be protected with pillows from rubbing against the side walls and fall down. The neck, occiput, and heels of intubated patients require special attention. The intervals between these nursing procedures should not exceed 2 h. It is helpful to establish a standard routine for inspecting or bedding obese patients [170, 171].

24.11.3 "Out of ICU" Procedures

Diagnostic procedures outside of the ICU, such as computerized tomography, angiography, or nuclear imaging for morbidly obese patients can be difficult or impossible because of their weight and size. Most radiology tables have weight limits of about 150–160 kg. Even though the CT scan can bear the weight, the nurse must measure the radius of the patient to see if the abdomen fits inside the scanner. Elective "out of ICU" procedures should be scheduled during normal business hours to ensure appropriate support in positioning the patient during the procedure. It is helpful to schedule elective and emergency procedures in collaboration with the team of the outlying department [169].

24.11.4 Special Devices

Facilities that treat morbidly obese patients need quite a number of special devices. Special beds rising to the level of operating-room tables are needed for obese ICU patients. Such a bed can also be used as a gurney. The operating-room table must be able to accommodate not only the weight of the obese patient, but also the size. Once the patient has been operated on, early mobilization and ambulation are extremely important to prevent perioperative morbidity. With a special bed obese patients can be easily mobilized either with help from the nurse or by themselves. The KCI-BariAir® provides the possibility to stand up over the foot end of the bed.

For critically ill obese patients it is essential to have a special lifting device which will bear their weight. With the HoverMatt® the patient can be lifted up in the bed or transferred from an examination table to the bed. This device is recommended for use with patients who cannot actively assist in lifting and turning, e. g., in the early postoperative period or for critically ill patients. Once the patient is mobilized, special attention must be paid to suitable chairs and even toilets. Wall-mounted toilets can be pulled out of the wall under the weight of an obese patient. However, it is not only the stability that must be considered, but also the width of the devices.

24.11.5 Employee Safety and Obesity Bias among Staff

The care of the immobile, morbidly obese patient includes manual turning for inspection, mobilization, and transport and poses an increased risk for employee safety. Purchasing adequate equipment for use with morbidly obese patients decreases the risk of injury and reduces the cost of workers' compensation for back injuries. Beyond special devices for lifting and transfer, it is essential to provide at least five people for the mobilization of an immobile obese patient: one person lifts the feet, one stands on each side of the bed, and one is solely responsible for the endotracheal tube. The final person stands behind the head of the patient and lifts the sheet from either side of the patient's head. The Trendelenburg position of the bed helps to move the patient. To prevent injuries the whole medical team should start the process in synchronization.

Even if all precautions are taken, annual performance competency of back safety techniques is helpful. Also back safety training by a physical therapist should be provided [169].

Once a bariatric surgery program is established, the entire staff needs concomitant education concerning the benefits of obesity surgery. This can be in the form of attending patient support groups, seminars given by the surgeon, or patient panel discussions [172].

References

1. Lobo DN, Bostock KA, Neal KR, et al (2002) Effect of salt and water balance on recovery of gastrointestinal function after elective colonic resection: a randomised controlled trial. Lancet 359:1812–1818
2. Grocott MP, Mythen MG, Gan TJ (2005) Perioperative fluid management and clinical outcomes in adults. Anesth Analg 100:1093–1106
3. Holte K, Kehlet H (2006) Fluid therapy and surgical outcome in elective surgery: a need for reassessment in fast-track surgery. Ann Am Coll Surg 202:971–981
4. Kehlet H (1997) Multimodal approach to control postoperative pathophysiology and rehabilitation. Br J Anaesth 78:606–617
5. Fearon KC, Ljungqvist O, Von Meyenfeldt M, et al (2005) Enhanced recovery after surgery: a consensus review of clinical care for patients undergoing colonic resection. Clin Nutr 24:466–477
6. Monner X, Rienzo M, Osman D, et al (2006) Passive leg raising predicts fluid responsiveness in critically ill. Crit Care Med 34:1402–1407
7. Vieillard-Baron A, Chergui K, Rabiller A, et al (2004) Superior vena caval collapsibility as a gauge of volume status in ventilated septic patients. Intensive Care Med 30:1734–1739
8. Bauer P, Reinhart K, Bauer M (2008) Significance of venous oximetry in the critically ill. Med Intensiva 32:134
9. van den Berghe G, Wouters P, Weekers F, et al (2001) Intensive insulin therapy in the surgical intensive care unit. N Engl J Med 345:1359–1367
10. Vanhoerebeek, I, De Vos R, Mesotten D, et al (2005) Protection of hepatocyte mitochondrial ultrastructure and function by strict blood glucose control with insulin in critically ill patients. Lancet 365:53–59
11. Yuill KA, Richardson RA, Davidson HI, et al (2005) The administration of an oral carbohydrate-containing fluid prior to major elective upper-gastrointestinal surgery preserves skeletal muscle mass postoperatively – a randomised clinical trail. Clin Nutr 24:32–37
12. Ljungqvist O, Nygren J, Thorell A (2002) Modulation of post-operative insulin resistance by pre-operative carbohydrate loading. Proc Nutr Soc 61:329–336
13. Soop M, Carlson GL, Hopkins J, et al (2004) Randomized clinical trail of the effects of immediate enteral nutrition on metabolic responses to major colorectal surgery in an enhanced recovery protocol. Br J Surg 91:1138–1145
14. Greisen J, Juhl CB, Grofte T, et al (2001) Acute pain induces insulin resistance in humans. Anesthesiology 95:578–584
15. Dixon JB, Pories WJ, O'Brien PE (2005) Surgery as an effective early intervention for diabesity: why the reluctance? (review). Diabetes Care 28:472–474
16. Mannan MA, Rahman MS, Siddiqui NI (2004) Obesity management in patients with type 2 diabetes mellitus (review). Mymensingh Med J 13:95–99
17. Ramaswamy A, Gonzales R, Smith CD (2004) Extensive preoperative testing is not necessary in morbidly obese patients undergoing gastric bypass. J Gastrointest Surg 8:159–164
18. Schricker T, Gougeon R, Eberhart L, et al (2005) Type 2 diabetes mellitus and the catabolic response to surgery. Anesthesiology 102:320–326
19. Blackstone R, Kieran J, Davis M, Rivera L (2007) Continuous perioperative insulin infusion therapy for patients with type 2 diabetes undergoing bariatric surgery. Surg Endosc 21:1316–1322
20. Fearon KC, Ljungqvist O, Von Meyenfeldt M, et al (2005) Enhanced recovery after surgery: a consensus review of clinical care for patients undergoing colonic resection. Clin Nutr 24:466–477
21. Ljungqvist O, Nygren J, Thorell A, et al (2001) Preoperative nutrition – elective surgery in the fed or the overnight fasted state. Clin Nutr 20 [Suppl]:167–171
22. Henriksen MG, Hessov I, Dela F(2003) Effects of preoperative oral carbohydrates and peptides on postoperative endocrine response, mobilization, nutrition and muscle function in abdominal surgery. Acta Anaesthesiol Scand 47:191–199
23. Hausel J, Nygren J, Thorell A, et al (2005) Randomized clinical trial of the effects of oral preoperative carbohydrates on postopera-

tive nausea and vomiting after laparoscopic cholecystectomy. Br J Surg 92:151–158

24. Weimann A, Braga M, Harsanyi L, et al (2006) ESPEN Guidelines on enteral nutrition: surgery including organ transplantation. Clin Nutr 25:224–244

25. Elmore MF, Gallagher SC, Jones JG, et al (1989) Esophagogastric decompression and enteral feeding following cholecystectomy: a controlled, randomized prospective trial. JPEN J Parenter Enter Nutr 13:377–381

26. Petrelli NJ, Stulc JP, Rodriguez-Bigas M, Blumenson L (1993) Nasogastric decompression following elective colorectal surgery: a prospective randomized study. Am Surg 59:632–635

27. Schwenk W, Bohm B, Haase O, et al (1998) Laparoscopic versus conventional colorectal resection: a prospective randomised study of postoperative ileus and early postoperative feeding. Langenbecks Arch Surg 383:49–55

28. ASPEN board of directors and the clinical guidelines task force (2002) Guidelines for the use of parenteral and enteral nutrition in adult and paediatric patients. JPEN J Parenter Enteral Nutr 26:1SA–138SA

29. Dannhauser A, Van Zyl JM, Nel CJ Preoperative nutritional status and prognostic nutritional index in patients with benign disease undergoing abdominal operations: part I. J Am Coll Nutr 1995 14:80–90

30. Rey-Ferro M, Castano R, Orozco O, et al (1997) Nutritional and immunologic evaluation of patients with gastric cancer before and after surgery. Nutritio 13:878–881

31. Meyer L, Meyer FR, Dralle H, et al for the East German Study Group for Quality Control in Operative Medicine and Regional Development in Surgery (2005) Insufficiency risk of esophagojejunal anastomosis after total abdominal gastrectomy for gastric carcinoma. Langenbecks Arch Surg 390:510–516

32. Watters JM, Kirkpatrick SM, Norris SB, et al (1997) Immediate postoperative enteral feeding results in impaired respiratory mechanics and decreased mobility. Ann Surg 226:369–377

33. Martignoni ME, Friess H, Sell F, et al (2000) Enteral nutrition prolongs delayed gastric emptying in patients after Whipple resection. Am J Surg 180:18–23

34. Lewis SJ, Egger M, Sylvester PA, Thomas S (2001) Early enteral feeding versus "nil by mouth" after gastrointestinal surgery: systematic review and meta-analysis of controlled trails. BMJ 323:773–776

35. Braunschweig CL, Levy P, Sheean PM, Wang X (2001) Enteral compared with parenteral nutrition: a meta-analysis. Am J Clin Nutr 74:534–542

36. Peter JV, Moran JL, Phillips-Hughes A (2005) Meta-analysis of treatment outcomes of early enteral versus parenteral nutrition in hospitalized patients. Crit Care Med 33:213-20

37. Feltis BA, Wells CL (2000) Does microbial translocation play a role in critical illness? Curr Opin Crit Care 6:117–122

38. Nieuwenhuijzen GAP, Goris R, Jan A (1999) The gut: "motor" of multiple organ dysfunction syndrome. Curr Opin Clin Nutr Metabol Care 2:399–404

38. Shikora SA (1997) Enteral feeding tube placement in obese patients: consideration for nutritional support. Nutr Clin Prac 12:S9–S42

39. Jorgensen H, Wetterslev J, Moiniche S, Dahl JB (2002) Epidural local anaesthetics versus opioide-based analgesic regiments on postoperative gastrointestinal paralysis, PONV and pain after abdominal surgery (Cochrane review). In: Cochrane Library, Issue 1. update software, Oxford

40. Ballantyne JC, Carr DB, deFerranti S, et al (1998) The comparative effects of postoperative analgesic therapies on pulmonary outcome: cumulative meta-analysis of randomized, controlled trails. Anesth Analg 86:598–612

41. Valentin N, Lombolt B, Jensen JS, et al (1986) Spinal or general anaesthesia for surgery of the fractured hip? A prospective study of mortality in 578 patients. Br J Anaesth 58:284–91

42. Beattie WS, Badner NH, Choi P (2001) Epidural analgesia reduces postoperative myocardial infarction: a meta-analysis. Anesth Analg 93:853–858

43. Kehlet H (1991) The surgical stress response: should it be prevented? Can J Surg 34:565–567

44. Holte K, Kehlet H (2002) Epidural anaesthesia and analgesia – effects on surgical stress responses and implications for postoperative nutrition. Clin Nutr 21:199–206

45. Pak WY, Thompson JS, Lee KK (2001) Effect of epidural anaesthesia and analgesia on perioperative outcome: a randomized, controlled Veterans Affairs cooperative study. Ann Surg 234:560–569

46. Rigg JR, Jamrozik K, Myles PS, and MASTER anaesthesia trial study group. (2002) Epidural anaesthesia and analgesia and outcome of major abdominal surgery: a randomized trial. Lancet 359:1276–1282

47. Peyton PJ, Myles PS, Silbert BS, et al (2003) Perioperative epidural analgesia and outcome after major abdominal surgery in high-risk patients. Anesth Analg 96:548–554

48. Kehlet H (1998). Modification of responses to surgery by neural blockade: clinical implications. In: Cousins MJ, Bridenbaugh PS (eds) Neural blockade in clinical anaesthesia and management of pain, 3rd edn. Lippincott-Raven, Philadelphia, pp 129–175

49. Walder B, Schafer M, Henzi I, Tramer MR (2001) Efficacy and safety of patient-controlled opioid analgesia for acute postoperative pain. A quantitative systematic review. Acta Aneasthesiol Scand 45:795–804

50. Charghi R, Backman S, Christou N, et al (2003) Patient-controlled iv analgesia is an acceptable pain management in morbidly obese patients undergoing gastric bypass surgery. A retrospective comparison with epidural analgesia. Can J Anesth 50:672–678

51. Brack A, Bottiger BW, Schafer M (2006) New aspects in postoperative pain therapy. Anesthesiol Intensivmed Notfallmed Schmerzther 41:184–192

52. Kehlet H (2004) Effect of postoperative pain treatment on outcome – current status and future strategies. Langenbecks Arch Surg 389: 44–249

53. Legeby M, Sandelin K, Wickman M, Olofsson C (2005) Analgesic efficacy of diclofenac in combination with morphine and paracetamol after mastectomy and immediate breast reconstruction. Acta Anaesthesiol Scand 49:1360–1366

54. Elia N, Lysakowski C, Tramer MR (2005) Does multimodal analgesia with acetaminophen, nonsteroidal antiinflammatory drugs, or selective cyclooxygenase-2 inhibitors and patient-controlled analgesia morphine offer advantages over morphine alone? Meta-analyses of randomized trials. Anesthesiology 103: 296–304

55. Marret E, Kurdi O, Zufferey P, Bonnet F (2005) Effects of nonsteroidal antiinflammatory drugs on patient-controlled analgesia morphine side effects: meta-analysis of randomized controlled trials. Anesthesiology 102:1249–1260

56. Romsing J, Moiniche S, Mathiesen O, Dahl JB (2005) Reduction of opioid-related adverse events using opioide-sparing analgesia with COX-2 inhibitors lacks documentation: a systematic review. Acta Anaesthesiol Scand 49:133–142

57. Romsing J, Moiniche S (2004) A systematic review of COX-2 inhibitors compared with traditional NSAIDs, or different COX-2

inhibitors for post-operative pain. Acta Anaesthesiol Scand 48:525–546

58. Garcia Rodriguez LA, Barreales Tolosa L (2007) Risk of upper gastrointestinal complications among users of traditional NSAIDS and coxibs in the general population. Gastroenterology 132:790–794

59. Peura DA, Goldkind L (2005) Balancing the gastrointestinal benefits and risks of nonselective NSAID. Arthritis Res Ther 7:7–13

60. Nau C, Schütler J (2008) Klinische Pharmakologie analgetischer Substanzen. In: Pogatzki-Zahn EM, Zahn PK (eds) Postoperative Schmerztherapie – Pathophysiologie, Pharmakologie und Therapie. Thieme, Stuttgart, pp 42–69

61. Whelton A (2006) Clinical implications of nonopioid analgesia for relief of mild-to-moderate pain in patients with or at risk for cardiovascular disease. Am J Cardiol 97:3E–9E

62. Warner TD, Mitchell JA (2008) COX-2 selectivity alone does not define the cardiovascular risks associated with non-steroidal anti-inflammatory drugs. Lancet 371:270–273

63. Hennekens CH, Borzak S (2008) Cyclooxygenase-2 inhibitors and most traditional nonsteroidal anti-inflammatory drugs cause similar moderately increased risks of cardiovascular disease. J Cardiovasc Pharmacol Ther 13:41–50

64. Schug SA, Camu F, Joshi GP, Pan S (2006) Cardiovascular safety of cyclo-oxygenase selective inhibitor parecoxib sodium: review of pooled data from surgical studies. Eur J Anaesthesiol 23:A-849

65. Joshi GP, Gertler R, Fricker R (2007) Cardiovascular thrombembolic adverse effects associated with cyclo-oxygenase-selective inhibitors and nonselective anti-inflammatory drugs. Anesth Analg 105:1793–1804

66. Bisgaard T (2006) Analgesic treatment after laparoscopic cholecystectomy: a critical assessment of the evidence. Anesthesiology 104:835–846

67. Batistich S, Kendall A, Somers S (2004) Analgesic requirements in morbidly obese patients. Anaesthesia 59:505–517

68. McCartney CJ, Sinha A, Katz J (2004) A qualitative systematic review of the role of M-methyl-D-aspartate receptor antagonists in preventive analgesia. Anesth Analg 98:1385–1400

69. Subramaniam K, Subramanian B, Steinbrook RA (2004) Ketamine as adjuvant analgesic to opioids: a quantitative and systematic review. Anesth Analg 99:482–495

70. Vandermeulen E (2006) Systemic analgesia and co-analgesia. Acta Anaesthesiol Belg 57:113–120

71. Carroll IR, Angst MS, Clark JD (2004) Management of perioperative pain in patients chronically consuming opioids. Reg Anesth Pain Med 29:576–591

72. Ho KY, Gan TJ, Habib AS (2006) Gabapentin and postoperative pain – a systematic review of randomized controlled trails. Pain 126:91–101

73. Hurley RW, Cohen SP, Williams KA, et al (2006) The analgesic effects of perioperative gabapentin on postoperative pain: a meta-analysis. Reg Anesth Pain Med 31:237–247

74. Seib RK, Paul JE (2006) Preoperative gabapentin for postoperative analgesia: a meta-analysis. Can J Anaesth 53:461–469

75. Turan A, Kaya G, Karamanioglu B, et al (2006) Effect of oral gabapentin on postoperative epidural analgesia. Br J Anaesth 96:242–246

76. Tiippana EM, Hamunen K, Kontinen VK, Kalso E (2007) Do surgical patients benefit from perioperative gabapentin/pregabalin? A systematic review of efficacy and safety. Anesth Analg 104:1545–1556

77. Bisgaard T, Klarskov B, Kehlet H, Rosenberg J (2003) Preoperative dexamethasone improves surgical outcome after laparoscopic cholecystectomy: a randomized double-blind placebo-controlled trail. Ann Surg 238:651–660

78. Romundstad L, Breivik H, Niemi G (2004) Methylprednisolone intravenously 1 day after surgery has sustained analgesic and opioide-sparing effects. Acta Anaesthesiol Scand 48:1223–1231

79. Sauerland S, Nagelschmidt M, Mallmann P, Neugebauer EA (2000) Risks and benefits of preoperative high dose methylprednisolone in surgical patients: a systematic review. Drug Saf 23:449–461

80. Zerah F, Harf A, Perlemuter L, et al (1993) Effects of obesity on respiratory resistance. Chest 103:1470–1476

81. Gaszynski T, Tokarz A, Piotrowski D, Machala W Boussignac (2007) CPAP in the postoperative period in obese patients. Obes Surg 17:452–456

82. Koenig SM (2001) Pulmonary complications in obesity. Am J Med Sci 321:249–279

83. Cooper KR, Phillips BA (1982) Effect of short-term sleep loss on breathing. J Appl Physiol 53:855–858

84. Gleeson K, Zwillich CW, White DP (1990) The influence of increasing ventilatory effort on arousal from sleep. Am Rev Respir Dis 142:295–300

85. Rapoport DM, Garay SM, Epstein H, Goldring RM (1986) Hypercapnia in the obstructive sleep apnoea syndrome: a re-evaluation of the "Pickwickian syndrome". Chest 89:627–635

86. Halaas JW, Gajiwala KS, Maffei SL, et al (1995) Weight-reducing effects of the plasma protein encoded by the obese gene. Science 269:543–546

87. Campfield LA, Smith FJ, Guisez Y, et al (1995) Recombinant mouse OB protein: evidence for a peripheral signal linking adiposity and central neural networks. Science 269:546–549

88. Erickson JC, Hollopeter G, Palmiter RD (1996) Attenuation of the obesity syndrome of ob/ob mice by loss of neuropeptide Y. Science 274:1704–1707

89. O'Donnell CP, Schaub CD, Haines AS, et al (1999) Leptin prevents respiratory depression in obesity. Am J Respir Crit Care Med 159:1477–1484

90. Phipps PR, Starrit E, Caterson I, et al (2002) Association of serum leptin with hypoventilation in human obesity. Thorax 57:75–76

91. Caro JF, Kolanczynski JW, Nyce MR, et al (1996) Decreased cerebrospinal fluid/serum leptin ration in obesity: a possible mechanism for leptin resistance. Lancet 348:159–161

92. Tweed WA, Phua WT, Chong KY, et al (1993) Tidal volume, lung hyperinflation and arterial oxygenation during general anaesthesia. Anaesth Intensive Care 21:806–110

93. Lamvu G, Zolnoun D, Boggess J, Steege JF (2004) Obesity: physiologic changes and challenges during laparoscopy. Am J Obstet Gynecol 191:669–674

94. McGlinch BP, Que FG, Nelson JL, et al (2006) Perioperative care of patients undergoing bariatric surgery. Mayo Clin Proc 81 [Suppl]:S25–S33

95. Eichenberger AS, Proietti S, Wicky S, et al (2002) Morbid obesity and postoperative pulmonary atelectasis: an underestimated problem. Anesth Analg 95:1788–1792

96. Kaw R, Michota F, Jaffer A, et al (2006) Unrecognized sleep apnoea in the surgical patient: implications for the perioperative setting. Chest 129:198–205

97. Berthon-Jones M, Sullivan CE (1987) Time course of change in ventilatory response to CO_2 with long-term CPAP therapy for obstructive sleep apnoea. Am Rev Respir Dis 135:144–147

98. Piper AJ, Sullivan CE (1994) Effects of short-term NIPPV in the treatment of patients with severe obstructive sleep apnea and hypercapnia. Chest 105:434–440

99. Block AJ, Boysen PG, Whynne JW (1979) Sleep apnoea, hypopnoea, and oxygen desaturation in normal subjects. N Engl J Med 300:513–517
100. Evans TW (2001) International Consensus Conference in Intensive Care Medicine: Non-invasive positive pressure ventilation in acute respiratory failure, organized jointly by the American Thoracic Society, the European Society of Intensive Care Medicine, and the Société de Réanimation de Langue Française, and approved by the ATS Board of directors, December 2000. Int Care Med 27:166–178
101. Huerta S, DeShields S, Shpiner R, et al (2002) Safety and efficacy of postoperative continuous positive airway pressure to prevent pulmonary complications after Roux-en-Y gastric bypass. J Gastrointest Surg 6:354–358
102. Nascimento J, Posner D, Rogers M, et al (2006) Risk of non-invasive positive pressure ventilation postoperatively in laparoscopic gastric bypass patients. Crit Care Med 33:A116
103. Jaber S, Delay JM Chanques G, et al (2005) Outcomes of patients with acute respiratory failure after abdominal surgery treated with non-invasive positive pressure ventilation. Chest 128.2688–2695
104. O'Rourke RW, Andrus J, Diggs BS, et al (2006) Perioperative morbidity associated with bariatric surgery: an academic centre experience. Arch Surg 141:262–268
105. Fernandez AZ jr, Demaria EJ, Tichansky DS, et al (2004) Multivariate analysis of risk factors for death following gastric bypass for treatment of morbid obesity. Ann Surg 239:698–702
106. Podnos YD, Jimenez JC, Wilson SE, et al (2003) Complications after laparoscopic gastric bypass: a review of 3464 cases. Arch Surg 138:957–961
107. Nguyen NT, Silver M, Robinson M, et al (2006) Result of a national audit of bariatric surgery performed at academic centres: a 2004 University HealthSystem Consortium Benchmarking Project. Arch Surg 141:445–449
108. Puzziferri N, Austrheim-Smith IT, Wolfe BM, et al Three-year follow-up of a prospective randomized trial comparing laparoscopic versus open gastric bypass. Ann Surg 2006; 243: 181-8
109. DeMaria EJ, Sugerman HJ, Kellum JM, et al (2002) Results of 281 consecutive total laparoscopic Roux-en-Y gastric bypasses to treat morbid obesity. Ann Surg 235:640–645
110. Nguyen NT, Paya M, Stevens CM (2004) The relationship between hospital volume and outcome in bariatric surgery at academic medical centers. Ann Surg 240:586–593
111. Courcoulas A, Schuchert M, Gatti G, Luketich J (2003) The relationship of surgeon and hospital volume to outcome after gastric bypass surgery in Pennsylvania: a 3-year summary. Surgery 134:613–621
112. Flum DR, Dellinger EP (2004) Impact of gastric bypass operation on survival: a population-based analysis. J Am Coll Surg 199:543–551
113. Tanaka S, Inoue S, Isoda F, et al (1993) Impaired immunity in obesity: suppressed but reversible lymphocyte responsiveness. Int J Obes Relat Metab Disord 17:631–636
114. Groszek DM (1982) Promoting wound healing in the obese patient. AORN J 35:1132–1138
115. Derzie AJ, Silvestri F, Liriano E, Benotti P (2000) Wound closure technique and acute wound complications in gastric surgery for morbid obesity: a prospective randomized trial. J Am Coll Surg 191:238–243
116. Mason EE, Renquist KE, Jiang D (1992) Perioperative risks and safety of surgery for severe obesity. Am J Clin Nutr 55 [2 Suppl]: 573S–576S
117. Forse RA, Karam B, MacLean LD, Christou NV (1989) Antibiotic prophylaxis for surgery in morbidly obese patients. Surgery 106:750–756; discussion 756–757
118. Wilson JA, Clark JJ (2003) Obesity: impediment to wound healing. Crit Care Nurs Q 26:119–132
119. McGlinch BP, Que FG, Nelson JL, et al (2006) Perioperative care of patients undergoing bariatric surgery. Mayo Clin Proc 81 [Suppl]:S25–S33
120. Topaloglu S, Avsar FM, Ozel H, et al (2005) Comparison of bariatric and non-bariatric elective operations in morbidly obese patients on the basis of wound infection. Obes Surg 15:1271–1276
121. Dindo D, Muller MK, Weber M, Clavien PA (2003) Obesity in general elective surgery. Lancet 361:2032–2035
122. Gonzalez R, Nelson LG, Gallagher SF, Murr MM (2004) Anastomotic leaks after laparoscopic gastric bypass. Obes Surg 14:1299–1307
123. Goldfeder LB, Ren CJ, Gill JR (2006) Fatal complications of bariatric surgery. Obes Surg 16:1050–1056
124. Kermarrec N, Marmuse JP, Faivre J (2008) High mortality rate for patients requiring intensive care after surgical revision following bariatric surgery. Obes Surg 18:171–178
125. Hamilton EC, Sims TL, Hamilton TT, et al (2003) Clinical predictors of leak after laparoscopic Roux-enY gastric bypass for morbid obesity. Surg Endosc 17:679–684
126. Merkle EM, Hallowell PT, Crouse C, et al (2005) Roux-en-Y gastric bypass for clinically severe obesity: normal appearance and spectrum of complications at imaging. Radiology 234:674–683
127. Madan AK, Stoecklein HH, Ternovits CA, et al (2007) Predictive value of upper gastrointestinal studies versus clinical signs for gastrointestinal leaks after laparoscopic gastric bypass. Surg Endosc 21:194–196
128. Rivers EP, Coba V, Whitmill M (2008) Early goal-directed therapy in severe sepsis and septic shock: a contemporary review of the literature. Curr Opin Anaesthesiol 21:128–140
129. Dellinger RP, Levy MM, Carlet JM, et al (2008) Surviving Sepsis Campaign: international guidelines for management of severe sepsis and septic shock: 2008. Crit Care Med 36:296–327
130. Bohnen J, Boulanger M, Meakins JL, McLean AP (1983) Prognosis in generalized peritonitis. Relation to cause and risk factors. Arch Surg 118:285–290
131. Seiler CA, Brugger L, Forssmann U, et al (2000) Conservative surgical treatment of intra-abdominal infection. Surgery 127:178–184
132. Heit JA, Mohr DN, Silverstein MD, et al (2000) Predictors of recurrence after deep vein thrombosis and pulmonary embolism: a population-based cohort study. Arch Intern Med 160:761–768
133. Geerts WH, Pineo G, Heit J, et al (2004) Prevention of venous thromboembolism: the 7th ACCP Conference on Antithrombotic and Thrombolytic Therapy. Chest 126 [Suppl]:338S–400S
134. Wells PS, Anderson DR, Bormanis J, et al (1999) Application of a diagnostic clinical model for the management of hospitalized patients with suspected deep vein thrombosis. Thromb Haemost 81:493–497
135. Kelly J, Hunt BJ (2003) A clinical probability assessment and D-dimer measurement should be the initial step in the investigation of suspected deep venous thromboembolism. Chest 124:1116–1119
136. Heim SW, Schectman JM, Siadaty MS, Philbrick JT (2004) D-dimer testing for deep venous thrombosis: a meta-analysis. Clin Chem 50:1136–1147
137. Kyrle PA, Eichinger S (2005) Deep vein thrombosis. Lancet 365:1163–1174

138. Quintavalla R, Larini P, Miselli A, et al (1992) Duplex ultrasound diagnosis of symptomatic proximal deep vein thrombosis of lower limbs. Eur J Radiol 15:32–36

139. Dolovich LR, Gnsberg JS, Douketis JD, et al (2000) A meta-analysis comparing low-molecular-weight heparins with unfractionated heparin in the treatment of venous thromboembolism. Arch Intern Med 160:181–188

140. Warkentin TE, Greinacher A (2004) Heparin-induced thrombocytopenia: recognition, treatment, and prevention. Chest 126:311S–317S

141. Monreal M, Lafoz E, Olive A, et al (1994) Comparison of subcutaneous unfractionated heparin with a low molecular weight heparin (Fragmin) in patients with venous thromboembolism and contraindications to coumarin. Thromb Haemost 71:7–11

142. Bounameaux H, de Moerloose P (2004) Is laboratory monitoring of low-molecular-weight heparin therapy necessary? No. J Thromb Haemost 2:551–554

143. Watson LI, Armon MP (2004) Thrombolysis for acute deep vein thrombosis (Cochrane Review). Cochrane Database Syst Rev 3:CD002783

144. White RH, Zhou H, Kim J, Romano PS (2000) Population-based study of the effectiveness of inferior vena cava filter use among patients with venous thromboembolism. Arch Intern Med 160:1033–1041

145. Kaufmann JA, Kinney TB, Streiff MB, et al (2006) Guidelines for the use of retrievable and convertible vena cava filters: report from the Society of Interventional Radiology multidisciplinary consensus conference. Surg Obes Relat Dis 2:100–112

146. Francis CW, Ginsberg JS, Berkowitz SD, et al (2003) Efficacy and safety of the oral direct thrombin inhibitor ximelagatran compared with current standard therapy for acute symptomatic deep vein thrombosis, with or without pulmonary embolism: the THRIVE treatment study. Blood 102:

147. Buller HR, Agnelli G, Hull RD, et al (2004) Antithrombotic therapy for venous thrombembolic disease: the 7th ACCP Conference on Antithrombotic and Thrombolytic Therapy. Chest 126 [Suppl]:401S–428S

148. Konstantinides SV (2008) Acute pulmonary embolism revisited. Heart 94:795–802

149. Le Gal G, Righini M, Roy PM, et al (2006) Prediction of pulmonary embolism in the emergency department: the revised Geneva score. Ann Intern Med 144:165–171

150. Wells PS, Anderson DR, Rodger M, et al (2000) Derivation of a simple clinical model to categorize patients' probability of pulmonary embolism: increasing the models utility with the SimpliRED D-dimer. Thromb Haemost 83:416–420

151. Righini M, Le Gal G, Aujeski D, et al (2008) Diagnosis of pulmonary embolism by, multidetector CT alone or combined with venous ultrasonography of the leg: a randomised non-inferiority trial. Lancet 371:1343–1352

152. Kyrle PA, Eichinger S (2008) New diagnostic strategies for pulmonary embolism. Lancet 371:1312–1315

153. Van Belle A, Büller HR, Huisman MV, et al for the Christopher Study Investigators (2006) Effectiveness of managing suspected pulmonary embolism using an algorithm combining clinical probability, D-dimer testing, and computed tomography. JAMA 295:172–179

154. Douma RA, Kamphuisen PW (2007) Thrombolysis for pulmonary embolism and venous thrombosis: is it worthwhile? Semin Thromb Hemost 33:821–828

155. European Society of Cardiology (2000) Guidelines on diagnosis and management of acute pulmonary embolism. Eur Heart J 21:1301–1336

156. British Thoracic Society (2003) Guidelines for the management of suspected acute pulmonary embolism. Thorax 58:470–483

157. McCotter CJ, Chiang KS, Fearrington EL (1999) Intrapulmonary artery infusion of urokinase for treatment of massive pulmonary embolism: a review of 26 patients with and without contraindications to systemic thrombolytic therapy. Clin Cardiol 22:661–664

158. Stock KW, Jacob AL, Schnabel KJ, et al (1997) Massive pulmonary embolism: treatment with thrombus fragmentation and local fibrinolysis with recombinant human-tissue plasminogen activator. Cardiovasc Intervent Radiol 20:364–368

159. Verstraete M, Miller GA, Bounameaux H, et al (1988) Intravenous and intrapulmonary recombinant tissue-type plasminogen activator in the treatment of acute massive pulmonary embolism. Circulation 77:353–360

160. Leacche M, Unic D, Goldhaber SZ, et al (2005) Modern surgical treatment of massive pulmonary embolism: results in 47 consecutive patients after rapid diagnosis and aggressive surgical approach. J Thorac Cardiovasc Surg 129:1018–1023

161. Quinlan DJ, McQuillan A, Eikelboom JW (2004) Low-molecular-weight heparin compared with intravenous unfractionated heparin for treatment of pulmonary embolism: a meta-analysis of randomized, controlled trials. Ann Intern Med 140:175–183

162. Büller HR, Davidson BL, Decousus H, et al (2004) Subcutaneous fondaparinux versus unfractionated heparin in the initial treatment of pulmonary embolism for the initial treatment of symptomatic deep venous thrombosis: a randomized trial. N Engl J Med 349:1695–702

163. Abir F, Bell R (2004) Assessment and management of the obese patient. Crit Care Med 32 [Suppl]:S87–S91

164. Sawyer RJ, Richmond MN, Hickey JD, Jarratt JAA (2000) Peripheral nerve injuries associated with anaesthesia. Anaesthesia 55:980–991

165. Warner MA, Warner ME, Martin JT Ulnar (1994) Neuropathy: incidence, outcome, and risk factors in sedated or anesthetized patients. Anesthesiology 81:1332–1340

166. Warner MA, Warner DO, Harper CM, et al (2000) Ulnar neuropathy in medical patients. Anesthesiology 92:613–615

167. Thaisetthawatkul P, Collazo-Clavell ML, Sarr MG, et al (2004) A controlled study of peripheral neuropathy after bariatric surgery. Neurology 63:1462–1470

168. Davidson JE, Callery C (2001) Care of the obesity surgery patient requiring immediate-level care or intensive care. Obes Surg 11:93–97

169. Gallagher SM (1993) Meeting the needs of the obese patient. AJN [Suppl]:3–14

170. Gallagher SM (1997) Morbid obesity: a chronic disease with an impact on wounds and related problems. Ostomy Wound Management 43:18–24

171. Davidson JE, Callery C (2000) Making the most of your time: the benefits of converting patient education programs into continuing nursing education. Obes Surg 10:482–483

Modern CT and MR Applications

Tobias Baumann, MD, Elmar Kotter, MD

25.1 Measurement of Body Fat Content and Distribution by Cross-sectional Imaging

Besides being used to diagnose a variety of diseases in adipose patients that can, but need not necessarily, be related to obesity, modern imaging modalities give rise to certain applications that are of special interest in obesity research. Both computed tomography (CT) and magnetic resonance imaging (MRI) provide three-dimensional data of the human body wherein the image contrast is related to the molecular composition of the observed tissues. This fundamental property renders cross-sectional imaging an advantageous way to study the body composition. The abnormalities in body composition in obesity, their detrimental effects on health, and their changes following bariatric surgery are of great importance. The following section presents an overview about a modern classification system for adipose tissue distribution derived mostly from findings in CT or MRI, provides some insight into the technical aspects of adipose tissue quantification, and addresses the observed changes in obesity and after surgery.

25.1.1 Definition and Classification of Adipose Tissue Deposits

The primary characteristic of obesity is an increased adipose tissue mass. Adipose tissue does not reflect a single compartment in the body, but anatomically different deposits can show diverse biological behavior. This insight is closely related to the discovery that adipose tissue not only represents a storage organ for fat, but also can be seen as an endocrine organ that reacts to and releases a broad pattern of cytokines, thereby influencing metabolic and inflammatory processes [1]. Although various methods are available to measure the quantity and distribution of adipose tissue in the human body – some of which will subsequently be discussed – it has been recognized that there is no uniform nomenclature for adipose tissue deposits and composition. Therefore, a classification system has recently been introduced to clarify the terminology used in body fat quantification [2].

Often the terms "fat" and "adipose tissue" are used as synonyms, but one should be aware that according to the medical context and the applied methods for quantification, adipose tissue does not consist solely of fat. Adipose tissue, a specialized, loose connective tissue that harbors abundant adipocytes, contains around 80% fat, whereas the other 20% comprise water, proteins, and minerals [3] in a standard body composition model.

On the other hand fat, although strictly regulated, is also present in other tissues and its accumulation has a severe pathophysiological impact, as will be discussed below. Therefore, body fat and amount of adipose tissue are closely correlated but not identical [4]. When cross-sectional imaging modalities are used for quantification, they normally address the amount of adipose tissue, while the quantification of intracellular lipid storage in other tissues can be achieved only indirectly or by means of spectroscopic analysis.

Whereas traditional classification systems for adipose tissue often represent a mixture of anatomical (subcutaneous, mammary, or organ-surrounding fat) and functional categories (e.g., white fat and brown fat) and are thus potentially ambiguous, a modern classification in cross-sectional imaging should rely on clearly visible fascial layers to differentiate between deposits of adipose tissue [2].

Total adipose tissue in this respect is considered to be the sum of adipose tissue, excluding head, hands, and feet. It can further be subdivided into subcutaneous and internal adipose tissue. Subcutaneous adipose tissue is defined as the layer between the dermis and the fasciae and aponeuroses of muscles, including mammary adipose tissue. Further discrimination can be made by utilizing a fascial layer in the lower trunk and gluteal region that divides the subcutaneous compartment into a superficial and a deep layer, with the superficial layer showing a rather homogeneous distribution around the body circumference, whereas the deep layer is located almost exclusively posteriorly (◘ Fig. 25.1).

It has been shown that those two layers exhibit different morphological and metabolic characteristics [5], and this subdivision can therefore be advocated in longitudinal studies. Internal adipose tissue can be divided further into visceral adipose tissue (VAT) and non-visceral adipose tissue comprising intra-, peri-, and intermuscular adipose tissue and parosseal adipose tissue.

Visceral adipose tissue, however, is again not a homogenous deposit, and furthermore, this term has been used with different definitions in the literature. In general, VAT can be regarded as the sum of intrathoracic (ITAT), intra-abdominal (IAAT), and intrapelvic (IPAT) adipose tissue. Intrathoracic adipose tissue, consisting of pericardial and extrapericardial tissue, has received less attention in the literature than the other two components of VAT, although pericardial fat has been suggested to be a potential buffer reducing the exposition of the heart itself to metabolic stress exerted by free fatty acids [6].

Most often, VAT is regarded as the sum of IAAT and IPAT measured between the diaphragm and the pelvic floor at the level of the femoral heads. When fascial

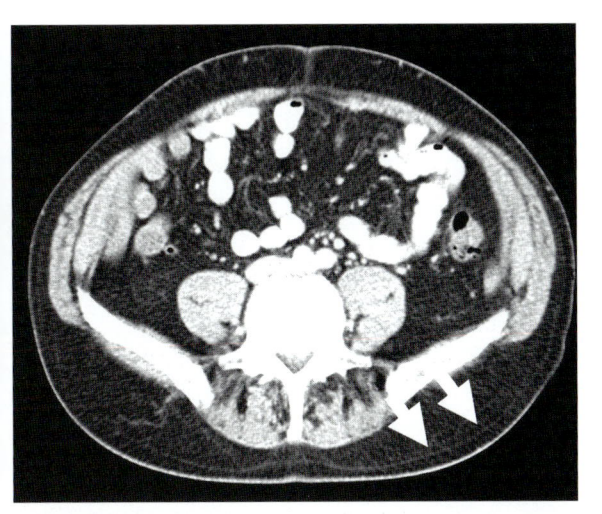

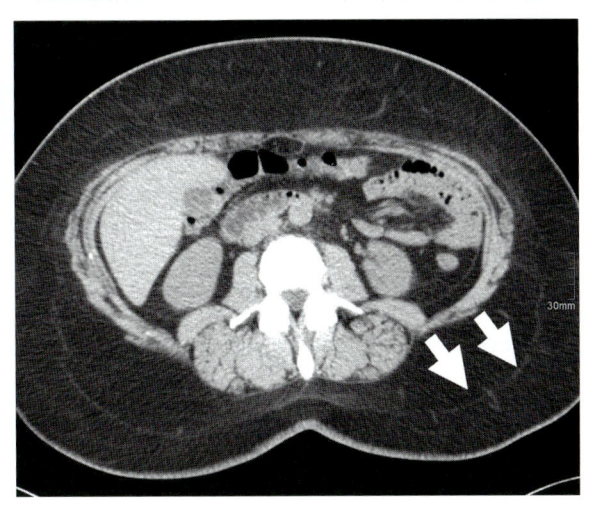

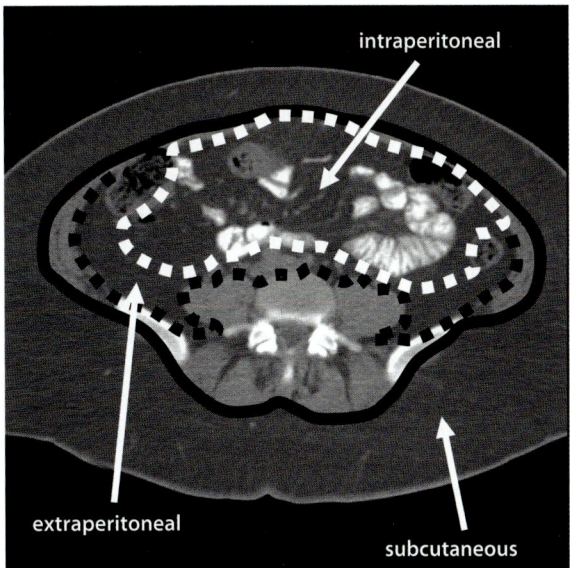

☐ **Fig. 25.2.** Subdivision of adipose tissue compartments. The subcutaneous compartment resides between the skin and the outer fascial layers of the muscular abdominal wall and the pelvic bone (*closed black line*). The intra-abdominal compartment is divided into the extraperitoneal part between the inner boundary of the abdominal wall posteriorly (*dotted black line*) and the peritoneum (*dotted white line*), which encompasses the intraperitoneal adipose tissue

☐ **Fig. 25.1.** Abdominal CT shows an additional fascial layer that subdivides the subcutaneous adipose tissue in the gluteal region (*arrows*). Note the different distribution of tissue in the two subjects presented

25.1.2 Aspects of Adipose Tissue Quantification

The most widely used parameter to determine obesity is the body mass index (BMI). However, it can neither distinguish between fat and lean mass nor provide information on tissue distribution [8]. Consequently, numerous techniques have been proposed for the quantification of adipose tissue and body fat content with and without the use of imaging. Multi-compartment models such as underwater weighing, dilution techniques, and dual-energy X-ray absorptiometry (DXA) are all reliable methods for obtaining accurate measures of total body fat [9]. Additionally, several anthropomorphic measures (e.g., waist circumference, waist-hip ratio, sagittal abdominal diameter, skinfold measurements) are employed in this respect. Although they serve as fast and inexpensive indicators of body composition and obesity, they provide little information on the exact distribution of adipose tissue, especially if more sophisticated anatomical classification systems are used, as outlined above, or if only regional analyses are intended.

Cross-sectional imaging modalities such as CT and MRI, on the other hand, can today provide high-resolu-

compartimentation and vascular territories are incorporated in the classification, this general definition is again subjected to further subdivision. In the abdomen adipose tissue resides intraperitoneally and extraperitoneally (☐ Fig. 25.2).

As the intraperitoneal part is drained via the portal vein directly to the liver, it has been hypothesized that release of free fatty acids from this compartment could have a pronounced effect on metabolism [7].

Although the ever more subtle distinction between different adipose tissue reservoirs appears, at least to some degree, very academic and lengthy, one should be aware of those definitions when reading the pertinent literature or – even more important – when planning further investigations.

tion data of all body regions, and even whole-body imaging can be achieved with a reasonable trade-off between acquisition time and resolution. Thus, these techniques can provide quantification of adipose tissue in combination with very accurate delineation of different deposits of adipose tissue, e.g., the differentiation between subcutaneous and visceral components. The following sections present the basic principles of these techniques and their applicability for creating a suitable image contrast between adipose tissue and its neighboring structures. Manual, semi-automatic, and fully automatic segmentation procedures that are needed for subsequent quantification are subsequently discussed.

Computed Tomography

In CT an X-ray source and its corresponding detector are oppositely mounted on a rotating gantry. By slice-wise detection of photon transmission during rotation the radiodensity of the examined object can be mapped to a two-dimensional image by means of back-projection. The linear attenuation coefficient of the investigated tissue is digitized and expressed in Hounsfield units (HU) ranging from -1000 to 3095, with the reference materials being water (0 HU) and air (-1000 HU).

Whereas most soft tissues comprising muscle, organs, and blood vessels exhibit attenuation values above 0 HU, fat shows a negative attenuation (-190 to -30 HU) (■ Fig. 25.3). This difference can be exploited to separate fat and water on CT images by means of post-processing. For sequential CT the patient table is at rest during exposure (single-slice acquisition) or is moved between image acquisitions (step-and-shot), while for helical CT the patient table is continuously moved simultaneous to gantry rotation, producing a helical-shaped sampling pattern of the examined volume. Today, helical CT is the standard acquisition mode for most applications as it can cover large body parts very fast. Depending on the number of detector rows (multi-detector CT), an abdominal CT examination, for example, can be accomplished in less than 10 s. Another advantage of helical CT is that it generates volumetric raw data that allow for image reconstruction in arbitrary planes and with low slice thicknesses and increments.

Relying on X-ray absorption as its basic principle of measure, CT always exposes the patient to ionizing radiation. Because the radiation dose inevitably increases with scan length, the application of CT as a whole-body technique for adipose tissue quantification must be considered carefully. Although CT is routinely applied to examine large parts of the human body due to its undoubted ability to depict a wide variety of disease manifestations,

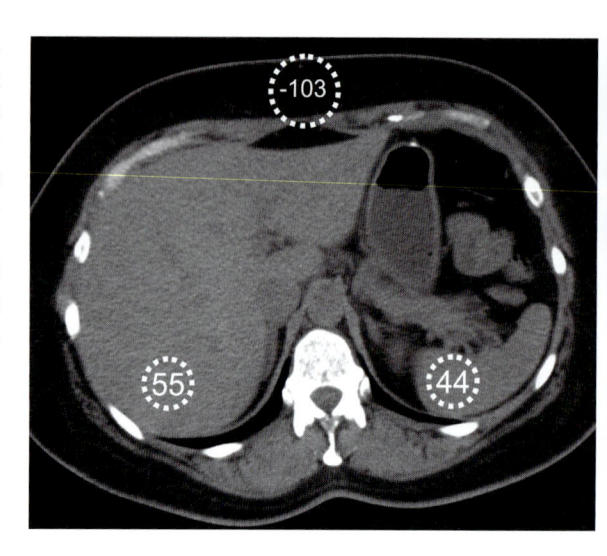

■ **Fig. 25.3.** Unenhanced abdominal CT scan shows representative attenuation values of the liver (*55 HU*), the spleen (*44 HU*), and adipose tissue (*-103 HU*)

its intentional use in volunteers or patients who would otherwise not receive an examination associated with X-ray exposure is not warranted.

Magnetic Resonance Imaging

Nuclei with an odd mass number exhibit a nuclear spin, thus generating magnetic properties. In MRI a large static magnetic field is applied in which these spins align their axis either parallel or antiparallel with this external field. In addition to this alignment they rotate around the field axis. This motion is called precession and its angular speed is determined by the Larmor frequency. The Larmor frequency depends on the nucleus and the magnetic field strength. If a radiofrequency pulse with the Larmor frequency is applied the spins are deflected from their precession axis, and at the same time they are focused to rotate in phase. After the end of the pulse, however, the spins return to their original alignment and lose their common phase. This process is called relaxation. Realignment with the outer field and the dispersion of phase are not immediate effects; they evolve over time until the original status has been re-established. The time constants at which these two processes occur are called T1 relaxation time and T2 relaxation time.

From this short summary of MR principles it becomes clear that at a given magnetic field strength inside the scanner (e.g. 1.5 Tesla) a pulse with a certain frequency will act on only a single type of nucleus. In clinical MR imaging parameters are always selected that aim at the ^{1}H proton. For investigational reasons, however, the scanners can be tuned to interact with other nuclei, e.g. [31]phosphorus or [13]carbon. The T1 and T2 relaxation times for ^{1}H nuclei are not constants, but are related to the molecular context of the protons and the presence of surrounding molecules. In MRI a series of pulses and local variations of the magnetic field (so-called gradients) are used to produce images in which the contrast is based on the different relaxation properties of the investigated tissues. Such a series of pulses and gradients is called an MR sequence. A multitude of different sequences are available, both commercially and scientifically, that provide different contrasts.

T1-weighted Imaging. Taking into account that image contrast is influenced by T1 and T2 relaxation times of the tissues in the field of view, it seems reasonable to choose a sequence that derives image contrast mainly from a parameter that shows unique values for adipose tissue. The T1 relaxation time of adipose tissue is ~250 ms, whereas the T1 relaxation time of most other tissues is much higher, e.g. ~900 ms for muscle (all times given for 1.5 Tesla systems) [10]. Thus, a sequence that translates differences in T1 relaxation times into image contrast should be able to distinguish between fat and its neighboring tissues. Such a sequence is called T1-weighted. Indeed, fat appears bright on T1-weighted images, whereas most other tissues appear darker (◘ Fig. 25.4).

Therefore, normal T1-weighted images have been widely applied in the determination of adipose tissue volume. It must be considered, however, that the absolute signal values in MRI depend on many factors and thus, in contrast to CT, fixed offset values to differentiate tissues cannot be employed. Furthermore, the signal values are subject to influence by inhomogeneities of the magnetic field and by the distance of a certain voxel to the receiver coil, which collects the MR signal. Hence, post-processing of T1-weighted images can be challenging. Techniques that do not rely on direct threshold-based classification of MR signal values in one T1-weighted image could therefore be more suitable for studying the amount of adipose tissue.

Fat-selective MRI. In clinical routine, most commonly not the depiction of fat but its selective suppression is of great importance to allow for better conspicuity of lesions, especially in contrast-enhanced MRI [11]. Many different techniques have been developed to achieve this goal. The most widely used technique is chemical-shift selective fat suppression. As described above, the Larmor frequency of a proton depends on the magnetic field it experiences. The external magnetic field (e.g. 1.5 Tesla) can, however, be partly shielded by electrons surrounding the protons

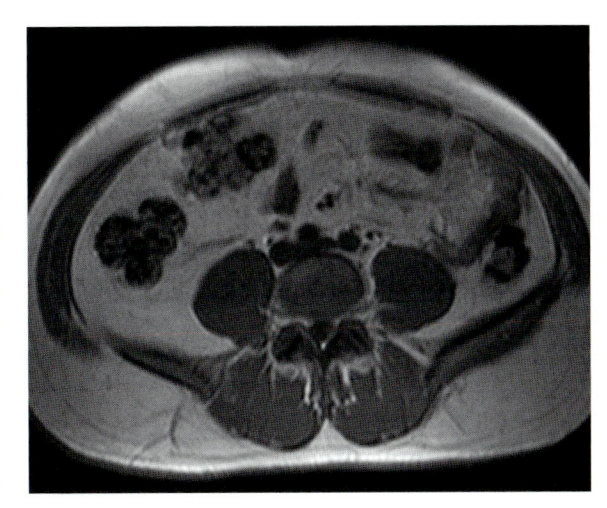

◘ **Fig. 25.4.** Abdominal T1-weighted image (gradient echo sequence) shows bright signal of adipose tissue, while almost all other tissues appear darker. Inhomogeneities are present in the MR signal intensity of fat, e.g., in the gluteal region

that are measured. Thus the local magnetic field and with it the Larmor frequencies of hydrogen nuclei in different molecules differ. The difference between the resonance frequencies of fat and water, the so-called chemical shift, is 3.5 ppm (220 Hz at 1.5 Tesla). Although this shift can be used to selectively suppress the signal from adipose tissue, it can also be exploited to calculate a "water image" and a "fat image" from two signal values for each voxel. In view of the fact that after the radiofrequency pulse the phase of the spins is initially aligned, it becomes evident that due to chemical shift the magnetic vector of fat and water protons inside the same voxel will rapidly dephase. After a certain time they will be displaced by 180° and after the same time span has passed again they will once more be aligned, and so forth. If an image is acquired when the spins of fat and water oppose each other, their signal will be at least partly cancelled, resulting in a decreased signal value for the whole voxel. Such images are termed "opposed-phase images". In contrast, if an image is reconstructed from time points when fat and water spins are aligned, their signal contribution for a whole voxel will be positively combined, leading to increased signal in the so-called in-phase image. The calculation of fat and water maps from in- and opposed-phase image was reported by Dixon in 1984 (◘ Fig. 25.5) [12].

Since its introduction, this technique has experienced many further refinements and variations, rendering it very stable against magnetic field inhomogeneities [13] and allowing for whole-body fat imaging [14]. Although other methods such as inversion recovery [15] or steady-state sequences with ramped flip angles (TIDE) [16] can

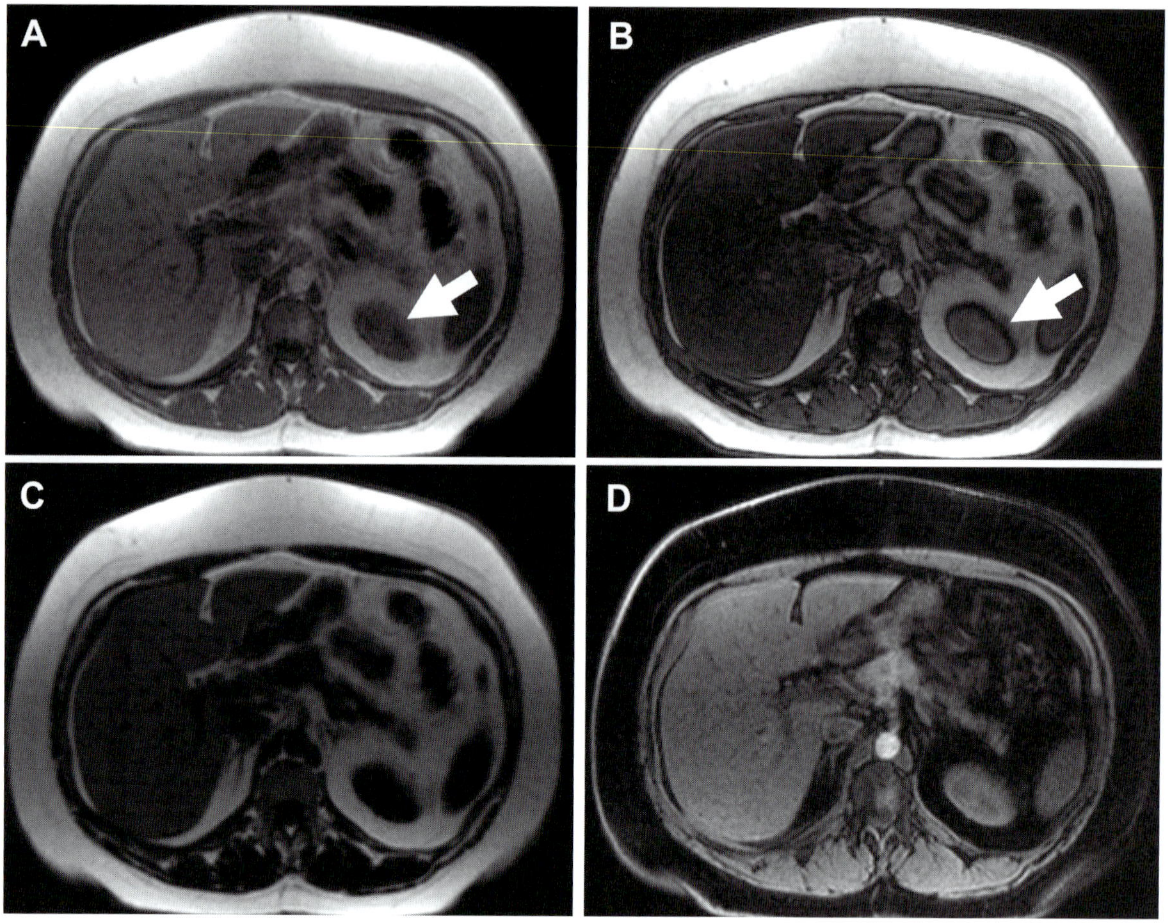

Fig. 25.5A–D. Images from an MR Dixon experiment. Both in-phase image (**A**) and opposed-phase image (**B**) show adipose tissue with bright signal intensity. Voxels that contain both fat and other tissues, e.g., at the boundary of the left kidney (*arrows*), appear bright on in-phase image and dark on opposed-phase image. Calculated "fat" (**C**) and "water" (**D**) images

also be applied to suppress or highlight adipose tissue, variants of the Dixon method are most frequently used and accepted in fat imaging.

Segmentation Techniques

Different segmentation methods can be applied to quantify the amount of adipose tissue from MR or CT images that differ in their degree of automation. In fully manual segmentation all areas being visually identified as consisting of adipose tissue have to be traced by a human operator. Although this approach can readily be performed on a variety of available software tools, it is very cumbersome and time-consuming. Additionally, it is subject to considerable user-dependent variation. On the other hand, the subdivision of adipose tissue in different compartments can easily be conducted by a human operator, whereas the differentiation of different adipose tissue deposits poses a serious challenge for automation. Semi-automatic techniques are therefore often applied in adipose tissue detection and classification. The advantage of the semiautomatic technique is that it makes use of time-saving and precise computer-automated procedures, while at the same time allowing for manual correction to achieve accuracy [17]. Histogram analysis identifies the composition of voxels solely on the basis of their signal value. Although in CT fixed thresholds could in principle be used to identify adipose tissue, in pathological conditions (e.g. lipodystropy) and for MRI in general, the correct threshold can vary between examination, slices, or even different regions within one slice. Region-growing algorithms can partly accommodate for this problem by using a combination of a signal threshold together with signal continuity. From a manually selected seed point all adjacent voxels or pixels are selected that fall in the predefined threshold around the signal of the seed point.

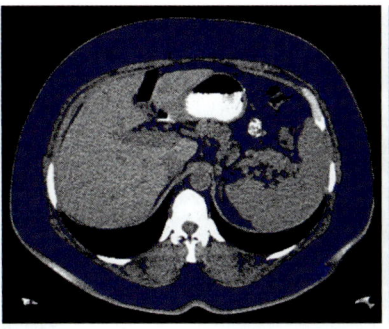 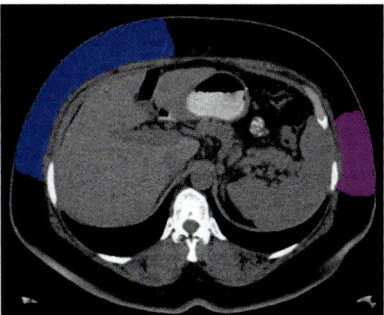 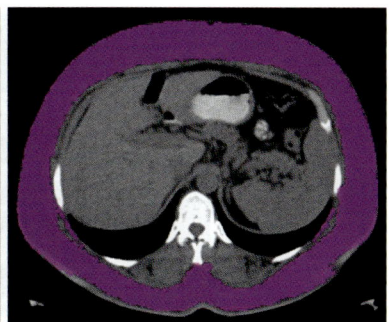

◘ Fig. 25.6. Different segmentation techniques can be applied or combined for adipose tissue quantification. In CT, threshold-based segmentation (*left*) can select the complete amount of tissue within an attenuation range between -200 and -30 HU (*dark blue overlay*). Region growing can be applied to select continuous tissue deposits based on attenuation and connectivity (*middle and right*). Light blue and *magenta* overlays show the segmentation in process started from two different seed points. Finally, in the *right* image the complete subcutaneous tissue compartment has been selected (*magenta*)

With this method contiguous parts of adipose tissue can easily be selected. If the signal variations exceed the threshold or if other tissues are interspersed, more than one seed point per slice is needed to identify the complete tissue compartment. Both histogram analysis and region growing are usually followed by a manual correction step to provide correct segmentation or further subdivision of the identified tissue components (◘ Fig. 25.6).

Several fully automatic approaches have been reported that aim at the segmentation of adipose tissue from CT and MRI data and at the same time differentiate between subcutaneous and visceral adipose tissue [18, 19]. Since, as has been addressed above, a fixed threshold between -190 HU and -30 HU is used for fat identification in CT, MRI data have to be corrected for inhomogeneities by advanced histogram analysis, clustering, and subsequent generation of a fat mask. The contours for subcutaneous and visceral adipose tissue are found mostly by active contour algorithms (◘ Fig. 25.7).

This kind of algorithm starts with many checkpoints confined to a circular contour clearly outside the object. Then the points on the contour move towards the center of the object until a step in signal intensity (from fat to non-fat) is encountered. At the same time, the curvature of the contour serves as a penalty term to ensure a smooth final contour that is less prone to outlier signal changes and insufficient local contour detection. At first the body outline is detected in this fashion. If the contour is allowed to move further inside the body and the criterion for the next signal step is inverted (from non-fat to fat), the contour of VAT can be found. Although these algorithms are very promising because they (a) do not require user interaction, (b) are fast, and (c) offer high reproducibility, they must still be considered prelimi-

nary, and further development and validation are needed before they can be advocated in large trials or clinical routine [20].

Comparison of Single-slice and Volume Measurements

Both MRI and CT can be used to measure single slices and volume datasets. Whereas quantification from volume datasets can be considered the most accurate measure, it is connected with considerably higher acquisition times, the necessity of correction methods for breathing or repeated breath-hold examinations, increased postprocessing effort and, in the case of CT, increased radiation exposure. Therefore, it has been suggested that the area of adipose tissue on one or a small number of axial slices be used as a measure of adipose tissue mass. If such an approach is intended, however, the positioning of the slices must be chosen to closely correlate with volumetric tissue amount. Many studies used the L4–5 level as slice position to quantify visceral and subcutaneous fat, but good correlation with volumetric measurement and the feasibility of detecting sex differences in adipose tissue distribution could not unequivocally be ascertained [21]. Shen et al. compared different single-slice areas of VAT with interpolated volumetric measurements in healthy volunteers with a mean BMI of 27 kg/m^2 and a maximum BMI of 40 kg/m^2. They found that a slice position 10 cm above L4–5 in men and 5 cm above L4–5 in women yielded the highest correlation with VAT volume. They concluded that the use of these corrected levels could increase the power of group comparison studies [22].

Based on these results, it seems sufficient to apply these single-slice measurements to quantify VAT.

25

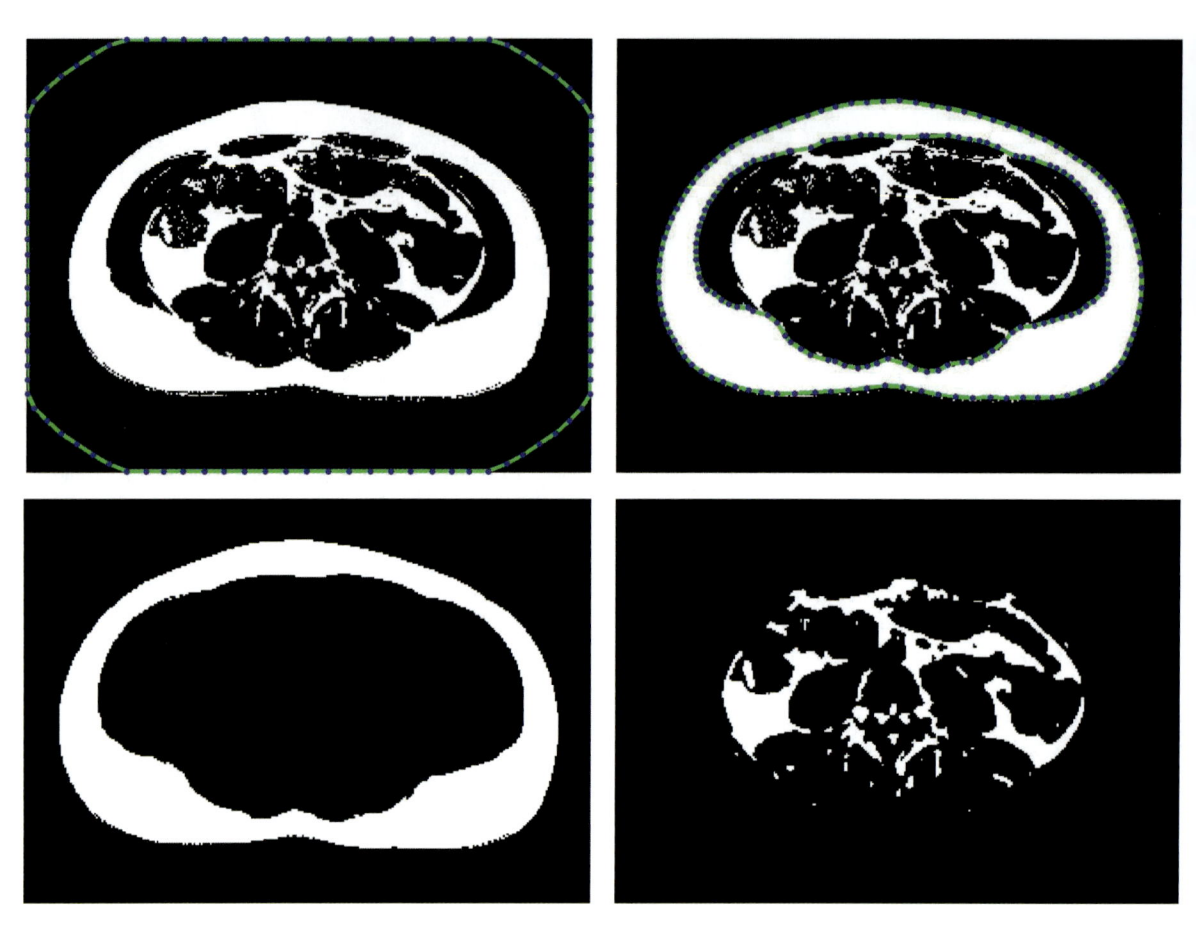

◻ Fig. 25.7. Segmentation with active contours. The procedure starts with many checkpoints located on a loose boundary around the body (*upper left*). Then the contour moves inward to find first the outer border of the body and subsequently the outer fascial contour (*upper right*). From an image that was already pre-segmented for the presence of adipose tissue the subcutaneous and visceral compartments can be calculated (*lower row*)

It should be kept in mind, however, that pathological conditions of fat distribution can interfere with the good correlation in healthy subjects. Commonly, single-slice measurements are also used to quantify other aspects of adipose tissue distribution such as amount of intraperitoneal fat or superficial vs. deep subcutaneous fat, although no established correlation exists between volume and single-slice measurements for categories other than VAT. It seems reasonable to use single-slice measurements for these purposes in interindividual or intergroup comparisons and correlation, but volumetric assessment might provide a more profound insight into the properties of these tissue deposits in the future.

The argument for using single-slice measurements is further strengthened by a good correlation with obesity-related risk parameters such as serum glucose or insulin levels in a large study population [23]. A comparative study between gastric bypass and vertical gastric banding employed single-slice-based adipose tissue areas as one outcome parameter and found no significant differences between the loss of subcutaneous and visceral adipose tissue 1 year after treatment, but there was a significantly higher reduction of adipose tissue areas in the bypass group [24].

Measurement of Ectopic Fat

In lipid homeostasis fat is stored in adipocytes, whereas lipid storage in the lean body mass is minimal and strictly regulated. When this regulation becomes disturbed, as is the case in obesity, intracellular lipids accumulate, for example in the liver, pancreas, muscle, and heart. These instances of intracellular lipid storage are of high pathophysiological interest, as they trigger a cascade of adverse effects that can lead to cell death (lipotoxicity) [25]. Although not readily accessible by standard imaging modalities due to their limited resolution, changes in echogenicity, radiodensity, and proton resonance frequencies can be used to non-invasively detect and measure these ectopic fat accumulations.

Intrahepatic Fat Accumulation. The accumulation of lipids in the liver can be the result of different pathological mechanisms. In obesity the most common form is non-alcoholic fatty liver disease (NAFLD). NAFLD has different stages, ranging from steatosis (non-alcoholic fatty liver, NAFL) to an intermediate form, called steatohepatitis, and finally to liver cirrhosis [26]. NAFLD is the most common cause of elevated liver enzymes in the United States [27] and constitutes the hepatic manifestation of the metabolic syndrome [28]. Insulin resistance, often associated with severe obesity, reduces the uptake of free fatty acids by adipocytes and at the same time leads to an increased synthesis of triglycerides in hepatocytes, accompanied by decreased oxidation of fatty acids. It is currently being discussed whether the formation of triglycerides from free fatty acids is part of the pathological process itself or can be considered a protective mechanism, as incorporation of fatty acids in triglycerides can have a detoxifiying effect [26].

The gold standard for measuring hepatic fat is biopsy, but the procedural risks comprise infection, hematoma, internal bleeding, and biliary leakage, as well the inherently large sampling error. Therefore, non-invasive methods for measuring fatty infiltration in the liver are generally used. Ultrasound, CT, MRI, and MR spectroscopy can be applied in this respect [29].

Ultrasound is widely used to evaluate hepatic steatosis. Fatty infiltration leads to an increased echogenicity of the liver parenchyma, which normally is assessed in visual comparison to the echogenicity of the cortex of the kidney. Ultrasound, however, cannot discriminate between fat accumulation and other causes of increased echogenicity, e.g. fibrosis. This has promoted the term "fatty fibrotic pattern". Although a sensitivity of 99% and a specificity of 94% have been reported to successfully detect this pattern [30], in general, the effectiveness of ultrasound is reduced in obese patients, resulting in a greatly decreased sensitivity of 49% and a specificity of 75% [31]. Furthermore, ultrasound seems to be less sensitive than other methods in determining the grade of steatosis, and it has been suggested that ultrasound is unlikely to correctly detect longitudinal changes in hepatic fat content between 20% and 40% due to successful intervention [32].

Computed tomography is very accurate in detecting steatosis, based on a difference of less than +4 HU between the liver and the spleen on unenhanced scans. With further decrease in hepatic radiodensity due to the accumulation of triglycerides and cholesterol, the vessels appear brighter than the surrounding parenchyma (◘ Fig. 25.8).

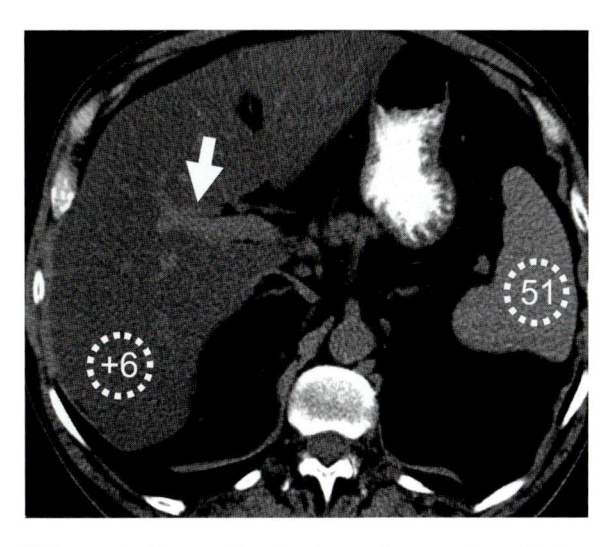

◘ **Fig. 25.8.** In this case of fatty liver disease the attenuation of the liver is decreased to only *6 HU*, resulting in the "bright" appearance of the intrahepatic vessels (*arrow*). In comparison, the spleen retains its normal attenuation values, resulting in a liver-spleen difference of *-45 HU*

Although the radiodensity of the liver itself, measured in HU, and the ratio between liver and spleen parenchyma have been shown to inversely correlate with the grade of steatosis in biopsy, it is still being debated whether CT is accurate enough to quantify hepatic fat content [29, 33].

In MRI the chemical shift can be exploited to create in-phase and opposed-phase images. Whereas in in-phase images the signals from water and fat hydrogen nuclei are positively combined, their signals partly cancel each other on opposed-phase images (see ◘ Fig. 25.5). This effect can be used to detect and quantify the fat content in the liver with good correlation to biopsy [32]. MRI may therefore evolve into a reliable tool to non-invasively measure steatosis without ionizing radiation.

MR spectroscopy can be used to directly measure the signal contributions of nuclei over a continuous range of chemical shifts in a predefined voxel. By comparing the area under the lipid peak with the area under the water peak in the resulting spectra, the fat content can be quantified. This percentage hepatic lipid content measured by MR spectroscopy has been shown to correlate with biopsy in patients with NAFLD [34], and MRS has been used to determine the presence of NAFLD in a large population study [35].

To date, several studies have shown the reduction of NAFLD associated with weight loss after bariatric surgery. It has been suggested that resolution of non-alcoholic steatohepatitis and the metabolic syndrome are correlated with the loss of fat mass and that malabsorptive interventions have more impact than restrictive methods [36–39].

To date, most studies rely on blood tests and liver biopsy to determine the presence and severity of NAFLD, but in a recent study that applied MRS and MRI a significant reduction of hepatic fat content was shown 3 months after gastric banding [40]. Changes in hepatic fat were more closely correlated with the reduction of serum gamma-glutamyl transferase than were anthropomorphic measures. The described imaging procedures, especially MRI and MRS, will allow for safe, accurate, and reliable measurement of hepatic steatosis in future longitudinal investigations.

Intramuscular Fat Accumulation. The increase in intramuscular triglycerides (IMTG) has been associated with obesity, aging, insulin resistance, and type-2 diabetes [41]. Although the term "intramuscular triglycerides" is generally used to describe fat accumulation in the skeletal muscle, it must be discriminated between storage of lipids in the myocytes themselves and adipose tissue interspersed between the muscle cells. In addition to the localization of lipids in the muscular tissue their composition must be determined. The amount of saturated and unsaturated fatty acids and the presence of metabolites such as ceramides have to be considered. It has been shown, for example, that ceramide content and the fraction of ceramides composed of saturated fatty acids was reduced in obese individuals after exercise training, whereas total IMTG content was unchanged [42]. Depending on the type of analysis, the term "intramyocellular lipids (IMCL)" should be preferred.

Although biopsy, histochemical staining, and electron microscopy are the methods of choice to extensively study IMTGs, imaging modalities such as CT, MRI, and MRS can contribute significantly to non-invasive measurement of IMTG content.

Computed tomography can detect adipose tissue that is interspersed in skeletal muscle on the basis of its high spatial resolution and the negative attenuation values of fat (-190 to -30 HU) compared with the positive attenuation of muscle itself. If lipids are incorporated in the muscle cells the attenuation of the muscle will decrease. It has been shown that the signal loss of muscle is correlated with its content of IMCL, as measured by MRS with excellent reliability [43].

Proton MRS can differentiate between intramyocellular and extramyocellular lipids based on the slight differences in chemical shift between lipid protons according to their surrounding tissue [44]. As it is non-invasive and does not use ionizing radiation, MRS is a suitable tool for longitudinal studies over time, with changes above 15% in IMTG content being detectable [45]. It should also be mentioned here that the use of proton MRS, as well as of ^{13}C and ^{31}P MRS, has significantly helped in determining the cellular mechanism of insulin resistance in type-2 diabetes [46]. The IMCL signal in MRS is dependent on the orientation of the muscle fibers, however, and great care must be taken to conduct the examination correctly. Furthermore, only certain muscle groups, especially in the lower leg, are accessible via MRS.

MRI using standard T1-weighted images with their inherently high signal intensity for fat can also be employed to determine adipose tissue in muscles, but it is limited by resolution and the lack of specificity of the signal intensity for fat. Special imaging techniques have been developed that allow for accurate fat mapping, however. Compared with MRS, correlation coefficients between 0.55 and 0.91 were achieved in the calf [47].

Adiposity of the Heart. Obesity is traditionally considered to be an indirect cause of heart disease. As obese individuals often present with several Framingham risk factors such as hypertension, dyslipidemia, and diabetes, they show an increased risk for myocardial infarction and ischemic cardiomyopathy. Additionally, obesity is related to increased stroke volume and heart rate, which in extreme obesity can progress to non-ischemic dilated cardiomyopathy.

However, it has been shown that besides these traditional explanations, the accumulation of lipids in the myocardium in obese individuals has a direct lipotoxic effect that eventually causes non-ischemic dilated cardiomyopathy [48]. As has been described for the liver and skeletal muscle, MRS can also be used to measure the triglyceride content in the myocardium. In comparison to the skeletal muscle, however, respiratory and cardiac motion is a major obstacle to this technique. Furthermore, the heart is surrounded by an epicardial fat pad that could interfere with accurate quantification. To overcome these limitations, triggering techniques are employed to accommodate for motion artifacts, and the volume of interest is placed in the septum to avoid epicardial influences. Measurement in the end-systole ensures that the septum exhibits its largest diameter during the cardiac cycle, thereby avoiding influences from the adjacent ventricles (◘ Fig. 25.9) [49].

In contrast to the liver, triglyceride levels were increased in the myocardium due to short-term caloric restriction, whereas a high caloric diet did not affect myocardial triglyceride content [50]. In obesity, which represents a long-term dyslipidemic condition, the myocardial fat content, however, increases progressively with BMI [49].

In 60 obese patients Roux-en-Y gastric bypass surgery led to a decrease of left ventricular wall thickness and concomitantly improved left ventricular function early and 3 years after surgery [51].

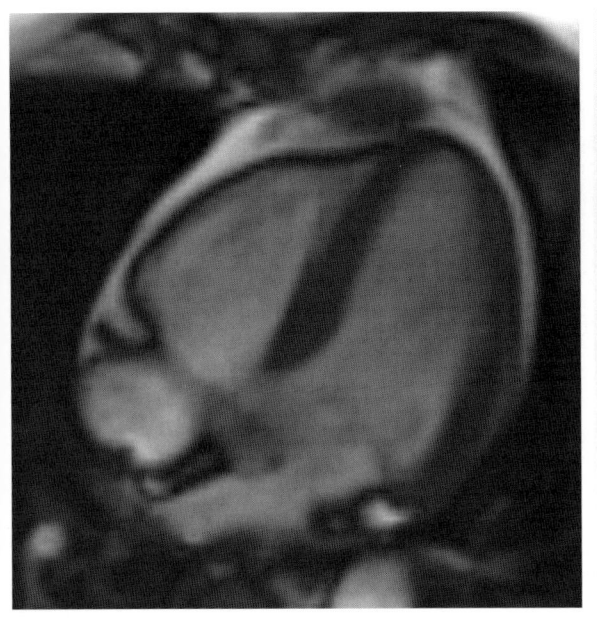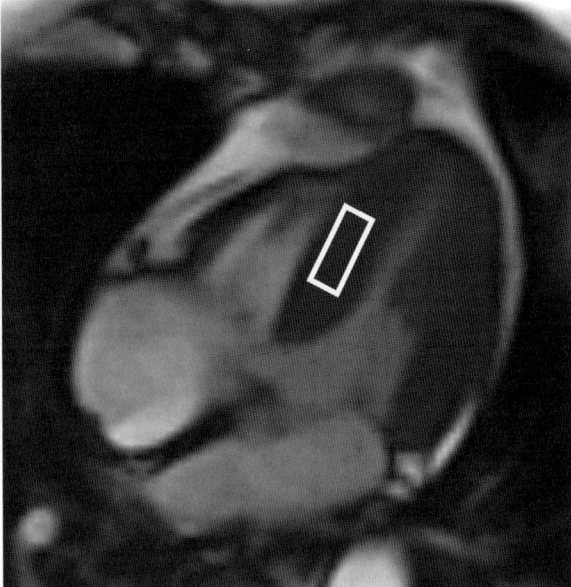

◘ Fig. 25.9. Images from a cine MR sequence of the heart during diastole (*left*) and systole (*right*). Note the thickened septum during systole. This is exploited to plan the region of interest for MR spectroscopy (*rectangle*) in order to avoid ventricular cross-talk

25.2 Abdominal Imaging after Metabolic Surgery

Besides quantification of adipose tissue by cross-sectional imaging modalities, imaging in bariatric patients is frequently performed after surgery either to rule out complications or to assess technical success criteria such as pouch size. Especially if weight regain or insufficient weight loss occur, imaging can provide information about whether restriction is still provided by the changes previously introduced to the gastrointestinal tract. Whereas the search for such complications as ileus or leakage, foremost early after surgery, is a well-known task for abdominal radiologists, the assessment of technical success criteria and some late complications requires good knowledge of the applied procedure and typical anatomical changes found after surgery.

25.2.1 Abdominal CT after Bariatric Surgery

If postoperative complications or technical failure of the procedure are clinically suspected, CT is applied to search for intestinal and extraintestinal complications at our institution. Although fluoroscopy is often applied after bariatric surgery, it suffers from considerable drawbacks. A routine upper gastrointestinal (UGI) series with water-soluble contrast material on the first day after surgery has been used extensively. The main reasons for this approach were to exclude leakage from the gastrojejunostomy and to assess the pouch size. However, the absence of extraintestinal contrast material on a fluoroscopy examination does not sufficiently rule out the presence of leakage, if clinical symptoms are indicative. Furthermore, the formation of the pouch is a highly standardized procedure at most bariatric surgery centers. If no problems during the procedure are reported by the surgeon, a markedly increased pouch size does not have to be expected early after surgery. Therefore, a routine UGI series is not performed at our institution.

For the CT examination oral contrast material should be applied in all cases, and an antiperistaltic agent is used to allow for better distension of the pouch and the Roux limb. Intravenous contrast material is mandatory in all cases of an acute clinical presentation or elevated inflammatory markers. If the examination is used only to assess the dimensions of the pouch during follow-up more than several weeks after surgery, the application of intravenous contrast material can be omitted. Image reconstruction should in all cases include axial images with a maximum slice thickness of 5 mm and coronal images. Images with a lower slice thickness (1–2 mm) offer the possibility of freely angulated multiplanar reconstructions and three-dimensional post-processing, both of which can be very helpful.

25

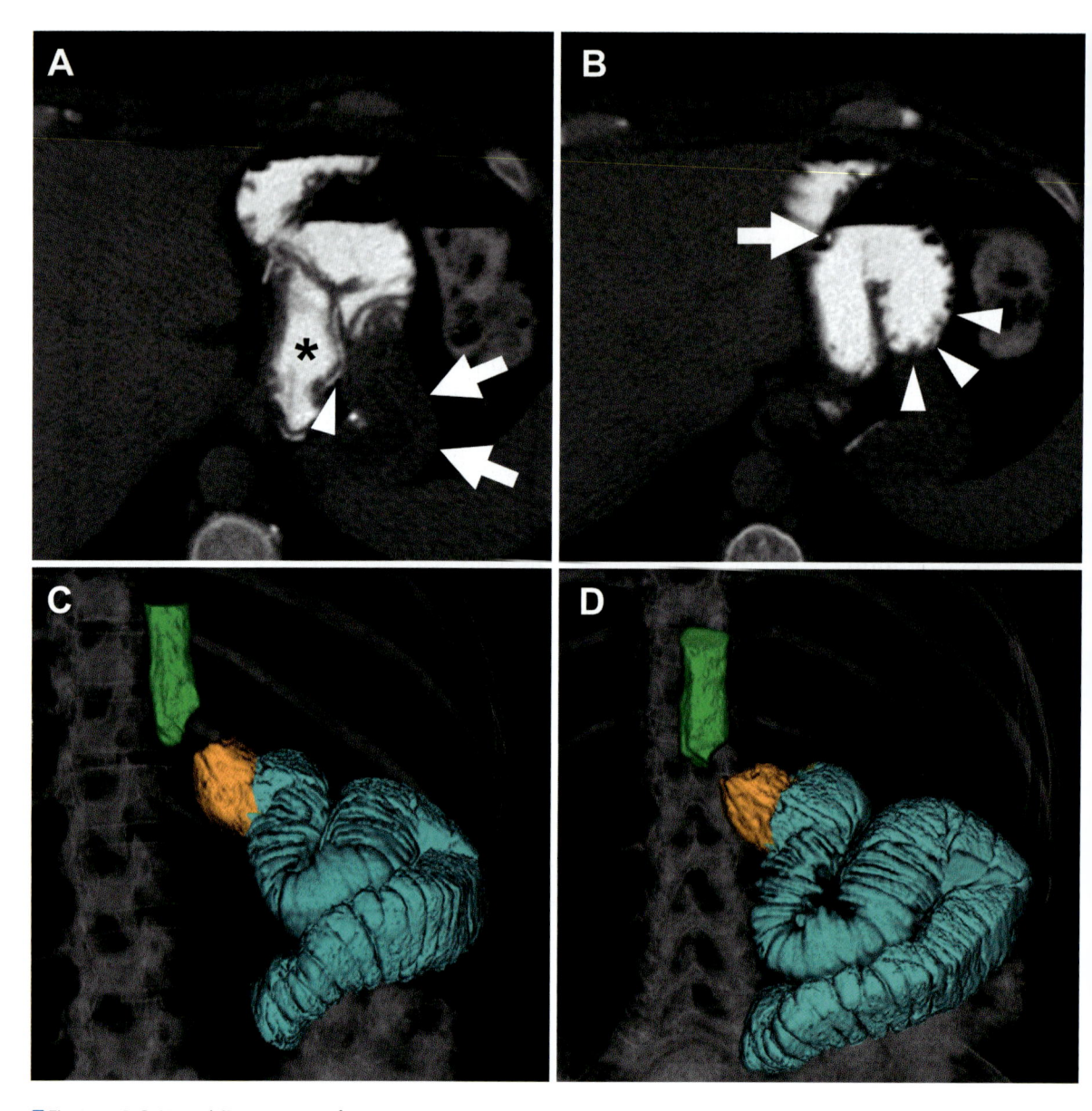

❏ **Fig. 25.10A–D.** Normal CT appearance after Roux-en-Y gastric bypass. **A** An axial slice at the level of the pouch (*asterisk*) shows the suture lines (*arrowhead*) that separate the pouch from the remnant stomach (*arrows*), which is not reached by oral contrast material. **B** Below the position of the first slice, the gastrojejunostomy can be seen. It is still partly surrounded by stapler lines (*arrow*). A small stump of the Roux-limb (*arrowheads*) is a normal finding. **C, D** Volume-rendering images in a different patient give a nice overview of the esophagus (*green*), the pouch (*orange*) and the jejunal limb (*cyan*)

Correct interpretation of imaging results in a given patient depends greatly on accurate information about the bariatric procedure performed and the reason for the examination. Therefore, in addition to general information on the current presentation of the patient and the actual question leading to the imaging test, a radiologist in a metabolic surgery team needs to have access to the following data:

- Which procedure was performed?
- When was the procedure performed?
- How were the anastomoses sewn (by hand or stapler)?
- Did the patient have prior abdominal surgery, especially other bariatric procedures?
- Have any complications occurred so far?
- Has the patient lost weight successfully?
- Has there been recent weight regain?

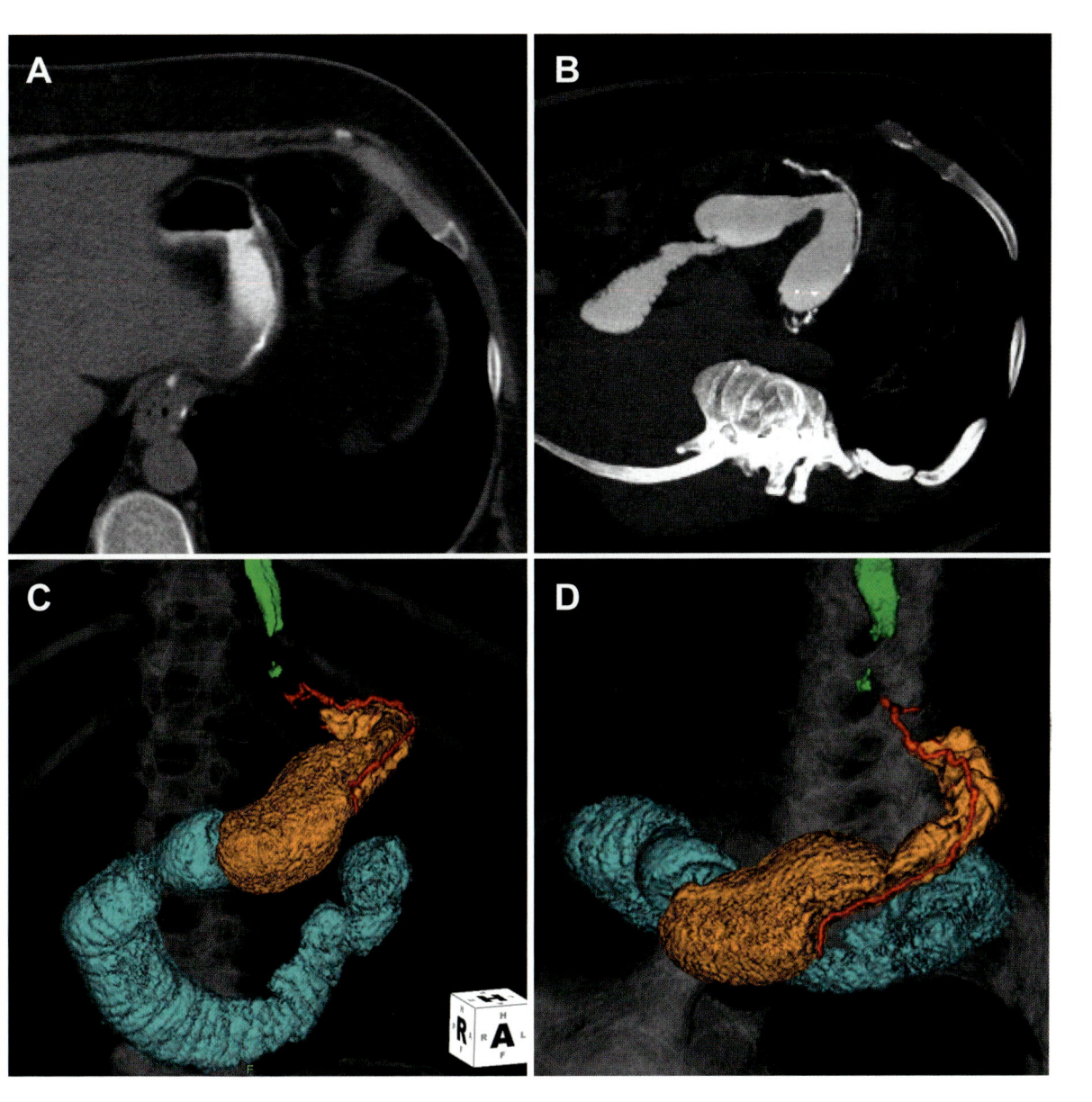

■ **Fig. 25.11A–D.** Normal CT appearance after sleeve gastrectomy. **A** An axial slice at the level of the corpus shows the narrow "Magenstrasse" delineated by the stapler line. As the stomach does not reside on one single plane inside the body, the sleeve is hard to capture on one slice. **B** A double-oblique MIP image shows the stomach in almost its full extent with the stapler line ending approximately 6 cm lateral to the pylorus. **C, D** Volume-rendering images in a different patient show a nice overview of the esophagus (*green*), the stomach (*orange*), the duodenum (*cyan*) and the stapler line (*red*)

— Does the patient suffer from repeated nausea or vomiting?
— Did the patient have a feeling of satiety after surgery, and is it still present or did it diminish over time?

■ Figure 25.10 shows the general appearance after gastric bypass, ■ Fig. 25.11 that after sleeve gastrectomy. Biliopancreatic diversion with duodenal switch basically exhibits

the same morphology as sleeve gastrectomy for the stomach, followed by an end-to-end gastrojejunostomy.

25.2.2 Pouch Size

Many bariatric procedures include restriction of the gastric volume by building a small stomach pouch or sleeve.

Adjustable gastric banding consists of an inflatable band around the stomach with creation of a small pouch with a narrow outlet [52]. Outlet diameter, but not stomach pouch size, can be controlled by saline injections into a subcutaneous reservoir. Dilatation of the pouch is inversely correlated with weight loss, and reduction of outlet diameter is less effective in patients with large pouches [53]. Concerning gastric bypass operations, the average volume of the gastric pouch should be 10–30 ml [54]. Roberts et al. have observed a negative correlation between pouch size and weight loss 6 and 12 months after the operation [55]. Pouch dilation has also been described as a late complication [56]. In sleeve gastrectomy the volume of the remaining sleeve should be about 100 ml, which is controlled by using a calibration tube during the procedure [57]. Krawczykowski found that weight reduction after biliopancreatic diversion (BPD), which in the case of duodenal switch (BPD DS) involves a sleeve gastrectomy, is strongly influenced by the volume of the sleeve (presentation, "sleeve gastrectomy" symposium & workshop, Elancourt, France 2008).

Apart from such patient-dependent factors as proper diet and regular sport activities, it is therefore crucial to assess whether restriction is still sufficient if insufficient loss of weight or even regain of weight occurs, because in case of insufficient restriction a re-operation may be necessary [58].

A variety of methods have been proposed for the measurement of pouch volume. In 1996, Flanagan employed the amount of ingested cottage cheese to estimate a functional pouch volume [59]. Endoscopic techniques have also been described. The oral-aboral extension of the pouch can be measured by retraction of the endoscope, while the transverse diameter can only be estimated. Forsell et al. presented a classification system in which pouch volume after gastric banding was estimated according to the visual aspect of the pouch and the distance between the cardia and the band. This system showed good correlations with MRI and barium swallow results [55]. An advantage of the endoscopic examination is the possibility of inspecting and diagnosing the pouch, the stoma, and the mucosa, as well as making a semi-quantitative measurement of the stoma diameter [37]. Most commonly, fluoroscopy is used to evaluate pouch size. This approach, however, is encumbered by projection of the sometimes complicated three-dimensional pouch volume in two planes or even a single plane, as lateral radiographs often cannot be taken due to the patient's size. Thus, although fluoroscopy is generally considered a standard method in patients after bariatric surgery, great care must be taken with this technique for a truly quantitative assessment. Consequently, inconsistent reports can be found

in the literature. While Roberts et al. found a correlation between pouch area in anteroposterior radiographs and excess weight loss after RnYGB [60, 61], other studies did not elucidate a correlation between pouch size on UGI contrast studies and postoperative weight loss [62].

Therefore, we developed a CT examination protocol that combines thin-section CT images acquired with oral contrast material and antiperistalis with state-of-the-art three-dimensional post-processing to accurately quantify the pouch volume and the area of the gastrojejunostomy. Early results demonstrate many cases of enlarged gastric pouches and a dilation of the gastrojejunostomy in patients with insufficient weight loss or weight regain [63]. The accurate depiction of the pouch and the adjacent intestinal structures not only allows for volumetric assessment but can also provide insight into the process of dilation and can influence the choice of eligible rescue procedures, although further studies are required for confirmation (◘ Fig. 25.12).

25.2.3 Stomach Motility

Although mechanical restriction and variation of the flow of food through the gastrointestinal tract is a hallmark of bariatric surgery, only little information is yet available on the influence of bariatric surgery on stomach motility. MRI has repeatedly been recognized as an ideal tool in this respect, because of three major advantages: (1) MRI offers high contrast between the stomach wall and fluid inside the stomach; (2) high temporal and spatial resolution can be achieved with modern MR imaging; and (3) due to the lack of radiation, repeated examinations can be performed. Steady-state free-precession (SSFP) sequences are most commonly applied in this respect, and recent advantages in parallel acquisition have further improved the temporal resolution.

Different parameters can be assessed by specialized MRI for the stomach. Multislice sequences are employed to study the volume of the stomach. Due to fast acquisition with single-shot or SSFP sequences, the entire stomach can be covered during a single breath-hold. This technique has been used to characterize the process of gastric emptying under different conditions [64]. Dynamic imaging with a temporal resolution of approximately 1 s allows for the repeated acquisition of up to three slices, producing a video-clip-like image series (◘ Fig. 25.13).

Either free breathing or repeated breath-hold scanning can be used to study the peristaltic waves in the stomach. Frequency, amplitude, width, occlusion, and speed of antral waves can be analyzed with this technique [65]. More advanced protocols have been used to study gastric relaxation and secretion.

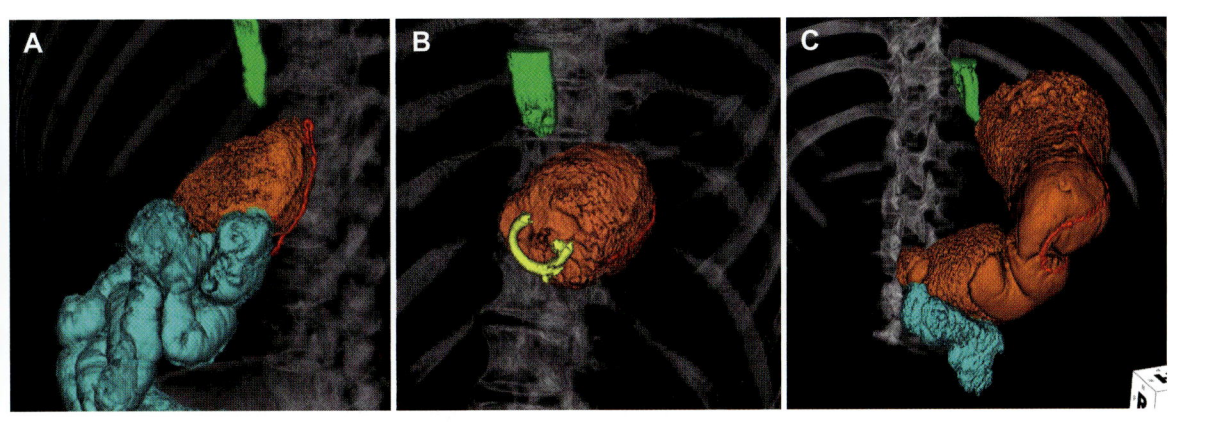

◻ **Fig. 25.12A–C.** Examples of pathological pouch conditions found during follow-up after bariatric surgery. Dilation of the pouch is most common, either as a single finding or combined with a widened gastrojejunostomy. **A** In the first case the pouch size was increased to 120 ml and the gastrojejunostomy showed a maximum diameter of 3.3 cm. **B** In the second case a Fobi ring was introduced to reinforce restriction following dilation to 90 ml pouch size. Follow-up shows an opening of the ring (*yellow*). **C** The last case shows a dramatically enlarged stomach. The *red* suture line and the course of the proximal bowel indicate that the patient had received prior sleeve gastrectomy and BPD-DS. Nevertheless, the stomach was re-enlarged, almost to its original size, with a volume >600 ml

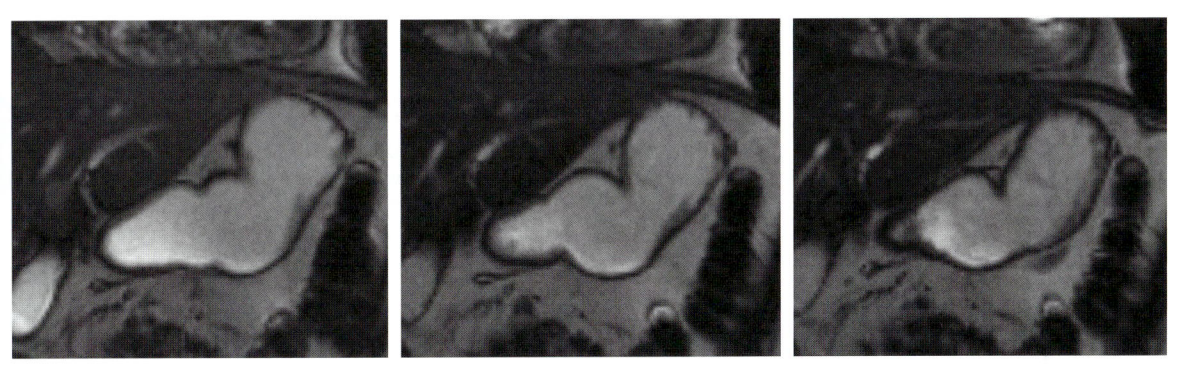

◻ **Fig. 25.13.** Representative images from a cine MR experiment. The patient drank 500 ml water before imaging and the time span between images is approximately 6 s. The propagation of the antral waves can be followed nicely

Given that these techniques render MRI a useful tool for the analysis of stomach motility, and despite the fact that bariatric surgery might dramatically affect this process, MRI has not yet been used in this respect. Interesting future insights into the effects of bariatric surgery can be expected.

References

1. Shuldiner AR, Yang R, Gong DW (2001) Resistin, obesity and insulin resistance – the emerging role of the adipocyte as an endocrine organ. N Engl J Med 345:1345–1346
2. Shen W, Wang Z, Punyanita M, et al (2003) Adipose tissue quantification by imaging methods: a proposed classification. Obes Res 11:5–16
3. Snyder WS, Cook MJ, Nasset ES, Karhausen RL, Howells GP, Tipton IH (1975) Report of the Task Group on Reference Man. In: Press UP, ed. ICRP Publication 23. Oxford, pp 40–45
4. Tothill P, Han TS, Avenell A, McNeill G, Reid DM (1996) Comparisons between fat measurements by dual-energy X-ray absorptiometry, underwater weighing and magnetic resonance imaging in healthy women. Eur J Clin Nutr 50:747–752
5. Kelley DE, Thaete FL, Troost F, Huwe T, Goodpaster BH (2000) Subdivisions of subcutaneous abdominal adipose tissue and insulin resistance. Am J Physiol Endocrinol Metab 278:E941–948
6. Marchington JM, Mattacks CA, Pond CM (1989) Adipose tissue in the mammalian heart and pericardium: structure, foetal development and biochemical properties. Comp Biochem Physiol B 94:225–232
7. Bjorntorp P (1990) "Portal" adipose tissue as a generator of risk factors for cardiovascular disease and diabetes. Arteriosclerosis 10:493–496

8. Jackson AS, Stanforth PR, Gagnon J, et al (2002) The effect of sex, age and race on estimating percentage body fat from body mass index: The Heritage Family Study. Int J Obes Relat Metab Disord 26:789–796

9. Snijder MB, van Dam RM, Visser M, Seidell JC (2006) What aspects of body fat are particularly hazardous and how do we measure them? Int J Epidemiol 35:83–92

10. Haacke EM, Brown RW, Thompson MR, Venkatesan R (1999) Magnetic resonance imaging: physical principles and sequence design. J. Wiley & Sons, New York

11. Frahm J, Haase A, Hanicke W, Matthaei D, Bomsdorf H, Helzel T (1985) Chemical shift selective MR imaging using a whole-body magnet. Radiology 156:441–444

12. Dixon WT (1984) Simple proton spectroscopic imaging. Radiology 153:189–194

13. Glover GH (1991) Multipoint Dixon technique for water and fat proton and susceptibility imaging. J Magn Reson Imaging 1:521–530

14. Sommer G, Fautz HP, Ludwig U, Hennig J (2006) Multicontrast sequences with continuous table motion: a novel acquisition technique for extended field of view imaging. Magn Reson Med 55:918–922

15. Bydder GM, Young IR (1985) MR imaging: clinical use of the inversion recovery sequence. J Comput Assist Tomogr 9:659–675

16. Paul D, Hennig J, Zaitsev M (2006) Intrinsic fat suppression in TIDE balanced steady-state free precession imaging. Magn Reson Med 56:1328–1335

17. Shen W, Chen J (2008) Application of imaging and other noninvasive techniques in determining adipose tissue mass. Methods Mol Biol 456:39–54

18. Ohshima S, Yamamoto S, Yamaji T, et al (2008) Development of an automated 3D segmentation program for volume quantification of body fat distribution using CT. Nippon Hoshasen Gijutsu Gakkai Zasshi 64:1177–1181

19. Positano V, Cusi K, Santarelli MF, et al (2008) Automatic correction of intensity inhomogeneities improves unsupervised assessment of abdominal fat by MRI. J Magn Reson Imaging 28:403–410

20. Bonekamp S, Ghosh P, Crawford S, et al (2008) Quantitative comparison and evaluation of software packages for assessment of abdominal adipose tissue distribution by magnetic resonance imaging. Int J Obes (Lond) 32:100–111

21. Sumner AE, Farmer NM, Tulloch-Reid MK, et al (2002) Sex differences in visceral adipose tissue volume among African Americans. Am J Clin Nutr 76:975–979

22. Shen W, Punyanitya M, Wang Z, et al (2004) Visceral adipose tissue: relations between single-slice areas and total volume. Am J Clin Nutr 80:271–278

23. Shen W, Punyanitya M, Chen J, et al (2007) Visceral adipose tissue: relationships between single slice areas at different locations and obesity-related health risks. Int J Obes (Lond) 31:763–769

24. Olbers T, Bjorkman S, Lindroos A, et al (2006) Body composition, dietary intake, and energy expenditure after laparoscopic Roux-en-Y gastric bypass and laparoscopic vertical banded gastroplasty: a randomized clinical trial. Ann Surg 244:715–722

25. Unger RH (2003) Minireview: weapons of lean body mass destruction: the role of ectopic lipids in the metabolic syndrome. Endocrinology 144:5159–5165

26. Choi SS, Diehl AM (2008) Hepatic triglyceride synthesis and nonalcoholic fatty liver disease. Curr Opin Lipidol 19:295–300

27. Angulo P (2002) Nonalcoholic fatty liver disease. N Engl J Med 346:1221–1231

28. Pagano G, Pacini G, Musso G, et al (2002) Nonalcoholic steatohepatitis, insulin resistance, and metabolic syndrome: further evidence for an etiologic association. Hepatology 35:367–372

29. Mehta SR, Thomas EL, Bell JD, Johnston DG, Taylor-Robinson SD (2008) Non-invasive means of measuring hepatic fat content. World J Gastroenterol 14:3476–3483

30. Needleman L, Kurtz AB, Rifkin MD, Cooper HS, Pasto ME, Goldberg BB (1986) Sonography of diffuse benign liver disease: accuracy of pattern recognition and grading. AJR Am J Roentgenol 146:1011–1015

31. Mottin CC, Moretto M, Padoin AV, et al (2004) The role of ultrasound in the diagnosis of hepatic steatosis in morbidly obese patients. Obes Surg 14:635–637

32. Fishbein M, Castro F, Cheruku S, et al (2005) Hepatic MRI for fat quantitation: its relationship to fat morphology, diagnosis, and ultrasound. J Clin Gastroenterol 39:619–625

33. Park SH, Kim PN, Kim KW, et al (2006) Macrovesicular hepatic steatosis in living liver donors: use of CT for quantitative and qualitative assessment. Radiology 239:105–112

34. Longo R, Pollesello P, Ricci C, et al (1995) Proton MR spectroscopy in quantitative in vivo determination of fat content in human liver steatosis. J Magn Reson Imaging 5:281–285

35. Browning JD, Szczepaniak LS, Dobbins R, et al (2004) Prevalence of hepatic steatosis in an urban population in the United States: impact of ethnicity. Hepatology 40:1387–1395

36. Barker KB, Palekar NA, Bowers SP, Goldberg JE, Pulcini JP, Harrison SA (2006) Non-alcoholic steatohepatitis: effect of Roux-en-Y gastric bypass surgery. Am J Gastroenterol 101:368–373

37. Frige F, Laneri M, Veronelli A, et al (2009) Bariatric surgery in obesity: changes of glucose and lipid metabolism correlate with changes of fat mass. Nutr Metab Cardiovasc Dis 19:198–204

38. Klein S, Mittendorfer B, Eagon JC, et al(2006) Gastric bypass surgery improves metabolic and hepatic abnormalities associated with nonalcoholic fatty liver disease. Gastroenterology 130:1564–1572

39. Nugent C, Bai C, Elariny H, et al (2008) Metabolic syndrome after laparoscopic bariatric surgery. Obes Surg 18:1278–1286

40. Phillips ML, Boase S, Wahlroos S, et al (2008) Associates of change in liver fat content in the morbidly obese after laparoscopic gastric banding surgery. Diabetes Obes Metab 10:661–667

41. Dube J, Goodpaster BH (2006) Assessment of intramuscular triglycerides: contribution to metabolic abnormalities. Curr Opin Clin Nutr Metab Care 9:553–559

42. Bruce CR, Thrush AB, Mertz VA, et al (2006) Endurance training in obese humans improves glucose tolerance and mitochondrial fatty acid oxidation and alters muscle lipid content. Am J Physiol Endocrinol Metab 291:E99–E107

43. Larson-Meyer DE, Smith SR, Heilbronn LK, Kelley DE, Ravussin E, Newcomer BR (2006) Muscle-associated triglyceride measured by computed tomography and magnetic resonance spectroscopy. Obesity (Silver Spring) 14:73–87

44. Boesch C, Slotboom J, Hoppeler H, Kreis R (1997) In vivo determination of intra-myocellular lipids in human muscle by means of localized 1H-MR-spectroscopy. Magn Reson Med 37:484–493

45. Torriani M, Thomas BJ, Halpern EF, Jensen ME, Rosenthal DI, Palmer WE (2005) Intramyocellular lipid quantification: repeatability with 1H MR spectroscopy. Radiology 236:609–614

46. Shulman GI (2004) Unraveling the cellular mechanism of insulin resistance in humans: new insights from magnetic resonance spectroscopy. Physiology (Bethesda) 19:183–190

47. Schick F, Machann J, Brechtel K, et al (2002) MRI of muscular fat. Magn Reson Med 47:720–727

48. McGavock JM, Victor RG, Unger RH, Szczepaniak LS (2006) Adiposity of the heart, revisited. Ann Intern Med 144:517–524

49. Szczepaniak LS, Dobbins RL, Metzger GJ, et al (2003) Myocardial triglycerides and systolic function in humans: in vivo evaluation by localized proton spectroscopy and cardiac imaging. Magn Reson Med 49:417–423

50. Lamb HJ, Smit JW, van der Meer RW, et al (2008) Metabolic MRI of myocardial and hepatic triglyceride content in response to nutritional interventions. Curr Opin Clin Nutr Metab Care 11:573–579

51. Ikonomidis I, Mazarakis A, Papadopoulos C, et al (2007) Weight loss after bariatric surgery improves aortic elastic properties and left ventricular function in individuals with morbid obesity: a 3-year follow-up study. J Hypertens 25:439–447

52. Favretti F, Segato G, De Marchi F, et al (2002) An adjustable silicone gastric band for laparoscopic treatment of morbid obesity – technique and results. Surg Technol Int 10:109–114

53. Forsell P (1996) Pouch volume, stoma diameter and weight loss in Swedish adjustable gastric banding (SAGB). Obes Surg 6:468–473

54. Madan AK, Harper JL, Tichansky DS (2008) Techniques of laparoscopic gastric bypass: on-line survey of American Society for Bariatric Surgery practicing surgeons. Surg Obes Relat Dis 4:166–172; discussion 172–163

55. Roberts K, Duffy A, Kaufman J, Burrell M, Dziura J, Bell R (2007) Size matters: gastric pouch size correlates with weight loss after laparoscopic Roux-en-Y gastric bypass. Surg Endosc 21:1397–1402

56. Schwartz RW, Strodel WE, Simpson WS, Griffen WO, jr (1988) Gastric bypass revision: lessons learned from 920 cases. Surgery 104:806–812

57. Johnston D, Dachtler J, Sue-Ling HM, King RF, Martin G (2003) The Magenstrasse and Mill operation for morbid obesity. Obes Surg 13:10–16

58. Flanagan L (1996) Measurement of functional pouch volume following the gastric bypass procedure. Obes Surg 6:38–43

59. Forsell P, Hellers G, Laveskog U, Westman L (1996) Validation of pouch size measurement following the Swedish adjustable gastric banding using endoscopy, MRI and barium swallow. Obes Surg 6:463–467

60. Nishie A, Brown B, Barloon T, Kuehn D, Samuel I (2007) Comparison of size of proximal gastric pouch and short-term weight loss following routine upper gastrointestinal contrast study after laparoscopic Roux-en-Y gastric bypass. Obes Surg 17:1183–1188

61. Madan AK, Tichansky DS, Phillips JC (2007) Does pouch size matter? Obes Surg 17:317–320

62. Karcz WK, Kuesters S, Marjanovic G, et al 3D-MSCT (2009) Gastric pouch volumetry in bariatric surgery – preliminary clinical results. Obes Surg 19:508–516

63. Goetze O, Steingoetter A, Menne D, et al (2007) The effect of macronutrients on gastric volume responses and gastric emptying in humans: A magnetic resonance imaging study. Am J Physiol Gastrointest Liver Physiol 292:G11–17

64. Kwiatek MA, Steingoetter A, Pal A, et al (2006) Quantification of distal antral contractile motility in healthy human stomach with magnetic resonance imaging. J Magn Reson Imaging 24:1101–1109

65. Treier R, Steingoetter A, Goetze O, et al (2008) Fast and optimized T1 mapping technique for the noninvasive quantification of gastric secretion. J Magn Reson Imaging 28:96–102

Laboratory Tests to Diagnose Nutritional Deficiencies

Julian Swierczynski, MD

The number of bariatric surgical procedures has increased markedly in the last years [1]. This phenomenon is strictly associated with increased knowledge among medical doctors about bariatric surgery indications, benefits, risks and prevention of the risks. This chapter focuses on the nutritional and metabolic complications associated with bariatric surgery and on recommended laboratory tests to diagnose these complications as early as possible. Moreover, to understand the pathophysiological mechanism of nutritional deficiencies after bariatric surgery, a short review of normal nutrient digestion, absorption and physiological role of these nutrients are also briefly discussed.

It is well established that bariatric surgery in morbidly obese subjects significantly ameliorates, reverses, or even eliminates obesity-related diseases including cardiac risk factors, diabetes mellitus type 2, hypertension, obstructive sleep apnea, and other complications presented in ◘ Table 26.1. These benefits usually occur in the majority of patients treated by bariatric surgery. Moreover, weight loss improves appearance, social and economic opportunities. After laparoscopic RYGB, life expectancy improves by approximately 11% compared to non-surgical treatment of obesity (treatment by diet and exercise) [2]. Moreover, some data indicate that morbidly obese patients had a 33% decreased hazard of death after gastric bypass [3]. Collectively, these beneficial effects markedly enhance quality of life and increase longevity after successful bariatric surgery [1]. Unfortunately, anatomical and physiological changes in the gastrointestinal tract caused by bariatric surgery lead to alterations in energy balance, enzyme secretion and enzyme action, food absorption and digestive track hormone secretion. Therefore, bariatric surgery may cause a variety of nutritional and metabolic alterations as presented in ◘ Table 26.1 [4-15]. These alterations can be mild with no apparent symptoms or cause life-threatening complications. These complications are the result of the extensive surgically-induced anatomical (exclusion of almost all of the stomach and the entire duodenum from the normal digestive process in some types of bariatric surgery) and consequently physiological (secretion of digestive enzymes and hormones) changes in the gastrointestinal tract, leading to both malabsorption and maldigestion of food as well as a decrease in uptake of nutrients.

These complications also depend on nutritional supplementation and dietary modification (changes in eating habits and food preference) after bariatric surgery. Although vitamin and mineral supplements are usually recommended as prophylaxis, daily multivitamin supplements often do not protect all patients from developing some deficiencies, including iron deficiency especially in young menstruating women [11]. Moreover, some data indicate that approximately 20% of the patients do not take dietary supplements after bariatric surgery [9]. Consequently, patients after bariatric surgery might develop deficiencies in some vitamins and minerals that are absorbed mainly in the upper part of the digestive tract [4,5,11,12,12]. Moreover, protein and fat malabsorption has also been observed in patients after bariatric surgery especially after BPD and RYGB [4,5,6,]. In general, these complications are predictable and consequently preventable and treatable. This requires careful clinical follow-up of patients after bariatric surgery. Prevention of nutritional and metabolic complications after bariatric surgery can be achieved by careful monitoring of patients and if necessary prophylactic nutrient supplementation should be provided. ◘ Table 26.2 compares the effect of different types of bariatric surgery on frequency of complications observed after surgical treatment of obesity. Most complications are rare (or not observed) after VBG. VBG is a restrictive type of bariatric surgery in which a small gastric pouch with small outlet is created. Because absorption from the entire small intestine is left intact, nutrient deficiencies after VBG are usually rare (◘ Table 26.2). Nutritional and metabolic complications are more common in malabsortive procedures (like BPD) which combine gastric volume reduction with a bypass of various lengths of small intestine (◘ Table 26.2). This is due due exclusion of important parts of the digestive tract from digestive continuity, which predispose patients to develop nutritional deficiency after bariatric surgery. The reduction in gastric volume, bypassing of the distal stomach, duodenum and proximal jejunum predispose patients who undergo RYGB to develop nutritional deficiency more often than after a VBG procedure (◘ Table 26.2). These complications are the result of loss of absorptive surface area and consequently reduction in absorptive capacity of nutrients, electrolytes and bile salt. Since complications depend on the categories of bariatric surgery (◘ Table 26.2), specific preventative measures should be performed in relation the type of the bariatric procedure.

Furthermore, considering that bariatric surgery is associated with both short- and long-term complications, clinical monitoring should be more frequent during the first two years after surgery. Later on, monitoring should be continued less frequently depending on the operative method (malabsorbtive or restrictive) and on clinical signs of vitamin, mineral and macronutrient deficiencies (see ◘ Table 26.3). According to Brolin and Leung [51], most surgeons do laboratory tests to investigate possible vitamin and mineral deficiencies. Laboratory tests and the percentage of surgeons who routinely do these laboratory tests are presented in ◘ Table 26.4. Moreover,

■ **Table 26.1** Beneficial effects of bariatric surgery and possible complications.

Beneficial effects	Ref.	Some complications	Ref.
1. Body weight and fat mass loss and BMI reduction	1,13,14, 35,37,40, 41,42, 44	1. Vomiting (many patients vomit during the first postoperative months). Persistent vomiting can cause hypokalemia which may lead to cardiac arrhythmias.	15,23
2. Recovery from type 2 diabetes	1,14, 35,44	2. Dumping syndrome (occurs in approximately 50% of patients after bariatric surgery) - postprandial symptoms that have been ascribed to rapid emptying of gastric contents.	15
3. Recovery from NAFLD	39, 42	3. Dehydration (results from multiple factors including vomiting and is associated with hypokaliemia and hypomagnesemia)	15
4.Reduction of biochemical cardiac risk factors: 1) Recovery from hyperlipidaemia: decrease in serum: a) total cholesterol, b) triacylglycerols, c) LDL-cholesterol and increase (after vertical banded gastroplasty or gastric banding) of HDL-cholesterol, 2) Decrease in C-reactive protein concentration, 3) Decrease in serum homocysteine concentration. 4) Decrease in serum Lp(a) concentration. 5) Decrease in serum hemoglobin A1c.	1,14, 33,34, 35,40, 41,42, 44	4. Protein malnutrition (frequently observed after malabsorptive surgical procedure and it is rare after gastric bypass	4,5,6,7,8, 10,12,15,37
5. Reduction of the prevalence of hypertension	1,14,35,	5. Hair loss (is observed usually 3-6 month after surgery and usually reverses without special intervention)	15
6. Reduction of the prevalence of obstructive sleep apnea	1,46	6. Gallstone formation (the incidence of gallstones after bariatric surgery vary between 22 to 71%)	7,8, 15,38
7. In patients with polycystic ovary syndrome, hirsuitism, hyperandrogenemia, ovulation and menstrual cycle significantly improved.	14	7. Vitamin deficiency. The frequency of vitamin B_{12} deficit is approx. 25% in the first 2 years after surgery and increases later on to 70%. Folate deficiencies is less frequent (about 20% at the end of 1 year) than deficiency of B_{12}. The deficiency of vitamin D can occur and is associated with hyperparathyroidism. The frequency of deficit in vitamins B_1, A, E and K after surgery are not significant.	4,6,7,10, 11,12,15, 22,30, 31,32, 36,37,
8. Improvement in quality of life	1,14	8. Iron deficiency (bypassing the distal part of the stomach hampers the absorption of iron, consequently iron deficiency can easily ensue for instance in menstruating women)	4,7,10 11 12,15,22, 31,32,
9. Reduction in mortality and morbidity	14,47	9. Bone demineralization (deficiencies in vitamin D and calcium after bariatric surgery can cause of hyperparathyroidism and consequently decrease in bone mass.	4,10,13,15, 16,17,18,19, 20,21,37,
10. Reduction in oxidative stress - one possible mechanism involved in the development of obesity-related co-morbidities	48, 49, 50	10. Zinc deficiency-low zinc serum concentration was described after gastroplasty as a results of reduced dietary intake	4,12, 28,
11. Decrease of inflammatory indicators (C-reactive protein and interleulin -6)	1,33, 43	11.Hypokalemia and hypomagnesaemia	23,24, 25,26,27,
12. Improvements in oxygen saturation, decreases in arterial carbon dioxide (CO_2) and increases in arterial oxygen content.	45, 46	12. Endogenous hyperinsulinemic hypoglycemia with nesidioblastosis (postprandial hyperinsulinemic hypoglycemia and hesidioblastosis in patients after Roux-en-Y gastric bypass was described	29
		13.Neurologic complications (the most common are peripheral neuropathy and encephalopathy)	55,71, 72
		14. Ocular complications (xerophthalmia, nyctalopia, ultimate blindness) of hypovitaminosis A.	58

Table 26.2 Some complications associated with different categories of bariatric surgery [7]

Complications	Vertical banded gastroplasty	Biliopancreatic diversion	Roux-enY gastric bypass
Severe malnutrition	Rare	Frequently observed	Less common
Fat malabsoroption	Not found	Frequently observed	Less common
Vitamin B12 deficiency	Not found	Frequently observed	Common
Iron deficiency	Rare	Frequently observed	Common
Folate deficiency	Not found	Frequently observed	Less common
Thiamine deficiency (vitaminB1)	Rare	Frequently observed	Common
Fat soluble vitamin deficiency	Not found	Frequently observed	Less common
Calcium deficiency	Rare	Frequently observed	Less common
Bone remodeling and decrease in bone mass	Rare	Frequently observed	Common
Cholelitiasis	Less common	Frequently observed	Common

according to Brolin and Leung [51], 22% of surgeons do these laboratory tests 3 months, 33% six months and 41% twelve months after RYGB. After BPD, 46% of surgeons perform the tests after three months, 33% after six months and 16% after twelve months [51].

Bernert et al. [4] proposed a nutritional check-up after 3 months, followed at 6–month intervals in the first 2 years, and then at least once per year after surgery. ◘ Table 26.5 presents the recommended laboratory test for patients undergoing bariatric surgery to diagnose the patient's nutritional state and possible nutritional deficiencies. Considering the frequency of the nutritional deficits among obese patients, especially deficiency in vitamins D3, B12, folates and iron, it is important to carry out a complete assessment before bariatric surgery (◘ Table 26.5) [4]. This procedure can identify patients with preexisting nutritional deficiencies. It is recommended that preexisting deficiencies be corrected before surgical treatment of obesity.

Nutrients are usually divided into two main groups: a) macronutrient like proteins, carbohydrates and lipids, and b) micronutrients such as vitamins, trace elements and minerals. Body weight maintenance and normal homeostasis depend on the digestion and absorption of all these nutrients. Altered digestion and absorption of nutrients after bariatric surgery result not only in weight loss, but also can lead to substantial nutrient deficiencies, sometimes with serious consequences. The most common nutritional deficiencies in patients after bariatric surgery are iron and vitamin B12 deficiency [4,11,12]. Other deficiencies are also reported in many papers,

including malnutrition that can lead to myopathy and to Wernicke's syndrome [4,5,6,11,12,13]. Disturbances in insulin homeostasis after bariatric surgery could lead to postprandial hyperinsulinemic hypoglycemia and nesidioblastosis. Postprandial hypoglycemia results from endogenous hyperinsulinemia from abnormal islets. Nesidioblastosis has been identified in researched resected specimens of the pancreas,. It seems that glucagon-like peptide -1 (and/or other beta cell trophic factors) contributes to the hypertrophy of pancreatic beta cells in these patients [28].

26.1 Macronutrient deficiencies

Proteins – are an essential structural component of all cells and the extracellular matrix. They are also needed for synthesis of almost all enzymes including digestive enzymes, synthesis and secretions of peptide or protein hormones, synthesis of plasma proteins, which in turn are essential for maintaining osmotic balance, transporting substances in the blood, maintaining immunity and blood coagulation. In the fasting state, when the breakdown of body proteins to amino acids is enhanced, the resulting amino acids are utilized for glucose production (gluconeogenesis), synthesis of non-protein nitrogenous compounds and for energy production (it should be noted that even in the fed state some amino acids formed during proteolysis are utilized for energy production). The recommended protein intake is 0.8 g per kg body weight per day for healthy subjects. This amounts to

◘ **Table 26.3** Clinical symptoms of vitamin or mineral deficiencies which can be observed after barriatric surgery [4] :

Vitamins or minerals	Clinical symptoms
Vitamin B12	**Hematopoiesis**: Megaloblastic anemia **Central Nervous System**: fatigue headaches, irritability, loss of vibration sensation, spinal cord degeneration, numbness, paresthesia **Intestinal tract**: diarrhea, constipation **Blood**: accumulation of homocysteine and methylmalonic acid
Folic acid (vitamin B9)	**Hematopoiesis**: Macrocystic anemia **Central Nervous System**: apathy, fatigue, headaches, insomnia, neural tube defects in fetus caused by inadequate folate levels in early stage of pregnancy, weakness **Intestinal tract**: loss of appetite, diarrhea **Blood**: hyperhomocysteinemia (appears to be a risk factor for cardiovascular disease)
Thiamin (vitamin B1)	**Cardiovascular system**: congestive heart failure **Central Nervous System**: mental confusion, irritability, memory loss, nervousness, numbness of hands and feet, pain sensitivity, poor coordination, weakness, ataxia. **Intestinal tract**: constipation, intestinal disturbances, loss of appetite **Eyes**: ophthalmoplegia (loss of eye coordination)
Vitamin B6 (pyridoxine)	**Skin and mucosa**: loss of hair, mouth lesions, facial oiliness, eye inflammation, acne **Other**: depression, dizziness, fatigue, impaired wound healing, irritability, loss of appetite, nausea **Hematopoiesis**: sideroblastic microcytic anemia (because B6 is required for synthesis of δ- aminolevulinic acid, a precursor of heme). **Blood**: hyperhomocysteinemia (appears to be a risk factor for cardiovascular disease)
Vitamin D	**Bone**: hyperparathyroidism, rickets (in young children), osteomalacia (in adults), osteoporosis, joint and bone pains
Vitamin K	**Hemostasis**: bleeding disorders due to increased coagulation time; Osteoporose
Vitamin A	**Eyes**: night blindness, xerophtalmia (keratinization of the cornea) **Skin:** follicular hyperkeratosis, xerosis, acne, dry hair
Iron	**Hematopoiesis**: anemia, microcytosis **Skin and mucosa**: brittle nails, inflamed tongue, mouth lesisons, pruritis **Intestinal tract**: constipation **Other**: confusion, depression, dizziness, fatigue, headaches
Calcium	In general symptoms of calcium deficiency resemble those of vitamin D deficiency, additionally muscle cramps (even tetany), tingling of the fingers and toes, numbness around the mouth are possible
Zinc	**Skin**: acne, eczema, white spots on nails, brittle nails, hair loss **Taste**: loss of sense of taste (decrease of food intake) **Other**: poor wound healing, depression, fatigue, immune impairment, amnesia, irritability, lethargy, male infertility
Magnesium	Weakness, tremors, hypertension, cardiac arrhythmias, myocardial infarction, hypokaliemia, hypokalcemia, osteoporosis
Selenium	Increased incidence of cancer, pancreatic insufficiency, immune impairment, male sterility
Copper	Anemia, neuronal degeneration, cardiac hypertrophy, impaired immune function, achromotrichia

approximately 56 g protein per day for a man weighing 70 kg. These recommendations need to be increased when breakdown of body protein is greatly accelerated (for instance in catabolic state induced by serious illness, major trauma, surgery). As far as normal adult protein requirements are concerned, it is important that essential amino acids (amino acids that cannot be synthesized by the human body) must be present in the diet. The human body can´t produce new proteins if only one of the essential amino acids is missing from the diet. Animal proteins usually contain all essential amino acids in the amounts needed by the human body. Vegetable proteins often lack

Table 26.4 Laboratory tests and the percentage of surgeons who do these laboratory tests after RYGB and BPD [51]

Laboratory test	Percentage of surgeons who routinely do laboratory tests after RYGB	Percentage of surgeons who routinely do laboratory test after BPD
Complete blood counts	95	96
Serum iron concentration	56 (estimated deficiency: 16%)	80 (estimated deficiency: 26%)
Serum vitamin B12 concentration	66 (estimated deficiency: 12%)	67 (estimated deficiency: 11 %)
Serum folate concentration	58	71
Serum electrolyte concentrations	76	88
Serum protein concentration	8	84
Serum fat soluble vitamin concentrations	-	46

one or more essential amino acids. For instance, corn is deficient in lysine, while legumes are deficient in methionine, but rich in lysine. This means that a combination of different vegetable proteins (vegetarian diets) can provide essential amino acids. In adults, proteins (molecules containing usually more than 100 amino acids residues), polypeptides (molecules containing 30-100 amino acids residues) and oligopeptides (chains of less than 30 amino acids residues) are not absorbed in appreciable amounts by the intestine. They must be hydrolyzed to free amino acids, dipeptides and tripetides by proteases including: pepsin, trypsin, chymotrypsin, elastase, carboxypeptidases, endopeptidases, aminopeptidase and dipeptidase. Gastric juice contains mainly HCL, which denatures proteins and pepsin (formed from pepsinogen at low pH), which hydrolyze proteins mainly into large peptides with some small peptides and free amino acids. The stomach absorbs negligible amounts of peptides and free amino acids. Most products of pepsin action move to the small intestine, where they are degraded by pancreatic digestive enzymes (produced as proenzymes) like trypsin, chymotrypsin, elastase and carboxypeptidases (A and B). Combined action of pepsin and pancreatic proteases result in formation of free amino acids (approximately 40%) and oligopeptides (approximately 60%) containing residue of up to 8 amino acids. These oligopeptides are further digested by endopeptidase, aminopeptidase and dipeptidase present on luminal surface of epithelial cells (brush border surface). The absorption of free amino acids, dipeptides and tripeptides (formed from proteins) takes place mainly in the duodenum (approximately 50%) and small intestine [5]. The exclusion of the duodenum and part of the intestine from digestion and absorption theoretically leads to protein deficiency. In general, the

reduction in dietary protein absorption after bariatric surgery is the result of: a) limited absorption surface (due to exclusion of important parts of digestive tract); b) decrease in stomach and pancreatic proteolytic enzyme secretion, and c) limited interaction between food containing proteins and proteolytic enzymes. Moreover, insufficient intake of meat (red meat is poorly tolerated by patients after bariatric surgery) or insufficient intake of alternative sources of proteins (dairy products, eggs, fish) can also cause protein deficiency after bariatric surgery. Protein deficiency may cause marasmus (due to inadequate intake of both protein and energy sources) and/or kwashiorkor (due to inadequate intake of proteins with adequate intake of energy). The patients with kwashiorkor often have edema, dry and brittle hair, diarrhea, dermatitis of various forms and hypopigmentation of the skin [4,5,6,7]. The most serious result of protein deficiency is the reduced ability to fight infection due to a reduced number of T-lymphocytes, defects in generation of phagocytic cells and synthesis of immunoglobulins, interferon and other important components of the immune system. Usually patients die from secondary infections rather than from starvation. Scopinaro et al. [52] suggested that the combination of hypoalbuminemia, anemia, edema, asthenia and alopecia is a reliable sign of protein malnutrition. Thus, careful clinical and nutritional follow-up is necessary to prevent these uncommon but potentially serious complications.

Protein–calorie malnutrition after RYGB appears to be very rare. Only few papers concerning this problem have been published so far [6,22]. For instance, Skroubis et al. [22] reported that the incidence of hypoalbuminemia was negligible in patients who underwent RYGB (found n only 1 of 79 patients). Faintuch et al. [6] ob-

◻ **Table 26.5** Recommendation for controls and diagnostic procedures after bariatric surgery (Freiburg, A. Engelhardt)

	Before surgery.	1 Month	3 month	6 month	12 month	18 month	24 month	Annually (more frequent if elevated or low)
Electrolytes Potassium, Na	+	+	+	+	+	+	+	+
Ca, PO4, Mg				+**	+		+	+**
Glucose***	+	+	+	+	+	+	+	+
BUN	+	+	+	+	+	+	+	+
Creatinin	+	+	+	+	+	+	+	+
Uric acid	+	+	+		+			(+)
Albumin	+			+**	+	+*	+	+
Liver enzymes	+	(+)	+	+	+	+	+	+
INR	+				+		+	+**
Blood cell count	+	+	+	+	+	+	+	+
Ferritin	+			+	+	+*	+	+
Transferin (transferin saturation)	+			+*	+	+*	+	+
Vit. A, E, K					+**		+*	+*
Vitamin D	+			+*	+*	+**	+	+
PTH				+*	+*	+**	+*	+*
Bone densitometry	+						+	+*
Vitamin B$_{12}$ Vit. B$_1$ Folic acid	+ +	((+)		+** ((+)	+ ((+) +**		+	+ ((+) (+)
Selenium				+*	+*		+	(+)*
Zinc,				+*	+			(+)*
Hemoglobin A1c	+				+			(+)
Insulin Resistance by DM t.2	+		+					
C-Peptid ***	+		+					+
Cholesterol and lipoprotein fractions (HDL, LDL, VLDL)	+			(+)	+			(+)
Urine analysis	+		+*		+*		+*	(+)

*   after BPD-DS or gastric bypass in Freiburg
**   after BPD
*** in Patients with Diabetes Mellitus ; postop frequent self control of blood glucose, until normal profile
( )   when serum level initially increased, or pathology in follow up controls
(( )   with frequent vomiting: control vit B1

served severe protein-calorie malnutrition in 11 patients among 236 (4.7%) treated by RYGB. Almost all these patients had a low serum concentration of albumin and hemoglobin. Widespread edema was observed in approximately 45% and extreme weakness in about 36 % of these patients [6]. These deficiency and clinical signs appeared mainly within the first 2 years after surgery. Severe forms of protein-calorie malnutrition with hypoalbuminemia, anemia and fatigue following BPD was more frequent than after RYGB [8,10]. For example some studies indicate that protein malnutrition is the most serious complication of BPD and occurred in almost 12% of patients [8]. It should be noted that hypoalbuminemia appeared as early as 1 year after BPD [8]. In other studies, hypoalbuminemia was found in almost 20% of patients after BPD [10].

Lipids. Triacylglycerols are the main lipids ingested by humans (constituting more than 90% of total lipids intake). Digestion of triacylglicerols starts in the upper intestine, absorption takes place in the distal intestine (ileum); it requires: a) hydrolysis of triacylglicerols to free fatty acids and 2-monoacylglycerols within the lumen of intestine; b) solubilization of lipids by bile acids and transport from the intestinal lumen into epithelial cells; c) resynthesis of triacylglicerol inside epithelial cells; d) packing of synthesized triacylglicerols into chylomicrons; e) exocytosis of chylomicrons from the epithelial cells into the lymphatic system (into the thoracic duct that enters the bloodstream through the left subclavian vein) and further to the blood. Pancreatic lipase present in pancreatic juice plays a key role in the hydrolysis of triacylglicerols. Pancreatic juice contains also unspecific lipid esterase, which hydrolyses cholesteryl esters to cholesterol and free fatty acids, and phospholipase A2 involved in the digestion of phospholipids. Bile acids and colipase, a small (12 kDa) protein present in pancreatic juice play an important role in the digestion and absorption of lipids. Colipase binds to pancreatic lipase and prevents inhibition of the lipase by bile acids. Absorption of triacylglicerols is significantly reduced in the absence of bile acids. Unabsorbed lipids are excreted with the stool (steatorrhea). In healthy subjects, ingested fat passes into the duodenum and causes an increase of CCK secretion. In turn, CCK stimulates the gallbladder to release bile (including bile acids) and the pancreas to release lypolytic enzymes. After a malabsorptive type of bariatric surgery (for instance after RYGB), the secretion of bile acids and pancreatic enzymes is reduced and lipids and proteins are not in contact with the enzymes because they do not pass through the duodenum. Consequently, delayed digestion (caused by too-low activity of pancreatic lipase) and the

delayed formation of mixed micelles (limited amount of bile acids) limit the amount of fat available for absorption. The malabsorption of lipids has not been observed after VBG, is rare after RYGB and observed mainly after jejunoileal bypass or biliopancreatic diversion [4,5,7]. This deterioration usually leads to steatorrhea, chronic diarrhea and reduced lipid soluble vitamin (A,D,E,K) absorption [12].

Carbohydrates – together with fatty acids (released from triacylglycerols) are an important source of energy for all organs/tissues of the human body and the sole energy source for red blood cells and the brain (except in starvation when keton bodies can be used as a source of energy for the brain). In the absence of adequate carbohydrate supply, fat and protein can be used directly as a source of energy for almost all tissues/organs of human body except red blood cells and the brain. Indirectly, proteins (amino acids) can be used as a substrate for glucose biosynthesis. In turn, glucose can be used as an energy substrate by brain and red blood cells. Consequently, a deficiency in carbohydrates can lead to a protein deficiency. The major carbohydrates in European diets are starch, sucrose (table sugar) and lactose (milk sugar). Monosaccharides, such as glucose and fructose, are usually present in the diet in small amounts. Starch, sucrose and lactose must be hydrolyzed to monosaccharides (glucose, fructose and galactose) before absorption. Starch is hydrolyzed by α-amylase of saliva and pancreas to glucose. Pancreatic α-amylase is secreted in large excess relative to starch intake and is more important for starch digestion than the salivary α-amylase. Combined action of salivary and pancreatic α-amylase results mainly in maltose (disaccharide), maltotriose (trisaccharide) and α-limit dextrins (oligosaccharides containing 8 glucose units with one or more α-1,6 glucoside bonds). Final hydrolysis of maltose, maltotriose and α-limit dectrins to glucose is carried out by the enzymes present on the luminal surface of the small intestinal epithelial cells like maltase (α-glucosidase), izomaltase (oligo-1-,6glucosidase) and glucoamylase (exo 1,4- α -glucosidase). Sucrose is hydrolyzed to glucose and fructose by sucrase (sucrose- α -glucosidase) and lactose is cleaved to glucose and galactose by lactase (β-galactosidase). Glucose (formed from starch, sucrose and lactose) and galactose (formed from lactose) are transported into the cells by sodium-dependent glucose (galactose) transporters (called: SGLT-1) located in the luminal membrane, which is strictly associated with the basolaterally located Na/K ATPase, that provides the driving energy for the transport system (transport of glucose and galactose into cells). Fructose is transported by separate, sodium- independent translocators located in the luminal membrane called GLUT 5. Transport of glucose, fructose and galactose from the intestinal cells into the blood involves the sodium-independent translocator called GLUT localized on the basolateral membrane. Carbohydrate absorption starts in the duodenum and is completed in the first 100 cm of the small intestine. Both sucrase and lactase are present on the luminal surface of small intestinal epithelial cells similarly as glucosidases. The capacity of α-glucosidases and sucrase in healthy subjects is usually much greater than needed for the complete digestion of starch and sucrose respectively. Contrary to this, lactase can be the rate-limiting enzyme for hydrolysis of lactose. Consequently, lactase is the most commonly deficient digestive enzyme, which is experienced as milk intolerance. In the case of lack of lactose hydrolysis in the upper small intestine, lactose becomes available for bacterial fermentation in the lower small intestine. Bacterial fermentation of lactose produces gas and osmotically-active substances that draw water into the intestinal lumen causing diarrhea. Theoretically, some types of bariatric surgery (for instance RYGB) might alter carbohydrate digestion and absorption due to combination of: a) decreased absorptive surface area; b) decreased pancreatic amylase secretion, and c) delayed interaction of amylase with starch. This can lead to carbohydrate balance disorder. It could cause a problem for patients with dumping syndrome, since the treatment of this syndrome includes a decrease in simple carbohydrate intake. In such a case, symptoms of a dumping syndrome can be eliminated/diminished by eating small-quantity, frequent meals containing fiber, proteins and complex carbohydrates with a minimal amount of simple sugars [53].

26.2   Micronutrient deficiencies

26.2.1   Vitamins

Vitamin B_{12} – In physiological conditions, vitamin B_{12} is supplied by animal products (mainly meat). After ingestion, vitamin B_{12} binds to proteins of the stomach. In the stomach, vitamin B_{12} is released from the protein by pepsin and hydrochloric acid (HCL). The released, free vitamin B_{12} is bound to haptocorrin, which is released from the salivary glands. In the small intestine, the haptocorrin is degraded by proteolytic pancreatic enzymes, vitamin B_{12} is released and transferred to the intrinsic factor (IF), a protein which is synthesized and secreted by the gastric parietal cells. The IF-vitamin B_{12} complex is internalized in the distal part of the small intestine by a specific receptor. Then the IF is degraded by proteolysis and vitamin B12 is released. The free vitamin B_{12} enters the systemic circulation, and is bound to transcobalamin. The complex vitamin B_{12} with transcobalamin (called holotranscobalamin) represents the biologically active form that is delivered to tissues. After cellular uptake of holotranscobalamin, transcobalamin is degraded and vitamin B_{12} released. In the cells (more precisely in cytosol), vitamin B_{12} (as methylcobalamin) functions as a coenzyme of methionine synthase, which catalyzes the conversion (methylation) of homocysteine to methionine in the presence of methyl-tetrahydrofolate. Since this reaction is strictly associated with methyltetrahydrofolate,which in turn is involved in the synthesis of thymidylate (one of the substrates for DNA synthesis) catalyzed by thymidylate synthase, vitamin B_{12} is necessary for normal DNA synthesis. Consequently, vitamin B_{12} deficiency results in impaired synthesis of DNA. In mitochondria, vitamin B_{12} (as 5'deoxyadenosylcobalamin, a derivative of vitamin B_{12}) is involved in the conversion of methylmalonyl-CoA (formed from propionyl- CoA, the end product of some amino acids, odd –chain fatty acids and the side chain of cholesterol) to succinyl-CoA catalyzed by methylmalonyl-CoA mutase. Considering that vitamin B_{12} is necessary for the conversion of homocysteine to methionine and methylmalonyl- CoA to succinyl-CoA, vitamin B_{12} deficiency can lead to accumulation of homocysteine and methylmalonic acids, metabolites considered as more sensitive indicators of vitamin B_{12} status than the plasma cobalamin concentration. Thus, serum homocysteine concentration can be used as a sensitive marker of the tissue concentration of functional abundance of vitamin B_{12} [7, 54]. But one has to remember that intracellular homocysteine metabolism and consequently serum homocysteine concentration depends not only on the vitamin B_{12}-dependent methionine synthase but also on the piridoxal phosphate (vitamin B6)-dependent cystationine beta-synthase [54]. An elevated plasma homocysteine concentration is associated with an increased cardiovascular risk, although it does not appear to be as important as diabetes, smoking, hyperlipidemia and hypertension. The typical symptoms of vitamin B_{12} deficiency are macrocystic anemia, glossitis and a neurological manifestation. Deficiency of vitamin B_{12} may be caused by insufficient intake (for instance in vegetarians, especially in vegans) or by malabsorption of vitamin of vitamin B_{12}. Malabsorption of vitamin B_{12} usually occurs in patients suffering from gastrointestinal conditions including decreased (or abolished) output of gastric intrinsic factor and/or hypo- or achlorhydia. Achlorhydia hampers the extraction of vitamin B_{12} from ingested protein. Intrinsic factor is necessary for the intestinal internalization of vitamin B_{12}. Lack of this protein results in impaired vitamin B_{12} uptake. Malabsorption of vitamin B_{12} can also occur in: a) pancreatic insufficiency, due to the lack of enzymes necessary to liberate vitamin B_{12} from haptocorrin (the protein that binds ingested vitamin B_{12}); b) patients with gastric or ileal resection and in patients with disorders of the small intestine (including celiac disease, Crohn's disease, ileitis). After RYGB, the secretion of HCL in the small gastric pocket is limited, the release of vitamin B_{12} from ingested proteins is also limited. Moreover, the exclusion of the stomach and the duodenum might disturb the link between the intrinsic factor and vitamin B_{12}. Consequently these events may lead to vitamin B_{12} deficiency after bariatric surgery [4,5,7,11,12]. The data reported so far indicate that the prevalence of vitamin B_{12} deficit occurs mainly after the first year following RYGB and is estimated between 12-70% [4]. Based on studies comprising approximately 1000 patients, the estimated frequency is about 25% in the first two years, and increased later on even to 70% [55]. The lower frequency of vitamin B_{12} deficit in the first year after surgery is probably due to relatively high body reserves of the vitamin (approx. 2000µg) versus daily needs (approx 2µg/day). Interestingly, megaloblastic anemia is very rare after bariatric surgery. Based on studies comprising approximately 350 patients, the estimated frequency of macrocytosis without anemia is below 1% [56]. Vitamin B_{12} deficiency is less likely after vertical banded gastroplasty (VBG), because there is no diminution of HCL production and the ingested food passes via the normal route. Nevertheless, determination of serum vitamin B_{12} concentration is recommended after any bariatric surgery (◘ Table 26.5).

Vitamin B_9 (Folates) – Plants are the key sources of dietary folates for humans. Absorption of folates takes place mainly in the proximal small intestine, but it may also occur through the whole intestine. Consequently a deficiency of dietary intake (fruits and vegetables) is the main cause of folate deficit. Folates play an important role in the one-carbon metabolism essential for biosynthesis of purines, tymidylate and consequently in DNA synthesis. Thus, folate deficiency inhibits synthesis of DNA by decreasing the availability of purines and tymidylate (dTMP). This leads to an arrest of cells in S phase, causing production of large macrocystic red blood cells. Thus, macrocystic anemia is characteristic of folate deficiency. Additionally, hyperhomocysteinemia (a risk factor for cardiovascular disease) is observed, because 5-methyltetrahydrofolate (formed from folate) serves as a methyl donor to homocysteine, which is converted to methionine, in a reaction catalyzed by vitamin B_{12}-dependent methionine synthase. This explains why vitamin B_{12} and folate deficiencies lead to hyperhomocysteinemia. Folate deficiency may also lead to an alteration in liver me-

tabolism leading to increased S-adenosylhomocysteine concentration and decreased choline concentration. A decreased choline concentration may cause liver damage. Folate deficiencies after bariatric surgery is less frequent than deficiencies of vitamin B_{12} and is estimated between 10–65 % (4,55).

Vitamin B_1 (Thiamine) – The food source of thiamine are cereals, meats (especially pork), fish, soy, dairy products, and finally fruits and vegetables. Thiamine is absorbed mainly in the duodenum and in the proximal small intestine by a translocator-mediated process (when concentration of vitamin is low) and by passive diffusion if high concentrations of the vitamin are present in the intestine (pharmacological doses of vitamin) [57]. In the cells, thiamine is rapidly converted to phosphate derivatives. Thiamine is a precursor of thiamine pyrophosphate (TPP), a coenzyme required for oxidative decarboxylation of pyruvate and 2-oxoglutarate catalyzed by pyruvate dehydrogenase and 2-oxoglutarate dehydrogenase, respectively and for the transketolase reaction of the pentose phosphate pathway (red blood cell transketolase is used for measuring thiamine status in the body). It is also a precursor of thiamine triphosphate, localized in peripheral nerve membranes, and functions in transmission of nerve impulses. Symptoms of thiamine deficiency involving the neural tissue and may result from the direct role of thiamine triphosphate in nerve transmission and/or from the accumulation of pyruvate and lactate (due to low activity of pyruvate dehydrogenase) in the neural tissue. Thiamine deficiency is mainly due to the combination of reduction in gastric acid secretion and food intake and is worsened by vomiting. Thus, theoretically vitamin B1 deficiency can be expected after bariatric surgery. The prevalence of vitamin B_1 deficiency is very low (approximately 1% at the end of 1 year after bariatric surgery) [55]. Considering, however, that the consequence of a deficiency of vitamin B_1 is very serious (Beri-Beri, irreversible polyneuropathy, Gayet-Wernicke's encephalopathy) vitamin B_1 deficiency must be suspected in case of even the slightest clinical symptoms, proven by vitamin B_1 measurement, and treated by the administration of vitamin B_1 [55].

Vitamin A – is derived from plant carotenoids, which are converted to retinol by animals and is stored in the liver as retinol palmitate. Carotenoids (especially beta carotene) have an important role as an antioxidant, which may reduce the risk of some diseases (including cancer) caused by reactive oxygen species. The active forms of vitamin A are retinol, retinal and retinoic acid. Retinol is converted to retinyl phosphate which plays a similar role as dolichol phosphate in the synthesis of glycoproteins and mucopolysaccharides needed for cell growth and mucus secretion. Retinoic acid binds to retinoic acid receptors (RARs) and retinoid X receptors (RXRs). These receptors bind to DNA and regulate the synthesis of proteins involved in the regulation of cell growth and differentiation. Retinal plays a key role in vision (becomes reversibly associated with opsin- the visual protein). Deficiency is rare in the general population (due to accumulation of the vitamin in the liver and the presence of vitamin A in foods like butter, milk, and vegetables) but it is a common consequence of severe liver damage or diseases associated with fat malabsorption. A decrease in serum retinol and β-carotene (in general vitamin A deficiency) concentrations was observed in obese patients before bariatric surgery compared to non-obese subjects [59]. Lower serum carotenoid concentrations in obese patients are probably associated with a dilution effect of carotenoids in the adipose tissue [60]. After bariatric surgery, a consistent and continuous decline in all carotenoids occurs, reaching almost undetectable levels in patients after BPD [61]. Le and coworkers [58] described patients with vitamin A deficiency and ocular complications (nyctalopia, bilateral conjunctival and corneal xerosis, bilateral corneal scarring) after a duodenal switch or gastric bypass surgery. Vitamin A deficiency has been observed by many bariatric surgeons and these data suggest that vitamin A deficiency (like other vitamin deficiencies) are more common after bariatric surgery than previously thought [62-68]. Thus, long-term nutritional monitoring is necessary after bariatric surgery, especially after malabsorptive operations.

Vitamin K – is found as K1 in vegetables and K2, which is synthesized by intestinal bacteria. Vitamin K is required for conversion of glutamic acid residues to gamma-carboxyglutamic acid residues in some proteins (proteins involved in blood clotting, noncollagen proteins in the bone, proteins involved in cell cycle regulation). Vitamin K deficiency occurs in patients with diseases leading to severe fat malabsorption and patients on long-term antibiotic therapy which may kill vitamin K-synthesizing bacteria in the intestine. The most easily detectable symptom of vitamin K deficiency in humans is an increased coagulation time. A vitamin K deficiency has been observed after bariatric surgery [68,69] with an incidence of 68% [68].

Vitamin E – is primariliy considered as a dietary factor which is important for normal reproduction. Vitamin E occurs in the diet as a mixture of tocopherols (α, β, γ, δ) and tocotrienols. All these compounds are naturally-occurring antioxidants. Tocopherols accumulate in circulating lipoproteins and cellular membranes where they act as scavengers for reactive oxygen species, protecting unsaturated fatty acids from peroxidation. It is assumed that the vitamin E content in the diet is high enough, so no major vitamin E deficiency diseases have been described. The disease that has been directly related to vitamin E deficiency is ataxia with familial isolated vitamin E deficiency (AVED). This is an uncommon autosomal recessive neurodegenerative disease. The clinical symptoms are similar to that of Friedreich ataxia. Epidemiological studies have indicated a probable involvement of vitamin E in the pathogenesis of atherosclerosis, diabetes, and some types of cancer. A low serum vitamin E concentration among overweight and obese persons has been reported [70]. This phenomenon may result from the increased systemic and adipose tissue-specific oxidative stress found in overweight persons, which may lead to an increased oxidative catabolism of vitamin E [70]. Theoretically, the absorption of vitamin E (like other fat soluble vitamins) would be lower after bariatric surgery due to fat malabsorption. Deficits in vitamin E after RYGB and BPD have been reported [4, 61,68,73]. It should be noted that some authors observed higher concentration of α-tocopherol 24 weeks after bariatric surgery than in patients before surgery [48].

Vitamin D3 (cholecalciferol) – is synthesized in the skin by UV irradiation of 7-dehydrochoelsterol. As long as the human body is exposed to sunlight (UV irradiation), there is no dietary requirement for vitamin D3. The best food sources of vitamin D3 are saltwater fish, mushrooms, dairy products, liver and egg yolk. Ingested cholecalciferol is transported with chylomicrons to the liver, where 25-hydroxycholecalciferol (25 (OH)D3, called calcidiol) is formed. From the liver, 25(OH)D3 is transported to the kidney, where it is converted into the biologically-active 1α, 25- dihydroxycholecalciferol (1,25(OH)2D3, called calcitriol). The 1,25 (OH)2D3 acts in the intestinal mucosal cells, where it increases the synthesis of proteins required for calcium absorption. In bone, 1,25(OH)2D3 and PTH act to promote bone resorption. In kidney, 1,25(OH)2D3 and PTH inhibit calcium excretion. Most cases of vitamin D3 deficiency result from fat malabsorption or severe liver and/or kidney diseases (where active forms of vitamin D3 are formed). Theoretically, the absorption of vitamin D3, similar to that of other fat soluble vitamins, would be lower after bariatric surgery due to fat malabsorption. After biliopancreatic diversion, approximately 26% of the patients were hypocalcemic, 50% had a low vitamin D concentration, 24% had elevated ALP, and 63% had an elevated PTH, despite taking multivitamins [74]. The deficiencies in calcium and vitamin D are less frequent and less severe after RYGB than after biliopancreatic diversion [16,17,66,75,]. However, hyperparathyroidism has been observed in patients after different types of bariatric surgery [16,17,76,77,78]. Moreover, hyperparathyroidism was more frequent in post-menopausal patients [16]. The consequence of hyperparathyroidism is an increase in bone remodeling and a decrease in bone mass [17]. For this reason, monitoring calcium, phosphate, PTH, alkaline phosphatase, vitamin D and its metabolites is essential after bariatric surgery. Some data suggest that the alterations in Ca homeostasis after RYGB-induced weight loss may be regulated primarily by the estradiol concentration [17]. To avoid bone loss, some authors recommended supplementation of calcium and vitamin D starting on 12th day after bariatric surgery [78]. It should be noted that morbid obesity itself is a significant risk factor for vitamin D depletion. This phenomenon is probably the consequence of sequestration of vitamin D in the adipose tissue [79]. For this reason, monitoring of serum vitamin D is essential before and after bariatric surgery. As already mentioned, the major potential impact of vitamin D depletion is a loss of bone mass. However, some data indicate that vitamin D may have substantial effects on the cardiovascular, immune and neuromuscular system as well as on cell proliferation, differentiation and apoptosis [80]. Recent studies suggest that serum vitamin D depletion is associated with increased blood pressure [79]. Thus, this finding is another reason why adequate vitamin D supplementation is necessary after bariatric surgery.

26.2.2 Microelements

Calcium – is the most abundant mineral in the human body (approximately 1 kg of calcium is present in an adult human). Most calcium is present in bone which plays an important role in calcium homeostasis. Bone is an active tissue that is constantly remodeled throughout life. Old bone is constantly removed by osteoclasts and new bone is formed by osteoblasts [81,82]. Bone resorption is controlled by many hormones and cytokines, which affect osteoclast formation and consequently osteoclast activity [80,82]. Parathormone and 1,25 (OH)2 D3 (calcitriol) increase bone resorption via a mechanism that is mediated by osteoblasts (osteoblast-producing IL-l, which increases osteoclast differentiation) [80,82]. Oestrogens have indirect negative impact on osteoclast differentiation. In fact, estrogen deficiency leads to increased osteoclast differentiation and bone resorption [83]. Cytokines like Il-1, Il-6 and TNFα are also known to increase bone resorp-

tion by stimulating osteoclast differentiation and activity [84]. The discovery of new members of the TNF receptor ligand family, the receptor activator of NF-κB (RANK), its ligand RANKL and the decoy receptor for RANKL, osteoprotegerin (OPG) has moved bone remodeling research into a new era. In summary, binding of RANKL to its receptor RANK caused osteoclast development from haematopoietic progenitor cell and consequently activated osteoclasts. OPG negatively regulated RANKL binding to RANK and therefore inhibited bone turnover by osteoclasts [81,82,84]. Besides the bone, the digestive tract and the kidney play an important role in overall calcium homeostasis. If adult ingests approximately 1000mg of calcium, about 350 mg is absorbed in the small intestine by mechanism stimulated by vitamin D3 (more precisely by 1,25 (OH)2 D3). It should be pointed out that net absorption of calcium in the intestine is approximately 200 mg per day, because pancreatic and other intestinal tract secretions contain approximately 150 mg of calcium. To maintain calcium balance, the kidneys must excrete the same amount of calcium that the intestinal tract absorbs. This is accomplished by a combination of filtration of calcium across the glomerular capillaries and subsequent reabsorption of most of the filtered calcium. This process is also controlled by PTH. The total blood calcium (10mg per dl) includes a fraction that is bound to plasma proteins (mainly albumin) and a fraction that is unbound to proteins, called ultrafilterable. The ultrafilterable fraction (approximately 60% of total plasma calcium) contains a fraction that is bound to aniona like phosphate and sulfate, and the remainder which is free ionized calcium (approx 50%). It should be noted that only free ionized calcium is biologically active. The changes in plasma protein concentrations are associated with changes in free ionized calcium concentrations. In blood, calcium is essential for blood coagulation. Calcium is also present in the extracellular space from which it can penetrate into the cells and regulate their most important activities like enzyme activity, hormone release, hormone action, muscle contractility, neuro-muscular irritability, cell proliferation, apoptosis. One can say that a few grams of calcium (of the approximately 1000 g of calcium that are in the human body) present in blood, extracellular space and in the cells might be insignificant quantitatively, but they are very significant qualitatively. Taken together, these facts suggest that calcium deficiency can result in a wide range of complications. On the other hand, considering that the calcium from food is mainly absorbed in the duodenum and proximal jejunum, bypassing these fragments of the intestine during bariatric surgery together with a reduced calcium and vitamin D3 intake (after bariatric surgery), can lead to calcium deficiency. It has been found that over a period of 4 years, the incidence of hypocalcemia increased from 15% to almost 50% in patients who had undergone BPD [12]. Moreover, hypocalcemia was associated in these patients with an increase in serum concentration of parathyroid hormone [12]. Loss of bone mass has been reported in patients undergoing other types of bariatric surgery [4, 12, 13, 14, 16, 17, 66, 74, 76, 77, 78]. In patients who underwent laparoscopic Roux-en-Y gastric bypass (LRYGB), decrease in bone mass and increase in markers of bone turnover (urinary N-telopeptide, cross-linked collagen 1) was observed [13]. All together, these data indicate that monitoring for calcium deficiency is recommended after bariatric surgery. Tests should include total serum concentration of calcium, serum concentration of phosphate, alkaline phosphatase, 25 (OH) D3 concentration and serum PTH level [4]. A bone mineral density examination can be performed in patients with either biochemical or clinical evidence of calcium deficiency [4].

Iron – In humans, iron is a component of heme in oxygen transport (hemoglobin) and oxygen storage (myoglobin) proteins and a constituent of heme, iron-sulfur containing centers in many oxidoreductases, including the components of the mitochondrial respiratory chin and ribonucleotide reductase involved in deoxyribonucleotide synthesis. Thus, iron as a component of proteins, has a pivotal role in energy metabolism, cell proliferation and DNA synthesis and repair. Severe cellular iron deficiency may result in inhibition of cell proliferation and cell death. On a systemic level, severe iron deficit causes anemia which impairs oxygen delivery to tissue. In mammals, absorption of dietary iron represents the only means to regulate body iron content. Iron can be absorbed from the intestine as non-heme iron or heme iron. Non-heme iron is absorbed through the action of the divalent metal transporter (DMT1, also called nRAMP2) and ferrireductase (DCYTB), both present at the apical membrane in the duodenum and proximal small intestine. It seems that ferrireductase donates electrons for the reduction of ferric iron (Fe +3) to the ferrous iron (Fe+2), which is transported by DMT1. The conversion of Fe +3 to Fe +2 is stimulated by hydrochloric acid (HCl). Heme iron is absorbed from the diet and is degraded by heme oxygenase and the iron released enters the intracellular non-heme iron (together with absorbed non-heme iron) pool. Export of iron from enterocytes to circulation requires special proteins called ferroportin (also called: FPN, IREG1 or MTP1) and a ferrooxidase to oxidize Fe+2 to Fe+3. Then two Fe+3 can be bound to apotransferrin forming holotransferrin, which transports iron to the cells including bone marrow where it is used for the formation of new red blood cells. Holotransferrin binds to the cell surface transferrin receptor and the complex formed is internalized through a receptor-mediated endocytosis. Iron release from holotransferrin to cytosol requires endosomal acidification, reduction of iron by ferrireductase, and ferrous iron export to the cytosol through the action of DMT1. Iron delivered to the cytosol can be used for formation of iron-containing proteins in the cytosol and mitochondria, where important steps of heme formation take place. Excess iron can be stored in ferritin. This protein can store several thousand iron atoms. Iron deficit may result from: a) deficiency of dietary iron intake; b) reduction of HCl secretion in the stomach; c) reduction of iron absorption in the duodenum and the proximal small intestine d) physiological (menstrual) and pathological (operative) blood loss. Thus, deficiency of iron after bariatric surgery can be expected. In fact, serum iron deficiency has frequently been observed in patients after bariatric surgery [4,11,12,22,25,37,85,86,87] with an incidence rate as high as approximately 50% [86]. The increased incidence of iron deficiency and anemia in women suggests that menstrual blood loss play a significant role [11,85]. It appears that operative blood loss was not a significant factor in the subsequent development of iron deficiency and anemia.

Potassium – hypokalemia has also been reported after bariatric surgery. In one study, the incidence of hypokalemia reached almost 60% [25]. In another study with 72 patients who underwent jejunoileal bypass because of morbid obesity, 8 patients presented with marked hypokalemia [24]. Moreover, one patient suffered from cardiac arrhythmias, which were likely evoked by hypokalemia due to persistent vomiting following laparoscopic adjustable gastric banding (LAGB) [23]. This stresses the need for frequent evaluation of serum potassium concentration after gastric restrictive surgery to avoid serious complications associated with hypokalemia.

Magnesium – is required for many enzyme activities (as activator), particularly those utilizing ATP as ATPMg complex and for neuromuscular transmission. The main symptoms of magnesium deficiency are weakness, tremor, and cardiac arrhythmia. The results concerning hypomagnesemia reported after bariatric surgery are conflicting. Some data indicate a relatively high occurrence of hypomagnesemia after bariatric surgery [4,24,25], however another study reported no significant effect of bariatric surgery on serum magnesium concentration [11].

Zinc – approximately 300 metalloenzymes, including DNA and RNA polymerases, contain zinc as a part of the catalytic center. Moreover, zinc forms zinc fingers (zinc coordinated to 4 amino acid residues present in several nuclear hormones receptors/transcription factors), which facilitates binding of the transcription factors to the DNA. In this way, zinc is involved in the regulation of transcription of many genes. Zinc is also present in gustin, a salivary polypeptide (produced in humans only by parotid saliva) that appears to be necessary for normal development of taste buds, so zinc deficiency leads to hypogeusia (decreased taste acuity). The contribution of zinc deficiency in hair loss remains under discussion. The absorption of zinc from the intestine is associated with absorption of lipids, which are reduced after bariatric surgery. Thus, theoretically a lower plasma zinc concentration after bariatric surgery can be expected. In fact, a low serum zinc concentration after bariatric surgery was observed [4,68]. Other studies indicate that the zinc erythrocyte and zinc urinary concentrations are the main changes 2 months after RYGB [28]. An abnormal serum zinc concentration in obese subjects was found both before and after RYGB [63]. It should be noted that zinc deficiency is postulated as a factor (along with iron and protein deficiencies) contributing to hair loss after bariatric surgery. Some data indicate reversal of hair loss after vertical gastroplasty when treated with zinc sulfate [88].

Copper – is a cofactor for several enzymes including: ceruloplasmin (which oxidizes iron to facilitate its binding to transferin), cytochrome c oxidase (important element of the mitochondrial respiratory chain), lysyl oxidase (responsible for oxidation of lysil residue to alylysil residue in procollagen to facilitate collagen cross-linking) superoxide dismutase (antioxidant enzyme) and desaturae (converting stearoilo-CoA to oleilo-CoA). The range of copper deficiency symptoms includes anemia, hypercholesterolemia, leucopenia, fragility of large arteries, demineralization of bone, and a demyelination of the neural tissue . In general, copper deficiency is rare in the population. Copper deficiency is associated with anemia, neutropenia and neurolological complications including myelopathy in patients after bariatric surgery [71,89,90]. Thus, for any patient with neurologic symptoms after bariatric surgery, evaluation of serum copper along with other minerals and vitamins is recommended.

References

1. Buchwald H, Avidor Y, Braunwald E, Pories W, Fahrbach K, Schoelles K. Bariatric Surgery. A systematic review and meta-analysis. JAMA 2004; 292: 1724-1737.
2. Patterson EJ, Urbach DR, Swanstrom LL. A comparison o diet and exercise therapy versus laparoscopic Roux-en-Y gastric bypass surgery for morbid obesity: a decision analysis model. J Am Coll Surg. 2003; 196: 379-384
3. Flum D, Dellinger E. Impact of gastric bypass operation on survival: a population-based analysis. J Am Coll Surg 2004; 199: 543-551
4. Bernet CP, Ciangura C, Coupaye M. Czernichow S, Bouillot JL, Basdevant A. Nutritional deficiency after gastric bypass: diagnosis, prevention anf treatment. Diabetes and Metabolism 2007; 33: 13-24
5. Ponsky TA, Brody F, Pucci E. Alterations in gastrointestinal physiology after Roux-en-Y gastric bypass I Am Coll Surg 2005; 2001: 125-131
6. Faintuch J, Matsuda M, Cruz M E L F, Silva MM, Teivelis M P, Garrido Jr A B, Gama-Rodrigues JJ. Severe protein-calorie malnutrition after bariatric procedures. Obes Surg 2004; 14: 175-181
7. Malinowski SS. Nutritional and metabolic complication of bariatric surgery. Am J Med Sci 2006; 331: 219-225
8. Byrne T K. Complications of surgery for obesisty. Surg Clin North Am 2001; 81:1181-1193
9. Dolan K, Hatzifotis M, Newbury L, Lowe N, Fielding G. A clinical and nutritional comparison of biliopancreatic diversion with and without duodenal switch. Ann Surg 2004; 240: 51-56
10. Marceau P, Hould F S, Lebel S, Marceau S, Biron S. Malabsortive obesity surgery Surg Clin North Am 2001; 81: 1113-1127
11. Amaral J F, Thompson W R, Caldwell M D, Martin H F, Randal HT. Prospective hematologic evaluation of gastric exclusion surgery for morbid obesity. Ann Surg 1985; 201: 186-193
12. Alvarez-Leite J I. Nutrient deficiencies secondary to bariatric surgery. Curr Opin Clin Nutr Metab Care 2004; 7:
13. Coates P S, Fernstrom J D, Fernstrom M H, Schauer P R, Greenspan S L. Gastric bypass surgery for morbid obesity leads to and ibcrease in bone turnover and a decrease in bone mass. J Clin Endocrinol Metab 2004; 89: 1061-1065
14. Bult M J F, van Dalen T, Muller A F. Surgical treatment of obesity Eur J Endocrinol 2008; 158: 135-145
15. Fujioka K. Follow-up of nutritional and metabolic problems after bariatric surgery Diabetes Care 2005; 28: 481-484
16. Goode L R, Brolin R E, Chowdhury H A, Shapses S A. Bone and gastric bypass surgery: Effects of dietary calcium and vitamin D. Obes Res 2004; 12: 40-47
17. Riedt C S, Brolin R E, Sherrell R M, Field M P, Shapses S A. True fractional calcium absorption is decreased after Roux-en-Y gastric bypass surgery. Obesity 2006; 14: 1940-1948
18. Sanchez-Hernandez J, Ybarra J, Gich I, De Leiva A, Rius X, Rodriguez-Espinoza J, Perez A. Effects of bariatric surgery on vitamin D status and secondary hyperparathyroidism: a prospective study. Obes Surg 2005; 15: 1389-1395
19. Johnson J M, Maher J W, Samuel I, Heitshusen D, Doherty C, Downs RW. Effects of gastric bypass procedures on bone mineral density, calcium parathyroid hormone, and vitamin D. J Gastrointest Surg 2005; 9: 1106-1110
20. Diniz Mde F, Diniz MT, Sanches SR, Salgado PP, Valadao MM, Araujo FC, Martins DS, Rocha AL. Elevated serum parathormone after Roux-en-Y gastric bypass. Obes Surg 2004; 14: 1222-1226
21. Shaker JL, Noton AJ, Woods MF, Fallon MD, Findling JW. Secondary hyperparathyroidism and osteopenia in women following gastric exclusion surgery for obesity. Osteoporos Int 1991; 1: 177-181
22. Skroubis G, Sakellaropoulos G, Pouggouras K, Mead N, Nikiforidis G, Kalfarentzos F. Comparison of nutritional deficiencies after Rouxen-Y gastric bypass and after billiopancreatic diversion with Roux-en-Y Gastric bypass. Obes Surg 2002; 12: 551-558
23. Reijnen MM, Janssen IM. Cardiac arrhythmias after laparoscopic banding. Obes Surg 2004; 14: 139-141
24. Rasmussen I, Enblad P, Arosenius KE. Jejunoileal bypass for morbid obesity. Report of a series with long-term results. Acta Chir Scand 1989; 155: 401-407

25. Halversen JD. Micronutrients deficiencies after gastric bypass for morbid obesity. Am Surg 1986; 52: 594-598

26. Hocking MP, Davis GK, Franzini DA, Woodward ER. Long-term consequence after jejunoileal bypass for morbid obesity. Dig Dis Sci 1998; 43: 2493-2499

27. Ramsey-Stewart G. The perioperative management of morbidly obese patients (a surgeon's perspective). Annaesth Intensive Care 1985; 13: 399-406

236. Cominetti C, Garrido AB Jr, Cozzolino SM. Zinc nutritional status of morbidly obese patients before and after Roux-en-Y gastric bypass: a preliminary report. Obes Surg 2006; 16: 448-453

28. Service GJ Thompson GB, Service FJ, Andrews JC, Collazo-Clavel ML, Lloyd RV. Hyperinsulinemic hypoglycemia with nesidioblastosis after gastric-bypass surgery. New Eng J Med 2005; 353: 249-54.

29. Brolin RE, Gorman JH, Gorman RC, Petschenik AJ, Bradley LB, Kenler HA, Cody RP. Prophylactic iron supplementation after Roux-en-Y gastric bypass. Arch Surg 1998; 133: 740-744

30. Parkes E. Nutritional management of patients after bariatric surgery. Am J Med Sci 2006; 331: 207-213

31. Crowley LV, Seay J, Mullin G. Late effects of gastric bypass for obesity. Am J Gastroenterol 1984; 79: 850-860

32. Williams DB, Hagedorn JC, Lawson EH, Galanko J A, Safadi B Y, Curet MJ, Morton JM. Gastric bypass reduces biochemical cardiac risk factors. Surgery for Obesity Related Diseases 2007; 3: 8-13

33. Jazet IM, de Groot GH, Tuijnebreyer WE, Fogteloo AJ, Vandenbroucke JP, Meinders AE. Cardiovascular risk factors after bariatric surgery: Do patients gain more than expected from their weight loss? Eur J Intern Med 2007; 18: 39-43

34. Borson-Chazot F, Teboul CHF, Labrousse F, Gaume C, Guadagnino L, Claustrat B, Berthezene F, Moulin P. J Clin Endocrinol Metab 1999; 84: 541-545

35. Rhode BM, Arseneau P, Cooper BA, Katz M, Gilfix BM, MacLean LD. Vitamin B-12 deficiency after gastric surgery for obesity Am J Clin Nutr 1996; 63: 103-109

36. Shah M, Simha V, Garg A. Review: Long-term impact of bariatric surgery on body weight, comorbidities, and nutritional status. J Clin Endocrinol Metab 2006; 91: 4223-4231

37. Wudel Jr L J, Wright JK, Debelak JP, Allos TM, Shyr Y, Chapman WC. Prevention of gallstone formation in morbidly obese patients undergoing rapid weight loss: Results of a randomized controlled pilot study. J Surg Res 2002; 102: 50-56

38. Clark JM, Alkhuraishi AR, Solga SF. Roux-en-Y gastric bypass improves liver histology in patients with non-alcoholic fatty liver disease Obes Res 2005; 13: 1180-1186

39. Zabrocka L, Raczynska S, Goyke E. BMI is the main determinant of the circulating leptin nn women after vertical banded gastroplasty. Obes Res 2004; 12: 505-512

40. Swierczynski J, Korczynska J, Goyke E et al. Serum hepatocyte growth factor concentration in obese women decreases after vertical banded gastroplasty Obes Surg 2005; 15: 803-808

41. Swierczynski J, Sledzinski T, Slominska E, Smolenski R, Sledzinski Z. Serum phenylalanine concentration as a marker of liver function in obese patients before and after bariatric surgery Obes Surg 2008 in press.

251. Gomez-Ambrosi J, Pastor C, Salvador J, Silwa C, Rotellar F, Gil Mj, Catal V, Rodriguez A, Cienfuegos JA, Fruhbeck G. Influence of waist circumstance on the metabolic risk associated with impaired fasting glucose: Effect of weight loss after gastric bypass Obes Surg 2007; 17: 585-591

42. Gorgen M, Arapis K, Limgba A, Schiltz M, Lens V, Azagra JS. Laparoscopic Roux-enY gastric byapass versus laparoscopic vertical banded gastroplasty: results of 2-year follow-up study. Surg Endosc. 2007; 21: 659-664

43. Rajala R, Partinen M, Sane T, Pelkonen R, Huikuri K, Seppalainen AM. Obstructive sleep apnea syndrome in morbidly obese patients J Intern Med 1991; 230: 125-129

44. Rasheid S, Banasiak M, Gallagher SF. Gastric bypass is an effective treatment for obstructive sleep apnea in patients with clinically significant obesisty. Obes Surg 2003; 13: 58-61

45. Christou NV, Sampalis JS, Lieberman M. Surgery decreases long term mortality, morbidity, and health care use in morbidly obese patients. Ann Surg 2004; 240: 416-423

46. Kisakol, G., Guney, E., Bayraktar, F., Yilmaz, C., Kabalak, T., and Ozmen, D. Effect of surgical weight loss on free radical and antioxidant balance: a preliminary report. Obes. Surg. 2002; 12:795-800

47. Uzun, H., Zengin, K., Taskin, M., Aydin, S., Simsek, G., and Dariyerli, N.. Changes in leptin, plasminogen activator factor and oxidative stress in morbidly obese patients following open and laparoscopic Swedish adjustable gastric banding. Obes. Surg. 2004; 14:659-665,

48. Uzun, H., Konukoglu, D., Gelisgen, R., Zengin, K., and Taskin, M. Plasma Protein Carbonyl and Thiol Stress Before and After Laparoscopic Gastric Banding in Morbidly Obese Patients. Obes. Surg. 2007.

49. Brolin RE, Leung M. Survey of vitamin and mineral supplementation after gastric bypass and biliopancreatic diversion for morbid obesity. Obes Surg 1999; 9: 150-154

50. Scopinaro N, Adami GF, Marinari GM et al. Bilipancreatic diversion: two decades of experience. In Deitel M, Cowan Jr GSM, eds Update: Surgery for the morbidly obese patient. Toronto:FD-Communication, 2000, 227-258

51. Carvajal SH, Mulvihill SJ. Postgastrectomy syndromes: dumping and diarrhea. Gastroenterol Clin North Am 1994; 23: 261-279

52. Hvas A-M, Nexo E Diagnosis and treatment of vitamin B12 deficiency. An update. Haematologica 2006; 91: 1506-1512.

53. Koffman BM, Greenfield LJ, Ali II, Pirzada NA. Neurologic complications after surgery for obesity Muscle Nerve 2006; 33: 166-176

54. Brolin RE, Gorman JH, Gorman RC, Petschenik AJ, Bradley LJ, Kenler HA, et al. Are vitamin B12 and folate deficiency clinically important after roux-en-Y gastric bypass? J Gastrointest Surg 1998; 2: 436-442

55. Rindi G, Ventura U. Thiamine intestinal transport. Physiol Rev 1972; 52: 821-826

56. Lee WB, Hamilton SM, Harris JP, Schwab IR. Ocular complications of hypovitaminosis A after bariatric surgery. Ophthalmology 2005; 112: 1031-1034

57. Pereira S, Saboya C, Chaves G, Ramalho A. Class III obesity and its relationship with the nutritional status of vitamin A in pre and postoperative gastric bypass. Obes Surg 2009 Jun;19(6):738–44

58. Rock CL, Swenseid ME. Plasma carotenoid levels in anorexia nervosa and in obese patients. Methods Enzymol 1993; 214: 116-124

59. Granado-Lorencio F, Herrero-Barbudo C, Olmedilla-Alonso B, Blanco-Navarro I, Perez-Sacristan B. Hypocarotenemia after bariatric surgery: A preliminary Study. Obes Surg 2009 Jul;19(7):879–82

60. Hatzifotis M, Dolan K, Newbury L, Fielding G. Symptomatic vitamin A deficiency following bilipancreatic diversion, Obes Surg 2003; 13: 655-657

61. Madan A Orth W, Tichansky D, Ternovits C. Vitamin and trace mineral levels after laparoscopic gastric bypass Obes Surg 2006; 16: 603-606

62. Chaves GV, Pereira SE, Saboya CJ, Ramalho A. Nutritional status of vitamin A in morbid obesity before and after Roux-en-Y gastric bypass. Obes Surg 2007; 17: 970-976

63. Lewandowski H, Breen TL, Huang EY. Kwashiorkor and an acrodermatitis enterropathica-like eruption after a distal gastric bypass surgical procedure. Endocr Pract 2007; 13: 277-282

64. Clements RH, Katasani VG, Palepu R, Leeth RR, Leath TD, Roy BP, Vickers SM. Incidence of vitamin deficiency after laparoscopic Roux-en-Y gastroc bypass in a university hospital setting. Am Surg 2006; 72: 1197-1202

65. Chae T, Foroozan R. Vitamin A deficiency in patients with a remote history of intestinal surgery. Br J Ophthalmol. 2006; 90: 955-956

66. Slater GH, Ren CJ, Siegel N, Williams T, Barr D, Wolfe B, Dolan K, Fielding GA. Serum fat-soluble vitamin deficiency and abnormal calcium metabolism after malabsortive bariatric surgery. J Gastrointest Surg 2004; 8: 48-55

67. Cone LA , Waterbor R, Sofonio MV. Purpura fulminans due to Streptococcus pneumoniae sepsis following gastric bypass. Obes Surg 2004; 14: 690-694

68. Kimmons JE, Blanck HM, Tohill BC, Zhang J, Khan LK. Associations between body mass index and the prevalence of low micronutrient levels among US adults MedGenMed 2006; 8: 59-68

69. Juhasz-Pocsine K, Rudnicki SA, Archer RL, Harik SI. Neurologic complications of gastric bypass surgery for morbid obesity. Neurology 2007; 68: 1843-1850

70. Kumar N. Nutritional neuropathies Neurol Clin 2007; 25: 209- 255

71. Evans DJ, Berney DM, Pollock DJ. Symptomatic vitamin E deficiency diagnosed after histological recognition of myometrial lipofuscinosis. Lancet 1995; 346: 545-546

72. Newbury L, Dolan K, Hatzifotis M, Low N, Fielding G. Calcium and Vitamin D depletion and elevated parathyroid hormone following biliopancreatic diversion. Obes Surg 2003; 13: 893-895

73. Nelson ML, Bolduc LM, Toder ME, Clough DM, Sullivan SS. Correction of preoperative vitamin D deficiency after Roux-en-Y bypass surgery. Surg Obes Relat Dis. 2007; 3: 437-437

74. Schweitzer DH. Mineral metabolism and bone disease after bariatric surgery and ways to optimize bone health Obes Surg 2007; 17: 1510-1516

75. Jin J, Robinson AV, Hallowell PT, Jasper JJ, Stellato TA, Wilhem SM. Increase in parathuroid hormone (PTH) after gastric bypass surgery appear to be of secondary nature. Surgery 2007; 142: 914-920

76. Avgerinos DV, Leitman IM, Martinez RE, Liao EP. Evaluation of markers for calcium homeostasis in a population of obese adults undergoing gastric bypass operations. J Am Coll Surg 2007; 205: 294-297

77. Carlin AM, Yager KM, Rao DS. Vitamin D depletion impairs hypertension resolution after Rou-en-Y gastric bypass. Am J Sur 2008; 195: 349-352

78. Holick MF. High prevalence of vitamin D inadequacy and implications for health Mayo Clinic Proc 2006; 81: 353-373

79. Raisz LG. Pathogenesis of osteoporosis: concepts, conflicts, and prospects. J Clin Invest 2005; 115: 3318-3325

80. Krishnan V, Bryant HU, MacDougald OA. Regulation of bone mass by Wnt signaling. J Clin Invest 2006; 116: 1202-1209

81. Oursler MJ, Landers JP, Riggs BL, Spelsberg TC. Oestrogen effects on osteoblasts and osteoclasts. Ann Med 1993; 25: 361-371

82. Wada T, Nakashima T, Hiroshi N, Penninger JM. RANKL-RANK signaling in osteoclastogenesis and bone disease. Trends Mol Med 2006; 12: 17-25

83. Love AL, Billet HH. Obesity, bariatric surgery, and iron deficiency: True, true, true and related. Am J Hematol 2008; 83: 403 – 409.

84. Brolin RE, LaMarca LB, Kenler HA, Cody RP. Malabsorptive gastric bypass in patients with superobesity. J Gastrointest Surg 2002; 6: 195-203

85. Mizon C, Ruz M, Csendes A, Carrasco F, Rebolledo A, Codoceo J, Inostroza J, Papapietro K, Pizarro F, Olivares M. Nutrition 2007; 23, 277-280

86. Neve HJ, Bhattti WA, Soulsby C, Kincey J, Taylor TV. Reversal of hair loss following following vertical gastroplasty when treated with zinc sulphate. Obes Surg 1996; 6: 63-65

87. Hayton BA, Broome HE, Lilenbaum RC. Copper deficiency-induced anemia and neutropenia secondary to intestinal malaobsorption Am J Hematol 1995; 48: 45-47

88. Kumar N, McEvoy KM, Ahlskog JE. Myelopathy due to copper deficiency following gastrointestinal surgery. Arch Neurol 2003; 60: 1782-1785

Life Quality Tests

Simon Kuesters, MD

Pregnancy

*Jarek Kobiela, MD, Wojciech Makarewicz, MD, Magdalena Wojanowska, MD,
Tomasz Stefaniak, MD, Lukasz Kaska, MD, A. J. Lachinski, MD*

About 25% of women meet the criteria for obesity, and one third of them are of reproductive age. Because of more frequently observed morbid obesity that requires surgical treatment, surgeons and gynecologists are facing new challenges. Not only the women's quality of life, but also the proper development of their children is important. This is a serious health and social-demographic problem because these women are at higher risk for medical problems. That is why complex perinatal care should be provided. This article reviews pregnancy and fertility issues in bariatric surgery patients.

28.1   Incidence and Implications of Obesity

Obesity, defined as a body mass index (BMI) of 30 kg/m^2 or greater, is a fast-growing health problem today, above all in industrial countries. It is becoming the main cause of preventable morbidity and mortality. Public health research has identified obesity as a leading cause of death in America, second only to tobacco-related diseases [1].

It is estimated that about 27% of the United States population is obese [2]. Obesity is increasing in all age groups and is observed to be more common among women than among men. About 25% of women meet the criteria for obesity, and one third of them are of reproductive age [3]. This is a serious health and social-demographic problem because these women are at higher risk for associated medical problems such as diabetes mellitus type 2, hypertensive disorders, coronary heart disease, stroke, depression, and sleep apnea [3, 4]. What is more, obesity also has an impact on their fertility performance and can cause complications in early pregnancy. Some studies have demonstrated that BMI increase is associated with a higher miscarriage rate, a lower mature oocyte yield, and a lower number of cryo cycles [5]. Furthermore, obese women who become pregnant have a greater risk of complications during pregnancy, delivery, and the postpartum period [2] (◘ Table 28.1). They are more likely to have gestational diabetes mellitus, chronic hypertension, preeclampsia, fetal macrosomia, cesarean section, and anesthesia-related complications in comparison to women with a normal BMI [6].

Obesity is a worldwide problem that results in approximately 300,000 deaths and costs of more than $100 billion per year [7]. Therefore, it should be kept in mind that it is cheaper to treat obesity than its complications and adverse medical outcomes.

◘ **Table 28.1** Maternal risks associated with obesity [2]

Period	Increased risk
Antenatal	Increased incidence of miscarriage Gestational diabetes mellitus Hypertension and preeclampsia Fetal anomalies Venous thromboembolism
Intrapartum	Failure of labor to progress Shoulder dystocia Fetal monitoring problems Emergency cesarean section Surgical complications
Postpartum	Wound infection Venous thromboembolism Postnatal depression

28.2   Treatment of Obesity: Bariatric Surgery

Treatment of obesity is difficult for patients. It is a long-term process that requires their patience and persistence in pursuing the goal, which is to lose weight. In the therapy of obese people a group of additional specialists including a nutritionist, a psychologist, and a rehabilitation therapist should be involved. Organizing the therapy this way makes it more effective.

At first, obese people are advised to change their lifestyle, which means dietary modifications and more physical activity. When this approach fails pharmacological therapy is initiated (involving agents affecting food intake or nutrient absorption, or increasing thermogenesis). Bariatric surgery is an option for carefully selected morbidly obese patients or patients with grade-2 obesity with co-morbid conditions when less invasive methods of weight loss have failed and the patient is at higher risk for obesity-related morbidity and mortality [8].

Considerations on pregnancy following bariatric surgery are dependent on the type of procedures performed. These are usually classified into two main groups, restrictive and malabsorptive, and sometimes into a third group of malabsorptive-restrictive procedures. Restrictive bariatric procedures induce weight loss by reducing stomach capacity, while malabsorptive operations diminish gastric volume and disrupt the proper absorption of ingested food and nutrients. Each category of procedures has its own impact on postoperative nutrition and pregnancy, but it is reported that malabsorptive procedures are connected with a higher risk of nutritional deficiency [3].

These procedures were introduced in Europe and America in the 1950s. The first technique was the jejunoileal bypass; 10 years later the jejunocolic bypass was performed, but because of severe complications it was abandoned. Later in the 1960s the first Roux-en-Y was performed and in the 1980s the open vertical banded gastroplasty procedure was pioneered by Mason and Kuzmak [9, 10]. The use of laparoscopy in these kinds of procedures has decreased the morbidity of gastric banding. Bariatric surgery is becoming an increasingly popular approach to treating obesity and is now one of the fastest growing fields of surgical practice. The number of procedures performed increases every year. It is estimated that more than 90% of these surgical interventions in Europe are laparoscopic adjustable gastric banding (LAGB) procedures [10].

28.3   Pregnancy after Bariatric Surgery

It is estimated that 87% of bariatric patients are women, most of them of reproductive age. Pregnancy after surgical bariatric treatment seems to be a complex medical challenge. It is necessary to inform women about special supplementation, additional laboratory tests and controls, possible complications, and the impact of bariatric surgery on their pregnancy. It is suggested that operated bariatric patients who become pregnant need to be examined and cared for by a group of specialists including a nutritionist, educated nursing staff, an obstetric caregiver, an endocrinologist, an internist, and the bariatric surgeon [11].

28.4   Preconception and Antepartum

Obese women have fertility problems. After bariatric procedures, when women are losing weight, their fertility performance improves. This may be effected by stabilizing the level of sexual hormones and by psychological factors: when women are losing weight they feel more sexually attractive. In the first period after the surgical procedure they should consider the use of contraceptives or another form of birth control [12]. Women should also be warned that oral contraceptives may not provide adequate levels in their blood, because of altered absorption from the gut, and other forms of contraception are therefore advisable, i.e., transdermal systems. Currently it is highly recommended that pregnancy be delayed for 12–18 months after surgery [13], because during the first year after a bariatric procedure patients go through a phase of rapid weight loss. This starvation state is a specific stress for the organism and may be dangerous for both the mother and the fetus [14]. If women becoming pregnant, as recommended, the malnutrition of mother and fetus is less dangerous than it would be during the first year after surgery.

28.4.1   Vomiting

Frequent problems faced by women who have undergone bariatric surgery are vomiting and nausea. Patients may experience persistent vomiting because they do not chew their food thoroughly or because they eat too rapidly. In the first trimester of pregnancy many women experience persistent vomiting, and if this is added to vomiting as an effect of a bariatric procedure it can be more difficult to handle [3, 15]. Pregnant women who have undergone adjustable gastric banding and are experiencing hyperemesis may have the fluid in the band reduced to facilitate pouch emptying, thus reducing the frequency of vomiting and providing some relief [13, 15].

28.4.2   Nutritional and Microelement Deficiencies

Following bariatric surgery, all patients have to take prescribed vitamins and minerals to prevent micronutrient deficiencies. Obviously, this problem is even more important when a woman who has undergone bariatric procedure is pregnant. Pregnancy would require additional supplementation. Ideally, micronutrient deficiencies should be prevented or treated before a woman becomes pregnant. Unfortunately, only 59% of women use a multiple vitamin supplement for a long period of time after bariatric surgery [16] and when they get pregnant they can be at a higher risk for some complications caused by micronutrient deficiencies, most frequently vitamin B_{12}, folic acid, calcium, and iron. Nutritional status during pregnancy and lactation may therefore be a contributing factor to maternal and infant morbidity and mortality.

A common issue following bariatric surgery is calcium deficiency caused by inadequate consumption or malabsorption. The bypass procedures frequently lead to calcium deficiency because they exclude the duodenum and proximal jejunum from calcium absorption [15]. It is recommended to take 1000–2000 mg of calcium citrate together with vitamin D (50–150 µg). The citrate form is optimal; it does not require an acidic stomach environment to be broken down and absorbed [15]. Inadequate calcium intake may result in maternal bone loss, reduced breast milk, Ca secretion, or inappropriate mineralization of the fetal skeleton. To prevent this complication fetus growth should be monitored regularly with ultrasound scans [15].

Another common problem of women after bariatric surgery is iron deficiency anemia. The pathogenesis is multifactorial and complex. It is related partially to a decreased intake of adequate quantities of iron-rich food such as red meat. Additionally after bariatric surgery, patients may develop achlorhydria which, leads to a reduction in iron absorption. Bypassing the duodenum and the proximal jejunum eliminates the first and main site of iron absorption [15, 17]. It is almost certain to occur after malabsorptive operations. Patients who have undergone restrictive operations do not experience iron deficiency, and routine supplementation for them may not be required. However, to verify iron sufficiency the serum levels of hemoglobin, serum iron, ferritin, and transferrin should be controlled regularly. Iron should be taken in ferrous form in a dose of 40–65 mg daily [15]. The supplementation should be modified after laboratory tests.

Attention should be paid as well to the next cause of anemia – vitamin B_{12} deficiency. Despite its being less common, almost every patient regularly receives cobalamin supplements. Following bariatric surgery the absorption of cobalamin may be disrupted at different levels depending on the type of procedure. Absence of an acid environment following gastric bypass surgery, inadequate secretion of intrinsic factor (IF), and finally malabsorption mean that too little vitamin B_{12}/IF is absorbed in the terminal ileum, leading to vitamin B_{12} deficiency [17]. The low level of cobalamin may result in elevated serum homocysteine levels, and hyperhomocysteinemia is related to early miscarriage. To avoid this complication the levels of homocysteine and vitamin B_{12} should be checked periodically. An inadequate level of vitamin B_{12} related to lower intake during pregnancy can result in neurobehavioral disorders in the infant with symptoms of decreased ability to concentrate, depression, problems with abstract thought, and memory impairment and confusion. Severe vitamin B_{12} deficiency can also result in infant anemia [18]. The recommended daily sublingual dose of cobalamin in pregnancy after bariatric surgery is 350 µg in easily absorbed crystalline form. This is generally sufficient to maintain adequate serum cobalamin levels, which will normalize the level of homocysteine [15]. Occasionally, when this therapy is not sufficient, intramuscular injections are recommended in monthly doses of 1000 µg [17]. We suggest the modern sublingual substitution, which is more comfortable for the patients.

During the past few years great emphasis has been put on folic acid and the prevention of fetal neural tube defects (NTDs), which occur when the brain, skull, spinal cord, and spinal column do not develop properly within 4 weeks after conception. The most common NTDs are anencephaly, which causes stillbirth and death soon after delivery, and spina bifida, which may result in a wide range of physical disabilities including partial and total paralysis [19]. If maternal folate stores are insufficient prior to conception, the risk of an adverse pregnancy outcome such as preterm delivery and birth defects in the following pregnancy is increased. That is why it is recommended that all women of childbearing age who are capable of becoming pregnant should supplement their folic acid intake. Following bariatric surgery, food rich in folate bypasses the duodenum or is not well-tolerated by the patients, so they are at higher risk of having folic acid deficiency and associated NTDs. However, supplementation with prenatal vitamins containing 1 mg of folic acid prior to and during pregnancy is usually sufficient to maintain adequate serum levels and reduce the risk of neural tube defects [20].

The next problem which should be considered is vitamin A deficiency. It is reported that it occurs in 10% of patients following gastric bypass. The exclusion of the duodenum results in delayed mixing of dietary fat (containing fat-soluble vitamins) with pancreatic enzymes and bile salts, with malabsorption and deficiency as the consequences [17]. Vitamin A plays an important part in reproduction and in cell differentiation and proliferation. An adequate level of vitamin A is necessary especially in the second and third trimesters of pregnancy for normal fetal lung development and maturation. Several studies have shown an increased risk of bronchopulmonary dysplasia (BPD) in preterm infants with insufficient vitamin A status [21]. Vitamin A deficiency also impairs iron status, increases susceptibility to respiratory infections and diarrhea, and increases morbidity and mortality. It has been suggested that the vitamin A status of pregnant women can influence vitamin A stores in the liver of the fetus [22]. To avoid this complication plasma retinol levels have to be checked periodically and if it is needed oral supplements should be prescribed, but special attention should be paid, because excessive amounts of retinol are teratogenic for the fetus [19]. Some studies recommend the intake of β-carotene (non-teratogenic) rather than retinol [21, 23]. An additional benefit of vitamin A supplementation in pregnant women is that it can increase hemoglobin concentrations [22].

Not only vitamin levels are disturbed in pregnancy or after bariatric procedures. Zinc levels can drop by about 30% during a 'normal' pregnancy, so it is important to have adequate supplies. This should be considered especially after malabsorptive bariatric operations. Low levels of zinc have been linked to premature deliveries, low birth weight, abnormal fetal development, and spina bifida. Cases of zinc deficiency during breastfeeding are accompanied by skin rashes or dermatitis as the main symptoms, often in combination with failure to thrive and irritability [24]. We suggest the optimal dose of zinc as 15 mg per day.

Magnesium supplementation during pregnancy may be able to reduce fetal growth retardation and preeclampsia and increase birth weight. Furthermore, it can help to prevent premature contractions by relaxing the muscles of the uterus. Studies show that magnesium levels are lower in women who have had premature labor, although there is not enough high-quality evidence to show that dietary magnesium supplementation during pregnancy is beneficial [25].

Little attention has been paid to the potentially important issue of antioxidant nutrient status in pregnancy. Oxidative stress caused by free radicals has been implicated in many studies of the etiology of preeclampsia. This is a very dangerous condition in pregnancy that in some cases can lead to poor growth of the baby and premature birth. There can also be serious complications for the woman, sometimes affecting the liver, kidneys, brain, or blood clotting system. Antioxidants, such as vitamin C, vitamin E, selenium, and lycopene, can neutralize free radicals. The current evidence does not support the use of antioxidants to reduce the risk of preeclampsia or other complications in pregnancy, but there are trials still in progress [26]. Moreover, selenium deficiency may be a factor in some early-pregnancy miscarriages. However, while adequate selenium is necessary for the normal development of a fetus, some evidence suggests that too much selenium may also cause a child to develop abnormally (nervous-system damage). Until the results of a randomized trial are published, it is not recommended that women take selenium supplements before or during pregnancy.

Summing up, in order to prevent complications in pregnancy after bariatric surgery in the form of micronutrient deficiencies and associated disorders, patients must be precisely informed about the necessity to take prescribed vitamins postoperatively. In addition, periodical serum examinations have to be done and if necessary the dose of prescribed vitamins should be changed for certain individuals. It is worth pointing out that recent studies of pregnancy after gastric-bypass surgery have shown no adverse perinatal outcomes associated with micronutrient deficiencies [27, 28].

28.4.3 Gestational Diabetes and Hypertension

With regard to pregnancy after bariatric surgery, it is important to emphasize that the incidence of gestational diabetes and hypertension is lower in pregnancies after bariatric procedures [17], and this is an undeniable benefit for the woman and the fetus. Standard testing for gestational diabetes in women following bariatric surgery is problematic. In pregnant women the glucose tolerance test can cause the dumping syndrome, with nausea, abdominal cramps, diarrhea, and heart palpitations [3]. In this special group of patients fasting blood sugar should be tested, or continuous glucose monitoring for several days should be performed [3, 15].

28.4.4 Weight Gain

Weight gain during pregnancy following bariatric surgery can vary. Women who have undergone adjustable gastric banding and sleeve gastrectomy present the highest variation in weight gain. It is reported that some of them lose weight during pregnancy while others gain more than is recommended. However, it is observed that women who delay pregnancy for at least 2 years following surgery are most likely to have a restricted or normal pregnancy weight gain [15]. Because of the potential for abnormal fetal growth, regular check-ups must be done, including ultrasound and a clinical examination [15]. In addition, those women, more frequently than the general population, are subjected to ultrasound scans every 4–6 weeks starting from the 24th week of gestation to monitor fetal growth [27]. The most recent information about outcomes after obesity surgery suggests that guidelines for weight gain during pregnancy after bariatric surgery should be revised. Commonly, it is recommended that normal-weight women with a BMI of 19.8–26 kg/m2 gain 11.5–16 kg, while those in the "high range" (BMI of 26.1–29 kg/m2) should have a "recommended target weight gain of at least 7 kg" according to the Institute of Medicine of the National Academy of Sciences.

28.5 Intrapartum

A normal and uncomplicated course of labor is expected in the post-bariatric surgery pregnant woman. It is reported that women whose weight is stabilized following bariatric surgery and who achieve nutritional balance usually experience less morbidity and mortality during pregnancy [3], because significant weight loss decreases the risk of intrapartum complications such as preeclampsia, large-gestational-age infant, operative delivery, and surgical wound infections [15], which are frequent in obese women.

However, there are some bariatric surgery-related complications which can appear during the perinatal period and have severe outcomes including fetal and/or maternal death. Following bariatric procedures, pregnant women may develop abdominal hernias, gallstones, gastrointestinal hemorrhage, or internal herniation of the bowel, all due to changes in nutrient absorption, changes in metabolism, and organ displacement as the uterus enlarges [3, 15]. There are three time periods when obstruction is more likely to occur: when the uterus becomes an abdominal organ, during labor, and during the postpartum period when the uterus involutes [29]. These complications are rare, but it is very important to inform pregnant women about the urgency of these conditions and to ask them to report the occurrence of severe pain, nausea, vomiting, fever, and flu-like symptoms [3].

28.6 Postpartum

As breastfeeding is recommended for at least 6 months, mothers after bariatric surgery should be encouraged to breastfeed their newborn children. It is obvious and undeniable that maternal nutrition has an impact on the quality of their milk. It should be not forgotten that the fetus may develop malnutrition, especially when the

mother has undergone a malabsorptive form of bariatric surgery. It is very important to maintain micronutrient supplementation after delivery and during breastfeeding to ensure the adequate intake of vitamins and minerals for the neonate and to prevent vitamin B deficiency, which can cause severe complications including failure to thrive, megaloblastic anemia, and development delays [3, 15]. Improvements in growth, development, and reversal of anemia have been observed following adequate vitamin B supplementation [15]. Mother and child should be under special medical care during the entire period of breastfeeding, just as during pregnancy. We perform medical controls of our pregnant and breastfeeding women every 3 months (Medical Universities in Gdansk and Freiburg). Micro- and macronutrient supplementation is provided as shown in ◘ Table 28.2 following adequate modification.

28.7 Conclusion

As obesity is a growing problem in modern societies, the number of women of childbearing age who become pregnant following bariatric surgery will be increasing in the course of time. Recent studies have shown that suitable medical care must be provided to prevent adverse medical outcomes during and after pregnancy following bariatric procedures. In addition, cooperation between the medical staff and well-informed pregnant women

◘ **Table 28.2** Suggested vitamin and mineral supplementation in patients after bariatric surgery procedures

	Gastric bypass	BPD	Sleeve gastrectomy
Calcium with vitamin D3	1000 mg (with 0.05 mg) daily	2000 mg (with 130 µg) daily	
Multivitamins and minerals	1 tablet daily	1 tablet daily	1 tablet daily
Fe^{+2}	1 tablet daily – for 1 week (3 weeks' break)	1 tablet daily 30 mg – for 1 week (3 weeks' break)	
Proteins	40–60 g daily	70–90 g daily	
Vitamin B_{12}	1000 µg i.m. or 25 000 units sublingually twice a week for 3 months	1000 µg i.m. or 25 000 units sublingually twice a week for 3 months	
Vitamin B_1	1 tablet 2.5 mg daily	1 tablet 2.5 mg daily	
Zinc	1 tablet 15 mg daily	1 tablet 15 mg daily	
Biotin, selenium	Daily for 4 months	Daily for 4 months	
Vitamin A	1 tablet 1 mg daily	1 tablet 1 mg daily	
Folic acid	400–800 µg	400–800 µg	

is very important and indispensable. Some studies have suggested that laparoscopic adjustable gastric banding (LAGB) or sleeve gastrectomy are more suitable for young women than Roux-en-Y gastric bypass or biliopancreatic diversion, but definitive studies comparing these two procedures have yet to be conducted. Following malabsorptive bariatric surgery, all pregnant patients should receive nutrient supplementation according to their individual needs. Patients should be informed about avoiding pregnancy in the first year after bariatric surgery and about the insufficiency of oral contraception. The period of pregnancy and breastfeeding should be correlated with laboratory test controls in each trimester and later every 3 months with appropriate supplement modification.

Bariatric surgery is the most rapidly growing area of surgical practice today. Therefore, we expect to face new long-term effects, with reproduction as one of the most important issues to be assessed.

References

1. Allison DB, Fonatine KR, Manson JE, et al (1999) Annual deaths attributable to obesity in the United States. JAMA 282:1530–1538
2. Brockelsby J, Dresner M (2006) Obesity and pregnancy. Curr Anaesth Crit Care 17:125–129
3. Edwards JE (2005) Pregnancy after bariatric surgery. AWHONN Lifelines 9:388–393
4. Sheiner E, Levy A, Silverberg D, et al (2004) Pregnancy after bariatric surgery is not associated with adverse perinatal outcome. Am J Obstet Gynecol 190:1335–1340
5. Esinler I, Bozdag G, Yarali H (2005) Does obesity have an adverse effect on conception rates with ICSI? Fertil Steril 84 [Suppl 1]:S256
6. Kumari AS (2001) Pregnancy outcome in women with morbid obesity. Int J Gynaecol Obstet 73:101–107
7. Klein S, Wadden T, Sugerman HJ AGA (2002) Technical review on obesity. Gastroenterology 123:882–932
8. National Institutes of Health (1998) Clinical guidelines on the identification, evaluation, and treatment of overweight and obesity in adults – the evidence report. Obes Res 6 [Suppl 2]: 51S–209S
9. Saber AA, Elgamal MH, McLeod MK (2008) Bariatric surgery: the past, present, and future. Obes Surg 18:121–128
10. O'Brien PE, Dixon JB, Brown W (2004) Obesity is a surgical disease: overview of obesity and bariatric surgery. ANZ J Surg 74:200–204
11. Deitel M (1998) Pregnancy after bariatric surgery. Obes Surg 8:465–466
12. Weiner RA (2006)Adipositaschirurgie Indikation und Therapieverfahren, Abs. 14 T.Fiebig. Sonderfall: Schwangerschaft, UNI-MED
13. Martin LF, Finigan KM, Nolan TE (2000) Pregnancy after adjustable gastric banding. Obstet Gynecol 95:927–930
14. Wittgrove AC, Jester L, Wittgrove P et al (1998) Pregnancy following gastric bypass for morbid obesity. Obes Surg 8:461–466
15. Woodard CB (2004) Pregnancy following bariatric surgery. J Perinat Neonatal Nurs 18:329–340
16. Dixon JB, Dixon ME, O'Brien PF (2001) Elevated homocysteine levels with weight loss after lap-band surgery: higher folate and vitamin B12 levels required to maintain homocysteine level. Int J Obes Relat Metab Disord 25:219–227
18. Decker GA, Swain JM, Crowell MD et al (2007) Gastrointestinal and nutritional complications after bariatric surgery. Am J Gastroenterol 102:2571–2580
19. Allen LH (1994) Vitamin B-12 metabolism and status during pregnancy, lactation and infancy. Adv Exp Med Biol 352:173–186
20. Williamson CS (2006) Nutrition in pregnancy. British Nutrition Foundation Nutrition Bulletin 31:28–59
21. Kushner R (2000) Managing the obese patient after bariatric surgery: a case report of severe malnutrition and review of the literature. JPEN J Parenter Enteral Nutr 24:126–132
22. Strobel M, Tinz J, Biesalski HK (2007) The importance of beta-carotene as a source of vitamin A with special regard to pregnant and breastfeeding women. Eur J Nutr 46 [Suppl 1]:11–20
23. van den Berg H (1996) Vitamin A intake and status. Eur J Clin Nutr 50 [Suppl 3]:S7–12
24. Conning DM (1991)Vitamin A in pregnancy. BNF Nutrition Bulletin 16
25. Lindsay HA (2005) Multiple micronutrients in pregnancy and lactation: an overview. Am J Clin Nutr 81:1206S–1212S
26. Makrides M, Crowther CA (1998) Magnesium supplementation in pregnancy. Cochrane Database of Systematic Reviews, issue 2
27. Rumbold A, Duley L, Crowther CA, Haslam RR (2005) Antioxidants for preventing pre-eclampsia. Cochrane Database of Systematic Reviews, issue 4
28. Dao T, Kuhn J, Ehmer D, et al (2006) Pregnancy outcomes after gastric-bypass surgery. Am J Surg 192:762–766
29. Bar-Zohar D, Azem F, Klausner J, et al (2006) Pregnancy after laparoscopic adjustable gastric banding: perinatal outcome is favorable also for women with relatively high gestational weight gain. Surg Endosc 20:1580–1583
30. Cunningham FG, Gant NF, Leveno KJ et al (2001) Williams obstetrics, 21st edn. McGraw-Hill, New York

V Secondary and Redo Operations

Principals of Metabolic Revisional Surgery

W. Konrad Karcz, MD, Waleed Bukhari, MD, Mark Daoud, MD, Simon Kuesters, MD

We do not know how many patients have undergone revisionary bariatric and metabolic surgery worldwide. Each clinic has its own percentage of re-operations, and the range is said to be between 2% and 20%. Parallel to the development of new methods, we now are increasingly aware of a number of patients who want revisionary surgery due to low EWL after the primary operation. The establishment of a central data bank for all metabolic patients would help us to investigate the real incidence of re-operations. The development and improvement of diagnostic procedures and guidelines prior to revisionary surgery is still one of our main objectives. Bariatric re-operations are technically demanding. Primary bariatric operations are relatively safe; a meta-analysis reports mortality of 0.02–1% [1]. However, the re-operation rate has been as high as 56% in some series [2, 3]. In this chapter were present various options for revisionary surgery and point out factors that ought to be considered when choosing the right procedure.

29.1 Indications for Revisional Surgery

Indications for revision operations can be divided into two categories: early and late post-operative complications. The first group includes hemorrhage (intraluminal, intra-abdominal, and others), suture insufficiency (pouch, remnant stomach, duodenum, intestine, GEA, DIA, JJA, and JIA), early herniation (mostly Littre's hernia), ileus, wound infections, intra-abdominal abscess, etc. These problems ought to be promptly and consistently solved according to general surgical principals. Late complications can be divided into three different clusters: (a) implant-related, (b) intestinal tract-related, and (c) metabolic with recurrence or aggravation of related disorders. Implant-related complications are directly associated with gastric banding, the Endo Barrier®, rings, etc. [4–6]. The three most common problems associated with implants are migration, dislocation, and infection. Also common are port-related problems in cases of adjustable gastric banding [5]. Alimentary tract-related postoperative complications usually lead to general and unspecific symptoms such as recurrent emesis, abdominal pain, pyrosis, or diarrhea. Correlating morphological diagnoses include stenosis (GEE, JJE), esophagus dilatation, biliary or acid reflux, ulcerations (pouch, remnant stomach, duodenum, GEA), and bowel obstruction. The most interesting group of late surgical complications includes the appearance, recurrence, or persistence of metabolic disorders. Here we include inadequate weight loss, weight regain, dumping syndrome (early and late), extensive malabsorption, problems related to malabsorption of medication [7], persistence of obesity-related diseases,

and recurrence of obesity-related diseases such as isolated diabetes (insulin required, oral drugs required), metabolic syndrome, or dyslipidemia. Up to now, the most common cause of re-operations following bariatric surgery has been insufficient weight loss or weight regain. However, the current changes and extension of indications for primary operations will probably lead to a shift of reasons for revisional operations [2, 3, 8–10].

Several indications for revisional surgery were established after bariatric and metabolic operations:

- Emergency operations – according to general surgical principles
- Weight regain – more than 2 kg per month for longer than 6 months
- Insufficient restriction – dilatation of GE, pouch, or sleeve; dysfunction of lower esophageal sphincter; band slippage
- Insufficient weight control – BMI >40 kg/m^2 2 years after the primary procedure
- Poor quality of life – BAROS score < 3 with corresponding complaints
- Recurrence of obesity-related diseases 1 year after primary surgery

In our opinion, the patient's physical activity should be assessed with objective measurements, for instance, resting energy expenditure (REE) or calorimetry to objectify the patient's muscle condition [12].

The information given by the patient is always subjective. Prior to a revisional operation the surgeon needs objective and detailed information about the stomach pouch volume. As a standard method, a two-dimensional X-ray with contrast medium is used to estimate the stomach pouch volume and its function [13–17]. Nevertheless, the pouch volume can often not be measured properly using this method. The volume of the pouch is reduced to two-dimensional areas which are measured semi-quantitatively. Furthermore, images can often be taken in only one plane due to the obese patient's body dimensions. It is also possible that different parts of the stomach pouch or sleeve are not placed in an optimal position; this results in an over-projection, especially if the pouch or sleeve is voluminous. The development of stomach pouch volumetry using multi-sliced computed tomography scans (MSCT) and special software for 3D-rendering allows precise estimation of pouch and sleeve volumes and also evaluation of related anatomical structures [18]. It also allows exact measurement of anastomoses, their shapes, and their positions after gastric bypass surgery. This directly influences revisions. Furthermore, other pathologies such as fistulas or internal herniations can be evaluated. Another essential examination is upper endoscopy with morphological inspection of the esophagus, the lower esophageal sphincter, the stomach pouch, anastomoses, and the upper intestine [19, 20].

All pathological changes should be subjected to histopathological inspection. The Helicobacter pylori test (f.i. HUT) needs to be performed prior to each revision procedure [21]. There is another group of functional examinations that can deliver useful informations: Esophageal and stomach pouch/sleeve 24-h manometry, pH-metry, and NMR dynamic stomach movement (NMR-DSM) [22, 23]. The role of the lower esophageal sphincter (LES) is especially important. It is responsible for keeping the pouch closed. After food enters the stomach, the region of the cardia is stretched, and as a consequence a feeling of satiety results. An insufficient LES is responsible for GERD after sleeve gastrectomy and partly responsible for a lack of satiety as well as for moderate esophagus dilatation after gastric banding, VBG, and sleeve or bypass procedures. The peristaltic NMR-DMS is able to recognize the speed of stomach emptying and peristaltic wave after sleeve gastrectomy and the function of the pylorus. Together with manometry, it delivers important pathophysiological data.

In the future, these examinations could influence the selection of the revisionary operation.

29.2 Contra-indications for revisional Surgery

All of us deliberate about when revisional surgery should be not performed. Patients without a follow-up history ought to first undergo a 3- to 6-month period of observation at a reference center. Detailed evaluation and adequate diagnostics are absolutely necessary. Patients who have not undergone full diagnostic evaluation should not be operated on; the risk of not choosing the optimal procedure is relatively high. All patients who do not receive approval from the associated consultants on the metabolic board should not be operated on. Without physical activity, a reduction of food intake leads to muscle atrophy. There are metabolic revision principles: avoid combining a very strong restriction with malabsoption, do not reduce the gastric pouch volume to under 10 ml, and do not reduce a common channel to shorter than 50 cm. Ignoring these principles leads to late complications and re-operations. We all agreed for the conclusion: no compliance, no revisional surgery.

29.3 Diagnostics Prior to Revision

One of the most important factors that should be evaluated in detail is the patient's eating habits. Eating protocols are very useful and ought to be analyzed by a professional

dietician and a psychologist specialized in eating disorders. All questions concerning volume and frequency of meals are very important for the surgeon. They lead directly to the functional stomach pouch restriction. In practice, we use the so-called pizza question, which gives us information about the gastric pouch volume. If the patient is able to eat more than half of a medium-size pizza, the restriction is probably no longer sufficient. This question should be asked in the course of evaluating the patient's eating habits. There are other tests as well, such as the cottage-cheese test, described by Flanagan [11]. Blood tests can objectively assess the patient's response to oral vitamin and micro-element supplementation. This, too, ought to influence selection of the revisional surgery procedure.

29.4 Revisional Surgery Following Obsolete Bariatric Operations

There are still patients who received a jejunoileal bypasses (■ Fig. 29.1), all of whom should undergo revisions. In the past, we performed such revisions mainly with an open technique. The laparoscopic approach can be very difficult because of intestinal adhesions, which can lead to a long operating time and intestinal lesions [24]. Almost all bariatric operations were performed as revisional operations after the JIB, from the physiological reconstruction to the Scopinaro operation [25–28]. Concerning the

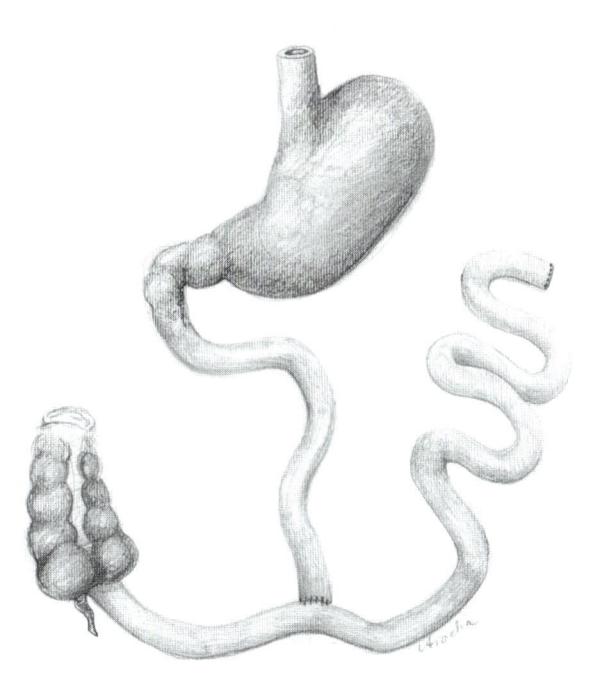

■ **Fig. 29.1.** Jejunoileal bypass

choice of the revisionary operation, the patient's BMI, the time after the primary operation, the length of follow-up, and individual patient needs should be considered.

The most conservative option is to transform the JIB into a BPD or BPD-DS. This can be done easily as an open procedure on the following conditions: the patient has no diarrhea, no hypoproteinemia, no liver disorder, and no deficiency of lipid-soluble vitamins. From a technical point of view, the procedure itself should be performed as a hybrid operation, with the upper part done laparoscopically (almost no adhesions there) and the intestinal part with open access through the old cicatrix. The operation begin laparoscopically in the upper abdominal cavity; a restriction is easy to achieve (sleeve or pouch formation). If possible, the intestinal preparation and reconstruction can also be done endoscopically. The GE (transformation to RYGB) or DE (transformation to DS) anastomosis is formed after the necessary preparation. If reconstruction of the intestine is difficult or if the anatomy is not clear, and 20 minutes of laparoscopic operation do not lead to progress, the reconstruction should be continue with a minilaparotomy.

A good option, especially for patients with malnutrition, severe flatulence, and diarrhea, is the conventional proximal gastric bypass. Another popular procedure is the physiological reconstruction of the intestine followed by gastric banding or sleeve gastrectomy to prevent weight regain. The isolated reconstruction of the intestine is done mostly in patients with extreme malabsorption. Patients with vertical banded gastroplasty and the Mill pro-

cedure are still frequently seen in clinical practice. Today, the VBG (◘ Fig. 29.2) and Mill procedures (◘ Fig. 29.3) are rarely performed due to disappointing long-term results and the availability of a variety of alternative metabolic operations [2, 29].

Frequent complications with the band and the vertical stapling line lead to a high re-operation rate after VBG [2, 30]. In the past, a common revision operation was the re-stapling of the vertical suture or the complete separation of the pouch and remnant stomach with a GIA stapler. There are still several clinics that perform a modified VBG with a Silastic ring and a complete stomach separation (◘ Fig. 29.4) in order to avoid gastro-gastric fistulas. In times of gastric banding and sleeve gastrectomy, the indication for Silastic ring gastroplasty (SRVG) should be carefully considered. We have found two main groups of patients with complications following VBG: those with strong restriction (length of the ring 5.5 cm, with vomiting more than once every day) and those without any restriction (mostly due to vertical stapling rupture and gastro-gastric fistula).

The anatomical and functional status of the stomach should be evaluated with gastroscopy, contrast medium, or, if possible, 3D MSCT, manometry, and pH-metry. If the patient regains weight or there is aggravation or recurrence of associated co-morbidities, it might be necessary to perform a conventional Roux-en-Y gastric bypass (CRYGB) (◘ Fig. 29.5) or a biliopancreatic diversion (BPD) (◘ Fig. 29.6) as a revisional operation [2, 29, 31–33]. In patients scheduled for CRYGB after VBG, Fobi

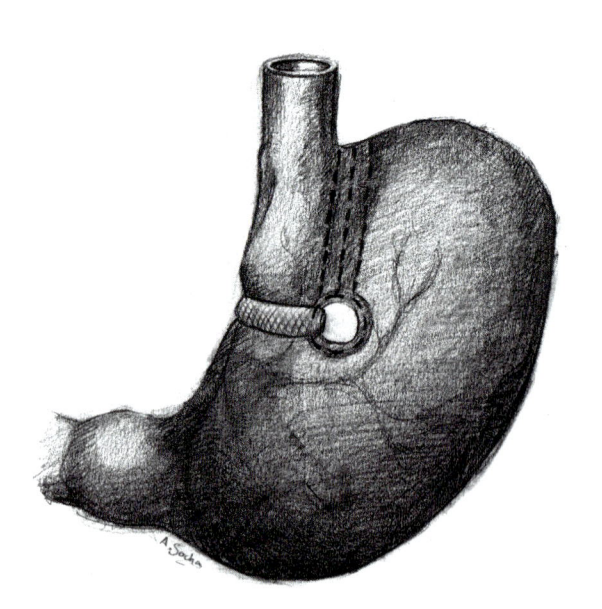

◘ **Fig. 29.2.** Vertical Banded Gastroplasty (VBG, E.E. Mason procedure)

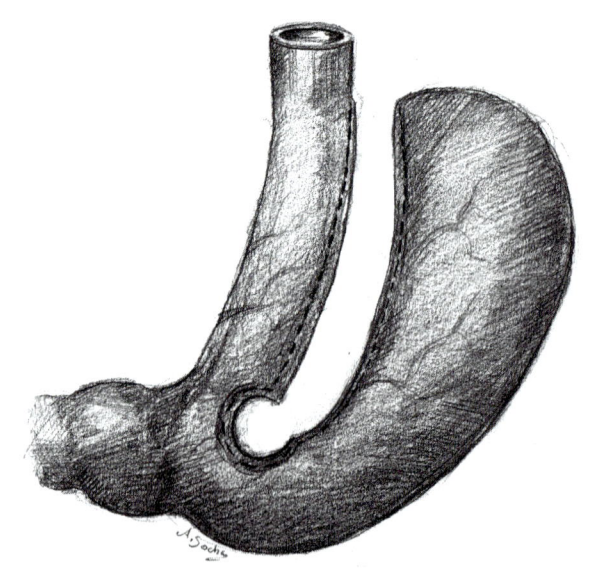

◘ **Fig. 29.3.** Magenstrasse and Mill procedure (M&M)

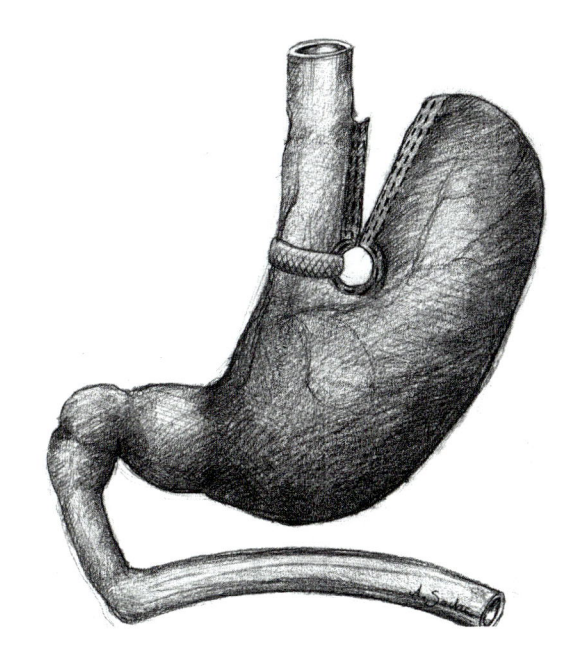

Fig. 29.4. Vertical Banded Gastroplasty with stomach pouch separation (MacLean procedure)

at al. left the pouch and band in place and performed the bypass distal to the VBG banding. This led to the development of the primary banded Roux-en-Y gastric bypass procedure [34, 35].

Nowadays, patients who do not suffer from strong restriction after VBG can be operated with a banded gastric bypass (BRYGB) (**Fig. 29.7**), but with a completely new stomach pouch formation. The first re-operations after VBG were done in open fashion. Now, we prefer to perform the operation laparoscopically. Following adhesiolysis, the dissection of the greater curvature and the opening of the bursa omentalis should be performed. The whole fundus should then be separated from the omentum majus with cutting of the short gastric arteries. The adhesions in the bursa omentalis are then much easier to identify and to separate, the banding is easier to identify, and the vertical TA90B Stapler suture is more clearly visible. Afterwards, the stomach should be horizontally dissected under the banding using a vertical linear Endo-GIA® (Covidien, Auto Suture, 60-mm staplers with green cartridge). Preparation of the lesser curvature and the left

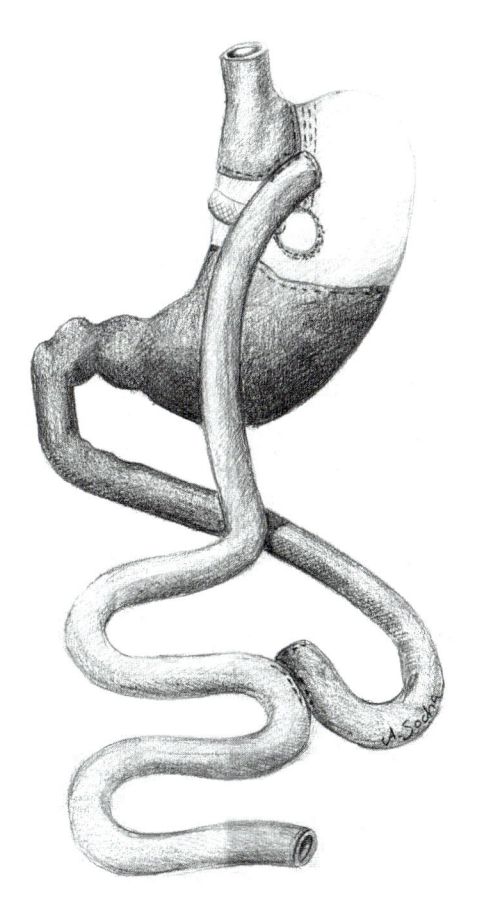

Fig. 29.5. Conventional Roux-en-Y gastric bypass, after VGB (Vertical Banded Gastroplasty)

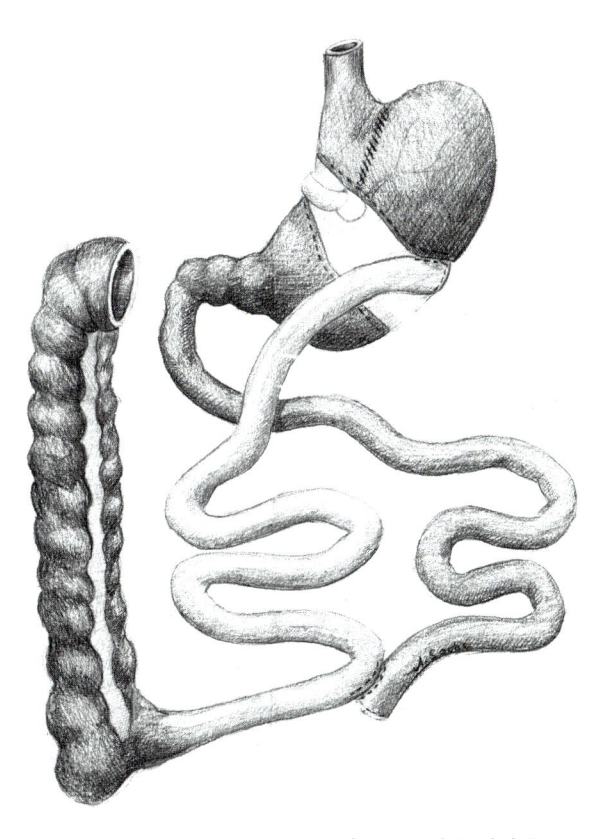

Fig. 29.6. Biliopancreatic Diversion after Vertical Banded Gastroplasty

29

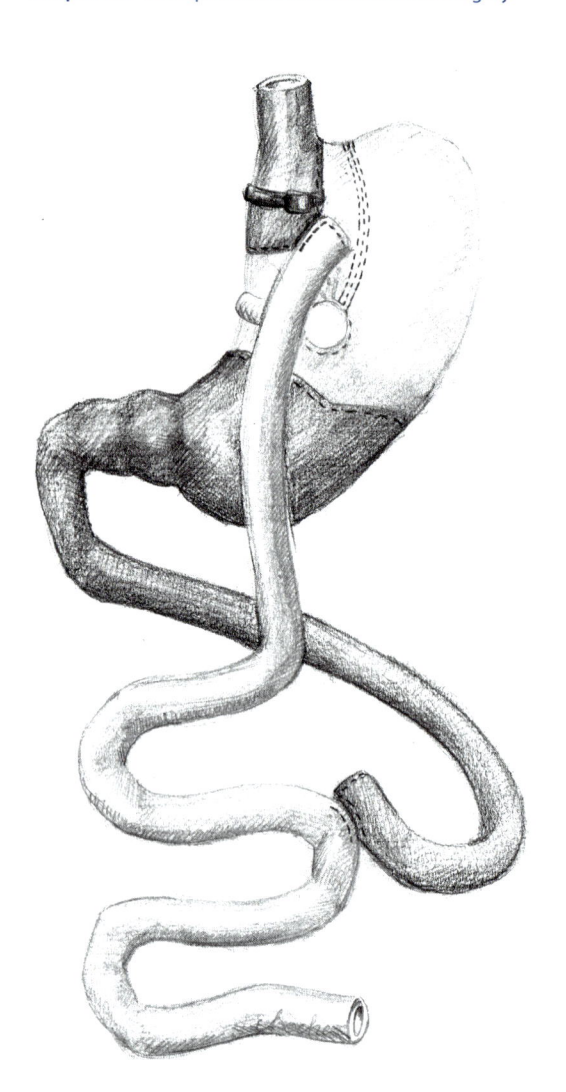

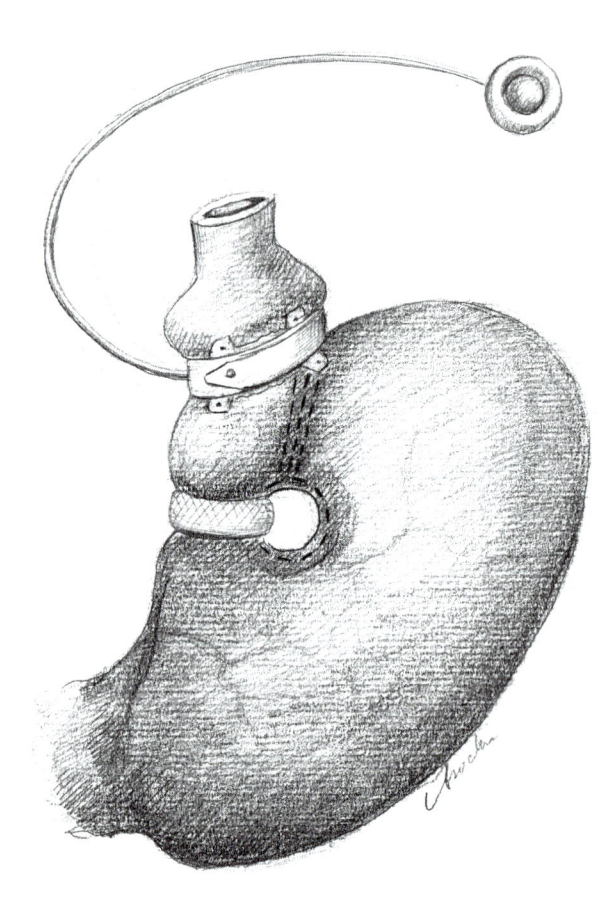

■ **Fig. 29.8.** Laparoscopic Adjustable Gastric Banding after Vertical Banded Gastroplasty

■ **Fig. 29.7.** Banded Roux-en-Y Gastric Bypass after Vertical Banded Gastroplasty

diaphragm crus is then easy to perform. Afterwards, the formation of the stomach pouch with a partial resection of the old dilated VBG pouch, fundus, and banding can be done. Weiner et al. proposed three conditions for performing the Scopinaro procedure after VBG: The distal stomach with the banding should be resected, the rejoining of the vertical VBG separation should be performed, and the patient's BMI should be over 50 kg/m² [36, 37].

To re-establish a sufficient restriction, several types of operations can be performed. Indications are: vertical staple line rupture, a good toleration of restriction, and relatively slow weight regain. There are several options: introduction of gastric banding (■ Fig. 29.8) or the sleeve gastrectomy with (■ Fig. 29.9) or without resection of the band (■ Fig. 29.10) [37]. This option has also led to a new primary technique: the banded sleeve resection

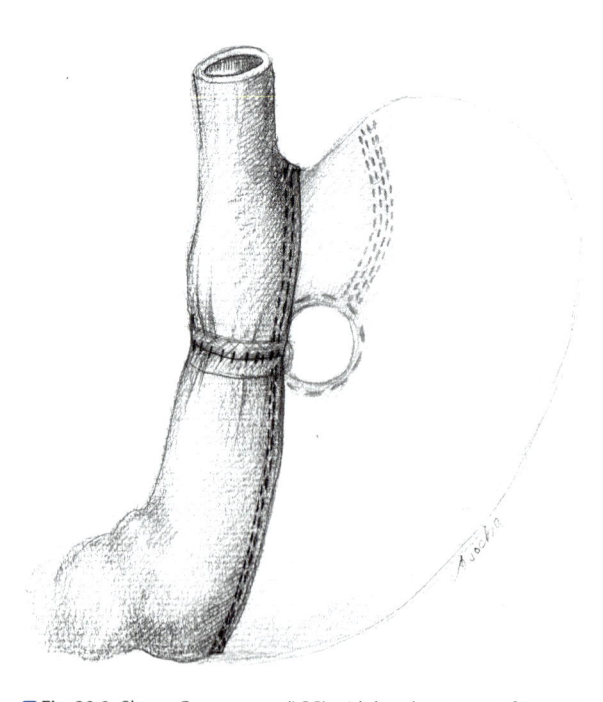

■ **Fig. 29.9.** Sleeve Gastrectomy (LSG) with band resection after Vertical Banded Gastroplasty

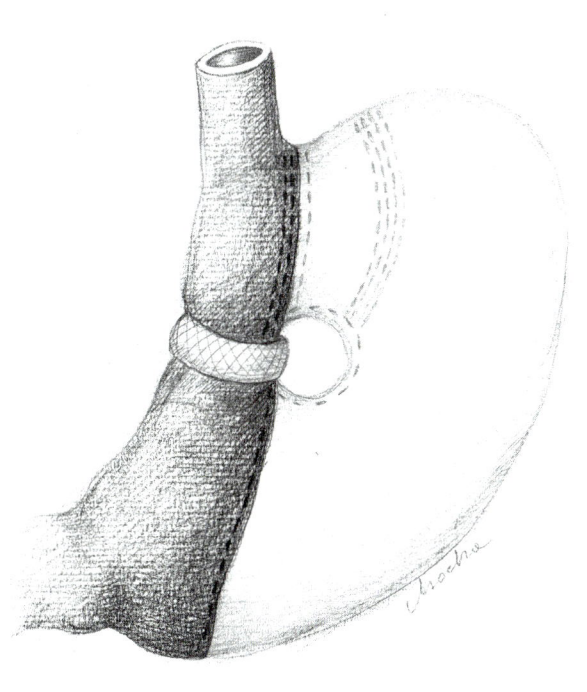

(■ Fig. 29.11) [38]. The BII gastric bypass, also called the mini-bypass, often leads to biliary reflux if it is performed as a one anastomosis bypass without Braun's anastomosis. Furthermore, stomach pouch and GEA dilatation are frequent because of the pouch formation technique, and the incidence of Petersen herniation is higher than after RYGB. There are almost no adhesions between the intestinal loop and the colon transversum. Prior to revision, the size of the stomach pouch should be carefully evaluated. The transformation into RYGB (■ Fig. 29.12) or

■ **Fig. 29.10.** Sleeve gastrectomy (LSG) without band resection after vertical banded gastroplasty

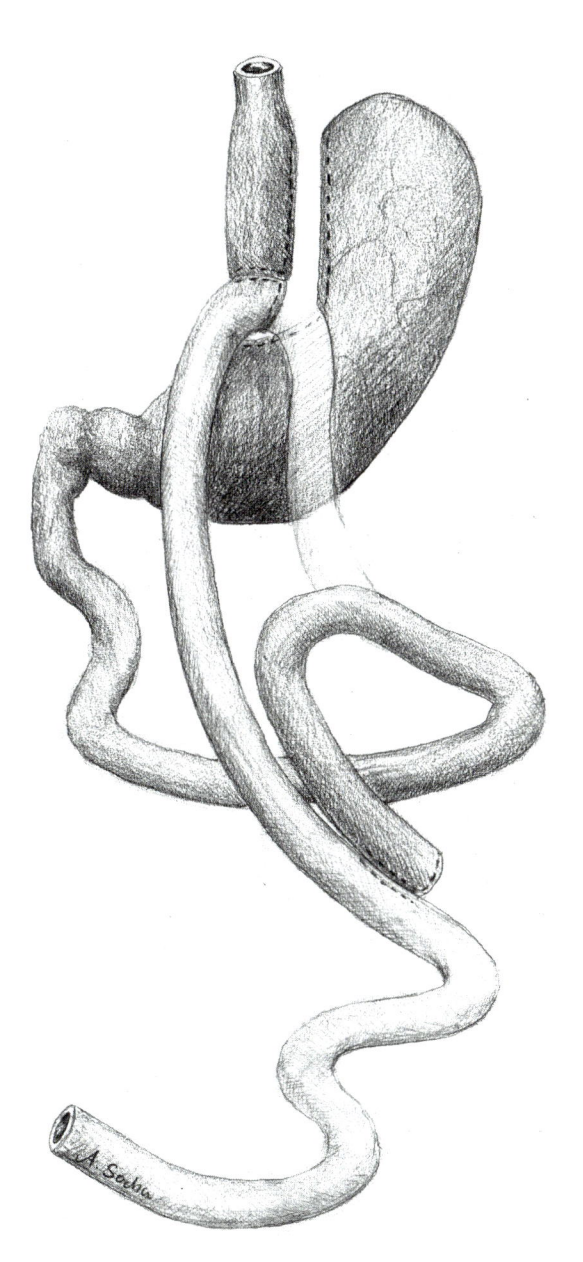

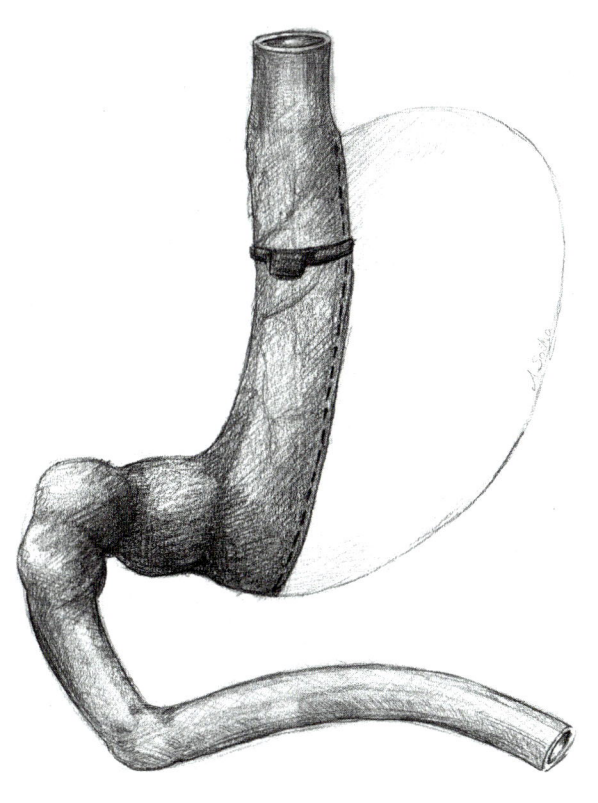

■ **Fig. 29.11.** Laparoscopic banded sleeve gastrectomy (LBSG)

■ **Fig. 29.12.** Transformation of one-anastomosis gastric bypass (BII gastric bypass, Mini-Bypass) into conventional Roux-en-Y Gastric Bypass

29

When the patient gains weight prior to the revision and the pouch is bigger than 150 ml, it is possible to perform a biliopancreatic diversion with a common channel (CC) of 75–100 cm. To perform a Scopinaro-standard CC the stomach pouch has to be bigger than 200 ml and the patient's BMI has to be >45 kg/m^2. If these conditions are not fulfilled the standard BPD-S operation with a short CC cannot be performed.

29.5 Restoration of Restriction

All bariatric procedures include gastric restriction by building a small pouch, sleeve, or upper stomach formation. The mechanical restriction and the neural sensation of satiety are the two main components of gastric restriction. In cases of insufficient weight loss or recurrent metabolic co-morbidities the anatomical aspects of the stomach pouch or sleeve inlet, outlet, and volume have to be evaluated [18, 39]. The proper functioning of the lower esophageal sphincter should also be assessed prior to operations. Revisions focus on the stomach pouch and it's outlet. In the case of LES dysfunction there will be no success if the revision is limited to the pouch size and pouch outlet.

The most popular metabolic operations are based mainly on restriction. These are laparoscopic adjustable gastric banding (LAGB), laparoscopic sleeve gastrectomy (LSG), and laparoscopic Roux-en-Y gastric bypass, if it is not performed as a distal bypass. If there is pouch dilation, the re-establishment of restriction leads to weight reduction and improvement of the metabolic disorders in most cases [17, 40]. The LABG was once a favored bariatric operation due to its low invasiveness and complete reversibility, but long-term observation showed a high rate of re-operations and an explantation rate of up to 40% [41–44]. Suter et al. presented a 33% rate of complications and a 20% revision rate [45].

These results demonstrate that correct implantation of the band is not an easy task. Regaining of weight after LAGB is due mostly to dislocation, migration, and pouch dilation. Other common reasons are infection and port-related problems [5]. There are many possibilities for re-establishing restriction after gastric banding, e.g., re-banding using the same or a new band or sleeve gastrectomy with or without band removal [46–48] (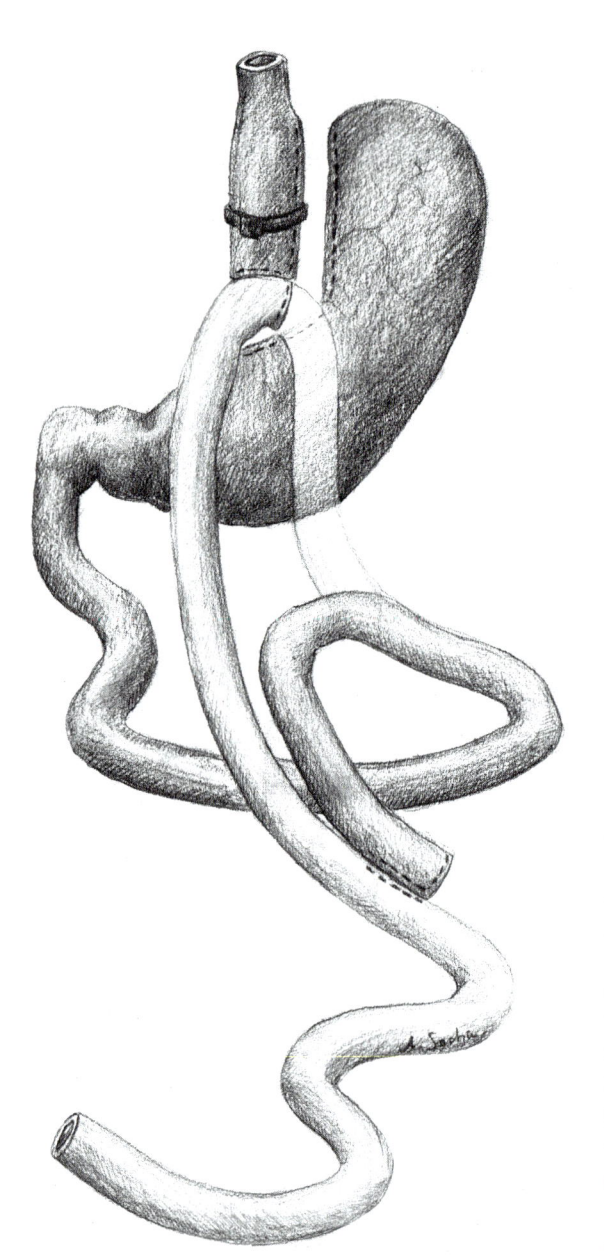 Fig. 29.14). The results published by Frezza et al. show that SG after LAGB is a real alternative to RYGB [50].

The option of a gastric bypass should be strongly considered for patients with persistent or recurrent metabolic diseases [46, 47]. Here, we also have the possibility of leaving the implant in the abdominal cavity. It should

Fig. 29.13. Transformation of one-anastomosis gastric bypass (BII gastric bypass, Mini-Bypass) into Banded Roux-en-Y Gastric Bypass

BRYGB (Fig. 29.13) is normally combined with a pouch reduction, a translocation of the biliopancreatic limb 80–100 cm below the GEA, and closing of the Petersen and Roux-en-Y apertures.

Those re-operations usually lead to weight stabilization and improvement of the local mucosa status. The procedure can be easily performed laparoscopically. The adhesions are normally not severe, and identification of anatomical structures is possible.

be said that the risk of an implant infection persists, es-pecially when there is contact with the open intestinal tract. In our opinion, the band should always be removed, and the bypass should be created as a one- or two-step procedure. The two-step procedure (band removal as a first and bypass formation as a second operation) could reduce the risk of a leakage caused by muscular atrophy underneath the band or doubling of the stomach wall in the staple line. Differences of thickness of the stomach wall lead to stapler suture insufficiencies. In our eyes, it is important to restore the anatomy by removing the band and performing the secondary operation 2 months later.

The sleeve gastrectomy (◘ Fig. 29.15) was a logical development after the vertical gastroplasty and the Ma-genstrasse procedure, but it was first performed in the context of BPD-DS [50, 51]. The volume of the remaining gastric sleeve should be roughly 100–120 ml. This can be controlled by using a calibration tube during the proce-dure [52, 53]. Nowadays, most bariatric surgeons use a 32- or 34-F bougie to form a proper-sized sleeve [54, 55]. A larger gastric tube seems to correlate with a higher risk of weight regain and sleeve dilatation [52]. We do not have long-term results yet, but it is already known that 50% of all patients undergo a secondary operation follow-ing SG. Nocca et al. reported a 6% rate of weight regain 2 years after SG [56]. We recommend performing a stom-ach 3D MSCT with volumetry prior to re-operation [18].

Restoration of restriction with a re-sleeve operation can lead to dysfunction of stomach motility, stenosis, and reflux with emesis or dysphagia. Such complications have to be treated with myotomy or resection of a stenosis [57]. Re-sleeve gastrectomy is therefore recommended only in cases of large sleeve dilations with a sleeve volume >500 ml [58]. There are two main causes of dilation after SG: an operative technique with a primary sleeve greater than 200 ml and patients who keep, or relapse into, vol-ume eating habits [56]. The re-sleeve operation can be used safely for patients who are scheduled for a second malabsorptive operation and still have a BMI over 50–60 and a volume of the primary sleeve >400 ml. A clear contra-indication for a re-sleeve operation is a volume of the sleeved stomach <150 ml.

Another option for creating a stronger restriction is the conversion to a gastric bypass. It is easy to transform the sleeve into a conventional or banded gastric bypass. The conventional gastric bypass does not lead to large weight changes, but the influence of metabolic disorders is larger compared with the SG [59, 60]. The gastric bypass, still considered the gold standard of bariatric surgery, leads to a regain of weight in up to 40% of pa-tients [61], but the revision rate is still lower than after VBG [2]. The long-term results presented by Christou et

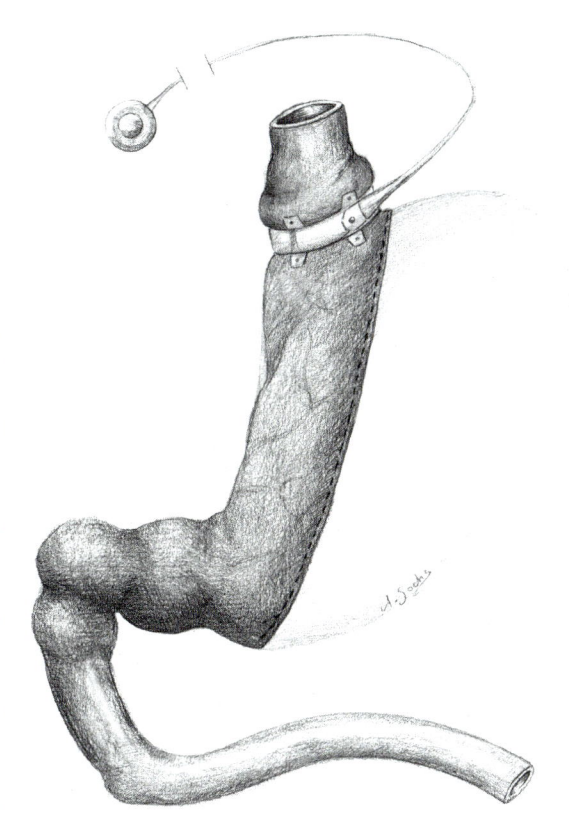

◘ **Fig. 29.14.** Transformation of Laparoscopic Adjustable Gastric Ban-ding into Sleeve Gastrectomy without gastric banding removal

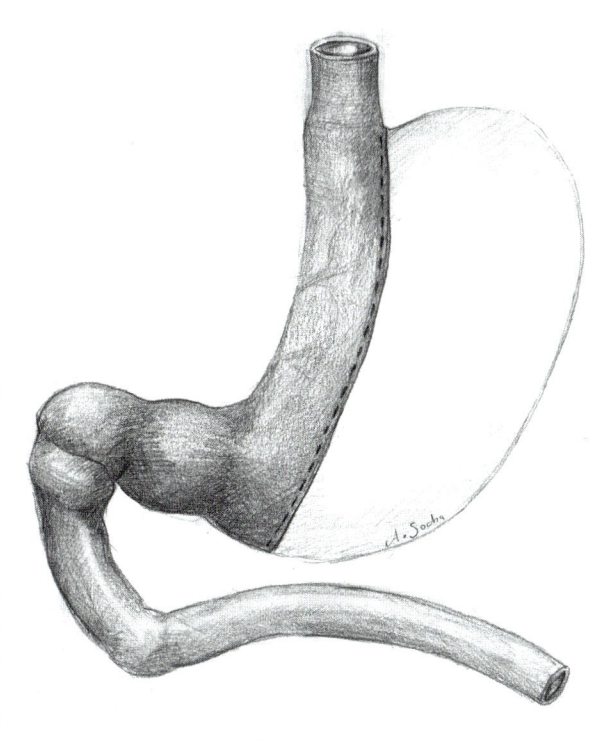

◘ **Fig. 29.15.** Laparoscopic Sleeve Gastrectomy

al. show that 35% of patients still have a BMI >35 kg/m² after RYGB [62]. Other authors report better results [60, 63]. It is unclear how many patients suffer from pouch dilatation or what the prevalence of GE dilatation is. We hope that 3D MSCT will give us more information in the future [18]. The volume of the gastric pouch should be between 15 and 30 ml [64]. Larger pouch volumes can be the result of wrong operating techniques or, secondarily, of eating habits. The width of the GEA also plays an important role: if it is too small, it can lead to stenosis and impaired emptying of the pouch, but if it is too large, a dilation of the first jejununal loop can result [14]. In this case the first jejunal loop can contribute to the functional stomach volume and thus enlarge it [18]. A precise evaluation of the diameter and area of the anastomosis allows the surgeon to choose the best revision strategy for the patient. It is known that GEA dilation can lead to insufficient weight control [65, 66].

If the patient tolerates well restriction, there are several options for revisional surgery. Endoscopic suturing to tighten a dilated gastric pouch is technically feasible and safe with Stomaphyx® as NOS (natural orifice surgery) and may lead to weight loss for certain patients [67]. Another logical option is to implant a GaBP ring in a revision maneuver, thus creating a banded bypass [34, 38]. An analogous procedure with gastric banding in addition to the RYGB was proposed by Bessler et al. (□ Fig. 29.16) [69]. It might be an easy and effective way to control the volume and outlet of the pouch. We recommend using rings of at least 6.5 cm in length in primary and 7.0 cm in re-operations (□ Fig. 29.17) [70, 71].

Some studies report better weight reduction after banded bypasses. Besides its restrictive role, the banding contributes to the reduction of undesirable side effects such as dumping syndrome and fetid flatulence. The banded bypass causes satiety and reduces caloric intake by delaying gastric emptying, even with low food intake. The silicone ring controls the diameter and area of the gastoenterostomy. After 2 years, the percentage of EWL ranged around 80%, and at 5 years' follow-up the EWL was roughly 75%. Only a slight weight regain of 2.5% or 5% is observed between the second and fifth postoperative year, whereas weight regain following LCRYGB is reported to be over 10% in the same period [68]. There are also patients who underwent BPD-DS procedures without the use of gastric tubes for sleeve calibration at the end of the 1990's and the beginning of the 21st century. Many of these patients now suffer from considerable stomach dilatation with ensuing recurrence of metabolic disorders or weight regain in cases where the CC is >100 cm. The stomach volume should then be reduced to about 200 ml to evoke a feeling of satiety again [58]. A

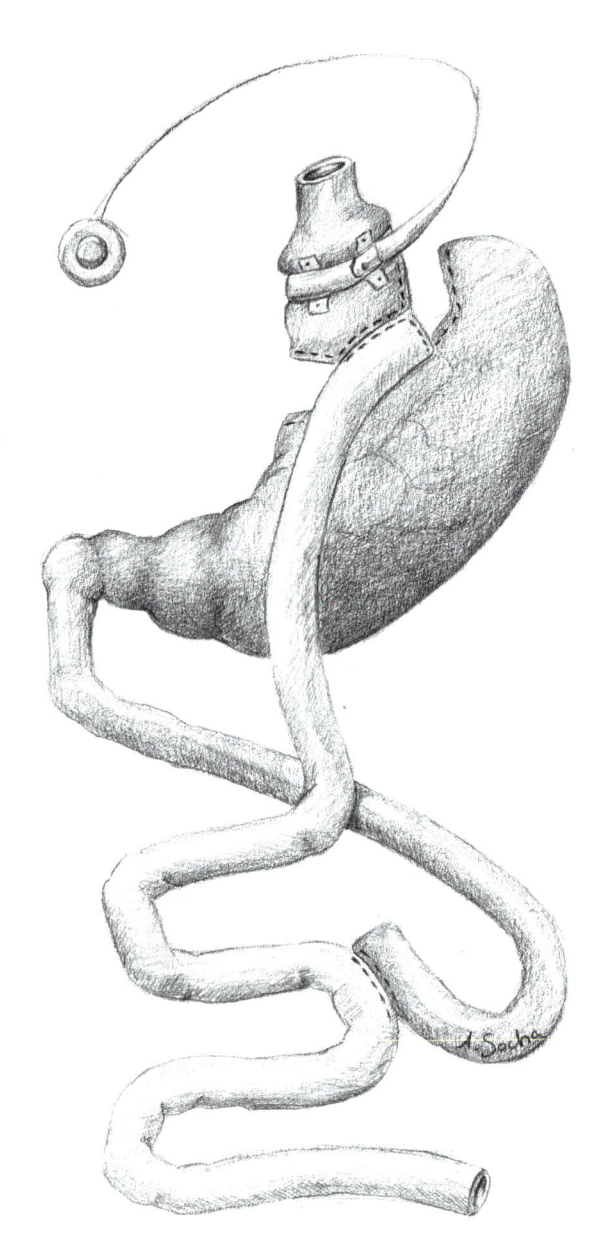

□ **Fig. 29.16.** Application of LAGB on Roux-en-Y Gastric Bypass (Bessler procedure)

similar constellation can be observed in a small group of BPD patients who present with an upper stomach dilatation, which can be treated with a fundus resection when necessary, thus reducing the stomach pouch to 150–200 ml (□ Fig. 29.18).

In case of malnutrition symptoms with severe hypoalbuminemia, liver dysfunction, severe diarrhea, and fetid flatulence and when the patient is not able to supplement adequately, it can be necessary to reduce malabsorption and to introduce a restrictive mechanism of weight or

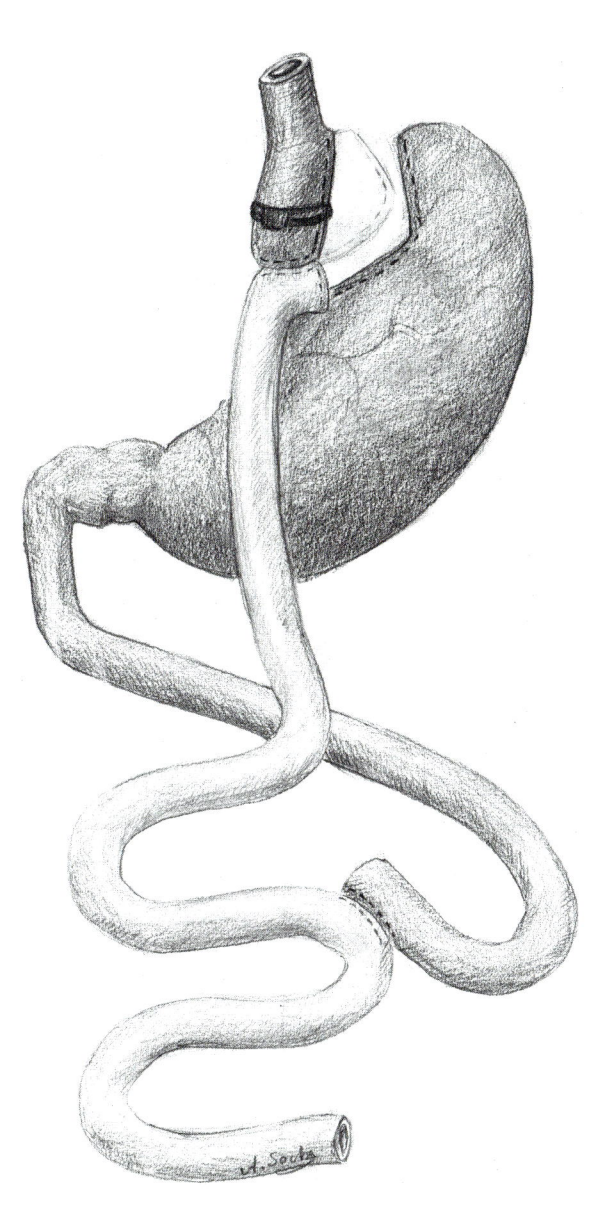

Fig. 29.17. Application of silastic ring on Roux-en-Y Gastric Bypass

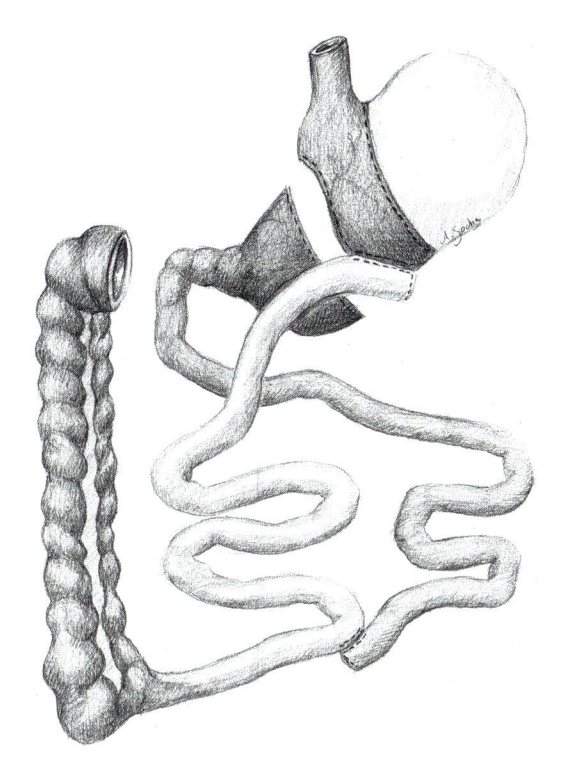

Fig. 29.18. Biliopancreatic Diversion with additional stomach fundus resection.

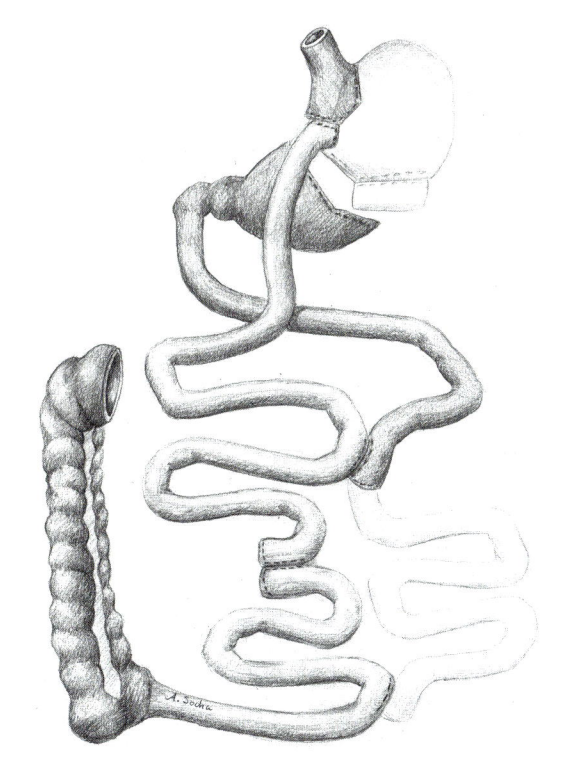

Fig. 29.19. Transformation of Biliopancreatic Diversion into Conventional Roux-en-Y Gastric Bypass

metabolic control. The introduction of the restriction with reduction of malabsoption is possible by transforming the BPD into a conventional or banded gastric bypass (■ Figs. 29.19, 29.20). Analogous procedures are BPD-DS to C- or B-RYGB transformations (■ Figs. 29.21, 29.22). The transformation of BPD to BPD-DS under the condition that distal gastrectomy was not performed is technically possible but not practicable. In our opinion, the artificial control of satiety is associated at least partly with the pouch volume. Hormonal and neural mechanisms also play an important role. Each year, several new hormonal or neurogenic active intestinal peptides (IP)

29

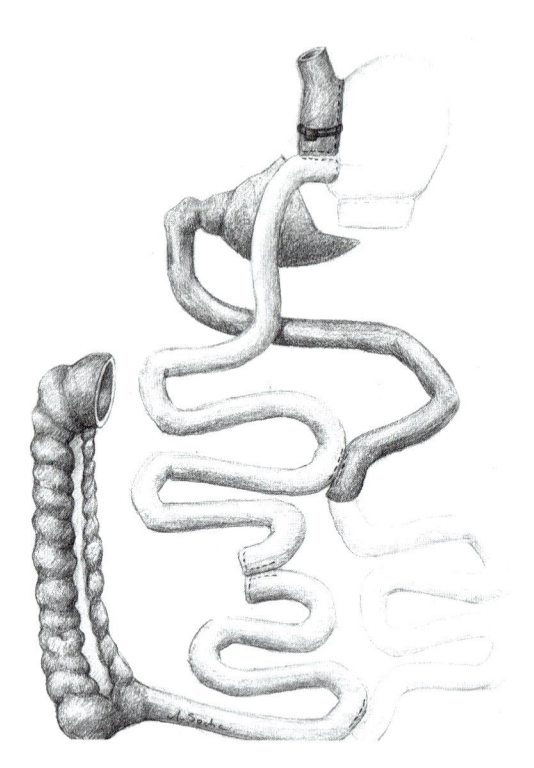

Fig. 29.20. Transformation of Biliopancreatic Diversion into Banded Roux-en-Y Gastric Bypass

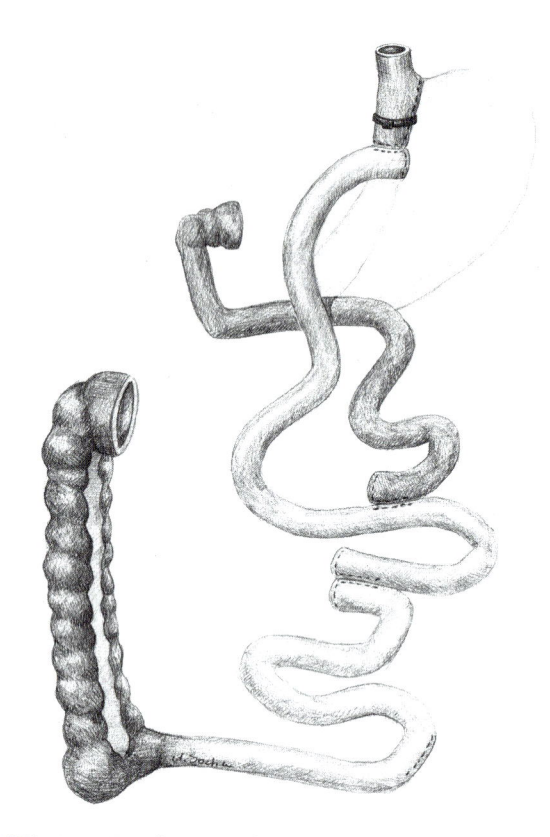

Fig. 29.22. Transformation of Biliopancreatic Diversion with Duodenal Switch into Banded Roux-en-Y Gastric Bypass

are identified. Also, the electrical stimulation alone of vagal nerves, pylorus stimulation, or stimulation of the duodenum leads to significant changes in the intestinal tract and body homeostasis [72]. In the future, restrictive surgery may be influenced by biologically active implants that react to physiological impulses from the intestinal tract and communicate directly or indirectly with central areas of hunger regulation.

29.6 Introduction of Malabsorption

Insufficient restriction quickly leads to metabolic disturbances, weight regain, and recurrence of associated diseases, especially in procedures based solely on food limitation. It is not easy to decide which method ought to be chosen in these cases. It is not always easy to decide in favor of revisional malabsorptive surgery. The most important question is whether the patient is capable of accepting the disadvantages of malabsorption. Artificial shortening of the intestine leads to chronic physiological changes. The recovery of sufficient restriction should therefore be considered first. An accurate diagnostic in-

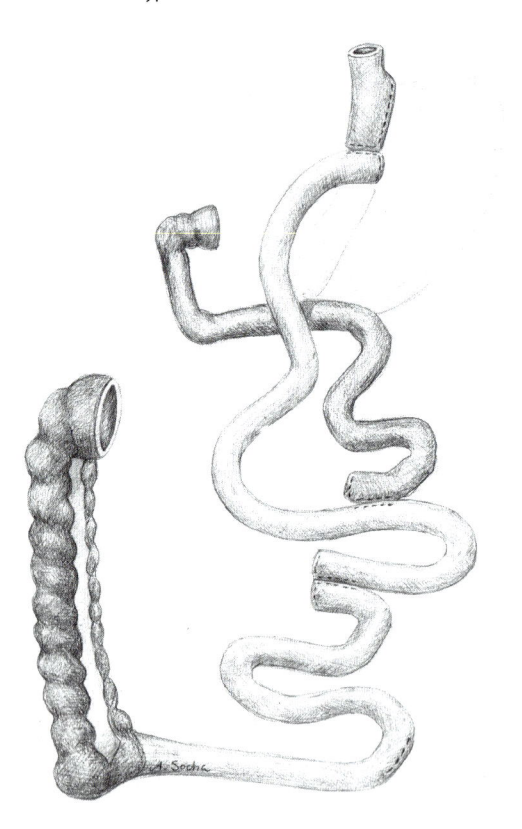

Fig. 29.21. Transformation of Biliopancreatic Diversion with Duodenal Switch into Conventional Roux-en-Y Gastric Bypass

vestigation may help to understand the mechanical situation of the intestinal tract, but is it a sufficient argument for introducing a malabsorptive component?

All cases that qualify for malabsorptive surgery ought to be discussed by an interdisciplinary board, following independent psychological, dietetic, and metabolic consultation. After the patient has been informed about the disadvantages of malabsorption and following pre-operative diagnostics and interdisciplinary consensus, the indication for malabsorptive surgery can be made. It must be said that there are clear contra-indications for secondary malabsorptive operations, such as a BMI under 35 after the primary metabolic procedure, a pre-existing malabsorptive state, malnutrition in vegetarians, pre-existing diarrhea, psychiatric diseases, and apparent lack of compliance. We exclude all patients with a history of major abdominal surgery with consecutive malabsorption, i.e., after ileum or colon resections for any reason; history of drug or alcohol abuse; history of recent or chronic steroid medication; auto-immune disease, inflammatory bowel disease, liver cirrhosis (CHILD B + C), serious active viral or bacterial diseases (e.g., HIV, hepatitis B and C, Tbc); pregnancy; history of any neoplasms in the past 5 years; need of long-term anticoagulation for any reason; and immunosuppression.

Proper selection of patients for malabsorptive procedures is a fundamental principle. The amount of malabsorption is directly associated with the length of the CC. The standard malabsorptive operations, i.e., the Scopinaro procedure and the duodenal switch (DS), have a CC of 50 and 75–100 cm [50, 73]. The incidence of malabsorptive complications is higher in patients with lower compliance. With all revision procedures, one should attempt a laparoscopic approach which is not difficult after LAGB. There are some possibilities for improving the metabolic outcome and influencing weight loss after LAGB by introducing malabsorption. It is known that over 40% of gastric banding patients undergo re-operations for different reasons. There are many clinics that perform the Scopinaro procedure after gastric banding (Fig. 29.23). The advantage of this technique is that it involves another "operating region" and a completely different mechanism of action. This option seems to be very good for patients with stress eating habits and a BMI over 50. The BPD-DS is not always easy to perform after LAGB because the band adhesion area is in the sleeve formation area, which can lead to local stapler insufficiencies and thus significantly increases the risk of complications. There is also the option of introducing malabsorption with a 100-cm CC as an isolated duodenal switch. The band has to be completely opened or, better, explanted during the procedure; a gastric resection is not done (Fig. 29.24). Such a

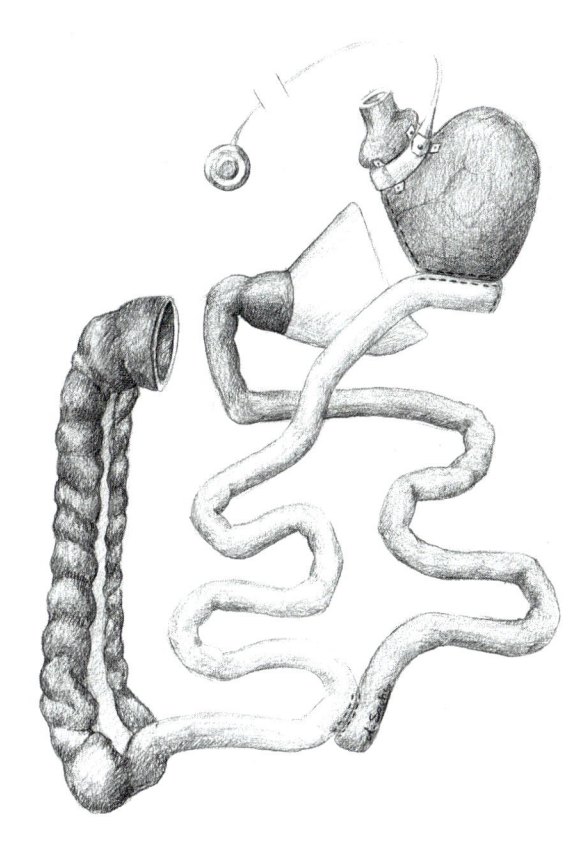

 Fig. 29.23. Biliopancreatic Diversion after gastric banding. The band is present here (it must always be explanted)

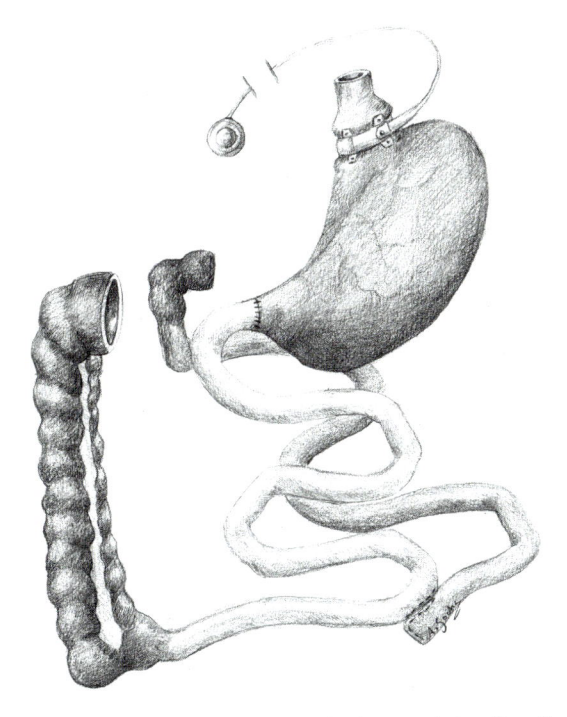

 Fig. 29.24. Isolated Duodenal Switch after gastric banding. The band is present here (it must always be explanted)

29

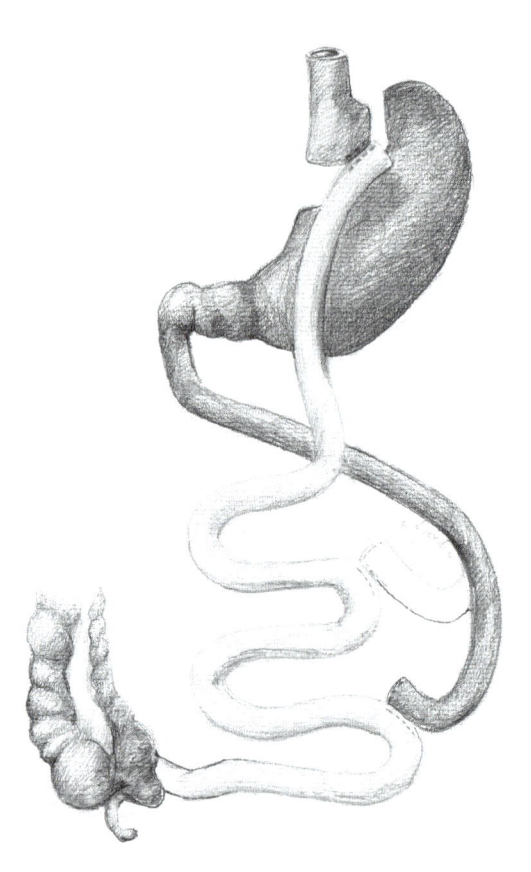

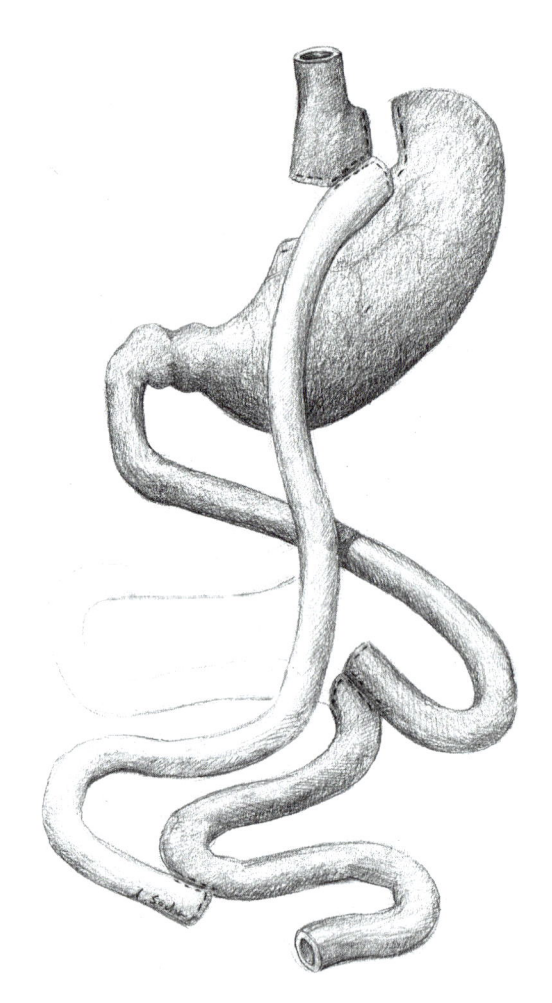

Fig. 29.25. Biliopancreatic limb distalization by conventional Rouxen- Y Gastric Bypass (Sugarman procedure)

procedure leads to roughly 60% of EWL [74]. The sleeve gastrectomy loses its restrictive effect in 50% of patients 5 years after the operation. These patients might require secondary malabsorptive procedures. Principally, there are two options: RYGB and DS. The recovery of restriction via RYGB leads to only very slight weight reduction in LSG patients. The introduction of malabsorption with a CC of 75–100 cm (longer CC in case of stronger restriction/smaller sleeve volume) with DS seems to be a much more effective method. In our series, almost all patients with super obesity weighed less than 100 kg 1 year after DS performed as a second-step operation.

The most interesting question is: What should be done in the case of insufficient weight control after a gastric bypass operation? If the introduction of a short intestine syndrome is not contra-indicated, we can introduce malabsorption. In our opinion, a patient scheduled for a re-operation should have a BMI >40 kg/m^2, a tendency to gain weight, or recurrence of associated morbidities to qualify for revisional malabsorption. The size of the stomach pouch must be measured prior to the operation. Knowledge of the pouch volume allows the surgeon to

Fig. 29.26. Alimentary limb distalization by conventional Roux-en-Y Gastric Bypass (Himpens-Lemmens procedure)

choose the revisional strategy and offers a criterion for introducing malabsorption. When the functional stomach volume is greater than 200 ml (summary of stomach pouch and first jejunal loop when the anastomosis is bigger than 2.5 cm) it is possible to perform the Sugarman operation with distalization of the biliopancreatic loop (Fig. 29.25) or relocation of the alimentary loop at about 100 cm from Bauhin's valve (Fig. 29.26) [75, 76]. Both of these operations are relatively easy to perform laparoscopically. The most difficult part is to disconnect the Roux-Y anastomosis, which can lead to stenosis or leakage. The ends of the transpositioned loops should always be resected to avoid suturing of the anastomosis in the scar tissue. Both operations lead to weight reduction and improvement of the metabolic situation. Another option proposed by Gagner et al. is to change the RYGB into a biliopancreatic diversion with duodenal switch [77]. Gagner also published a 40% failure rate af-

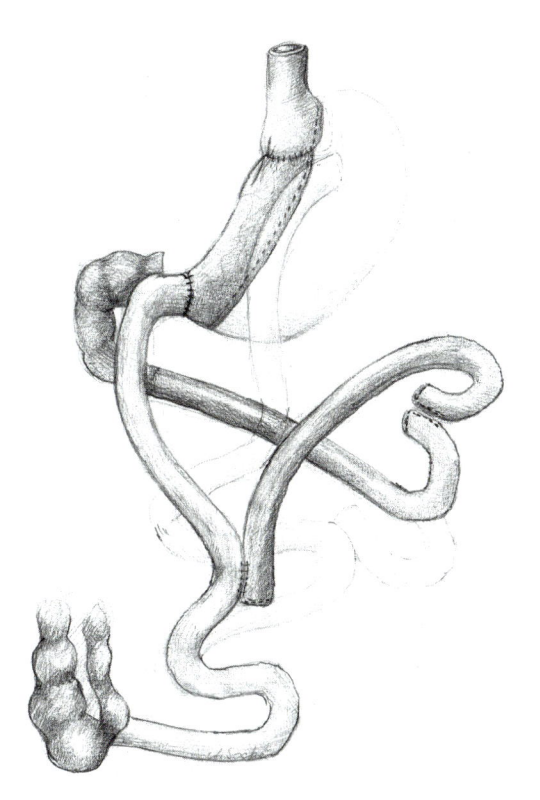

Fig. 29.27. Transformation of conventional Roux-en-Y Gastric Gypass procedure into Biliopancreatic Diversion with Duodenal Switch

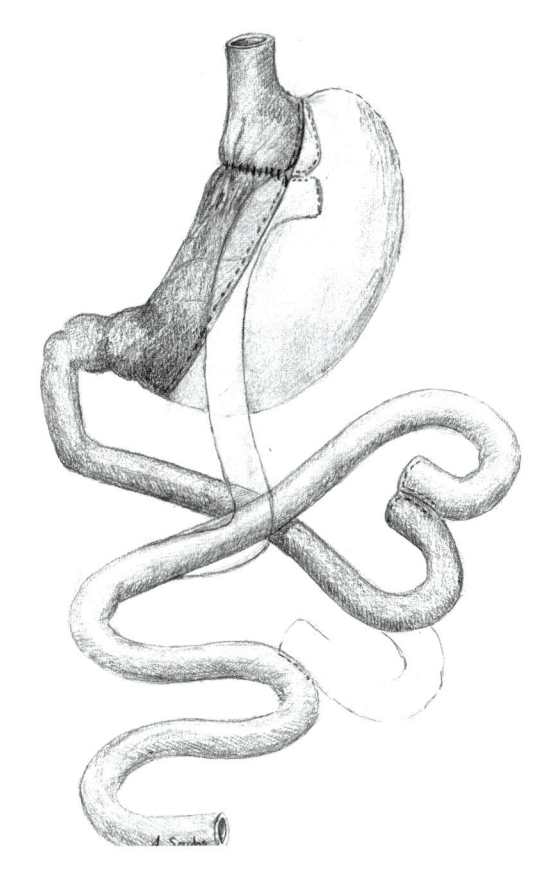

Fig. 29.28. Transformation of conventional Roux-en-Y GB procedure into Sleeve Gastrectomy with intestinal tract reconstruction

ter RYGB; these patients were successfully treated with a BPD-DS [61]. The transformation to a duodenal switch is a technically difficult and has many potential complications (**Fig. 29.27**). The reconstruction of the bypassed stomach by a gastro-gastrostomy and the following sleeve resection are the most difficult parts of the operation. The second half is very similar to the standard duodenal switch procedure. Performing the whole transformation during one operation is sometimes very difficult and leads to very long operating times [61, 77].

We have introduced a straightforward criterion for when to perform a one-step operation: If the reconstruction of the stomach and the sleeve resection take less than 120 min, we perform the whole operation at once. Usually, however, it is easier to divide the operation into two separate parts. This reduces the complication rate (**Fig. 29.28**). The recovery of restriction and introduction of malabsorption usually lead to an improvement of weight loss and metabolic status in little time [61]. Since mortality and morbidity are relatively low and excess weight loss is relatively good after malabsorption, this option ought to be considered in addition to procedures based solely on restriction. Furthermore, we believe that this option should be offered to patients when restriction has failed.

Continued surveillance of patients after any type of metabolic procedure is of greatest importance. There are still not enough data in the literature comparing the different techniques, especially in terms of long-term results. Prospective randomized trials are needed to compare different procedures. The group of patients with a revisional operation due to recurrent or persistent metabolic disorders is growing. Reasons might be the limited spectrum of primary bariatric and metabolic procedures performed in some clinics and the lack of good indication guidelines. A systematic analysis of indications for different metabolic procedures needs to be discussed. It is probable that this could lead to a lower re-operation rate. At the moment, there seems to be no gold-standard operation in the growing area of metabolic surgery.

There are many other procedures that have not been mentioned in this chapter on revisional surgery. There are many new procedures, e.g., the duodenal bypass, the loop duodenal switch, the ileal transposition, the banded sleeve resection, that are currently performed in small

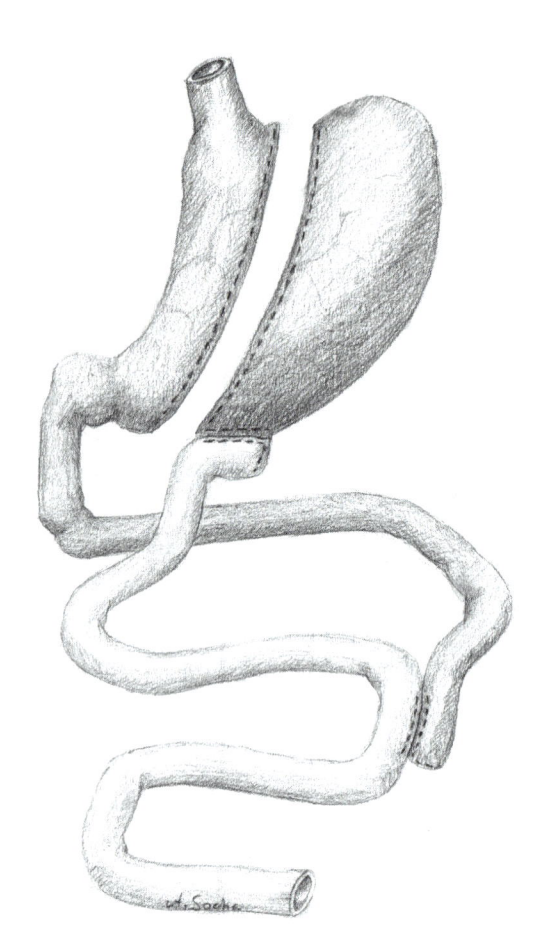

■ **Fig. 29.29.** Vertical stomach separation with Roux-en-Y remnant stomach drainage

series, and vagus, stomach, or duodenal pacemakers, or procedures that are still in the process of development such as the vertical stomach separation (■ Fig. 29.29) [38, 72, 78–80]. Certainly, new primary and revisionary operations will be developed as a result of better understanding of the pathophysiology of metabolic processes. Furthermore, new methods implementing bio-active implants, genetically modified "symbionts", gene therapy, or new drugs will undoubtedly have a significant impact on metabolic surgery in the future.

References

1. Maggard MA, Shugarman LR, Suttorp M, Maglione M, Sugerman HJ, Livingston EH, et al (2005) Meta-analysis: surgical treatment of obesity. Ann Intern Med 142:547–559
2. van Gemert WG, van Wersch MM, Greve JW, Soeters PB (1998) Revisional surgery after failed vertical banded gastroplasty: restoration of vertical banded gastroplasty or conversion to gastric bypass. Obes Surg 8:21–28
3. Gawdat K (2000) Bariatric re-operations: are they preventable? Obes Surg 10:525–529
4. Fobi M, Lee H, Igwe D, Felahy B, James E, Stanczyk M, et al (2001) Band erosion: incidence, etiology, management and outcome after banded vertical gastric bypass. Obes Surg 11:699–707
5. Weiss HG, Kirchmayr W, Klaus A, Bonatti H, Muhlmann G, Nehoda H, et al (2004) Surgical revision after failure of laparoscopic adjustable gastric banding. Br J Surg 91:235–241
6. Fishman E, Melanson D, Lamport R, Levine A (2008) A novel endoscopic delivery system for placement of a duodenal-jejunal implant for the treatment of obesity and type 2 diabetes. Conf Proc IEEE Eng Med Biol Soc 2008:2501–2503
7. Padwal R, Brocks D, Sharma AM (2009) A systematic review of drug absorption following bariatric surgery and its theoretical implications. Obes Rev 2010 Jan;11(1):45–50
8. Martin MJ, Bennett S (2007) Pretransplant bariatric surgery: a new indication? Surg Obes Relat Dis 3:648–651
9. Pillai AA, Rinella ME (2009) Non-alcoholic fatty liver disease: is bariatric surgery the answer? Clin Liver Dis 13:689–710
10. Schulman AP, Del GF, Sinha N, Rubino F (2009) Metabolic surgery for the treatment of type 2 diabetes. Endocr Pract 20:1–24
11. Flanagan L (1996) Measurement of functional pouch volume following the gastric bypass procedure. Obes Surg 6:38–43
12. de Castro CM, de Lima Montebelo MI, Rasera I jr., de OA jr., Gomes Gonelli PR, Aparecida CG (2008) Effects of Roux-en-Y gastric bypass on resting energy expenditure in women. Obes Surg 18:1376–1380
13. Nishie A, Brown B, Barloon T, Kuehn D, Samuel I (2007) Comparison of size of proximal gastric pouch and short-term weight loss following routine upper gastrointestinal contrast study after laparoscopic Roux-en-Y gastric bypass. Obes Surg 17:1183–1188
14. Roberts K, Duffy A, Kaufman J, Burrell M, Dziura J, Bell R (2007) Size matters: gastric pouch size correlates with weight loss after laparoscopic Roux-en-Y gastric bypass. Surg Endosc 21:1397–1402
15. Madan AK, Tichansky DS, Phillips JC (2007) Does pouch size matter? Obes Surg 17:317–320
16. Forsell P, Hellers G, Laveskog U, Westman L (1996) Validation of pouch size measurement following the Swedish adjustable gastric banding using endoscopy, MRI and barium swallow. Obes Surg 6:463–467
17. Langer FB, Bohdjalian A, Felberbauer FX, Fleischmann E, Reza Hoda MA, Ludvik B, et al (2006) Does gastric dilatation limit the success of sleeve gastrectomy as a sole operation for morbid obesity? Obes Surg 16:166–171
18. Karcz WK, Kuesters S, Marjanovic G, Suesslin D, Kotter E, Thomusch O, et al (2008) 3D-MSCT gastric pouch volumetry in bariatric surgery – preliminary clinical results. Obes Surg 2009 Apr;19(4):508–16
19. Munoz R, Ibanez L, Salinas J, Escalona A, Perez G, Pimentel F, et al (2009) Importance of routine preoperative upper GI endoscopy: why all patients should be evaluated? Obes Surg 19:427–431
20. de Moura AA, Cotrim HP, Santos AS, Bitencourt AG, Barbosa DB, Lobo AP, et al (2008) Preoperative upper gastrointestinal endoscopy in obese patients undergoing bariatric surgery: is it necessary? Surg Obes Relat Dis 4:144–149
21. Hartin CW, Jr., Remine DS, Lucktong TA (2009) Preoperative bariatric screening and treatment of Helicobacter pylori. Surg Endosc 2009 Nov;23(11):2531–4
22. Klaus A, Weiss H (2008) Is preoperative manometry in restrictive bariatric procedures necessary? Obes Surg 18:1039–1042
23. Merrouche M, Sabate JM, Jouet P, Harnois F, Scaringi S, Coffin B, et al (2007) Gastro-esophageal reflux and esophageal motility

disorders in morbidly obese patients before and after bariatric surgery. Obes Surg 17:894–900

24. Gentileschi P, Lirosi F, Benavoli D, Sica G, Di LN, Venza M, et al (2009) Laparoscopic reoperative approach after open bariatric surgery. Chir Ital 61:137–141

25. Raftopoulos I, Courcoulas AP (2008) Revision of jejunoileal bypass to Roux-en-Y gastric bypass: technical considerations and outcomes from 2 cases. Surg Obes Relat Dis 4:198–201

26. Hanni CL, Pool LR, Dean RE, Cronquist JC (1984) Treatment of jejunoileal bypass failure by reanastomosis and gastroplasty in a single-stage procedure. Review of 47 cases. Am Surg 50:354–357

27. Junker K, Jensen JB, Jensen HE (1981) Simultaneous small-intestinal reconstruction and gastric partitioning as treatment for complications after jejunoileal bypass for morbid obesity. Scand J Gastroenterol 16:433–436

28. LaFave JW, Alden JF (1979) Gastric bypass in the operative revision of the failed jejunoileal bypass. Arch Surg 114:438–444

29. Schouten R, van Dielen FM, van Gemert WG, Greve JW (2007) Conversion of vertical banded gastroplasty to Roux-en-Y gastric bypass results in restoration of the positive effect on weight loss and co-morbidities: evaluation of 101 patients. Obes Surg 17:622–630

30. Marsk R, Jonas E, Gartzios H, Stockeld D, Granstrom L, Freedman J (2008) High revision rates after laparoscopic vertical banded gastroplasty. Surg Obes Relat Dis 2009 Jan-Feb;5(1):94–8

31. Behrns KE, Smith CD, Kelly KA, Sarr MG (1993) Reoperative bariatric surgery. Lessons learned to improve patient selection and results. Ann Surg 218:646–653

32. Sanchez H, Cabrera A, Cabrera K, Zerrweck C, Mosti M, Sierra M, et al (2008) Laparoscopic Roux-en-Y gastric bypass as a revision procedure after restrictive bariatric surgery. Obes Surg 18:1539–1543

33. Daskalakis M, Scheffel O, Theodoridou S, Weiner RA (2009) Conversion of failed vertical banded gastroplasty to biliopancreatic diversion, a wise option. Obes Surg 2009 Dec;19(12):1617–23

34. Fobi MA, Lee H (1998) The surgical technique of the Fobi-Pouch operation for obesity (the transected Silastic vertical gastric bypass). Obes Surg 8:283–288

35. Fobi MA (2005) Placement of the GaBP ring system in the banded gastric bypass operation. Obes Surg 15:1196–1201

36. Menon T, Quaddus S, Cohen L (2006) Revision of failed vertical banded gastroplasty to non-resectional Scopinaro biliopancreatic diversion: early experience. Obes Surg 16:1420–1424

37. Elazary R, Hazzan D, Appelbaum L, Rivkind AI, Keidar A (2008) Feasibility of sleeve gastrectomy as a revision operation for failed Silastic ring vertical gastroplasty. Obes Surg 2009 May;19(5):645–9

38. Alexander JW, Martin Hawver LR, Goodman HR (2009) Banded sleeve gastrectomy – initial experience. Obes Surg 2009 Nov;19(11):1591–6

39. Kuesters S, Marjanovic G, Karcz WK (2009) Redo operations after bariatric and metabolic surgery [in German]. Zentralbl Chir 134:50–56

40. Muller MK, Wildi S, Scholz T, Clavien PA, Weber M (2005) Laparoscopic pouch resizing and redo of gastro-jejunal anastomosis for pouch dilatation following gastric bypass. Obes Surg 15:1089–1095

41. DeMaria EJ, Sugerman HJ, Meador JG, Doty JM, Kellum JM, Wolfe L, et al (2001) High failure rate after laparoscopic adjustable silicone gastric banding for treatment of morbid obesity. Ann Surg 233:809–818

42. Angrisani L, Furbetta F, Doldi SB, Basso N, Lucchese M, Giacomelli M, et al (2002) Results of the Italian multicenter study of 239 super-obese patients treated by adjustable gastric banding. Obes Surg 12:846–850

43. O'Brien PE, Dixon JB (2003) Lap-band: outcomes and results. J Laparoendosc Adv Surg Tech A 13:265–270

44. Weiner R, Blanco-Engert R, Weiner S, Matkowitz R, Schaefer L, Pomhoff I (2003) Outcome after laparoscopic adjustable gastric banding - 8 years experience. Obes Surg 13:427–434

45. Suter M, Calmes JM, Paroz A, Giusti V (2006) A 10-year experience with laparoscopic gastric banding for morbid obesity: high long-term complication and failure rates. Obes Surg 16:829–835

46. Weber M, Muller MK, Michel JM, Belal R, Horber F, Hauser R, et al (2003) Laparoscopic Roux-en-Y gastric bypass, but not rebanding, should be proposed as rescue procedure for patients with failed laparoscopic gastric banding. Ann Surg 238:827–833

47. Lanthaler M, Mittermair R, Erne B, Weiss H, Aigner F, Nehoda H (2006) Laparoscopic gastric re-banding versus laparoscopic gastric bypass as a rescue operation for patients with pouch dilatation. Obes Surg 16:484–487

48. Acholonu E, McBean E, Court I, Bellorin O, Szomstein S, Rosenthal RJ (2009) Safety and short-term outcomes of laparoscopic sleeve gastrectomy as a revisional approach for failed laparoscopic adjustable gastric banding in the treatment of morbid obesity. Obes Surg 2009 Dec;19(12):1612–6

49. Frezza EE, Torre EJ, Enriquez C, Gee L, Wachtel M, Corvala JA (2008) Laparoscopic sleeve gastrectomy after gastric banding removal: a feasibility study. Surg Innov 2009 Mar;16(1):68–72

50. Hess DS, Hess DW, Oakley RS (2005) The biliopancreatic diversion with the duodenal switch: results beyond 10 years. Obes Surg 15:408–416

51. Johnston D, Dachtler J, Sue-Ling HM, King RF, Martin G (2003) The Magenstrasse and Mill operation for morbid obesity. Obes Surg 13:10–16

52. Weiner RA, Weiner S, Pomhoff I, Jacobi C, Makarewicz W, Weigand G. (2007) Laparoscopic sleeve gastrectomy - -influence of sleeve size and resected gastric volume. Obes Surg 17:1297–1305

53. Gagner M, Deitel M, Kalberer TL, Erickson AL, Crosby RD (2009) The Second International Consensus Summit for Sleeve Gastrectomy, March 19–21, 2009. Surg Obes Relat Dis 5:476–485

54. Deitel M, Crosby RD, Gagner M (2008) The First International Consensus Summit for Sleeve Gastrectomy (SG), New York City, October 25–27, 2007. Obes Surg

55. Baltasar A, Serra C, Perez N, Bou R, Bengochea M, Ferri L (2005) Laparoscopic sleeve gastrectomy: a multi-purpose bariatric operation. Obes Surg 15:1124–1128

56. Nocca D, Krawczykowsky D, Bomans B, Noel P, Picot MC, Blanc PM, et al (2008) A prospective multicenter study of 163 sleeve gastrectomies: results at 1 and 2 years. Obes Surg 2008 May;18(5):560–5

57. Dapri G, Cadiere GB, Himpens J (2009) Laparoscopic seromyotomy for long stenosis after sleeve gastrectomy with or without duodenal switch. Obes Surg 19:495–499

58. Gagner M, Rogula T (2003) Laparoscopic reoperative sleeve gastrectomy for poor weight loss after biliopancreatic diversion with duodenal switch. Obes Surg 13:649–654

59. Rosenthal R, Li X, Samuel S, Martinez P, Zheng C (2009) Effect of sleeve gastrectomy on patients with diabetes mellitus. Surg Obes Relat Dis 5:429–434

60. Pories WJ, Swanson MS, MacDonald KG, Long SB, Morris PG, Brown BM, et al (1995) Who would have thought it? An operation proves to be the most effective therapy for adult-onset diabetes mellitus. Ann Surg 222:339–350

61. Trelles N, Gagner M (2009) Revision bariatric surgery: laparoscopic conversion of failed gastric bypass to biliopancreatic diversion with duodenal switch. Minerva Chir 64:277–284

62. Christou NV, Look D, Maclean LD (2006) Weight gain after short- and long-limb gastric bypass in patients followed for longer than 10 years. Ann Surg 244:734–740

63. Fobi M, Lee H, Igwe D, Felahy B, James E, Stanczyk M, et al (2002) Gastric bypass in patients with BMI <40 but >32 without life-threatening co-morbidities: preliminary report. Obes Surg 12:52–56

64. Madan AK, Harper JL, Tichansky DS (2008) Techniques of laparoscopic gastric bypass: on-line survey of American Society for Bariatric Surgery practicing surgeons. Surg Obes Relat Dis 4:166–172

65. Naslund I (1984) A method for measuring the size of the gastric outlet in obesity surgery. Acta Chir Scand 150:399–404

66. Loewen M, Barba C (2008) Endoscopic sclerotherapy for dilated gastrojejunostomy of failed gastric bypass. Surg Obes Relat Dis 4:539–542

67. Thompson CC, Slattery J, Bundga ME, Lautz DB (2006) Peroral endoscopic reduction of dilated gastrojejunal anastomosis after Roux-en-Y gastric bypass: a possible new option for patients with weight regain. Surg Endosc 20:1744–1748

68. Fobi MA, Lee H, Felahy B, Che K, Ako P, Fobi N (2005) Choosing an operation for weight control, and the transected banded gastric bypass. Obes Surg 15:114–121

69. Bessler M, Daud A, Kim T, DiGiorgi M (2007) Prospective randomized trial of banded versus nonbanded gastric bypass for the super obese: early results. Surg Obes Relat Dis 3:480–484

70. Crampton NA, Izvornikov V, Stubbs RS (1997) Silastic ring gastric bypass: a comparison of two ring sizes: a preliminary report. Obes Surg 7:495–499

71. Stubbs RS, O'brien I, Jurikova L (2006) What ring size should be used in association with vertical gastric bypass? Obes Surg 16:1298-–1303

72. Miller K, Hoeller E, Aigner F (2006) The implantable gastric stimulator for obesity: an update of the European experience in the LOSS (Laparoscopic Obesity Stimulation Survey) Study. Treat Endocrinol 5:53–58

73. Marceau P, Hould FS, Potvin M, Lebel S, Biron S (1999) Biliopancreatic diversion (doudenal switch procedure). Eur J Gastroenterol Hepatol 11:99–103

74. Slater GH, Fielding GA (2004) Combining laparoscopic adjustable gastric banding and biliopancreatic diversion after failed bariatric surgery. Obes Surg 14:677–682

75. Fobi MA, Lee H, Igwe D, Jr., Felahy B, James E, Stanczyk M, et al (2001) Revision of failed gastric bypass to distal Roux-en-Y gastric bypass: a review of 65 cases. Obes Surg 11:190–195

76. Sugerman HJ, Kellum JM, DeMaria EJ (1997) Conversion of proximal to distal gastric bypass for failed gastric bypass for superobesity. J Gastrointest Surg 1:517–524

77. Parikh M, Pomp A, Gagner M (2007) Laparoscopic conversion of failed gastric bypass to duodenal switch: technical considerations and preliminary outcomes. Surg Obes Relat Dis 3:611–618

78. Wang TT, Hu SY, Gao HD, Zhang GY, Liu CZ, Feng JB, et al (2008) Ileal transposition controls diabetes as well as modified duodenal jejunal bypass with better lipid lowering in a nonobese rat model of type II diabetes by increasing GLP-1. Ann Surg 247:968–975

79. Mason EE (1999) Ileal [correction of ilial] transposition and enteroglucagon/GLP-1 in obesity (and diabetic?) surgery. Obes Surg 9:223–228

80. Salvi PF, Brescia A, Cosenza UM, D'Urso R, Cardelli P, Badiali M (2009) Gastric pacing to treat morbid obesity: two years' experience in four patients [in Italian]. Ann Ital Chir 80:25–28

Plastic Surgery after Massive Weight Loss

Björn Stark, MD, Gunther Felmerer, MD

procedure to be able to estimate substitution of vitamins and proteins. If this is not respected, wound healing complications can occur, in hypoproteinemia there may be formation of seromas, and edema is more extensive.

30.3 Body Contouring Procedures

30.3.1 Abdominoplasty

When laparotomy is planned for non-laparoscopic bariatric surgery, incision planning should be done together with the plastic surgeon of the obesity center team, as this may be combined with a primary adjuvant palliative reduction of a fat apron. More importantly, it can help to avoid scars that may impede the supply of blood to the skin in later standard abdominoplasty procedures. Excess abdominal skin and laxity of the abdominal muscles commonly are the most striking stigmas after weight loss, in some cases the skin overhangs the genitalia as far down as to the knee. The standard abdominoplasty (■ Figs. 30.2, 30.3) with an anterior low transverse incision, mobiliza-

tion of a skin flap to the xyphoid, resection of its inferior portion, and implantation of the umbilicus into the flap was introduced by Pitanguy more than 30 years ago [9]. Later modifications included the addition of liposuction, the level and dimensions of dissection, and a W-shaped incision.

Regnault's open-W incision [10, 11] is still popular, but the modern trend is to modify the angle of the lateral limbs based on bathing-suit preferences and to preserve the maximum blood supply to the abdominoplasty flap. Liposuction and/or posterior standard incisions in continuity with the abdominoplasty may be used to achieve a more circumferential reduction of the trunk [12].

High lateral tension at the level of the skin suture will also have some tightening effect on the flanks, will concentrate skin tension laterally, and will reduce scar length and the impairment of circulation of the median flap tip [13]. Except in patients with a pre-existing median laparotomy scar, a reversed T-dermolipectomy is rarely indicated today.

As after pregnancy, tissue relaxation may also include abdominal wall muscles and rectus diastasis. Wide ab-

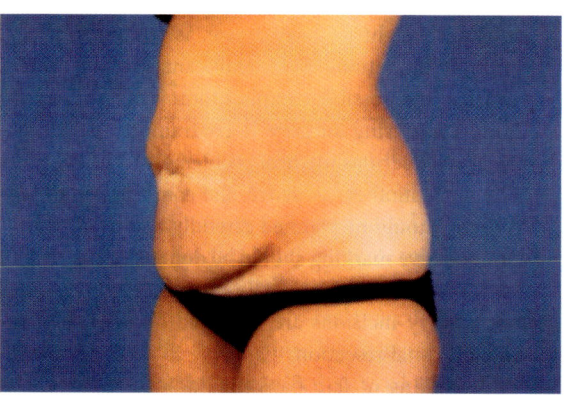

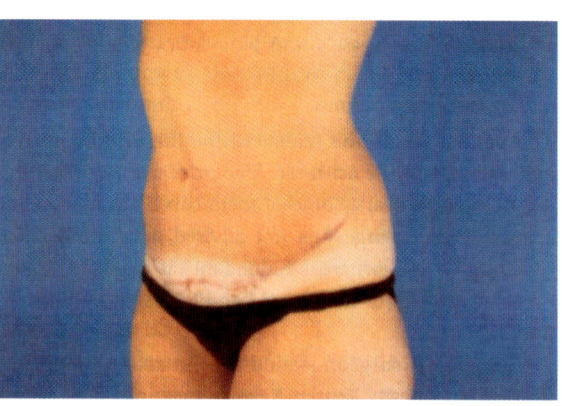

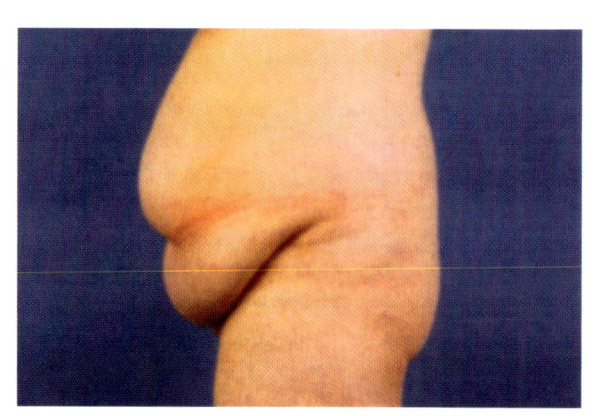

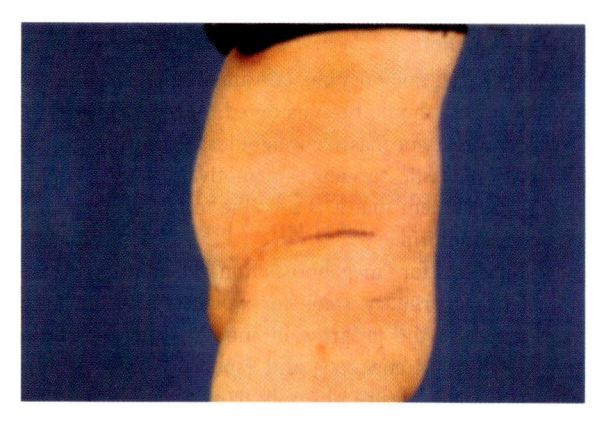

■ **Fig. 30.2.** Pre- and postop (right): standard abdominoplasty after loss of 35 kg and birth of twins

■ **Fig. 30.3.** High lateral tension abdominoplasty in a 48-year-old patient with vertical and horizontal excess skin: (left) preop, (right) result 6 months postop

dominal rectus muscle plication (WARP) [14] addresses this problem and is a standard procedure adjunctive to abdominoplasty. With a running strong non- or slowly resorbable suture the midline between both rectus muscles is reinforced; the waist is accentuated by this procedure [13]. Frequently, these patients will also present with umbilical hernia; this is reinforced by the WARP procedure, which replaces the rectus muscles into their median parallel position. Abdominoplasty (*after* weight loss) is a relatively benign procedure, which now has to be weighed against a much more extensive total lower circular "body lift".

Multiple striae distensae are to be found as a sign of rupture of the connective tissue. This overexpanded skin cannot shrink after plastic surgery and must be excised. Striae distensae ("pregnancy scars") caused by distension of the dermis, most frequently on the lower trunk, will be partially removed with the resected skin, but they have otherwise escaped effective treatment so far (◘ Fig. 30.2).

Regular abdominoplasty techniques can be applied after minor weight loss and in patients with good skin quality. The scars are then short, and lateral redundant skin is not an issue. Minor fat deposits can be treated by liposuction.

A longer scar is not avoidable if the patient's skin quality is poor (◘ Fig. 30.3). Unfortunately, this is most often the case, since we see more and more patients who have lost more than 50 pounds after modern bariatric surgery. Thus the short-scar techniques in breast reduction or abdominoplasty that are in the repertoire of modern plastic surgery cannot be applied in the more severe cases. The only choice is to keep the scars in an area where they can easily be hidden – in the bikini area.

If non-laparoscopic visceral bariatric surgery is planned, a plastic surgeon should be involved in planning the location of incisions, and even an initial moderate dermolipectomy may be combined with laparotomy for severe excess skin reduction.

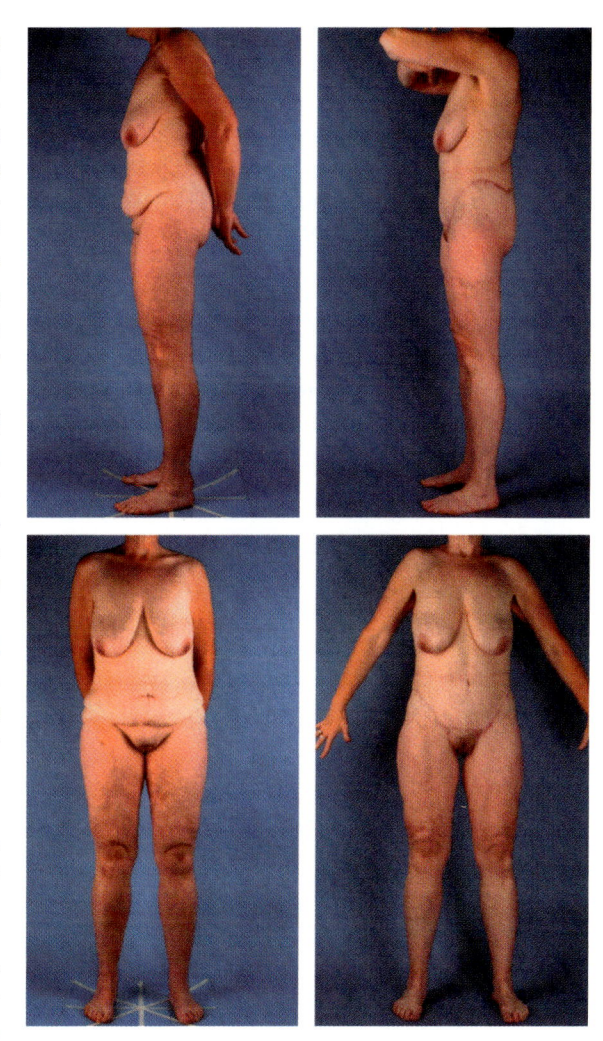

◘ **Fig. 30.4.** Belt lipectomy preop (left), postop (right); note the much better accentuated waist area

30.3.2 Belt Lipectomy

If redundant skin is found more in the abdomen, flanks, and buttocks and less in the legs a belt lipectomy is a good option. A circumferential "belt" of skin and fat is removed along the waist area. Undermining of adjacent areas (outer aspects of legs, flank rolls) is sometimes needed, but not to such an extent as in body lifts [15].

Belt lipectomy procedures are excellent to restore the waist area and lead less than body lifts to the tent phenomenon (◘ Fig. 30.4). In body lifts the whole weight of the legs is suspended on the skin of the back and the ab-

domen, and the vectors therefore pull the tissues downward more than in belt lipectomies [16].

30.3.3 Thigh Lift

The extent of deformity seen in the thighs of patients after massive weight loss varies considerably. Some patients who had a large amount of fat deposited in the legs may come to surgery with excellently deflated legs. It is ideal to operate on these patients. Some still have minimally deflated legs with larger deposits of fat. Then liposuction is performed first, or in adjunct to a thigh lift if the fat deposits are only moderate. In patients with massive weight loss a thigh lift is usually part of a lower body lift. When it is performed as a single operation the abdominal and inguinal region should be treated first since relaxed skin in these areas influences considerably the amount of redundant leg skin.

During preoperative evaluation the decision can be made as to whether a vertical lifting after Lockwood [17] (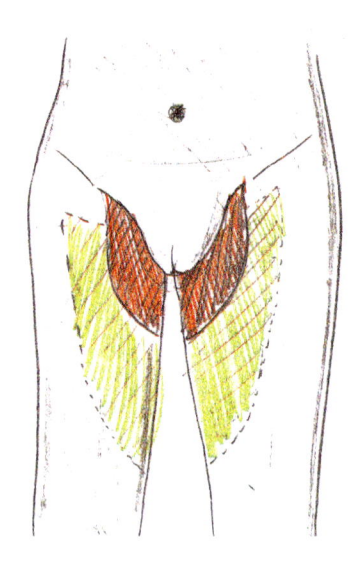 Fig. 30.5) or a more traditional leg lift [18] with a horizontal reduction and therefore a T-shaped scar would be appropriate.

If there is a history of thrombosis or embolism, a vascular examination with color Doppler is mandatory. Varicose veins with insufficiency should be addressed at least 6 months prior to a thigh lift. Patients with a persistent occlusion of the deep veins of the thigh should be excluded from thigh lifts. Care must be taken to preserve

Fig. 30.5. The leg lift after Lockwood. Undermining is in yellow, resection is in red

the deep lymphatic ducts that drain the leg. Preoperative ankle swelling must be recognized.

During the operation the anchoring technique is advised at Colles' fascia near the pubic bone, as described by Lockwood [17]. The right placement of scars and the avoidance of too much tension on the skin can lead to satisfactory results.

30.3.4 Body Lift

Also a misnomer, as it addresses only the lower trunk, buttocks, and thighs, the circular "body lift" in one of its modifications has become a comprehensive option for postbariatric patients. It offers the possibility to solve several problems at one time, though at the price of a much more extensive procedure with higher morbidity.

Lockwood [19–22] believes that sagging above the level of the umbilicus occurs primarily from horizontal skin relaxation. Because of adherence of the superficial fascia, the least amount of vertical laxity occurs in the anterior midline. Lockwood [19, 22] described an extensive procedure that combines transverse resection of redundant skin and fat from the lower trunk with repair of the superficial fascia to lift the flanks, thighs, and buttocks.

The preoperative markings are very important to obtain a perfectly symmetrical result. The position of the patient's underwear is marked first. This is followed by the future scar position, which should easily be hidden by the underpants. After that the primary incision line is marked in a different color, at the gluteal region, 2–4 cm cranial from the future scar line at the midaxillary line; dorsally, it then follows the scar line cranially (see 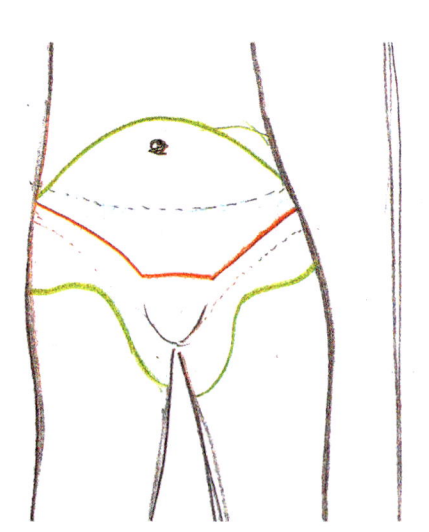 Fig. 30.6). In the front view the future scar line is drawn

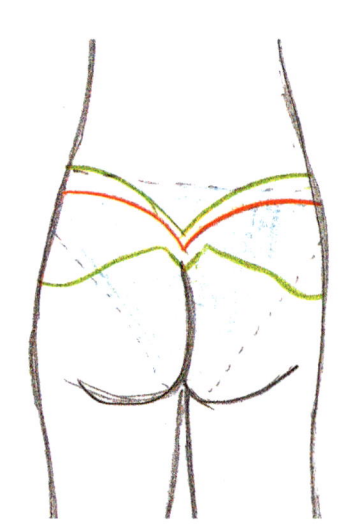

Fig. 30.6. Preop markings in a body lift: the red line indicates the future scar; between green lines is the redundant tissue which needs to be resected. Blue indicates shape of the undergarment

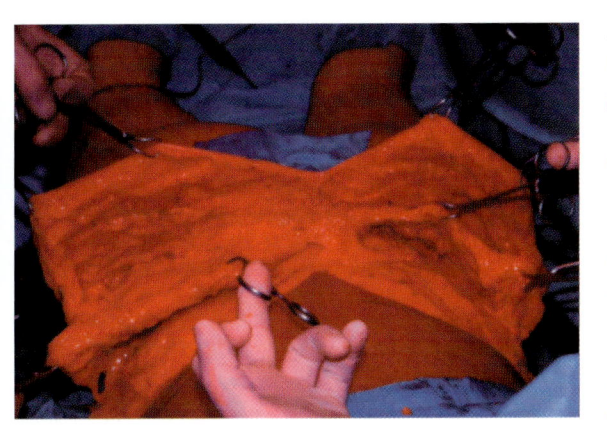

Fig. 30.7. The superficial fascia of the buttock area is held by clamps during a lower body lift procedure

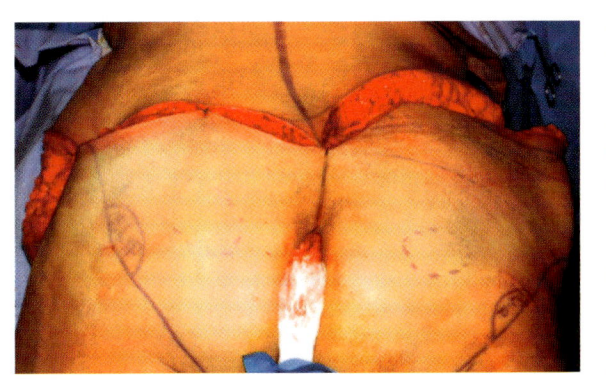

Fig. 30.8. Dorsal aspect in body lift; the trochanteric zone of adherence is already dissected

again, joining the dorsal scar line at the midaxillary line. Further lines are drawn from the medial leg fold to the pubic area.

The operation begins with the patient in prone position. Figure 30.7 shows the posterior undermining of skin flaps; the superficial fascia system (SFS) is held with a clamp. The attachments of the SFS at the trochanteric region are released to permit maximum lift (Figs. 30.7, 30.8).

This is followed by complete suture of both the SFS and the dermal layers for lasting suspension of the rearranged tissues. When indicated, Lockwood uses adjunctive liposuction to equalize the thickness of the skin flaps at the line of closure. Thereafter, the patient is turned onto her back. The resection is extended anteriorly and inferiorly on either side of the pubis to include a medial thigh lift in one lower body lift (Fig. 30.9). If needed, a complete abdominoplasty is performed. Non-absorbable sutures are placed at the inner aspect of the thigh and anchored at Colles' fascia (perineal fascia) to prevent vulvular distortion by too much tension on the skin. After the operation the patient should ambulate as soon as she is able to prevent venous thrombosis.

30.3.5 Buttock Lift

The buttocks are generally addressed in a lower body lift. While it is rarely a functional problem, hanging buttocks are a severe cosmetic problem for many patients after they have lost weight.

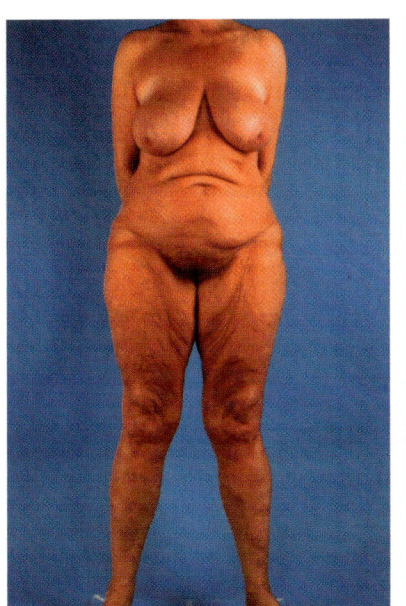
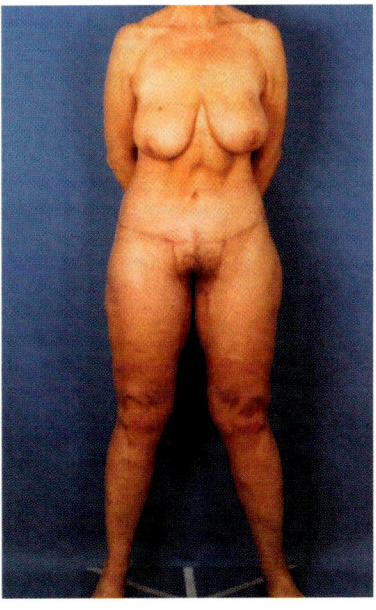

Fig. 30.9. A 52-year-old patient after 32 kg weight loss, before (left) and after (right) lower body lift

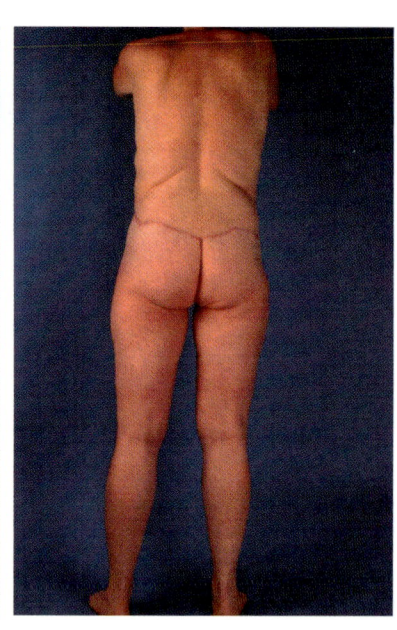

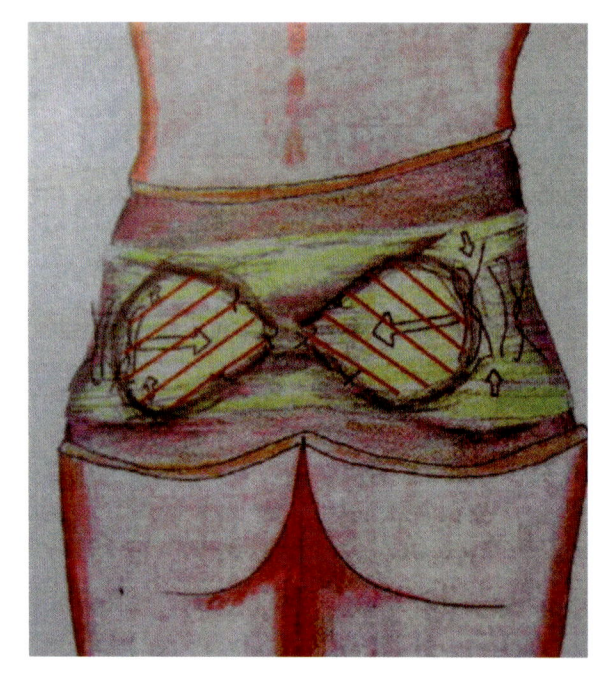

■ **Fig. 30.10.** Buttock lift in a combined belt lipectomy; (left) preop, (right) postop

■ **Fig. 30.11.** Sutured augmentation of the posterior fascia by Richter [16]; the red hatched area is the region with maximum projection

Prior to surgery, the patient wears his or her favorite underwear and the marks for future scars are placed under the clothing. The lower border of the resection is marked, but during the operation a little less is sometimes resected. Symmetrical resection is mandatory. The resection figure is like a seagull and the buttocks are not only cranially lifted but also rotated. It is important to double the fascia in the midline of the buttock, as described by Richter et al. [16], or to create a subcutaneous flap [23, 24]; otherwise the result is a flat buttock area (■ Figs. 30.10, 30.11).

30.3.6 Brachioplasty

The goal of brachioplasty is to eliminate tissue redundancy and reduce the circumference of the arm. Upper arm flabbiness is the direct result of a loosening of the connections of the arm's SFS to the axillary fascia, as well as of relaxation of the axillary fascia itself, with age, weight fluctuations, and gravitational pull yielding a 'loose hammock' effect, resulting in significant ptosis of the posteromedial arm [25].

Because circular excisions at the level of the axilla result in highly visible scars and limited correction, most authors recommend direct elliptical excision of the redundant tissue and place the incision medially along a line connecting the axillary dome to the medial epicondyle (■ Fig. 30.12). We often modify this to an L-shaped incision with a shorter transverse excision in the axilla. Patients whose skin is less elastic may require an extended thoracobrachioplasty, as described by Pitanguy [18]. In moderate cases without laxity of the lateral chest wall, L-shaped incisions are recommended [26].

30.3.7 Mastopexy – Reduction Mammoplasty

The average female breast consists of 50–70% adipose tissue [27]. The psychological and somatic side effects of primary juvenile hyperplasia itself can have a negative effect on adolescent eating habits. Isolated gigantomastia may be a cause of impairments including effects on the skeletomuscular system (neck and shoulder pain), peripheral nerve compression, breast pain, and intertrigo [28]. Following massive weight loss, frequently some hypertrophy and usually considerable ptosis will persist.

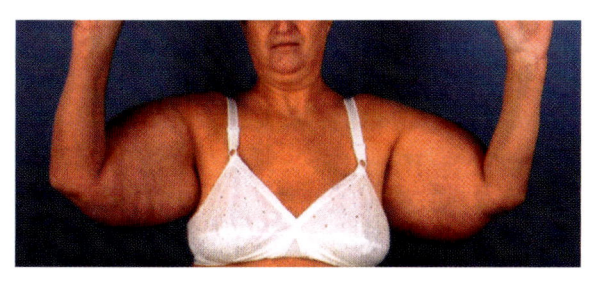
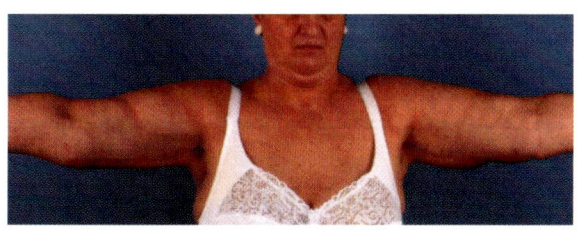

□ Fig. 30.12. This patient suffered from Madelung's disease and was treated with liposuction and brachioplasty; (above) preop, (below) 5 months postop

The goals of reduction mammaplasty and mastopexy are to:
- Improve symptomatology
- Reduce the volume of breast tissue while maintaining the vascular and neural integrity of the nipple areola
- Reposition the nipple-areolar complex in its anatomically correct position
- Create a predictable, stable, and better breast shape
- Provide parenchymal support to the breast for longevity of the result
- Eliminate excess skin while reducing tension on the closure (avoid using the skin to create the breast shape)
- Minimize scars

A myriad of surgical techniques have been described. Most accepted procedures for mastopexy as well as for reduction mammaplasty now follow the principles outlined as early as 1919 [29] by Lexer: the nipple-areolar complex is transposed on dermal de-epithelialized cranial and bilateral pedicle skin and volume reduction is performed in the lower quadrants, resulting in a periareolar and inverted T-scar [30, 31]. Lejour [27] has to be credited for adding liposuction, suspending sutures, and fixation of the remaining gland on the pectoralis fascia. In many cases also a vertical scar avoids the inframammary incision [32] (□ Fig. 30.13).

In case of massive ptosis after weight loss, skin excesses may extend along the inferior axilla onto the lateral chest. In these cases the lateral inferior inframammary skin resection can be extended onto the lateral chest (see Sect. 5.2.3.9).

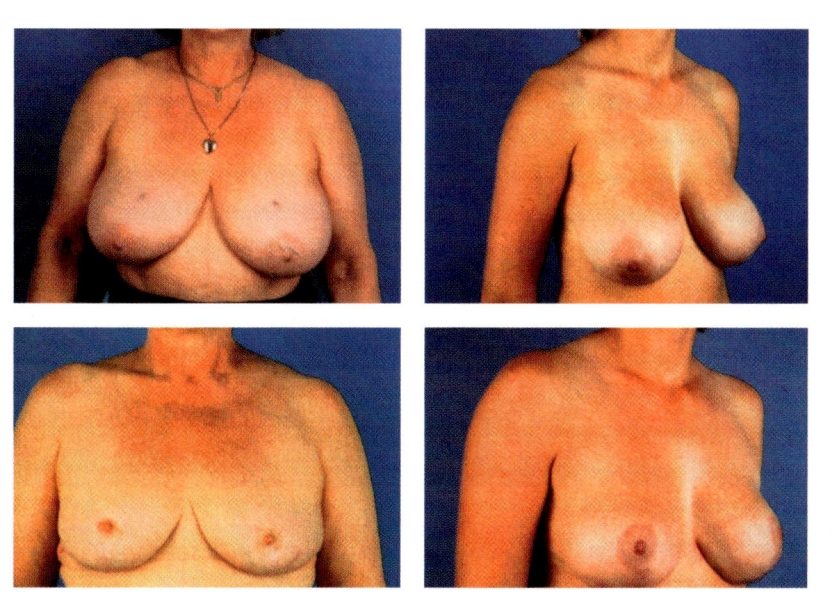

□ Fig. 30.13. Two typical types of breast reduction: (left) Höhler's method with an inverted T-shaped scar; (right) vertical scar-reduction technique after Lejour

30.3.8 Corrections for Gynecomastia

Gynecomastia denotes enlargement of the male breast. The condition is common during puberty secondary to proliferation of breast parenchyma but usually abates after progression for 3–18 months. Multiple medications, hormonal imbalances, systemic conditions (i.e., obesity, hyperthyroidism, liver disease), and exogenous hormones have all been implicated in the development of gynecomastia. Gynecomastia is classified into four grades on the basis of breast volume and degree of ptosis [33]. This female appearance of the breasts may be due to an abundance of skin and adipose and glandular tissue and is common in manifest obesity, but it frequently persists after weight loss, causing considerable discomfort. Historical techniques for correction by transverse amputation of the breast with replantation of the nipple-areolar complex should be obsolete.

Liposuction with or without ultrasound may be sufficient in many cases, taking advantage of a surgically induced retraction of excessive skin. Even if a firm gland requires incisional subcutaneous mastectomy, this should be combined with liposuction to taper the contour transition from the excisional defect to the surrounding chest skin [29, 34, 35]. When skin is too excessive a doughnut-shaped circumareolar skin resection is combined with liposuction and gland excision, care being taken to plan the inner margin well within and not at the margin (peri-areolar) of the areola, as the remaining areola will always widen postoperatively. In severe Simon grade-IV ptotic gynecomastia an inverted T-scar reduction mastectomy analogous to reduction mammaplasty in women will be necessary. If the skin redundancy goes beyond the breast into the axilla and lateral chest a chest lift is a valuable adjunct or alternative (see below).

30.3.9 Chest Lift

Skin redundancy of the chest wall leads to an unaesthetic breast: Lifting of the arms causes the skin to be pulled upward and the inframammary crease to disappear. At the same time, the nipple-areolar complex is lifted up in a more natural lateral position, so that the breast shape and appearance become more harmonious. Chest lifting avoids noticeable scarring on the frontal view of the chest (◘ Fig. 30.14) [36, 37]. Often a chest lift is combined with a mastopexy and a brachioplasty. ◘ Figure 30.14, lower left, shows the incision line and ◘ Fig. 30.14, lower right, the resulting scars after a combined chest lift with bra-

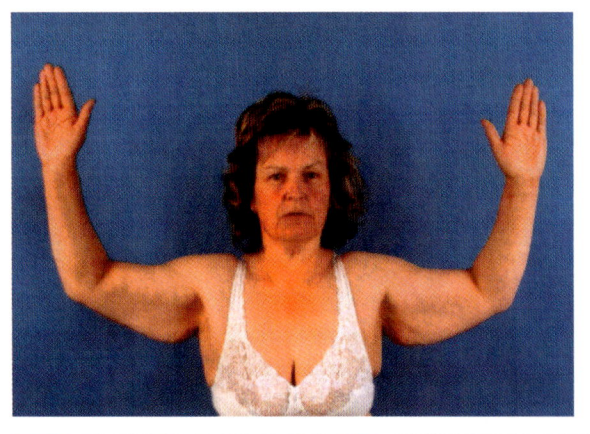
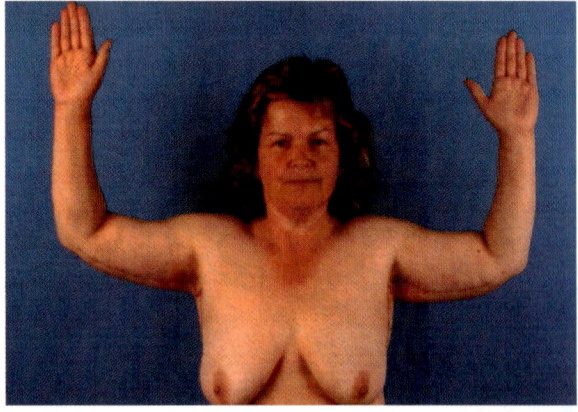
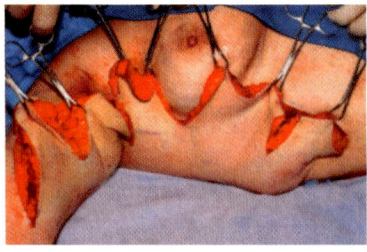
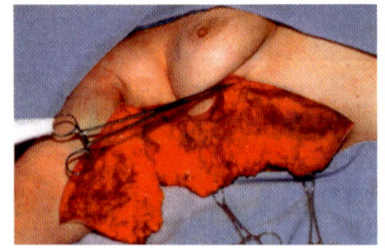
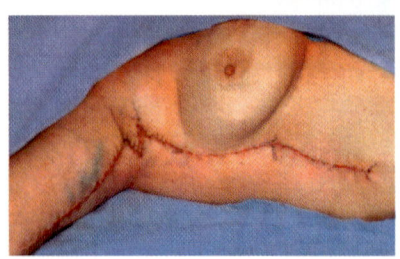

◘ **Fig. 30.14.** Chest lift combined with brachioplasty: (upper left) preop, (upper right) 6 months postop. (lower left): a considerable amount of tissue can be resected. (lower middle): a clamp is holding the lateral submammary fold cranially where it must be fixed to the periosteum of the third rib. lower middle: A Z-plasty is sometimes needed to prevent scar contraction

chioplasty. The clamp in 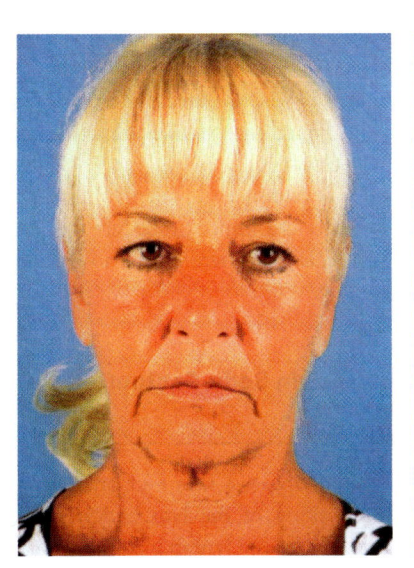 Fig. 30.14, lower middle, shows the repositioning of the lateral submammary fold, which also needs to be repositioned by a non-absorbable suture to the periosteum of the third rib laterally.

30.3.10 Facial and Cervical Rhytidectomy (Face-Neck Lift)

When patients achieve considerable weight loss, they are happier. However, volume loss in the face may result in an unfavorable change of their facial appearance, as the resulting ptosis and rhytidosis of the face may include all the stigmas of premature facial aging and tiredness. Besides mid- and lower facial ptosis, this includes relaxation of the neck with platysmal bands, brow ptosis, blepharochalasis, and tear troughs. Correction of these residua of the obese past may considerably improve patients' self-image and can also be considered reconstructive rather than "cosmetic".

Facial aging involves the loss of deep-layer support as attenuation of facial retaining fibrous connections occurs because of the previous distension by abundant fat. These deep-layer changes manifest as ptotic malar fat pads with deepening of nasolabial folds, marionette lines, jowl formation, platysmal bands, and cervical skin laxity (Fig. 30.15). The deep-layer technique for face lifting predictably and safely alters the superficial musculoaponeurotic system (SMAS) and facial retaining ligaments to produce facial rejuvenation by creating vectors of deep-layer support that reposition ptotic tissues. Precise excision of redundant skin allows a close-to-normal skin tension closure, minimizing scar detectability [38].

Taking these three-dimensional changes into account, it is obvious that only superficial "mini-lift" skin techniques will not achieve a natural-looking and longstanding reconstructive result. Individual evaluation has to be performed with close consultation between the patient and the plastic surgeon to discuss adjunct procedures, such as blepharoplasty, (endoscopic) forehead lifts, lip lift, and skin rejuvenation procedures.

30.3.11 Liposuction

Aspiration lipectomy (liposuction) is the most frequent and "popular" procedure in aesthetic surgery, but it is neither trivial nor a primary tool for body weight reduction. Liposuction with vacuum cannulae traumatizes the subcutaneous compartment and causes fluid shifts and blood loss, with sharply increasing complications, when the volume suctioned exceeds 5 l. Prior to the successful advent of bariatric surgery, serial "megaliposuction", aspirating up to 15 l of fat per session, was advocated by some [4, 5] for morbid obesity but is considered only rarely as an adjunct today.

Liposuction is a very valuable tool in non-obese patients with localized fat depots as exemplified by the typical "saddlebags" of some women. Cosmetic results vary greatly according to localization and individual factors (age, skin quality), as it relies largely on the elastic ability of the skin to retract after the volume has been reduced. This makes it obsolete as a singular procedure for most patients after weight loss. Nevertheless, liposuction may be a very helpful adjunct to many resection dermolipectomies and "lifts" (Fig. 30.16).

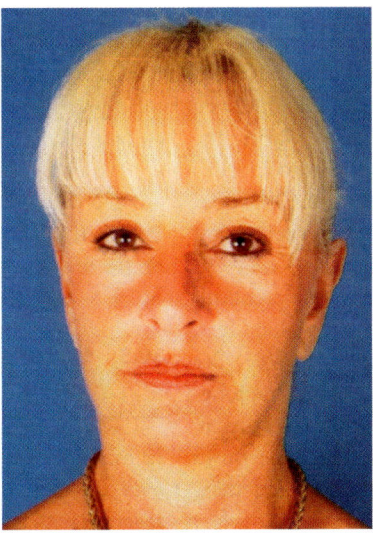

 Fig. 30.15. Neck lift: patient with 30 kg weight loss, (left) before and (right) after face lift

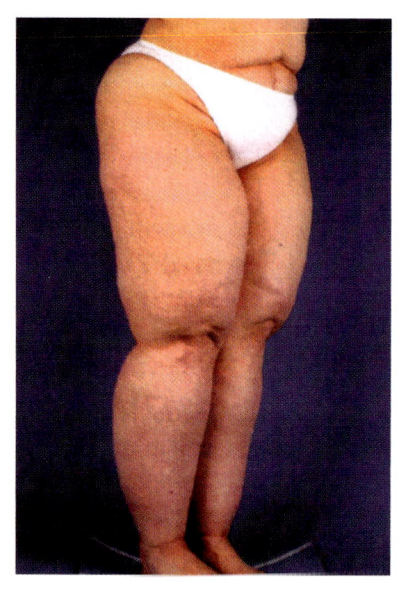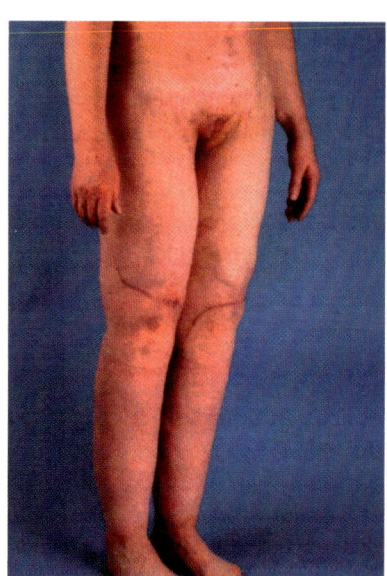

☐ **Fig. 30.16.** A 43-year-old patient with severe lipedema of both legs, (left) before treatment and (right) after three sessions of liposuction (9 l on each leg), body lift, and knee lift

30.4 Complications

The tension created in body-forming procedures can lead to wound separation, even with a thorough reconstruction of the superficial fascial system. Minor areas of delayed wound healing are commonly seen in thigh plasties. Wound healing problems are found more often in the thighs than in other regions. These areas are often contaminated and moist because of the adjacent perineal area. The wounds heal by secondary intention and do not have long-term negative effects.

In smokers wound healing problems almost always occur in body lifts. Many surgeons refrain from operating on patients who smoke. The patient should stop smoking at least 2 weeks in advance and for 3 weeks after surgery.

Infection, as with any surgery, might also be seen in body-contouring surgery. For longer procedures such as body lifts the risk of bacterial contamination rises. Antibiotic prophylaxis should be maintained during the first postoperative days. Severe infection of subcutaneous tissue is very rare in body-contouring surgery; if it does occur, it needs to be treated aggressively by debridement and drainage.

Large undermining and operations in adjacent regions as in lower body lifts can lead to greater blood loss, even if meticulous hemostasis is performed [19]. For legal reasons, patients have to be informed about autohemotherapy and the possible need for blood transfusion. Blood transfusion is rarely seen in one-area procedures such as abdominoplasty, thigh lift, arm lift, and mastopexy.

Because of the prolonged operating time the risk of thrombosis and pulmonary embolism increases. Therefore, it is recommended to administer low-dose heparin (weight adapted) during the hospital stay. Ambulation should be encouraged from the first postoperative day; anti-embolism stockings or elastic bandaging are recommended. The total risk of pulmonary embolism is less than 0.1% according to Lockwood [20].

Seroma formation is the most common problem after plastic dermolipectomy surgical procedures [39]. It is far more often observed in the legs and flanks than in the breasts or arms. It is not very clear where these seromas come from. One theory is that during surgery the lymphatic trunks are harmed, and because lymphatic fluid has the tendency to coagulate very slowly, the cut vessels stay open and lymphatic fluid drains into the wounds.

To prevent seromas it is wise to leave drains in place for a prolonged period. Sometimes seroma puncture on an outpatient basis is necessary.

Widening of scars is common, and patients should be advised that a scar revision as a minor procedure may be indicated and worthwhile, as later there will be no tension on the revision suture line.

30.5 Lymphatic Issues in Body-Contouring Surgery

In morbidly obese patients massive skin folds may hang over the knees. This kinking of the lymphatic vessels together with excessive weight and lymph load may cause a vicious circle of combined lipomatosis and stasis lymphedema and be an indication for dermolipectomy before weight reduction has been achieved [40]. Even after massive weight loss, sagging of skin in the leg can lead to considerable localized lymphedema. Patients with lymphedema of the leg are not excluded from surgery, but to prevent further aggravation the anatomical location of the superficial thigh collectors must be respected surgically, and such procedures are optimally embedded in an interdisciplinary lymphological-surgical concept, with preoperative decongestion.

It is recommended to provide custom-fitted compression garments to prevent such lymphatic complications as edema and lymphoceles. They need to be worn for at least 6 weeks, sometimes for 6 months. Swelling in the legs and in the anterior abdominal wall is seen quite often postoperatively and cannot be predicted.

Candidates with preoperative orthostatic edemas are more often prone to postoperative edema. Very rarely, chronic lymphedema occurs.

30.6 Conclusions: Plastic Surgery in a Comprehensive Treatment Plan

Morbid obesity is a disease with catastrophic consequences for the patient's physical and mental health and social well-being. Both visceral surgery and medical concepts have dramatically improved the somatic treatment options to reduce the underlying caloric imbalance. This does not necessary correspond proportionally to an improved body image, due to persisting stigmas. The plastic surgeon performs the final surgical step. The patient now expects a body shape restored to normal.

Besides some somatic morbidity of inelastic and redundant skin, the aesthetic concerns of these patients, who have gone to great effort to improve their lives, must be taken seriously from the beginning. Obesity is a multifactorial pathological entity requiring an interdisciplinary approach that focuses on the individual patient. Specialized plastic surgery can offer a lot, even if this becomes relevant only further down the line, and this prospect must be included in the concept of a comprehensive obesity center.

References

1. Markman B, Barton FE jr (1987) Anatomy of the subcutaneous tissue of the trunk and lower extremity. Plast Reconstr Surg 80:248–254
2. Sarwer DB, Fabricatore AN (2008) Psychiatric considerations of the massive weight loss patient. Clin Plast Surg 35:1–10
3. Sarwer DB, Thompson JK, Mitchell JE, Rubin JP (2008) Psychological considerations of the bariatric surgery patient undergoing body contouring surgery. Plast Reconstr Surg 121:423e–434e
4. Dhami LD, Agarwal M (2006) Safe total corporal contouring with large-volume liposuction for the obese patient. Aesthetic Plast Surg 30:574–588
5. Alegria Peren P, Barba Gomez J, Guerrero-Santos J (1999) Total corporal contouring with megaliposuction (120 consecutive cases). Aesthetic Plast Surg 23:93–100
6. Zook EG (1975) The massive weight loss patient. Clin Plast Surg 2:457–466
7. McCraw LH jr (1974) Surgical rehabilitation after massive weight reduction. Case report. Plast Reconstr Surg 53:349–352
8. Davis TS (1984) Morbid obesity. Clin Plast Surg 11:517–524
9. Pitanguy I (1975) Abdominal lipectomy. Clin Plast Surg 2:401–410
10. Regnault P (1975) Abdominoplasty by the W technique. Plast Reconstr Surg 55:265–274
11. Regnault P (1989) About the W abdominoplasty. Plast Reconstr Surg 83:1084
12. Dubou R, Ousterhout DK (1978) Placement of the umbilicus in an abdominoplasty. Plast Reconstr Surg 61:291–293
13. Momeni A, Torio-Padron N, Bannasch H, Borges J, Stark GB (2008) A new method for reducing postoperative complications and scar length in abdominoplasty. Plast Reconstr Surg 121:227e–228e
14. Toranto IR (1990) The relief of low back pain with the WARP abdominoplasty: a preliminary report. Plast Reconstr Surg 85:545–555
15. Aly AS, Cram AE, Chao M, Pang J, McKeon M (2003) Belt lipectomy for circumferential truncal excess: the University of Iowa experience. Plast Reconstr Surg 111:398–413
16. Richter DF, Stoff A, Velasco-Laguardia FJ, Reichenberger MA (2008) Circumferential lower truncal dermatolipectomy. Clin Plast Surg 35:53–71; discussion 93
17. Lockwood TE (1988) Fascial anchoring technique in medial thigh lifts. Plast Reconstr Surg 82:299–304
18. Pitanguy I (2000) Evaluation of body contouring surgery today: a 30-year perspective. Plast Reconstr Surg 105:1499–1514; discussion 1515–1516
19. Lockwood T (1993) Lower body lift with superficial fascial system suspension. Plast Reconstr Surg 92:1112–1122; discussion 1123–1125
20. Lockwood T (1995) High-lateral-tension abdominoplasty with superficial fascial system suspension. Plast Reconstr Surg 96:603–615
21. Lockwood TE (1991) Superficial fascial system (SFS) of the trunk and extremities: a new concept. Plast Reconstr Surg 87:1009–1018
22. Lockwood TE (1991) Transverse flank-thigh-buttock lift with superficial fascial suspension. Plast Reconstr Surg 87:1019–1027
23. Centeno RF (2006) Autologous gluteal augmentation with circumferential body lift in the massive weight loss and aesthetic patient. Clin Plast Surg 33:479–496
24. Centeno RF, Mendieta CG, Young VL (2008) Gluteal contouring surgery in the massive weight loss patient. Clin Plast Surg 35:73–91; discussion 93
25. Lockwood T (1995) Brachioplasty with superficial fascial system suspension. Plast Reconstr Surg 96:912–920
26. Hurwitz DJ, Holland SW (2006) The L brachioplasty: an innovative approach to correct excess tissue of the upper arm, axilla, and lateral chest. Plast Reconstr Surg 117:403–411; discussion 412–413

27. Lejour M (1994) Vertical mammaplasty and liposuction of the breast. Plast Reconstr Surg 94:100–114
28. Horch RE, Jaeger K, Stark GB (1999) Quality of life after breast reduction-plasty [in German]. Handchir Mikrochir Plast Chir 31:137–142
29. Lexer E (1921) Corrección de los pechos pendulos (Mastoptose). San Sebastian Guipuzcoa Medica 63:213
30. Höhler H (1977) Reduction mammoplasty in hyperplasias of the female breast [in German]. Chirurg 48:377–383
31. Pitanguy I (1967) Surgical treatment of breast hypertrophy. Br J Plast Surg 20:78–85
32. Lejour M (1993) Vertical mammaplasty. Plast Reconstr Surg 92:985–986
33. Simon BE, Hoffman S, Kahn S (1973) Classification and surgical correction of gynecomastia. Plast Reconstr Surg 51:48–52
34. Stark GB, Grandel S, Spilker G (1992) Tissue suction of the male and female breast. Aesthetic Plast Surg 16:317–324
35. Voigt M, Walgenbach KJ, Andree C, Bannasch H, Looden Z, Stark GB (2001) Minimalinvasive, chirurgische Therapie der Gynäkomastie – Liposuktion und Exhärese Technik. Chirurg 72:1190–1195
36. Finckenstein JG, Wulf H (2006) Chest lifting. Aesthetic Plast Surg 30:286–293
37. Hurwitz DJ, Neavin T (2008) L brachioplasty correction of excess tissue of the upper arm, axilla, and lateral chest. Clin Plast Surg 35:131–140; discussion 149
38. Connell BF (1981) Surgical technique of cervical lift and facial lipectomy. Aesthetic Plast Surg 5:43–50
39. Shermak MA, Rotellini-Coltvet LA, Chang D (2008) Seroma development following body contouring surgery for massive weight loss: patient risk factors and treatment strategies. Plast Reconstr Surg 122:280–288
40. Felmerer G, Torio-Padron N, Momeni A, Földi E, Stark GB (2004) Reduction procedures in lymphedema and associated obesity adjuvant to CDP. Lymphology 37 [Suppl 1-717]: 467–467 (Progress in Lymphology XIX), Földi E, Földi M, Witte MH (eds)

Hernias after Bariatric Surgery

Robert E. Brolin, MD

Hernias are among the most common late (>30 days) complications of operations performed for treatment of morbid obesity. Incisional hernia is the most frequent late complication in many large series of open bariatric operations. Conversely, laparoscopic bariatric operations are associated with a significantly higher rate of internal/mesenteric hernias in comparison to the open approach [1]. This chapter covers all types and aspects of hernias that develop after both open and laparoscopic bariatric operations.

31.2 Open Procedures

The incidence of incisional hernia after open bariatric operations ranges from 5% to 35% [2, 3]. Most large published series with follow-up greater than 2 years report an incidence in the 15–20% range [1]. There is surprisingly little detailed information on incisional hernias after open bariatric operations. The risk factors for incisional hernia in this situation are the same as after nonbariatric operations and include postoperative wound infection, malnutrition, immunosuppressive drugs, older age, and diseases associated with increased intra-abdominal pressure, e.g., small bowel obstruction. Several studies have shown that morbid obesity is associated with a high baseline intraabdominal pressure [4]. Thus, severe obesity is an inherent risk for postoperative incisional hernia. There is virtually no information regarding the relative contributions of the various risk factors to development of incisional hernia after open abdominal operations. Sugerman et al. compared the incidence of postoperative hernia in two high-risk groups, one including patients on prednisone who had total abdominal colectomy for inflammatory bowel disease and the other patients who had open Rouxen-Y gastric bypass (RYGB) [2]. The hernia rate was significantly higher after RYGB (20%) than after colectomy (4%). The consistently high rate of incisional hernia after open bariatric operations suggests that morbid obesity is among the most powerful risk factors for development of this late complication.

Several reports have focused on techniques for closure of the primary incision and their relationship to the incidence of incisional hernia. Those who favor use of a continuous closure cite the benefit of equalization of pressure over the entire length of the incision [5]. Those who favor use of interrupted sutures cite the consequences of failure of a single suture, which may be inconsequential if only one or two individual interrupted sutures fail [5, 6]. Conversely, acute fascial dehiscence can occur after failure of a long continuous closure. Although the continuous versus interrupted closure controversy re-

mains unresolved as regards bariatric patients, the author performed a prospective, randomized comparison using continuous double-stranded absorbable monofilament suture versus a braided polyfilament permanent suture of the same diameter.

In that study, there was a significantly lower hernia rate 2 years postoperatively in the continuous-closure group [3]. One drawback of the study was the fact that two different types of suture were used. Hence, the influence of suture material may have played a role in the outcome. The 10% incidence of hernia with a minimum 2-year follow-up in our continuous-closure patients is lower than reported in most large series of open bariatric operations.

Other types of hernias are relatively rare after open bariatric operations. The incidence of internal hernia is not reported in most published accounts of open bariatric operations.

I am aware of only three patients who developed internal hernias in a personal series of more than 1600 open primary RYGBs. Umbilical hernias are incidentally present in as many as 5% of patients who undergo bariatric surgery. In the author's experience, the recurrence rate of umbilical hernias repaired during a primary open operation is substantially higher in patients whose closure of the upper midline incision includes the umbilical defect than in patients whose umbilical hernia repairs are not incorporated in closure of the incision.

31.3 Laparoscopic Procedures

Multiple studies have shown that the incidence of wound problems is significantly lower after laparoscopic operations compared with their open counterparts [1, 7]. Incisional hernias after laparoscopic operations almost invariably occur at the port sites. The incidence of port site hemia after laparoscopic Roux-en-Y gastric bypass (LRYGB) is reported in the range of 0–1.7% [1, 7, 8]. In the early era of minimally invasive bariatric surgery, there was considerable debate regarding the need to close port sites at the conclusion of the procedure. Improvements in trocar technology have likely reduced the need to close ports of <12 mm diameter. Most surgeons still close port sites of 15 mm or greater. The author is aware of three port site hernias (0.4%) in a personal series of 730 primary LRYGBs. This percentage could be divided by 6 since we use at least six ports per operation. Two of these hernias were probably related to the trauma associated with replacement/reinsertion of multiple trocars at the same site. Multiple same-site trocar insertions should probably be considered an indication for closing that site.

Most bariatric surgeons believe that patients with pre-existing abdominal wall hernias who undergo laparoscopic bariatric operations should have concomitant repair of the hernia. Exceptions to this algorithm might include umbilical hernias that are too small to entrap bowel and large, broad-based hernias that require prosthetic mesh for definitive repair. Abdominal insufflation is tremendously compromised by large abdominal wall hernias. Repair of large, broad-based abdominal wall hernias should either precede a laparoscopic bariatric procedure or be performed concomitantly with an open bariatric operation. On several occasions I have used absorbable mesh to temporarily repair a large ventral hernia in conjunction with an open RYGB. Subsequent definitive repair of such hernias is facilitated by substantial weight loss.

The most dangerous hernias associated with laparoscopic bariatric operations occur within spaces created by dividing the mesentery of the small bowel. Internal hernia after LRYGB is almost invariably associated with small bowel obstruction (SBO). Because acute SBO is potentially life-threatening, prevention of internal hernias has become a highly relevant issue in minimally invasive bariatric surgery. In the early era of LRYGB, many surgeons made no attempt at the closure of spaces created by dividing the jejunal mesentery. However, a rash of cases of SBO after LRYGB caused a number of surgeons to reevaluate their position on this issue.

The anatomy of the potential defects created during LRYGB is shown in ◘ Figs. 31.1 and 31.2. Of the three potential spaces created during retrocolic LRYGB, Petersen's space between the mesentery of the Roux limb and transverse mesocolon is the most common site for internal herniation according to most clinical reports, with mesocolic hernias running a close second [9–11]. Conversely, the so-called jejunojejunostomy defect is the most common site for internal hernias after antecolic LRYGB [10, 11]. Many surgeons who perform antecolic LRYGB, including the author, place the jejunojejunostomy on the transverse colon or upper mesocolon, which, for all practical purposes, consolidates Petersen's space and the jejunojejunostomy defect into a single large space [12].

It seems eminently logical that closure of spaces created by transecting the jejunum and constructing the Roux-en-Y would decrease the incidence of internal hernia. However, there are conflicting data regarding reduction in the incidence of internal hernia and closure of

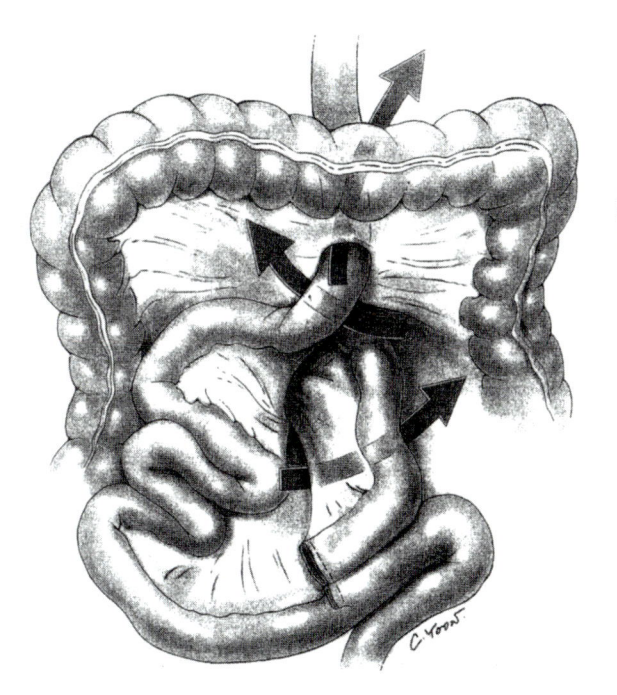

◘ Fig. 31.1. Three potential spaces created in retrocolic Roux-en-Y reconstruction including mesocolic (*upward arrow through transverse mesocolon*), Petersen's (*arrow towards patient's right side beneath mesentery of Roux limb*), and the so-called jejunojejunostomy defect (*arrow towards patient's left side beneath mesentery of the biliopancreatic limb*)

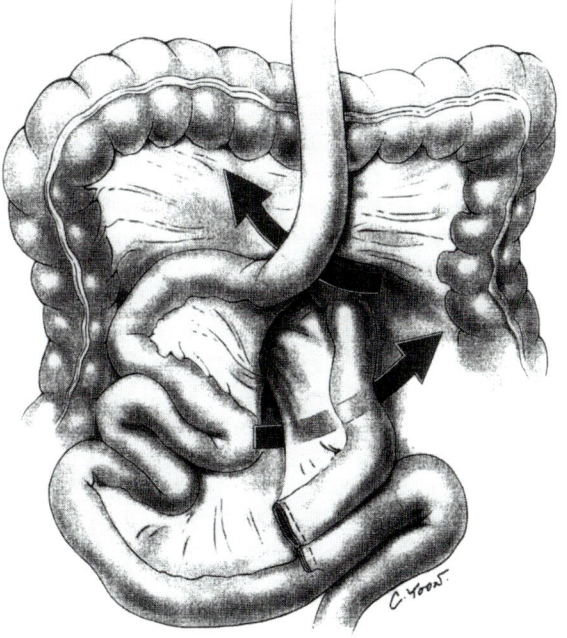

◘ Fig. 31.2. Two potential spaces created in antecolic Roux-en-Y reconstruction including Petersen's space (*arrow towards patient's right*) and the jejunojejunostomy space (*arrow towards patient's left*). Placement of the jejunojejunostomy on the transverse colon essentially eliminates Petersen's space

these mesenteric spaces. Champion and Williams were the first to compare both Roux limb position and closure versus nonclosure of mesenteric spaces in a large series of patients who had LRYGB [13]. In that series, there was no difference in the incidence of internal hernia between the closure (4.1%) and nonclosure (4.7%) groups after retrocolic LRYGB. Conversely, Carmody et al. noted a significant reduction in hernias after routine closure (0.6%) compared with nonclosure (7.5%) of mesenteric defects after retrocolic LRYGB [9]. In this report, there was no difference in the incidence of internal hernia between the patients in the ante- and retrocolic groups who did not have closure of mesenteric defects. However, none of the patients had antecolic LRYGB with closure of the mesenteric spaces.

Several recent publications have suggested that specific techniques used for creation of the jejunojejunostomy can virtually eliminate internal hernia after antecolic LRYGB. Quebbemann and Dallal suggest that a leftward orientation of the Roux limb in LRYGB will result in a significantly lower rate of internal hernia [14]. Cho et al. claim that not dividing the small bowel mesentery is the key to preventing internal hernia [12], while Finnell et al. believe that a long "triple-stapled" jejunojejunostomy is the critical feature of their technique [15]. Both groups perform a side-to-side stapled anastomosis. At the conclusion of each group's LRYGB, the jejunojejunostomy rests on the transverse colon. Neither group closed the mesenteric defects. Mean follow-up in the two series was 11 and 18 months, respectively. The author's initial technique of antecolic LRYGB was very similar to that of Cho et al., who reported a <1.0% incidence of internal hernia with <12 months' follow-up [12, 16].

Our first internal hernia was recognized 18 months postoperatively. However, after 5 years, we noted 15 internal hernias (2.4%) that resulted in acute SBO with our initial technique of mesenteric closure. The relatively sudden increase in SBO following LRYGB has also led to a debate regarding the preferred position of the Roux limb. The great majority of clinical reports suggest that the incidence of bowel obstruction secondary to internal hernia is greater in patients with a retrocolic Roux limb. Two recent meta-analyses of hernia after LRYGB cite retrocolic positioning of the Roux limb as a risk factor for internal hernia [10, 11]. Champion and Williams reported a significantly lower incidence of SBO in patients who had an antecolic (0.43%) than in those who had a retrocolic (4.5%) Roux limb orientation [13]. There are conflicting data regarding Roux limb position that evoke other important issues. Two important variables that are inconsistently reported in papers that focus on SBO after LRYGB are the technique used for closure of potential

mesenteric defects and the mean duration of postoperative follow-up. Several publications describe a transition from nonclosure to closure of potential defects without allowing for sufficient follow-up to capture cases of SBO in the closure group [9, 17, 18]. Most clinical reports with a <2% incidence of SBO from internal hernia have mean follow-up times of <18 months [12, 15]. Conversely, virtually all published series with >5% incidence of SBO after LRYGB have mean follow-up intervals of >2 years [19, 20]. In my own series, the mean time between LRYGB and acute obstruction caused by internal hernia was 20 months. Likewise, Carmody et al. reported a significantly lower internal hernia rate after LRYGB in patients with the shortest duration of follow-up after LRYGB [9].

Although the preponderance of recent literature tends to support closure of potential mesenteric defects after LRYGB, there is surprisingly little emphasis on the technical aspects of closure. Several authors have used absorbable suture material for closure of these spaces, with mixed results. I seriously question the use of absorbable suture to achieve "permanent" closure of potential mesenteric defects. Would these surgeons use absorbable suture to repair an incisional hernia? Use of a continuous rather than interrupted sutures for closure appears to be the preferred technique in most published reports. However, there are no prospective published reports that simultaneously compare more than one method of closure of mesenteric defects during LRYGB. In my view, closure of these mesenteric defects can be quite challenging in super-obese LRYGB patients who have a large omentum and a thick layer of mesenteric fat. It behooves bariatric surgeons to learn a comfortable and technically sound method for closure of these defects. Several surgeons, including the author, have noted a relationship between internal hernias and successful weight loss after LRYGB [21, 22]. Since the great preponderance of the weight loss after RYGB is fat rather than lean body mass, it seems likely that potential hernia defects will gradually enlarge as the mesenteric fat disappears. Since most RYGB patients reach the nadir of weight loss between 18 and 24 months postoperatively, one would expect that a minimum follow-up in excess of 24 months were required in order to reliably determine the incidence of internal hernia after LRYGB. Twelve of my 15 patients who developed SBO due to internal hernia had a BMI of <30 kg/m^2 at the time of presentation. Preoperative diagnosis of internal mesenteric hernia is difficult after LRYGB [17, 23]. Plain abdominal radiographs are frequently normal or nondiagnostic. Abdominal CT scanning with oral contrast is the best diagnostic test [23, 24]. Although CT scans in this setting are usually reliable in the diagnosis of mechanical SBO, the presence of internal hernia is more difficult to establish. Internal hernias typically result in a closed-loop obstruction, which may rapidly progress to strangulation. Strangulation obstruction of the small bowel is life-threatening. Volvulus of the bowel, which has even greater propensity for strangulation, is commonly associated with internal hernia after LRYGB. The author and others recommend diagnostic laparoscopy in pursuit of symptoms suggestive of partial SBO. Laparoscopy in this setting has been consistently rewarding in the discovery of internal hernias (100%) and volvulus (33%) [22]. These operations can be performed with a 24-h stay and minimal morbidity. Repair of internal hernias is technically straightforward and should be performed with nonabsorbable sutures. Volvulus associated with internal hernia and SBO creates considerably more problems. Because detorsion of the mesentery is frequently difficult using laparoscopic instruments, conversion to an open procedure is common in this setting. Conversely, volvulus associated with internal hernia in the absence of acute SBO can usually be managed via laparoscopy [22].

31.4   Conclusion

In summary, internal hernia is a relatively common complication of LRYGB. Because internal hernia is the most common cause of SBO in LRYGB patients, it seems appropriate to operate upon all patients who present with acute SBO after LRYGB. This philosophy represents a paradigm shift from the open RYGB era, when the most common cause of SBO was adhesions that frequently could be treated successfully by tube decompression alone. There is little evidence that closed-loop obstruction can be treated successfully by tube decompression. Delay in operating is the most commonly cited reason for increased morbidity and mortality in large series of patients with SBO. Because internal hernia and volvulus are frequently associated with strangulation, there is no reason to postpone an operation in patients who present with SBO after LRYGB. I am hopeful that overcoming the learning curve associated with this new procedure will result in a lower incidence of SBO as a consequence of internal hernia.

References

1. Podnos YD, Jimenez JC, Wilson SF, et al (2003) Complications after laparoscopic gastric bypass. A review of 3464 cases. Arch Surg 138:957–961
2. Sugerman HJ, Kellum JM, Reines HD, DeMaria EJ, Newsome HH, Lowry JW (1996) Incisional hernia: greater risk with morbidly obese than steroid-dependent patients; low recurrence rate with prefascial polypropylene mesh repair. Am J Surg 171:80–84
3. Brolin RE (1996) Prospective, randomized evaluation of midline fascial closure in gastric bariatric operations. Amer J Surg 172:328–331
4. Sugerman H, Windsor A, Bessos M, Wolfe L (1997) Intra-abdominal pressure, sagittal abdominal diameter, and obesity co-morbidity. J Intern Med 241:71–79
5. Richards PC, Balch CM, Aldrete JS (1983) Abdominal wound closure: a prospective randomized study of 571 patients comparing continuous vs interrupted suture techniques. Ann Surg 197:238–243
6. Poole GV jr, Meredith JW, Kon ND, et al (1984) Suture technique and wound bursting strength. Am Surg 50:569–572
7. Nguyen NT, Goldman C, Rosenquist J, et al (2001) Laparoscopic vs. open gastric bypass: a randomized study of outcomes, quality of life and costs. Ann Surg 234:279–291
8. Higa KD, Boone KB, Ho T (2000) Complications of the laparoscopic Roux-en-Y gastric bypass: 1,040 patients – what have we learned? Obes Surg 10:509–513
9. Carmody B, DeMaria EJ, Jamal M, et al (2005) Internal hernia after laparoscopic Roux-en-Y gastric bypass. Surg Obes Rel Dis 188:543–548
10. Koppman JS, Li C, Gandsas A (2008) Small bowel obstruction after laparoscopic Roux-en-Y gastric bypass: a review of 9527 patients. J Am Coll Surg 206:571–584
11. Iannelli A, Facchiano E, Gugenheim J (2006) Internal hernia after laparoscopic Roux-en-Y gastric bypass for morbid obesity. Obes Surg 16:1265–1271
12. Cho M, Pinto D, Corrodeguas L, et al (2006) Frequency and management of internal hernias after laparoscopic antecolic Roux-en-Y gastric bypass without diversion of the small bowel mesentery or closure of mesenteric defects: review of 1400 consecutive cases. Surg Obes Rel Dis 2:87–91
13. Champion JK, Williams M (2003) Small bowel obstruction and internal hernias after laparoscopic Roux-en-Y gastric bypass. Obes Surg 13:596–600
14. Quebbemann BB, Dallal RM (2005) The orientation of the antecolic Roux limb markedly affects the incidence of internal hernias after laparoscopic gastric bypass. Obes Surg 15:766–770
15. Finnell CW, Madan AT, Tichansky DS, Ternovits C, Taddeucci RJ (2007) Nonclosure of defects during laparoscopic Roux-en-Y gastric bypass. Obes Surg 17:145–148
16. Suggs WJ Kouli W, Lupovici M, et al (2007) Complications at gastrojejunostomy after laparoscopic Roux-en-Y gastric bypass: comparison between 21- and 25-mm circular staplers. Surg Obes Rel Dis 5:508–514
17. Higa KD, Ho T, Boone KB (2003) Internal hernias after laparoscopic Roux-en-Y gastric bypass: incidence, treatment and prevention. Obes Surg 13:3504
18. Nguyen NT, Huerta S, Gelfand D, Stevens M, Jim J (2004) Bowel obstruction after laparoscopic Roux-en-Y gastric bypass. Obes Surg 14:190–196
19. Escalona A, Devand N, Perez G, et al (2007) Antecolic versus retrocolic alimentary limb in laparoscopic Roux-en-Y gastric bypass: a comparative study. Surg Obes Rel Dis 3:423-427
20. Capella RF, Iannace VA (2006) Bowel obstruction after open and laparoscopic gastric bypass surgery for morbid obesity. J Am Coll Surg 203:328–335
21. Ahmed AR, Richards G, Husain S, et al (2007) Trends in internal hernia incidence after laparoscopic Roux-en-Y gastric bypass. Obes Surg 17:1563–1566
22. Gandhi A, Brolin RE (2009) Elective laparoscopy for herald symptoms of mesenteric/internal hernia after laparoscopic Roux-en-Y gastric bypass. Surg Obes Relat Dis 2009 Mar-Apr;5(2):144–9

23. Onopchenko A (2005) Radiological diagnosis of internal hernia after Roux-en-Y gastric bypass. Obes Surg 15:606–11
24. Blachar A, Federle MP (2002) Gastrointestinal complications of laparoscopic Roux-en-Y gastric bypass surgery in patients who are morbidly obese: findings on radiography and CT. Am J Roentgenol 179:1437–1442

31

Chronic Venous Insufficiency and Venous Ulcers in the Obese

Carolin Kayser, MD

Chronic venous insufficiency (CVI) and venous ulceration are major health issues in developed countries. CVI is estimated to be present in 0.1–0.2% of the population at risk in Western countries [1] and is thought to be the underlying cause of 70–90% of all leg ulcers [2]. Ulcer healing rates can be poor, with only 50% healing at 4 months [3], 20% remaining open at 2 years, and 8% remaining open at 5 years [4]. Additionally, the annual recurrence rate varies from 6% to 15% [5, 6]. From an economic point of view, leg ulcerations are responsible for the loss of 2 million working days and treatment costs of approximately $3 billion per year in the United States [7]. The association between obesity and varicosis has been confirmed, especially in female patients [8], but the role of obesity in more severe stages of CVI is not well-established. For example, increased intra-abdominal pressure has been implicated as a factor in CVI. Additionally, several factors contributing to CVI are also associated with morbid obesity. Both conditions can be regarded as chronic diseases, both are diseases of civilization, and both can cause large treatment costs over a prolonged period of time. Therefore, patients suffering from both conditions always need combined and multimodal therapy to achieve positive therapeutic results.

32.1 Definition

Chronic venous insufficiency is a combination of symptoms caused by venous hypertension and the resultant structural and functional changes taking place in the affected veins. The venous hypertension itself can result from venous valvular incompetence, venous obstruction, or a combination of both [9]. The most frequent causes are primary abnormalities of the venous wall and/or the valves or secondary changes due to previous thrombosis leading to reflux and obstruction [10]. Congenital malformations are a rare cause of CVI.

32.2 Etiology and Risk Factors

CVI and venous ulcers seem to be associated with leg injuries, obesity, deep vein thrombosis, and pulmonary embolism. They also appear to be more prevalent in women, and the risk of ulcers increases consistently with age in both genders [11–15]. Additionally, the factors listed in ▫ Table 32.1 seem to be correlated to the development of venous ulcers, although the evidence to date is insufficient [16, 17]:

In many cases, there is recurrence of the venous ulcer. The incidence of recurrent ulceration after complete healing was reported as 28% at 2 years, 38% at 3 years, and 57% at 4 years [20, 21] in several clinical studies.

32.3 Pathophysiology

CVI develops at pathologically high venous blood pressure. Normal values range from 20 to 30 mmHg, but they can increase up to 60–90 mmHg due to thrombosis, pathological findings in the venous valves, or weakened muscle pump. The increased intravenous pressure leads to pathological changes in the venous wall, which are responsible for subsequent complications.

32.3.1 Changes in the Major Veins in CVI

Varicose veins are the most frequent manifestation and symptom of CVI. Primary varicosis results from venous dilatation without previous thrombosis, trauma, or other disturbances of the venous blood flow. Some research suggests that the venous walls are more distensible in patients with primary varicosis than in other patients [22]. Secondary varicosis follows deep vein thrombosis and recanalization that gives rise to incompetent deep and perforating veins. In both forms, valvular incompetence leads to elevated venous pressure, which leads to further destruction of the venous valves, thus forming a vicious

▫ **Table 32.1** Risk factors for CVI

Varicose veins	Diabetes mellitus	Number of pregnancies
Lack of physical activity or inappropriate activity [18, 19]	Family history of CVI, especially maternal side	Standing and sitting position during work or leisure time
Renal disease	Heart failure	Use of hormones (women)
Rheumatoid arthritis	Hypertension	Tight undergarments
Smoking	Constipation	

circle which can continue even after elimination of the underlying cause.

The varicosis usually starts in the area of connection of the deep and superficial venous systems (saphenofemoral junction, saphenopopliteal junction, and perforating system). In some cases, the junctions and perforators are not affected, and valvular incompetence arises simply from valvular varices resulting in reflux. This is more common in women who have symptoms suggestive of pelvic congestion after several pregnancies, and such symptoms are also found in obese patients.

The lack of venous drainage and the resulting venous hypertension also increase the pressure in the capillary area and thus the transmural pressure in postcapillary vessels. This leads to capillary damage, fluid exudation, edema, and tissue malnutrition and maloxygenation. Inflammation, infection, thrombosis, and tissue necrosis with lipodermatosclerosis follow, finally resulting in ulceration.

The main cause of secondary varicosis is a former deep vein thrombosis and the subsequent changes in the venous system. An incomplete recanalization can lead to outflow obstruction and damage to surrounding valves with reflux, which is regarded as responsible for most cases of post-thrombotic syndrome. An early recanalization, on the other hand, is associated with valvular competence [23]. The changes in venous hemodynamics develop with time: 35–69% of patients suffer from post-thrombotic syndrome after 3 years, 49–100% after 5–10 years [24, 25]. These figures also depend on localization and extent of the thrombosis: Proximal thrombosis leads to a higher incidence of post-thrombotic syndrome.

32.3.2 Changes in Microcirculation

Since new non-invasive techniques have made it possible to study changes in the microcirculation of the skin, the severe impairment of capillary function in CVI is known to lead to the well-known skin changes seen in affected patients. In cases of mild CVI, these changes may be minimal. Especially in areas of visible skin changes, the capillaries are seen to be dilated, elongated, and twisted. These findings occur most often in patients with deep vein insufficiency and damage to the perforating veins [26–29]. Capillary thromboses lead to maloxygenation and malnutrition of the skin. Later in the course there is damage to the capillary system and ulcerations occur [30]. Additionally, microedema and pericapillary fibrin appear, possibly increasing the malnutrition and maloxygenation [31]. After fibrinogen leaks into the interstitial space, fibrin polymers form around the capillaries, building a cuff which may interfere with the diffusion of oxygen and nutrients and trap growth factors necessary for wound healing [32, 33]. A minimal trauma may lead to a chronic wound. Similar changes take place in the lymphatic vessels of the lower limb, contributing to the lack of drainage [34].

Other authors emphasize the trapping and activation of white blood cells in the endothelial wall of capillary beds exposed to high venous pressure. Following attachment to intracellular adhesion molecules, the white blood cells are activated and high levels of cytokines and free radicals occur [35, 36]. An inflammatory reaction follows, leading to injury of venous and surrounding tissue and predisposing to ulceration. However, these suggested steps in the development of ulcerations need to be elucidated in further investigations [37].

32.3.3 Associated Changes

Many studies with patients suffering from CVI indicate changes in fibrinogen and impaired fibrinolysis. Increased levels of plasma fibrinogen have been reported regularly [38]. Also degradation products and lymphatic fibrinogen are elevated, indicating a high turnover of molecule and plasma leakage in the capillary area [39]. Consequently, rheological changes of altered viscosity and red cell aggregation [40] occur, but the impact of these findings on the course of the disease is not well-known. The role of inflammatory cells and that of the fibrin cuff mentioned above also need to be subjected to further investigation.

32.3.4 Influence of Obesity

Increased intra-abdominal pressure has been implicated as a factor in CVI. In 1997, a correlation between intra-abdominal pressure and venous stasis was found [41], and Danielsson and co-workers measured significantly elevated femoral venous pressure in obese patients with elevated bladder pressure (indirectly measured intra-abdominal pressure) [42]. Padberg et al. [43] were able to show that patients with morbid obesity had severe limb symptoms typical of CVI, but approximately two thirds of the limbs showed no anatomical evidence of venous disease. The authors also came to the conclusion that the obesity itself contributed to the morbidity. A large overhanging pannus is also said to decrease the venous flow from the lower extremities and therefore to increase CVI. Other factors such as lack of physical activity could also impair the venous emptying of the leg.

Avascularity in excessive fatty tissue decreases the tissue oxygen level [44]. Additionally, the elevated body mass needs an elevated cardiac output, which leads to relative or absolute heart failure. The skin in the periphery of the blood stream therefore suffers from chronic hypoperfusion and hypo-oxygenation. Due to the lowered tidal volume and vital capacity of the lung, the oxygen in the arterial blood is also reduced. Proteins and nutrient levels are also lowered in the periphery of the body, causing a lack of auxiliary factors for tissue remodeling and renewal, and thus decreasing wound-healing capacity. The adipose tissue also interferes with the lymphatic system, causing secondary lymphedema. Lymphedema itself leads to chronic inflammation of skin, subcutaneous tissue, and the lymphatic network. In combination, this can lead to cellulitis, which further decreases the lymphatic transport and therefore elevates the risk of future episodes of cellulitis. The resulting lymphostasis leads to an accumulation of protein in the interstitial space, infiltration of neutrophils, macrophages and fibroblasts, deposition of collagen and further destruction of the lymphatic network.

32.4 Clinical Findings

There are various symptoms of CVI, and the history and clinical findings often do not reveal the underlying cause. Patients' complaints range from aching, heaviness of the legs and feet, cramps, itching, burning sensations, edema, visible and prominent superficial veins, skin changes such as pigmentation, ulceration, lipodermatosclerosis, and eczema to restless legs syndrome and severe changes in the shape of the leg. Over the past 30 years, many classifications of chronic venous disease have been generated, beginning with that of Widmer in 1978 (see ◘ Table 32.2) [45].

Most of these classifications lacked the necessary completeness to be appropriate for scientific use. In 1994, the American Venous Forum presented the CEAP classification, which includes clinical, etiological, anatomical, and pathophysiological aspects of CVI [46, 47]. Some authors and clinicians criticize the CEAP classification because of its complexity, but practical use of this classification does not require that every patient undergo the full range of diagnostic methods. A common classification with highly defined stages of CVI seems to be mandatory, especially in research reports. A short overview of the CEAP classification is given in ◘ Table 30.3.

As an example, a patient with symptomatic varicose veins that extend throughout the whole territory of the long saphenous vein and with swelling, pain, and lipodermatosclerosis associated with incompetent perfora-

◘ **Table 32.2** Classification of CVI according to Widmer [45]

Stage	Clinical findings
I	Reversible edema
	Corona phlebectatica
	Peri-malleolar varicosis
II	Persistent edema
	Hemosiderosis
	Purpura of the lower leg
	Dermatosclerosis and Lipodermatosclerosis
	Atrophie blanche
	Eczema
	Cyanosis of the skin
III	Venous ulceration

tors in the calf with a normal deep system is denoted C2,3,4s-Ep-As2,3,p18-Pr [10]. Additionally, severity and disability can be noted.

32.5 Diagnostics

The diagnosis of CVI can be made on the basis of clinical findings alone in most patients. To determine the underlying cause and therapeutic options, a further diagnostic workup is necessary. A wide number of tests and procedures have been developed to reveal a calf muscle pump dysfunction or the anatomical extent of obstruction or reflux. Especially in patients with risk factors such as obesity and/or thrombosis, it is difficult to decide which test to perform at a given point in the clinical examination.

A careful clinical history and examination are mandatory. Genetic disposition, other underlying medical conditions, drugs, risk factors, work-related factors, sports, operations or trauma in the medical history of the lower limb, number and course of pregnancies, phlebitis, and thrombosis should be evaluated. During the clinical examination, a gross inspection of the whole body, a close inspection of the skin at the lower limb, palpation, examination of arterial and venous vascular status including peripheral pulses, and a gross neurological and orthopedic examination should be performed. The tourniquet test provides information about the sites of deep-to-superficial reflux but depends on the prominence of varicose veins; no statement can be made about obstruction or reflux in the deep veins.

⬛ **Table 32.3** CEAP classification according to Nicolaides et al. [10]

The CEAP classification of CVI		
C: Clinical signs	0	No visible/palpable signs
	1	Telangiectases or reticular veins
	2	Varicose veins
	3	Edema
	4	Skin changes (pigmentation, eczema, lipodermatosclerosis)
	5	Skin changes and healed ulceration
	6	Skin changes with active ulceration
E: Etiology	E_C	Congenital
	E_P	Primary, undetermined cause
	E_S	Secondary, known cause (post-thrombotic, post-traumatic, other)
A: Anatomical distribution	1	**Superficial veins A_S** Telangiectases/reticular veins Greater saphenous
	2	above knee
	3	below knee
	4	Lesser saphenous
	5	Nonsaphenous
	6	**Deep veins A_D** Inferior Vena cava / Iliac
	7	Common
	8	Internal
	9	Extenal
	10	Pelvic-gonadal, broad ligament, other Femoral
	11	Common
	12	Deep
	13	Superficial
	14	Popliteal
	15	Crural – anterior tibial, posterior tibial, peroneal (all paired)

⬛ **Table 32.3** *Continued*

The CEAP classification of CVI		
	16	**Muscular – gastrocnemial, soleal, other Perforating veins A_P**
	17	Thigh
	18	Calf
P: Pathophysiological	P_R	Reflux
	P_O	Obstruction
	$P_{R,O}$	Reflux and obstruction
Clinical Score	Pain	0: None 1: Moderate, not requiring analgesics 2: Severe, requiring analgesics
	Edema	0: None 1: Mild / moderate 2: Severe
	Venous claudication	0: None 1: Mild / moderate 2: Severe
	Pigmentation	0: None 1: Localized 2: Extensive
	Lipodermatosclerosis	0: None 1: Localized 2: Extensive
	Ulcer - size	0: None 1: <2 cm diameter 2: >2 cm diameter
	Ulcer - duration	0: None 1: <3 months 2: >3 months
	Ulcer - recurrence	0: None 1: Once 2: More than once
	Ulcer - number	0: None 1: 1, single 2: Multiple
Disability Score	0	Asymptomatic
	1	Symptomatic, can function without support device
	2	Can work 8-h day only with support device
	3	Unable to work even with support device

The "typical" venous ulcer presents in the gaiter area associated with hyperpigmentation and lipodermatosclerosis, but an estimated 21% of patients with venous ulcers suffer from concomitant arterial insufficiency [2]. Palpation of pulses in the affected lower leg may be difficult or even impossible due to edema. However, an additional arterial disease can be estimated easily by measuring arterial closing pressure with a conventional hand-held Doppler transducer and determining the ankle-brachial index or toe-brachial index. Compression therapy, which may be planned for after completion of the examination, can have contrary effects when exceeding arterial pressure.

Malignant degeneration may take place in chronic ulcerations. The presence of squamous cell or basal cell carcinoma in a classic venous ulcer has been described in the literature. To exclude a different underlying cause or malignant transformation, a biopsy should be acquired after 6 months of ineffective causal therapy. If vasculitis is assumed or has to be ruled out, the biopsy should be taken at the edge of the ulcer.

32.5.1 Radiography

Ascending Phlebography. Ascending phlebography used to be the diagnostic method of choice in venous insufficiency. Definition of anatomy and detection of insufficient major veins, detection of incompetent perforator veins, and the distinction between primary and secondary affection were the goals of this invasive method. Additionally, it was possible to diagnose a deep vein thrombosis, and the differentiation of early and late thrombosis was possible. In principle, a contrast medium is injected into a vein at the dorsal side of the foot and followed until it reaches the inferior vena cava. The velocity of the filling of veins can be influenced by tourniquets or positioning of the patient [48, 49].

The limitation of this diagnostic method lies in the lack of functional assessment. Although a thrombosis can be identified, no assessment of severity or of the adequacy of collateral veins can be made [50].

Descending Phlebography. The aim of descending phlebography is to demonstrate venous reflux, either from the pelvis to the lower limb or from deep to superficial veins, or in the area of venous valves. The contrast medium, which has to be heavier than the blood itself, is injected into the major veins either popliteal or femoral, and the functional assessment of parts below the injection level is possible. The Valsalva maneuver is used to close the venous valves, and different positioning of the

patient can lead to different assessments [51–55]. Continuous or intermittent registration has to be obtained, and the reflux can be rated in five grades [56–58].

Since the introduction of duplex scanning, use of the invasive and rather expensive technique of descending phlebography has decreased and is now limited to certain indications (deep vein reconstruction, incongruence of duplex findings).

Varicography. With varicography, the contrast medium is injected directly into the varicose vein itself. Its purpose is mostly to detect the connection of recurrent varicose veins to deeper veins [59]. Especially during operations, it can guide the surgeon to affected veins with minimal incisions for precise vascular surgery [60, 61].

32.5.2 Duplex Scanning

Duplex scanning can be used in the detection of deep vein thrombosis, obstruction, and reflux. Also, the description of anatomical changes in CVI is possible [62, 63]. Color flow imaging can provide information about velocity and direction of blood flow in both superficial and deep veins. With this imaging method, it has become conventional to show central flow as blue and recurrent flow as red. The advantages of duplex scanning are the low price, the vivid imaging, and the different levels of examination, but the findings of a duplex scan depend greatly on the operator, the compliance of the patient, and several other premises such as body weight and the extent of edema in the lower limb. In the case of obese patients, phlebography is sometimes the better choice [64–66].

The use of duplex scanning has been expanded in recent clinical studies. Serial examinations indicated that duplex scanning was the ideal method for following the natural course of thrombosis and post-thrombotic syndrome. The progressive development of reflux and the recanalization of veins even after complete thrombosis were shown in such serial scans. It was also shown that the organization process and rate of thrombolysis differ greatly from patient to patient, leading to the possibility of detecting patients with a high risk of post-thrombotic complications. In general, the resolution of a thrombus follows a three-step sequence [23, 67–69]:

- Rapid spontaneous thrombolysis, preservation of valvular function, restoration of the vein to normal appearance
- Increasing echogenicity, indicating fibrosis
- Slow recanalization, causing valve destruction, reflux, and post-thrombotic symptoms

Data suggest that there is a strong correlation between the severity of CVI and the anatomical extent and distribution of reflux. Since duplex scanning is a very sensitive method of detecting reflux in any anatomical region and to any extent, patients at high risk for long-term complications of CVI can be detected with a simple diagnostic tool [70]. Due to different classifications and reporting methods, the clinical studies available were not able to prove a direct correlation, and further studies should therefore be performed.

Detection and validation of gastrocnemial reflux can be easily detected via a duplex scan. Detection is mandatory, because successful treatment of this reflux, which is the cause of some forms of primary venous insufficiency and a common cause of recurrence, can easily be achieved with surgical ligation.

32.5.3 Liquid Crystal Thermography

After a tiptoe exercise, thermography easily detects insufficient perforator veins, described as hot spots in the registration, with a sensitivity of 94% [71]. With the development of liquid crystal plates, the method has been simplified and can be used as a screening test. Compared with duplex scanning, the positive predictive value of thermography is 91% [72]. Relatively cost-effective, simple, and accurate, liquid crystal thermography seems to be suitable for use in the preoperative marking of incompetent perforating veins.

32.5.4 Air Plethysmography

Air plethysmography (APG) is able to measure all venous functions responsible for CVI: reflux, obstruction, and muscle pump dysfunction [73]. In general, changes in the volume of the examined limb are measured by air displacement in a cuff surrounding the calf. Maneuvers to empty and fill the venous system are performed during the measurement. The following parameters and measurements are part of the standard diagnostics:

— Venous outflow rapid cuff deflation, elevated limb, proximal venous occlusion
— Venous refill dependent limb position after venous outflow measurement, determination of the venous filling index
— Calf muscle pump measurement after a single and after ten contractions (tiptoe maneuver); determination of the ejection capacity

Overall, APG provides quantitative information about several aspects of venous function. It is the diagnostic tool of choice prior to interventions or assessment of interventional success. A pathological venous filling index in APG has been found to correlate with the severity of CVI [74, 75]. The venous filling index, with a sensitivity of up to 80% [75], may be the best parameter for detecting venous reflux, and complications of CVI such as ulcerations have been shown to correlate with measurements of ejection capacity [10, 73, 74].

32.5.5 Photoplethysmography

Photoplethysmography (PPG) can be used to confirm the diagnosis of CVI [76]. A PPG probe is placed on the foot, maneuvers to empty the venous system with calf muscle contraction are performed, and the return of blood is detected by increased backscatter of light. The refill time may be calculated as the time required for the PPG tracing to return to 90% of the baseline after emptying of the venous system by contraction. These measurements have been shown to correlate with invasive measurements to diagnose CVI [77]. Depending on the position of the patient, a venous refill time of less than 18–20 s is indicative of CVI; in the same setting a refill time of more than 20 s can be regarded as normal. To differentiate between deep or superficial venous insufficiency and to define local functional changes, a tourniquet or pressure cuff can be used, but these measurements are not quantitative; although a short refill time suggests more severe disease, the correlation remains poor [10]. In conclusion, PPG can help to rule out CVI but provides no further detailed information [78].

32.5.6 Ambulatory Venous Pressure

Measurement of ambulatory venous pressure (AVP) is regarded as the hemodynamic gold standard in assessing CVI. A pressure transducer needle is injected into the pedal vein and measurements are made at rest and during and after exercise. Usually, tiptoe maneuvers are used. Additionally, pressure can be registered before and after the placement of an ankle cuff to differentiate between deep and superficial venous reflux. The clinically most important parameters obtained with this technique are mean AVP and refill time [79, 80]. Both provide information about the global competence of the venous system, but some authors question the accuracy of the measurements regarding the deep system [80]. Overall, this technique is not commonly used, owing to its invasiveness and the availability of alternative diagnostic modalities. Attempts have been made to obtain venous pressure by means of non-invasive methods, but this needs to be investigated further [81].

32.5.7 Studies of Microcirculation

Microvascular investigations seem to be limited to scientific purposes and can determine the pathogenesis of skin lesions in CVI. Their clinical value seems doubtful. But the possibility of quantifying early changes of the skin in CVI may give such examinations and tests a prognostic value that should be objectified in clinical studies [10].

Skin Biopsy. Following excision or punch biopsy in regions of interest, various staining methods can be applied. In clinical routine, malignancies or vascular changes due to vasculitis must be ruled out [82, 83]. Additionally, this method has been widely used in researching skin changes in CVI.

Capillaroscopy. Capillaroscopy remains a research tool. Although knowledge of the pathophysiology of venous ulcerations has been enlarged by studies using capillaroscopy, its clinical value in the management of patients suffering from CVI is very limited [10]. It was shown that the capillaries in patients with CVI are coiled and dilated, that the number of capillaries is reduced, and that capillaries are lacking in areas with atrophie blanche [84, 85].

Laser Doppler Fluxometry (LDF). This technique is currently employed in clinical microvascular research but is also limited in its clinical use [86]. LDF is used to identify relative changes in local blood flow as a response to stimuli such as orthostasis or thermal stress [10]. For example, the effect of compression therapy on local blood flow can be measured. It was shown that elastic or pneumatic compression tended to normalize the blood flow in limbs with CVI and induce normal vasomotion [86, 87].

Transcutaneous Oxygen Tension. Transcutaneous oxygen tension can be defined as a measure of the surplus oxygen available for diffusion to the skin surface from the capillaries. Usually, these measurements are made under hyperthermic conditions. Most patients with CVI show a significantly decreased oxygen tension, and this worsens as the disease progresses[88, 89].

Fluorescence Microlymphography. This technique is the only method for analyzing the structure and function of the lymphatic tissue of the skin. Following injection of a lymphophilic dye, the dynamics and extent of dye spread and the morphology of the lymphatic network are recorded and analyzed. In a state of CVI with morphological changes of the skin, changes of the lymphatic network also occur and the network of lymphatic vessels is interrupted [90].

Interstitial Pressure Measurements. The measurement of interstitial pressure is useful for studying the evolution of CVI, but several limitations reduce its clinical applications. There are high costs associated with this test, and two operators have to be trained and have to take part in the test at the same time.

32.5.8 Selection of Diagnostic Methods

Unfortunately, there is no method available that provides all the needed information for diagnosis and therapy in a single testing. The clinical aim remains the acquisition of all the needed information with a minimum of expense and inconvenience to the patient.

The initial examination of a patient suffering or assumed to be suffering from CVI should determine the presence or absence of obstruction and reflux. This includes a detailed medical history and pocket Doppler ultrasound examination. In most cases (up to 90%), the underlying pathological condition can be identified by these means. The Doppler examination is also adequate to localize obstruction or reflux. Phlebography may be necessary in a few cases. Plethysmography to measure AVP can follow for quantification of reflux and obstruction.

Nicolaides et al. [10] suggest adapting the diagnostic means to the clinical stages following the CEAP classification. The authors also suggest dividing the diagnostic methods into three levels, according to practicality, cost-effectiveness, and invasiveness:

- Level I: Clinical examination and history
  Doppler examination
- Level II: Duplex scanning
  Plethysmography
- Level III: Phlebography
  Varicography
  Pressure measurements

An overview of the diagnostic features in the different clinical stages is given in ▫ Table 30.4.

Selection of the suitable diagnostic method can be even more difficult with obese patients than with other patients. In general, Doppler and duplex scanning can deliver inaccurate or false results due to the amount of subcutaneous fatty tissue and fluid collections. Reticular veins are widened and disturb the acquired signal. Pl-

□ Table 32.4 Level of diagnostic methods recommended in different clinical classes of CVI according to the CEAP classification (modified according to [10])

Class 0/1	Level I	Most cases
	Level II	Duplex scanning in symptomatic disease
Class 2	Level I	Varicose veins confined to the long saphenous system with reflux at the saphenofemoral junction Absence of reflux in the popliteal fossa
	Level II	Varicose veins involving the short saphenous system Reflux in the popliteal fossa Suspected incompetent thigh or calf perforating veins Recurrent varicose veins and history of DVT
	Level III	Deep venous reflux or obstruction
Class 3	Level I	All patients
	Level II	Determination of deep venous reflux and obstruction
	Level III	Pathological findings in level II
Classes 4–6	Level I	All patients
	Level II	All patients
	Level III	Patients in preparation for deep venous reconstruction

ethysmography also provides inaccurate findings in cases of morbid obesity. In these patients, phlebography is indicated early in the diagnostic process and can provide exact results, although the examination is inconvenient and semi-invasive.

32.6 Therapy

Different types of treatment have to be considered in the therapy of CVI and venous ulcerations. Local wound care should include debridement and infection control, the use of modern wound dressings to provide a moist environment, and pain management. For non-healing wounds, autologous skin grafting and the use of human skin equivalents should be considered. For symptomatic and causal treatment of CVI, compression therapy applied by wraps, stockings, and compression pumps and venous surgery are the methods of choice [1]. Edema and trophic disturbances must be eliminated and the aggravation of the CVI grade must be prevented. Postural adjustments such as elevating the legs to minimize edema and reducing intra-abdominal pressure should be made. In general, most physicians prefer the conservative approach and opt for surgical methods only after prolonged duration of treatment. For the obese patient, therapy should be multimodal, composed of compression therapy, mild exercise, local therapy, and weight reduction if possible. Mere treatment of the CVI will not result in a satisfying outcome.

32.6.1 Mechanical Compression Therapy

Mechanical compression therapy provides the basis for non-invasive CVI therapy and can be used alone or in combination with other methods. It can be applied in all clinical stages of the disease. Its effectiveness is due to the assistance of the muscle pump, and walking or other physical activity is recommended to enhance the therapeutic effect. A pressure gradient is provided from the ankle to the knee or thigh, with the highest pressure achieved at the ankle. The functional loss of damaged valves and veins can thus be adjusted and the capillary pressure is lowered. This promotes skin perfusion and elevation of the blood velocity and lymph flow. Some authors also suggest an elevated fibrinolysis and resultant decrease of changes in the capillary walls. Edema and ulcerations are decreased.

Compression stockings are provided for different grades, depending on the pressure exerted at the ankle. In general, 20–30 mmHg is recommended for patients with mild symptoms, such as varicose veins, mild edema, and pressure sensations in the leg; 30–40 mmHg is recommended for patients with severe varicosis or moderate CVI; 40–50 mmHg and more than 60 mmHg may be used in patients with severe CVI and resulting complications. If a high rate of compliance can be achieved, treatment with compression stockings reaching 30–40 mmHg can result in significant improvement in pain, swelling, skin pigmentation, activity, and well-being [91]. In case of venous ulceration, graded compression stockings are effective in both healing and preventing recurrence, and in up to 93% of patients healing of the ulcer can be achieved within a mean of 5.3 months [92].

At the beginning of compression therapy, knee-high stockings, which are better tolerated than full-length stockings, should be prescribed for the patient [93]. The tension needed for effective treatment is based on the clinical class of disease according to the CEAP classification: In classes 2 and 3, 20–30 mmHg is sufficient, in classes 4–6, 30–40 mmHg is needed, and in case of recurrent ulceration, 40–50 mmHg should be achieved [78]. Most problems with compression therapy occur in the daily routine. Elderly and physically impaired patients lack the ability to put on the stockings and take them off, especially if chronic wounds are present and the stockings have to be applied over wound dressings. Some companies provide devices to help the patients put on and remove the stockings, but these devices also require a certain physical ability. Additionally, compression therapy has the anticipated effect only when the stockings, etc. are properly adjusted. In some cases, elastic wraps may provide certain benefits, but dislocation of the wraps can be seen in most patients in clinical routine.

With obese patients, compression therapy is even more difficult to apply effectively. The inability to put on the garment and take it off reduces its use, and even specially prescribed garments do not fit properly due to the irregular shape of the extremities. In severe obesity, compression pumps can be used to support the effects of compression stockings. Data imply that the use of a pneumatic pump improves venous return and fibrinolytic activity, therefore reducing the fibrin cuff around the capillary bed [94]. Multicompartmented pumps show a greater effect on edema mobilization with compression from the ankle up to the thigh. The patients have to wear compression stockings between treatments with the compression pump, Clinical data suggest that the combination of stockings and pumps leads to good results in ulcer healing time [95].

Prior to the beginning of compression therapy, the arterial perfusion status and neurological status of the leg should be determined, since low perfusion and peripheral neuropathy are absolute or relative contraindications to compression. Some authors reject the use of compression therapy for patients with signs of invasive infection at an ulcer site [1]. In our opinion, mild compression in combination with antibiotic agents can be applied without any risk of severe systemic infection or worsening of the local infection.

32.6.2   Local Skin and Wound Care

CVI leads to compromised skin integrity; therefore, extensive skin care has to be maintained. Dry areas must be kept moist to prevent micro-injuries due to small cracks, with subsequent infection. A topical steroid has to be applied in case of stasis dermatitis.

Moist treatment is regarded as the state of the art in the treatment of chronic wounds. Dry wound dressings are reserved for palliative treatment of tumor wounds or necrotic tissue prior to surgical intervention.

At the beginning of treatment, necrotic and severely infected tissue should be removed. Debridement can be achieved with the patient under local anesthesia, while general anesthesia should be considered for painful wounds and large wound areas. To remove superficial necrotic parts and decrease the bio-burden, a high-pressure micro-stream pump filled with water or antiseptic detergent can be used. Despite the relatively high pressure of the fluid stream (up to 300 mmHg), painless wound cleaning can be performed.

A wide variety of modern wound dressings are available to achieve moist wound treatment. Many physicians face the problem of choosing the appropriate dressing. A short overview of modern wound dressings is given in ◘ Table 30.5. Adverse effects of wound dressings are not common and include maceration of the surrounding skin, the development of irritant contact dermatitis, and allergic dermatitis.

In obese patients, several additional factors favor the onset and prolongation of wound infections and chronic wounds: Morbidly obese patients have a 20% incidence of type-2 diabetes [96–98]. This increases the risk of bacterial infections of the skin; colonization of wounds by bacteria (forming of bio-burden) can contribute to the inflammatory process and therefore slow down wound healing [99]. The maintenance of adequate personal hygiene is limited by the patients' physical limitations and redundant skin folds. Especially in the intertriginous areas, there is constant fluid collection due to perspiration, and this favors fungal infection. Local therapy is even more important in these situations and sometimes depends on daily professional assistance.

32.6.3   Systemic Medical Therapy

Medical therapy of CVI is strictly symptomatic and therefore limited. Diuretics seem to be the most commonly used drugs, with the reduction of intravascular fluid and mobilization of fluid in the interstitial space as the main targets. But the use of diuretics in this indication can be

□ Table 32.5 Modern wound dressings

Dressing	Characteristics	Indications	Limitations
Paraffin gauze	Does not stick to surface	Flat, shallow wound	No exudation management
	Exudate passes through to secondary dressing		
Semi-permeable adhesive films	Permeable to air and water vapor	Closure of superficial, partial thickness wounds	Low exudation management
	Barrier to fluids and bacteria	Difficult anatomical sites	Maceration of the surrounding skin
	Left in place for several days, transparent for wound check		
Hydrocolloids	Adhesive, water and gas impermeable	Wounds with light to heavy exudate	Limited exudation management
	Forming gel	Rehydration of necrotic wounds	Gel may be mistaken for infection
	Protection of pressure areas		
Alginate	Production of hydrophilic gel	Lightly contaminated wounds and cavities	Dry wounds
	Adsorption of non-cellular components	Enhances debridement	Necrosis
			Non-adhesive, another dressing needed for fixation
Hydrogels	Provide moisture	Dry, necrotic wounds	Little exudation management
	Encourage debridement		
Hydrofiber	Forms gel in contact with exudates	Deep wounds with moderate to high exudation	Dry wounds
Hydrocellular or polyurethane foam	Highly absorbent	Large exudation volumes	Dry wounds
	Transmits moisture vapor and oxygen	Available as cavity-dressing	No enhancement of debridement
	Thermal insulation		
Silver-coated	Silver in ionic or nanocrystalline form	Colonized or infected wounds	Invasive infections (additional antibiotic systemic therapy required)
	Antimicrobial agent		
Activated charcoal	High exudation management	Palliative wound treatment	No curative treatment
	Odor control		

achieved only with simultaneous compression therapy; diuretics alone do not have the necessary effect.

Chronic ulcers show colonization by bacteria. Colonization of wounds (formation of bio-burden) can contribute to the inflammatory process and therefore slow down wound healing [99]. If there is evidence of invasive infection, the use of antibiotics is mandatory. Some authors advise basing the therapy on bacterial cultures and determination of bacterial sensitivities [1].

Some authors also favor the use of rheological and venotonic agents. Pentoxifylline alters the microcirculation in

CVI and was tested in many trials in the treatment of venous ulceration. It also may prevent white blood cell activation and therefore decrease the level of cytokines and improve oxygenation in the ischemic tissue [100]. As in diuretic therapy, combination with compression therapy is necessary. Venotonic agents, such as Daflon, are also recommended by different authors to increase the tone in abnormally dilated veins. With increased tone, the capillary leak may be reduced and microcirculation may accelerate [101].

Some other agents, such as Aspirin and platelet-derived growth factor, have been reported to promote ulcer healing and reduce recurrence rates, but these effects need to be further investigated in clinical trials.

32.6.4 Local Medical Therapy

Sensitization to locally applied substances, including corticosteroids and wound dressings, occurs in up to 80% of patients with CVI, depending on the duration and severity of the illness. In addition, non-allergic reactions of the surrounding tissue can occur. Therefore, indications for external drugs and dressings are limited.

32.6.5 Physical Therapy and Exercise

Since dysfunctions in the calf and foot muscle pump play a major part in the pathophysiology of CVI, muscle training and controlled exercise can contribute to the reduction of disease symptoms and aggravation. Padberg et al. [102] randomized patients in a small clinical trial to either routine daily activity or structured calf muscle exercise and came to the conclusion that structured exercise may prove beneficial as supplemental therapy. Additionally, classical components of physiotherapy can also have beneficial effects, such as controlled walking training, mobilization in the lower ankle joint, manual lymph drainage, and intermittent technical compression, as mentioned above.

In morbid obesity, lack of exercise and elevated intra-abdominal pressure aggravate CVI. Theoretically, mild exercise and weight reduction could improve the venous function in the legs. In daily routine, however, weight loss is not possible by conservative means and exercise cannot be performed because of the physical limitations. The treating physician has to consider other options, such as mild aquarobics to minimize pressure on the bones and joints and to lower the effective body weight during exercise. In 1998, Melissas et al. [103] showed that weight reduction led to an improvement in the condition of the lower legs in obese patients. This weight reduction was obtained through bariatric surgery.

32.6.6 Interventional Therapy

Sclerotherapy. This therapeutic option is indicated mainly in obliterating telangiectases, varicose veins, and venous segments with reflux. It may be used as primary treatment or in combination with surgical procedures. There are different sclerosing agents available, including

hypertonic solution of sodium chloride, detergents (sodium tetradecyl sulfate, etc.), and other compounds such as sodium iodide and chromated glycerine. In smaller veins, the agent used has to be diluted to prevent tissue inflammation and necrosis. The most common adverse effect of sclerotherapy is hyperpigmentation of the surrounding skin due to hemosiderin degradation. A randomized multicenter study carried out in 2003 [104] showed that microthrombectomy 1–3 weeks after the initial therapy resulted in less pigmentation and pain, but this has not yet become part of clinical routine.

Ablative Therapy with Endovascular Radiofrequency and Laser. This technique is frequently used for great saphenous vein reflux as an alternative to stripping. Thermal energy in the form of radiofrequency or laser is used to obliterate the veins. The heat generated causes a local thermal injury to the vein wall, leading to thrombosis and eventual fibrosis. Although this technique is less invasive than conventional stripping, potential complications include saphenous nerve injury and deep vein thrombosis in up to 16% of subjects [105].

Endovascular Therapy. Endovascular therapy has gained importance in restoring the outflow of the venous system and providing relief of obstruction. Prior to the introduction of endovascular therapy, iliac vein stenosis and obstruction were treated with surgical procedures such as venous bypass und reconstruction with prosthetic materials. Nowadays, these procedures are performed only infrequently, thanks to venous stenting. In 33% of cases, complete resolution of edema and in 55% of patients with venous ulcerations, complete healing of the ulcerations were shown in a large single-center series in 2002 [106], but close follow-up is mandatory because approximately 23% of patients suffer from in-stent restenosis [107].

Surgical Therapy. Surgical options should be considered if CVI is refractory to medical and invasive therapy. It includes excision of insufficient areas of the epifascial venous system and their links to the deep venous system (crossectomy, resections, and ligation of perforating veins).

Additionally, local surgical therapy in ulcus cruris and rare therapeutic options such as valve reconstructions and transpositioning operations should be considered.

Ligation, Stripping, Phlebectomy / Miniphlebectomy. For many patients suffering from CVI, phlebectomy of the saphenous vein with high ligation of the saphenofemoral junction is regarded as the treatment of choice [108]. Additional venous pathologies, such as large venous varicose clusters, can be removed at the same time. Stripping and ligation of the great saphenous vein can be applied in classes 2–6 of CVI, according to the CEAP classification, and have been shown to significantly improve venous hemodynamics, reflux, symptoms, and ulcer healing [109, 110]. The effect on ulcer healing in combination with compression therapy was proven in a study in 2004 that examined 500 patients [111]. Miniphlebectomy is the treatment of choice for obese patients. As with conventional stripping, affected veins are removed, but the removal is strictly limited. Thanks to the limitation of the operative procedure, it can be performed under local anesthesia with lower perioperative morbidity, and the small incisions cause a much lower rate of wound infections and impaired wound healing.

Subfascial Endoscopic Perforator Surgery. The ligation of perforator veins in patients with an incompetent perforating system has been a surgical principle for many years. Benefits were shown especially in patients with advanced CVI. Difficulties were encountered in traditional surgical procedures due to the tissue damage in the affected areas, but subfascial endoscopic surgery offers the advantage of an operative access distant to the pathological site, thus avoiding areas of lipodermatosclerosis or ulcers. This surgical method can be combined with superficial vein ablation, leading to a 91% ulcer healing rate after 2.9 months [112] and can be applied in severe cases of CVI.

Valve Reconstruction. Incompetence of the venous valves due to injury or primary dysfunction contributes to the development and progression of CVI. Reconstruction of the deep vein valves can be considered for selected patients with advanced CVI and recurrent ulceration with disabling symptoms. The techniques of both open and closed valvuloplasty have been described as showing 59% competency and 63% ulcer-free status at 30 months [113, 114]. Due to the necessity of postoperative anticoagulation, bleeding is regarded as a frequent complication after these procedures, and DVT, pulmonary embolism, wound infections, and ulcer recurrence are also reported, but these operative procedures are not regarded as standard therapeutic means. Additional operations such as transposition of the profunda femoris vein or saphenous vein valve; and axillary vein valve transplantation to the popliteal or femoral vein are performed in selected cases, but these procedures have often resulted in early thrombosis, poor patency and competency, and high patient morbidity. Therefore, valvular reconstruction methods are still not regarded as primary interventions.

There are limited therapeutic options for the obese patient. Usually, compression and miniphlebectomy are regarded as the therapies of choice. As mentioned above, compression therapy faces limitations and problems in daily routine, exercise and weight loss are hard to achieve, and invasive methods are accompanied by elevated perioperative morbidity and mortality. Despite all obstacles, a multimodal therapy should be planned and followed to grant the most benefit for the patient.

32.7 Prophylaxis and Aftercare

Because most of the risk factors for CVI cannot be treated or removed in a patient, recurrence of the condition is possible at all times, even if the former therapy was completely sufficient. To detect a recurrence of the illness as early as possible, examination of the venous status is recommended on a regular basis. If a dysfunction of the venous hemodynamics cannot be treated fully at one point, continuous conservative therapy is reasonable. It is also recommended that the patient's CEAP class be determined on a regular basis to notice changes due to therapeutic interventions or even aggravation of the disease in case of therapy failure.

32.8 Conclusion

Morbid obesity and CVI are both chronic conditions and closely linked to each other. Sooner or later, an obese patient will suffer from permanent damage to the veins of the lower extremities. Impaired wound healing due to hypo-oxygenation and structural changes in the skin aggravate the risk for CVI-associated complications such as infections and chronic wounds.

Sufficient therapy of the CVI alone is not possible; a multimodal therapy has to be planned and implemented. The main parts of this concept must be sufficient compression therapy, weight reduction, exercise or elevation of mobility, nutritional consulting, and psychological assistance. Constant clinical evaluation and examination are also necessary. Additionally, constant teaching of the patient and achievement of a high level of compliance should be part of the routine.

References

1. Weingarten MS (2001) State-of-the-art treatment of chronic venous disease. Clin Infect Dis 32:949–954
2. Capeheart JK (1996) Chronic venous insufficiency: a focus on prevention of venous ulceration. J Wound Ostomy Continence Nurs 23:227–234
3. Skene AI, Smith JM, Dore CJ, et al (1992) Venous leg ulcers: a prognostic index to predict time to healing. BMJ 305:1119–1121
4. Callam MJ, Harper DR, Dale JJ, Ruckley CV (1987) Chronic ulcer of the leg: clinical history. Br Med J (Clin Res Ed) 294:1389–1391

5. Hansson C, Andersson E, Swanbeck G (1987) A follow-up study of leg and foot ulcer patients. Acta Derm Venereol 67:496–500
6. Mayberry JC, Moneta GL, DeFrang RD, Porter JM (1991) The influence of elastic compression stockings on deep venous hemodynamics. J Vasc Surg 13:91–99; discussion 99–100
7. Bergan JJ, Schmid-Schonbein GW, Smith PD, et al (2006) Chronic venous disease. N Engl J Med 355:488–498
8. Brand FN, Dannenberg AL, Abbott RD, Kannel WB (1988) The epidemiology of varicose veins: the Framingham Study. Am J Prev Med 4:96–101
9. Kistner RL (1996) Definitive diagnosis and definitive treatment in chronic venous disease: a concept whose time has come. J Vasc Surg 24:703–710
10. Nicolaides AN (2000) Investigation of chronic venous insufficiency: a consensus statement (France, March 5–9, 1997). Circulation 102:E126–163
11. Wienert V (1999) Epidemiology of leg ulcers. Curr Probl Dermatol 27:65–69
12. Boccalon H, Janbon C, Saumet JL, et al (1997) Characteristics of chronic venous insufficiency in 895 patients followed in general practice. Int Angiol 16:226–234
13. Nelzen O, Bergqvist D, Lindhagen A, Hallbook T (1991) Chronic leg ulcers: an underestimated problem in primary health care among elderly patients. J Epidemiol Community Health 45:184–187
14. Moffatt C (1998) Issues in the assessment of leg ulceration. J Wound Care 7:469–473
15. Scott TE, LaMorte WW, Gorin DR, Menzoian JO (1995) Risk factors for chronic venous insufficiency: a dual case-control study. J Vasc Surg 22:622–628
16. Cornwall JV, Dore CJ, Lewis JD (1986) Leg ulcers: epidemiology and aetiology. Br J Surg 73:693–696
17. Nelzen O, Bergqvist D, Lindhagen A (1991) Leg ulcer etiology – a cross-sectional population study. J Vasc Surg 14:557–564
18. Elbeze Y HdFY, Chalabi A, et al (1995) Echo-Doppler veineux au repos et a léffort chez le sportif de bon niveau. Phlébologie 48:445–450
19. Berard A, Abenhaim L, Platt R, et al (2002) Risk factors for the first-time development of venous ulcers of the lower limbs: the influence of heredity and physical activity. Angiology 53:647–657
20. Marston WA, Carlin RE, Passman MA, et al (1999) Healing rates and cost efficacy of outpatient compression treatment for leg ulcers associated with venous insufficiency. J Vasc Surg 30:491–498
21. Erickson CA, Lanza DJ, Karp DL, et al (1995) Healing of venous ulcers in an ambulatory care program: the roles of chronic venous insufficiency and patient compliance. J Vasc Surg 22:629–636
22. Zsoter T, Cronin RF (1966) Venous distensibility in patients with varicose veins. Can Med Assoc J 94:1293–1297
23. Killewich LA, Bedford GR, Beach KW, Strandness DE jr (1989) Spontaneous lysis of deep venous thrombi: rate and outcome. J Vasc Surg 9:89–97
24. Lindner DJ, Edwards JM, Phinney ES, et al (1986) Long-term hemodynamic and clinical sequelae of lower extremity deep vein thrombosis. J Vasc Surg 4:436–442
25. O'Donnell TF jr., Browse NL, Burnand KG, Thomas ML (1977) The socioeconomic effects of an iliofemoral venous thrombosis. J Surg Res 22:483–488
26. Belcaro G, Laurora G, Cesarone MR, et al (1995) Microcirculation in high perfusion microangiopathy. J Cardiovasc Surg (Torino) 36:393–398
27. Leu AJ, Franzeck UK, Bollinger A (1991) Microangiopathies in chronic venous insufficiency (CVI) [in German]. Ther Umsch 48:715–721
28. Leu AJ, Leu HJ, Franzeck UK, Bollinger A (1995) Microvascular changes in chronic venous insufficiency – a review. Cardiovasc Surg 3:237–245
29. Shami SK, Cheatle TR, Chittenden SJ, et al (1993) Hyperaemic response in the skin microcirculation of patients with chronic venous insufficiency. Br J Surg 80:433-5
30. Bollinger A, Leu AJ (1991) Evidence for microvascular thrombosis obtained by intravital fluorescence videomicroscopy. Vasa 20:252–255
31. Browse NL, Burnand KG (1982) The cause of venous ulceration. Lancet 2:243–245
32. Rudolph DM (1998) Pathophysiology and management of venous ulcers. J Wound Ostomy Continence Nurs 25:248–255
33. Falanga V, Eaglstein WH (1993) The "trap" hypothesis of venous ulceration. Lancet 341:1006–1008
34. Bollinger A, Isenring G, Franzeck UK (1982) Lymphatic microangiopathy: a complication of severe chronic venous incompetence (CVI). Lymphology 15:60–65
35. Takase S, Bergan JJ, Schmid-Schonbein G (2000) Expression of adhesion molecules and cytokines on saphenous veins in chronic venous insufficiency. Ann Vasc Surg 14:427–435
36. Dormandy JA (1997) Pathophysiology of venous leg ulceration – an update. Angiology 48:71–75
37. Veraart JC, Verhaegh ME, Neumann HA, et al (1993) Adhesion molecule expression in venous leg ulcers. Vasa 22:213–218
38. Boisseau MR, Seigneur M, et al (1995) Relationship between age, fibrinogen and clinical status in 313 patients with CVI. Biorheology 32:279
39. Leach RD (1984) Venous ulceration, fibrinogen and fibrinolysis. Ann R Coll Surg Engl 66:258–263
40. Ernst E MA, Marshall M (1989) Limited blood fluidity as a contributory factor of venous stasis in chronic venous insufficiency. Phlebology 4:107–111
41. Sugerman H, Windsor A, Bessos M, Wolfe L (1997) Intra-abdominal pressure, sagittal abdominal diameter and obesity comorbidity. J Intern Med 241:71-9
42. Danielsson G, Eklof B, Grandinetti A, Kistner RL (2002) The influence of obesity on chronic venous disease. Vasc Endovascular Surg 36:271–276
43. Padberg F jr, Cerveira JJ, Lal BK, et al (2003) Does severe venous insufficiency have a different etiology in the morbidly obese? Is it venous? J Vasc Surg 37:79–85
44. Topaloglu S, Avsar FM, Ozel H, et al (2005) Comparison of bariatric and non-bariatric elective operations in morbidly obese patients on the basis of wound infection. Obes Surg 15:1271–1276
45. Widmer LK (1978) Peripheral venous disorder: prevalence and socio-medical importance: observation in 4529 apparently healthy persons: Basle III Study. Hans Huber, Bern, pp 1–90
46. Nicolaides AN EB, Bergan JJ, et al (1995) Classification and grading of chronic venous disease in the lower limb: a consensus statement. Phlebology 10:42–45
47. Porter JM, Moneta GL (1995) Reporting standards in venous disease: an update. International Consensus Committee on Chronic Venous Disease. J Vasc Surg 21:635–645
48. Nicolaides AN, Kakkar VV, Field ES, Renney JT (1971) The origin of deep vein thrombosis: a venographic study. Br J Radiol 44:653–663

49. Hach W (1985) Varicose veins of the deep perforating veins – a typical phlebologic disease picture [in German]. Vasa 14:155–157

50. Raju S, Fredericks R (1991) Venous obstruction: an analysis of one hundred thirty-seven cases with hemodynamic, venographic, and clinical correlations. J Vasc Surg 14:305–313

51. Kistner RL, Kamida CB (1995) 1994 update on phlebography and varicography. Dermatol Surg 21:71–76

52. Perrin M, Bolot JE, Genevois A, Hiltband B (1988) Dynamic popliteal phlebography [in German]. Phlebologie 41:429–440

53. Cid Dos Santos J (1948) The diagnosis and treatment of vascular obstruction. Gaz Med Port 1:631–643

54. Luke JC (1951) The deep vein valves: a venographic study in normal and postphlebitic states. Surgery 29:381–386

55. Gullmo A (1956) On the technique of phlebography of the lower limb. Acta Radiol -46:603–620

56. Herman RJ, Neiman HL, Yao JS, et al (1980) Descending venography: a method of evaluating lower extremity venous valvular function. Radiology 137(1 Pt 1):63–69

57. Ackroyd JS, Lea Thomas M, Browse NL (1986) Deep vein reflux: an assessment by descending phlebography. Br J Surg 73:31–33

58. Kistner RL, Ferris EB, Randhawa G, Kamida C (1986) A method of performing descending venography. J Vasc Surg 4:464–468

59. Stonebridge PA, Chalmers N, Beggs I, et al (1995) Recurrent varicose veins: a varicographic analysis leading to a new practical classification. Br J Surg 82:60–62

60. Hobbs JT (1980) Peroperative venography to ensure accurate sapheno-popliteal vein ligation. Br Med J 280:1578–1579

61. Thomas ML, Bowles JN (1985) Incompetent perforating veins: comparison of varicography and ascending phlebography. Radiology 154:619–623

62. Szendro G, Nicolaides AN, Zukowski AJ, et al (1986) Duplex scanning in the assessment of deep venous incompetence. J Vasc Surg 4:237–242

63. Rollins DL, Semrow CM, Friedell ML, Buchbinder D (1987) Use of ultrasonic venography in the evaluation of venous valve function. Am J Surg 154:189–191

64. Franco G (1993) Doppler pulsed and color echography of the inferior vena cava [in German]. Phlebologie 46:389–392; discussion 402–403

65. Messina LM, Sarpa MS, Smith MA, Greenfield LJ (1993) Clinical significance of routine imaging of iliac and calf veins by color flow duplex scanning in patients suspected of having acute lower extremity deep venous thrombosis. Surgery 114:921–927

66. Dupas B, el Kouri D, Curtet C, et al (1995) Angiomagnetic resonance imaging of iliofemorocaval venous thrombosis. Lancet 346:17–19

67. Meissner MH, Caps MT, Bergelin RO, et al (1995) Propagation, rethrombosis and new thrombus formation after acute deep venous thrombosis. J Vasc Surg 22:558–567

68. Markel A, Manzo RA, Bergelin RO, Strandness DE jr (1992) Valvular reflux after deep vein thrombosis: incidence and time of occurrence. J Vasc Surg 15:377–382; discussion 383–384

69. O'Shaughnessy AM, Fitzgerald DE (1997) Natural history of proximal deep vein thrombosis assessed by duplex ultrasound. Int Angiol 16:45–49

70. Labropoulos N, Giannoukas AD, Nicolaides AN, et al (1996) The role of venous reflux and calf muscle pump function in non-thrombotic chronic venous insufficiency. Correlation with severity of signs and symptoms. Arch Surg 131:403–406

71. Elem B, Shorey BA, Williams KL (1971) Comparison between thermography and fluorescein test in the detection of incompetent perforating veins. Br Med J 4:651–652

72. Kalodiki ECL, Geroulakos G, et al (1995) Liquid crystal thermography and duplex in the preoperative marking of varicose veins. Phlebology 10:110–114

73. Christopoulos D, Nicolaides AN, Szendro G (1988) Venous reflux: quantification and correlation with the clinical severity of chronic venous disease. Br J Surg 75:352–356

74. Harada RN, Katz ML, Comerota A (1995) A noninvasive screening test to detect "critical" deep venous reflux. J Vasc Surg 22:532–537

75. Criado E, Farber MA, Marston WA, et al (1998) The role of air plethysmography in the diagnosis of chronic venous insufficiency. J Vasc Surg 27:660–670

76. Nicolaides AN, Miles C (1987) Photoplethysmography in the assessment of venous insufficiency. J Vasc Surg 5:405–412

77. Abramowitz HB, Queral LA, Finn WR, et al (1979) The use of photoplethysmography in the assessment of venous insufficiency: a comparison to venous pressure measurements. Surgery 86:434–441

78. Eberhardt RT, Raffetto JD (2005) Chronic venous insufficiency. Circulation 111:2398–2409

79. Nicolaides AN, Hussein MK, Szendro G, et al (1993) The relation of venous ulceration with ambulatory venous pressure measurements. J Vasc Surg 17:414–419

80. Neglen P, Raju S (2000) Ambulatory venous pressure revisited. J Vasc Surg 31:1206–1213

81. Fronek A, Kim R, Curran B (2000) Non-invasively determined ambulatory venous pressure. Vasc Med 5:213–216

82. Harris B, Eaglstein WH, Falanga V (1993) Basal cell carcinoma arising in venous ulcers and mimicking granulation tissue. J Dermatol Surg Oncol 19:150–152

83. Gosain A, Sanger JR, Yousif NJ, Matloub HS (1991) Basal cell carcinoma of the lower leg occurring in association with chronic venous stasis. Ann Plast Surg 26:279–283

84. Fagrell B (1982) Microcirculatory disturbances – the final cause for venous leg ulcers? Vasa 11:101–103

85. Speiser DE, Bollinger A (1991) Microangiopathy in mild chronic venous incompetence (CVI): morphological alterations and increased transcapillary diffusion detected by fluorescence videomicroscopy. Int J Microcirc Clin Exp 10:55–66

86. Belcaro G, Gaspari AL, Legnini M, et al (1988) Evaluation of the effects of elastic compression in patients with chronic venous hypertension by laser-Doppler flowmetry. Acta Chir Belg 88:163–167

87. Belcaro G, Grigg M, Rulo A, Nicolaides A (1989) Blood flow in the perimalleolar skin in relation to posture in patients with venous hypertension. Ann Vasc Surg 3:5–7

88. Franzeck UK, Bollinger A, Huch R, Huch A (1984) Transcutaneous oxygen tension and capillary morphologic characteristics and density in patients with chronic venous incompetence. Circulation 70:806–811

89. Neumann HA, van Leeuwen M, van den Broek MJ, Berretty PJ (1984) Transcutaneous oxygen tension in chronic venous insufficiency syndrome. Vasa 13:213–219

90. Thomas PR, Nash GB, Dormandy JA (1988) White cell accumulation in dependent legs of patients with venous hypertension: a possible mechanism for trophic changes in the skin. Br Med J (Clin Res Ed) 296:1693–1695

91. Motykie GD, Caprini JA, Arcelus JI, et al (1999) Evaluation of therapeutic compression stockings in the treatment of chronic venous insufficiency. Dermatol Surg 25:116–120

92. Mayberry JC, Moneta GL, Taylor LM jr, Porter JM (1991) Fifteen-year results of ambulatory compression therapy for chronic venous ulcers. Surgery 109:575–581

93. Choucair M, Phillips TJ (1998) Compression therapy. Dermatol Surg 24:141–148
94. Tarnay TJ, Rohr PR, Davidson AG, et al (1980) Pneumatic calf compression, fibrinolysis, and the prevention of deep venous thrombosis. Surgery 88:489–496
95. Smith PC, Sarin S, Hasty J, Scurr JH (1990) Sequential gradient pneumatic compression enhances venous ulcer healing: a randomized trial. Surgery 108:871–875
96. Schauer PR, Burguera B, Ikramuddin S, et al (2003) Effect of laparoscopic Roux-en Y gastric bypass on type 2 diabetes mellitus. Ann Surg 238:467–484; discussion 484–485
97. Scott SK, Rabito FA, Price PD, et al (2006) Comorbidity among the morbidly obese: a comparative study of 2002 U.S. hospital patient discharges. Surg Obes Relat Dis 2:105–111
98. Pontiroli AE, Folli F, Paganelli M, et al (2005) Laparoscopic gastric banding prevents type 2 diabetes and arterial hypertension and induces their remission in morbid obesity: a 4-year case-controlled study. Diabetes Care 28:2703–2709
99. Niezgoda JA, Mendez-Eastman S (2006) The effective management of pressure ulcers. Adv Skin Wound Care 19 [Suppl 1]:3–15
100. Falanga V, Fujitani RM, Diaz C, et al (1999) Systemic treatment of venous leg ulcers with high doses of pentoxifylline: efficacy in a randomized, placebo-controlled trial. Wound Repair Regen 7:208–213
101. Ibegbuna V, Nicolaides AN, Sowade O, et al (1997) Venous elasticity after treatment with Daflon 500 mg. Angiology 48:45–49
102. Padberg FT jr, Johnston MV, Sisto SA (2004) Structured exercise improves calf muscle pump function in chronic venous insufficiency: a randomized trial. J Vasc Surg 39:79–87
103. Melissas J, Christodoulakis M, Spyridakis M, et al (1998) Disorders associated with clinically severe obesity: significant improvement after surgical weight reduction. South Med J 91:1143–1148
104. Scultetus AH, Villavicencio JL, Kao TC, et al (2003) Microthrombectomy reduces postsclerotherapy pigmentation: multicenter randomized trial. J Vasc Surg 38:896–903
105. Hingorani AP, Ascher E, Markevich N, et al (2004) Deep venous thrombosis after radiofrequency ablation of greater saphenous vein: a word of caution. J Vasc Surg 40:500–504
106. Neglen P, Raju S (2002) Intravascular ultrasound scan evaluation of the obstructed vein. J Vasc Surg 35:694–700
107. Neglen P, Raju S (2004) In-stent recurrent stenosis in stents placed in the lower extremity venous outflow tract. J Vasc Surg 39:181–187
108. Sarin S, Scurr JH, Coleridge Smith PD (1994) Stripping of the long saphenous vein in the treatment of primary varicose veins. Br J Surg 81:1455–1458
109. Padberg FT, Jr., Pappas PJ, Araki CT, et al (1996) Hemodynamic and clinical improvement after superficial vein ablation in primary combined venous insufficiency with ulceration. J Vasc Surg 24:711–718
110. MacKenzie RK, Allan PL, Ruckley CV, Bradbury AW (2004) The effect of long saphenous vein stripping on deep venous reflux. Eur J Vasc Endovasc Surg 28:104–107
111. Barwell JR, Davies CE, Deacon J, et al (2004) Comparison of surgery and compression with compression alone in chronic venous ulceration (ESCHAR study): randomised controlled trial. Lancet 363:1854–1859
112. Bianchi C, Ballard JL, Abou-Zamzam AM, Teruya TH (2003) Subfascial endoscopic perforator vein surgery combined with saphenous vein ablation: results and critical analysis. J Vasc Surg 38:67–71
113. Kistner RL (1975) Surgical repair of the incompetent femoral vein valve. Arch Surg 110:1336–1342
114. Raju S, Berry MA, Neglen P (2000) Transcommissural valvuloplasty: technique and results. J Vasc Surg 32:969–976

Perspectives of Metabolic Surgery

Goran Marjanovic, MD, W. Konrad Karcz, MD

The number of bariatric operations performed each year is growing continuously and it is to be assumed that this trend will continue during the coming years. Furthermore, we will probably experience a surge of metabolic operations in the near future [1-4].

33.1 Present conservative therapeutic strategies

Overweight and obese individuals have four choices: accept their weight as it is with additional relevant co-morbidity, change their diet and physical activity behaviours, use a weight loss medication, or have weight loss surgery with a possible influence on metabolism. Those options extend from low risk/less effectiveness to higher risk/ better effectiveness. Experimental and clinical data now support the use of a range of dietary strategies including low-carbohydrate, low-fat and high protein diets which can show a marginal weight loss. The main problem seems to be a relatively low long-term acceptance leading to high drop-out rates up to 45% even in well-published studies [6-8]. Increases in physical activity can produce measurable benefits and support weight loss strategies and fitness of obese patients [9]. But studies fail to show a positive effect of exercise on obesity-related comorbidities and hard end points such as cardiovascular complications. Furthermore, the recommendation for enhancement of physical activity should be made thoroughly in every individual patient, since inadequate activity involves serious problems especially in patients with high cardiovascular comorbidity and obesity-related joint disorders. In the last decade, medical therapy of obesity and metabolic disorders has aroused much public interest, especially with the introduction of a class of drugs blocking the cannabinod 1 receptor. Rimonabant (Sanofi Aventis) was the first one of this class to be approved. In a meta-analysis of more than 4000 patients, *Christensen et al.* could show a significant effect of about 5% weight loss, but this was accompanied by serious, especially neuropsychiatric, side effects [10]. In the last few years new enthusiasm was raised by novel pharmaceutical targets like neuropeptide YY 1-36 and NPY5 receptor anatagonist [11-14] or the discovery of the satiety molecule Nesfatin-1, but this evaporated rapidly with the absence of clinical success. Low effectiveness, high risk and relatively high costs are the main reasons for the failure of medical therapy of obesity both in clinical practice and in the world- wide health insurance system.

33.2 Change in faith: from conservative to bariatric surgery

Most patients are not able to lose weight by changing behaviour by conservative medical therapy. Currently, surgical therapy offers the greatest likelihood of the highest degree of weight loss and thus has evolved rapidly as the most effective option for treatment of obesity worldwide. Established procedures are classified as restrictive [15-20] and combined [21-26], implementing a more or less pronounced malabsorption, and malabsorptive. The metabolic components, which are as a matter of fact introduced at the same time with the operation, change the organs' physiology and the homeostasis of the intestinal tract (local hormonal homeostasis, different vagal stimulation, food digestion and absorption modification). Initially, however, questions have persisted about whether bariatric surgery has long-term beneficial effects on mortality. This special issue was impressively addressed in the prospective controlled SOS study (Swedish Obesity Study) 2007. More than 4000 individuals were randomized either to weight loss surgery or medical therapy. Different operative techniques were applied (gastric banding, vertical gastroplasty, gastric bypass) and many patients in the surgical arm underwent an older gastric restriction procedure that is not used any more because it had lower levels of efficacy and greater risk than currently- used approaches. Despite the limited surgical procedures, this study, for the first time, could prove a significant 30% reduction of mortality of the surgically- treated patients compared to the conservative group [27]. In a similarly-impressive study by Adams et al. [28], the same issue was examined in a retrospective cohort design, in which mortality rates of almost 10`000 individuals with gastric bypass were compared to a control group identified through driver`s license records. In a follow-up of more than 7 years, a 40% reduction of overall mortality was shown. The incidence of diabetes mellitus was reduced by 92% and tumor-associated mortality by 60%, thus being comparable to the results of the SOS study. Current population data from the Swedish Health Care Registry regarding frequency and sort of bariatric procedures and especially perioperative mortality are presented in the study by *Sundbom* and *Karlson* [29]. They found a 27% increase of bariatric procedures in 10 years. Initially, restrictive procedures like gastric banding were preferred with about 80%; these are now being performed only in 20% of the cases. In contrast, gastric bypass now clearly dominates with about 79% of all bariatric procedures. However, the main result of this analysis is the relatively low perioperative mortality of only 0.16% of over 8,000 performed procedures. Despite the growing complexity of the procedures performed now, bariatric surgery seems to have a relatively high reliability.

33.3 Change in thinking: Development of metabolic surgery

"Who would have thought it? An operation proves to be the most effective therapy for adult-onset diabetes mellitus" – this was the title of the study by *Pories et al.* in 1995 which was published in *Annals of Surgery* [30]. This was a report of a series of 608 patients with morbid obesity, in whom a gastric bypass was performed. Of these patients, 54% had a manifest diabetes mellitus type II or impaired glucose tolerance. Nearly all patients had a long-term follow-up of more than 14 years. The main information of this study was not that diabetes mellitus resolved in 91% of the patients, but that one single surgical procedure could keep it under control for a time of 14 years - which so far seemed to be progressive and incurable. Another important finding was that serum glucose improved just a few days after surgery – i.e. at a time where a significant weight loss could not have been reached. The independence of metabolic implications of a gastric bypass procedure on the serum glucose was confirmed by a constant course of serum glucose over time, even if most of the patients remained at mean 50% over their ideal weight despite an initially significant weight loss. Different assumptions were made to explain the metabolic effects of gastric bypass, including a reduced calory supply / intake and especially an endocrine effect of the gastrointestinal tract in form of so-called incretines, which are excreted after contact of food to bowel wall mucosa and may have an effect on insulin secretion and action. Further studies followed and could prove, not only for the gastric bypass but also for biliopancreatic diversion, which the metabolic effect initiates rapidly and strongly affects the diabetic status, independent of weight loss [24, 31]. However, the effect of reduced calory supply / intake does not seem to play a crucial role, since serum glucose remains stable in patients after biliopancreatic diversion, even if they reach a normal or raised eating volume with time [24]. However, the assumption of the endocrine activity of the gastrointestinal tract was confirmed by the hypothesis about incretins and anti-incretins by *Franceso Rubino's* research group [32]. They proposed that gastric bypass and biliopancreatic diversion differ significantly considering the operative procedure, but that in both procedures, a by-passing of the duodenum and the proximal jejunum is performed. In this area, cells are presumed to exist excreting the so-called incretins (GIP, GLP-1, IGF) and on the other hand cells excreting unknown anti-incretin factors

in equilibrium. They speculated that type II diabetes is a consequence of an imbalance between incretin and anti-incretin secretion, assuming that anti-incretins lead to reduced insulin secretion and insulin action. When by-passing the duodenum and the proximal jejunum, the secretion of especially anti-incretins is reduced, whereas the direct contact of undigested food with the mucosa of the distal jejunum and ileum promote the secretion of incretins and thus the insulin concentration and action. A few years later, the same group published animal experimental data supporting their hypothesis. They have shown that exclusion of the duodenum and of the first 10 cm of the jejunum in rats significantly and rapidly ameliorates glucose tolerance. The reversion of duodenal exclusion again led to aggravation of glucose homeostasis. This effect was independent of food intake, body weight, malabsorption or direct contact of food with the distal small bowel [33]. Even if detailed molecular mechanisms have to be examined in future, Rubino's work provides further important and very interesting aspects for the understanding of the pathophysiology of type II diabetes and puts the gastrointestinal tract and it endocrine function in the foreground.

33.4 Refinement of metabolic surgery techniques and new directions

This new insight into the endocrine activity of the "enteroinsular axis" [34] and the incretin factors like GIP, GLP-1 and Ghrelin [35] account for better comprehension of different effects of different bariatric procedures on weight loss and especially on the diabetic metabolic status.

33.5 Improving restriction

The knowledge of endocrine factors such as Ghrelin was one important factor allowing gastric sleeve resection to develop to an accepted independent bariatric procedure with good mid-to-long-term effects [17, 36]. The explanation for the success of this method seems to be not only pure restriction but also an effect on satiety, since ghrelin may stimulate the appetite and main parts of ghrelin production in the fundus are resected at sleeve resection. In laparoscopic sleeve gastrectomy (LSG), the stomach is reduced to a narrow tube which can dramatically reduce the stomach volume and influence the gastric peristaltic wave. Significantly better results have been reached in extended weight loss (EWL) using a 32 F gastric tube for the resection, than in patients without or with less restrictive calibration [37]. The main problem in restrictive procedures in the further course seems to be the dilatation of the gastric remnant, such as the gastric tube in LSG or the gastric pouch and its gastro-enteroanastomosis in laparoscopic gastric bypass (LRYGB) which may be a potential source of therapy failure. An attempt to prevent dilatation of the gastric pouch in LRYGB procedure by placing a silastic ring at the outlet of the created pouch has brought promising results [38]. The banded gastric bypass operation for morbid obesity is a serendipitous evolution from both the Mason gastric bypass and the vertical banded gastroplasty (VGB) operations [39, 40]. Failed VGB operations were converted to a gastric bypass and constructed distal to the band, because it was unsafe to remove the Marlex mesh band. Thus, leaving the band above the gastrojejunostomy was found to provide better weight loss compared to patients with VGB operations [41-43]. This GaBP Ring System™ (Benetec Medical Inc, USA) is a pre-manufactured set with a prosthetic autolocking band (GaBP ring) and a radiopaque marker. It is made of silicone rubber. The ends of the band have a plastic one-way locking mechanism. As it is premanufactured, the band provides for better standardisation and quality control than surgeon-fashioned bands or rings. When considering LSG, the study by *Langer et al.* [44] was the first study on the incidence of gastric tube dilatation following LSG. Dilatation was diagnosed by upper GI contrast studies in the patients with a follow-up of over 12 months. Consequently, adding a silastic band to sleeve gastrectomy might increase the success rate by preventing gastric tube dilatation (W.K. Karcz et al. Banded Sleeve Gastrectomy. Congress of Advanced Laparoscopy, Athene, June 2008). To date, studies and reports of series are lacking and would be of great interest. However, it must be mentioned that, compared to conventional LSG, additional potential complications may occur using LBSG, such as silicone band migration, dislocation or infection and dysphagia-related symptoms. All of those disadvantages have been observed in VGB and Fobi banded gastric bypass, but at low rates [45,46]. Another technique to prevent dilatation of the gastric tube after sleeve gastrectomy was recently examined in a pig model. A sleeve gastrectomy with wrapping using polytetrafluoroethylene dual mesh was designed and tested for 8 weeks. It was shown to be feasible and weight gain was reduced in the porcine model [47]. This technique may prevente, not only dilatation of the gastric tube but also the peristaltic wave of the gastric remnant. Once again, further studies are required to improve the satiety effect through more extensive restriction. An important issue for future studies will be the postoperative changes

in the gastric peristaltic wave, exploring the gastric tube emptying time and thus giving further important information about the effect of gastric metabolic surgery. Developments have also been made in the refinement of laparoscopic gastric banding. *Weiner et al.* [48] presented data on a new type of band which was adjusted telemetrically without the need for an access port. This electromechanical gastric banding device uses an external control unit to supply both power and control information to adjust the band. This Easyband Telemetrically Adjustable Gastric Band (Endoart, Switzerland) does not contain batteries or hydraulic components like in common adjustable bands, but it consists of an annular band connected through a flexible cable to a small, flat internal antenna. For band adjustment, the external antenna is placed over the patient's skin where the internal antenna is located. Furthermore, a patient-specific microchip memory card is used to store the band's diameter after the last adjustments. Early results indicate clinical safety and efficacy compared to other commercially-available gastric bands. In superobese patients, placement of an intragastric balloon is often needed as first-stage therapy in preparation for bariatric surgery. There is no general recommendation for the filling volume of the balloons, so a fixed regime (i.e. about 700ml) is used in most patients [49]. In this regard, new techniques are being developed to have the possibility to change the filling volume of the balloon individually during therapy and thus improve restriction when necessary. This could give further important information with special regard to potential success in weight loss restrictive surgery. Studies on these techniques are lacking thus failing to establish a more invasive conservative therapy, since astrostomy with potential complications seems to be necessary to achieve the goal.

33.6 Improving the function of the lower oesophageal sphincter

When discussing new techniques to improve restriction of the gastric remnant in sleeve gastrectomy or gastric bypass, one should consider the function of the lower esophageal sphincter. If a higher restriction is reached, a significantly higher reflux into the esophagus might occur as a consequence, with potential esophageal dilatation in the further course. A reduced satiety effect might be the result with concomitant therapy failure and inadequate weight loss. Here it could be helpful to use the magnetic band for the supporting UOS. Studies are running currently on to support the GERD patients. When the method will be successful it will find its place also in the metabolic surgery. Furthermore, the development of a Barret esophagus might be evoked. Hence, the choice for the restrictive procedures should be based on the preoperative measurement of lower esophageal sphincter function, especially before following operations: Gastric Banding, (Conventional or Banded) Sleeve Gastrectomy and Banded Gastric Bypass [50]. In the future better solution would be an "intelligent" band which can change its diameter according to the volume and consistency of the food passage. Similar, especially microelectronically-based, developments are being made in the treatment of end-stage fecal incontinence with microsystems technology providing the German Artificial Sphincter System GASS with a remote-controlled artificial bowel sphincter [51]. These new directions inaugurate a wide field of interdisciplinary research for which paths still have to be explored.

33.7 Improving satiety through neural stimulation

Different possibilities to exert influence on the feeling of satiety on a neuro-muscular basis (gastric /duodenal stimulation, vagal nerve stimulation, deep brain stimulation) exist and have been examined during the last decade. They display greater understanding of eating behavior in mammals and raise new options for patients with obesity. They have in common an electrical stimulation of nerve structures with a consequent effect on satiety and movement of the gastrointestinal tract. Gastric and duodenal stimulation was in special focus, since the stomach and the duodenum seem to play a central role in eating behaviour. In animal studies, acute electrical stimulation of the stomach or the duodenum was shown to decrease appetite-stimulating gut hormones and to increase appetite-inhibiting gut hormones in gastric and duodenal tissues. Gastric and duodenal stimulation may decrease ghrelin levels in the gastric fundus [52]. Alterations in the synthesis and secretion of these satiety-related peptides may contribute to the understanding of alterations in eating behaviour in clinical studies. It PET imaging analyses in a series of obese patients, it could be proven that gastric stimulation induced activation of cerebral regions previously shown to be involved in drug craving in addicted subjects (orbitofrontal cortex, cerebellum, striatum and especially the hippocampus). This suggests that similar brain circuits underlie the enhanced motivational drive for food and drugs seen in obese and drug-addicted patients [53]. A further study confirmed these results concerning the central involvement of the hippocampus and additionally proposed neuronal nitric oxide synthesis in the central mediation

of gastric stimulation therapy for obesity [53-55]. Several studies or case series were presented in recent years with relatively low numbers of patients (8-101 patients) with a BMI of 30 – 47 kg/m². Gastric stimulation appeared to be associated with weight loss, decrease in blood pressure in hypertensive patients and with a reduction or elimination of symptoms in those who had a gastroesophageal reflux disease, but the results were inconsistent [56-66]. Even though implantable gastric stimulation has been proposed as a first-line treatment for severely obese patients, a recent prospective, randomized, placebo-controlled, double-blind, multicenter study of 190 patients failed to show the aforementioned beneficial effects. The control group lost 11.7% of EWL and the treatment group 11.8% of EWL according to an intent-to-treat analysis [67]. The results of this study are contradictory to studies mentioned above and do not support the application of implantable gastric stimulation. Additional research is indicated to understand the physiology and potential benefits of this therapy. As well as for gastric stimulation, animal data exist which provide evidence of an effect of vagal nerve stimulation on satiety, food intake and body weight [68]. The metabolism rate does not seem to be affected [69]. Clinical data are rare since only a serendipitous observation was made in 14 patients who were treated with vagal nerve stimulation for severe treatment-resistant depression. This treatment was accompanied by significant gradual weight loss despite the patients' report of not dieting or exercising. The weight loss was proportional to the initial BMI, that is, the more severe the obesity, the greater the weight loss. The authors discussed a modulation of eating behaviour through the activity of the vagal nerve and proposed further controlled studies in the treatment of obesity [70]. Deep brain stimulation is an accepted procedure in the treatment of Parkinson disease and has an established safety profile. To date, only a few animal studies give us important information about the effect of deep brain stimulation on weight loss in obese subjects. It has been shown that continuous bilateral stimulatory inhibition of the rat lateral hypothalamic nucleus was feasible and led to significant decrease in food intake and subsequent sustained weight loss [71]. Appetite modulation in conjunction with enhancement of the metabolic rate by means of hypothalamic lesions has been widely documented in animal models and even in humans. It appears that these effects can be reproduced by deep brain stimulation and the titratability and reversibility of this procedure, in addition to its well-established safety profile, make hypothalamic deep brain stimulation an appealing option for obesity treatment. Chronic stimulation of the Nucleus accumbens may allow modulation of reward sensation and dietary preferences. Inhibition of food reward may lead to significant weight reduction [72]. Nevertheless, these appealing hypotheses have to be proven in future animal studies and especially in obese human subjects.

33.8 Change in development: Synthesis of new metabolic operative techniques

With increasing understanding of metabolic surgery, new interventional and surgical methods are being developed aimed not only at the treatment of obesity but especially obesity-related diseased like type II diabetes mellitus or hypertriglyceridemia. The role of duodenal bypass as an underlying mechanism of action in gastric bypass surgery has received considerable attention. Similar results as in duodenal bypass surgery are found with a 60-cm fluoropolymer sleeve that is deployed totally endoscopically via a coaxial catheter system into the jejunum and fixed in the proximal duodenum with a Nitinol anchor. The system creates a proximal biliopancreatic diversion of food and digestion enzymes and provides a significant weight loss, and at the same time a new treatment option for patients with type II diabetes. This sleeve was tested in a pig model for 90-120 days and seemed to have a good tissue response [73,74]. The same research group published data of the first human experience with the GI Dynamics Endobarrier™ (Lexington, Massachusetts, USA) system, which was applied in an obese patient in the USA. The patient lost 9 kg weight in three months - at that time point, the sleeve could be explanted without problems [75]. Encouraging results of the "duodeno-jejunal bypass with sleeve" have been obtained in a prospective case series of 12 patients (mean BMI 43 kg/m²) with a 12- week follow-up. The mean weight loss was 23% in 10 patients, in whom the system was left for the whole follow-up period. In all four patients with type II diabetes, the serum glucose was in a normal range throughout this period. Only few, rather small side effects, like nausea, vomiting or abdominal pain occurred during the first two weeks [76]. A recent open label, prospective, randomized controlled trial of an endscopic duodeno-jejunal bypass sleeve versus low calorie diet provides further evidence of a short-term (12 weeks) efficacy regarding weight loss, and long-term results are being pursued [77]. But despite of the encouraging results of this new technique, potential and serious complications like upper GI bleeding or sleeve obstruction or difficulties in explantation after therapy should be kept in mind. An interposition of an ileal segment on a proximal IT location or gastro-, duodenoileostomy, lead to higher and especially much faster secretion of GLP-1 and polypeptide YY (3-36) and

thus increase the insulin secretion / action and accelerate the feeling of satiety. When a sleeve gactrectomy is performed in addition to these procedures, the Ghrelin effect is diminished and satiety further increased. In South America, these procedures are combined and used by patients. In a 2-year follow-up the results are similar to the established bariatric procedures with respect to both weight loss and improvement of comorbidities like type II diabetes [78]. In these studies, different independent procedures have been combined which are being examined further in recent animal studies by expert groups in the field. Sleeve gastrectomy with ileal transposition (SGIT) or single ileal transposition (IT) have been studied by *Gagner* and his team in a porcine model and compared to gastric bypass and a sham group. They found SGIT to be as effective as gastric bypass in terms of weight loss in a short follow-up. Single IT procedure seemed to be less effective than the combination of sleeve gastrectomy and ileal transposition [79]. Once again, based on the hypothesis that the gut hormones play a central role in weight control, SGIT is a procedure that combines low levels of orexigenic peptides such as ghrelin and creates an early exposure of undigested nutrients to the distal gut by transposing an ileal segment, which enhances early release of anorexigenic peptides such as PYY (3-36) and GLP-1. Furthermore, 10 years ago, *Mason* [80] already stated that it appeared from all that was known about GLP-1, that single ileal transposition would be an ideal operation for treatment of type II diabetes mellitus.

33.9 Change of paradigm: Setting new Barriers

This new comprehension of the metabolism of bariatric surgery leads to new therapeutic solutions for obesity and especially for obesity-related comorbidities like diabetes mellitus II, thus breaking accepted concepts and barriers regarding the BMI limit for surgical indication. Finally, regarding the known clinical impact of variable bariatric procedures on the successful surgical therapy of type II diabetes, an exciting question arises: would these surgical procedures be as effective in only overweight or slightly obese patients (BMI < 35 kg/m²), in whom a bariatric procedure has always been contraindicated, up to now? Cohen et al [81] have performed a duodeno-jujunal bypass in two only overweight patients (BMI 22-34kg/m²) with type II diabetes mellitus. One year after surgery, the patients still had normal HbA1C levels without significant weight loss. In 1997, Mingrone published the case of a young diabetic woman with normal body weight. She underwent biliopancreatic diversion because of a chylomicronemia. Her level of serum insulin and serum glucose normalised within three months, although she has gained weight in the same period [82]. Further bariatric procedures in patients with a BMI lower than 34kg/m² have been presented by other authors, too [81,83]. Even if some proposed that the etiology of type II diabetes mellitus in obese patients differs significantly from that in non-obese patients [84], this could not be confirmed by other studies [85,86]. It was reported that the extent of insulin resistance correlates with the degree of obesity up to a BMI of 30 kg/m2 and that there are no changes in higher BMI levels [87]. These observations suggest that bariatric procedures could achieve control of serum glucose at least in patients with slight obesity (BMI < 30kg/m²). Considering that more than 60% of the patients with type II diabetes mellitus have a BMI greater than 28 kg/m² [88], an enormous potential exists for metabolic surgery. Nevertheless, evidence and experience of metabolic surgery in patients with overweight only (BMI < 30kg/m²) are still not sufficient to recommend breaking old BMI barriers; but the time has come to set new limits. We will in the future operate the patients with metabolic indications without BMI restrictions using new technical equipment, like 3D Laparoscopy (◘ Fig. 33.1), what will lead to understand the pathophysiological pathways and accelerate the development of new medications.

References

1. Levy P, Bonsignore MR, Eckel J. Sleep, sleep-disordered breathing and metabolic consequences. Eur Respir J 2009; 34:243-60.
2. Redon J, Cifkova R, Laurent S, et al. The metabolic syndrome in hypertension: European society of hypertension position statement. J Hypertens 2008; 26:1891-900.
3. Valdivielso P, Sanchez-Chaparro MA, Calvo-Bonacho E, et al. Association of moderate and severe hypertriglyceridemia with obesity, diabetes mellitus and vascular disease in the Spanish working population: Results of the ICARIA study. Atherosclerosis 2009.
4. Temelkova-Kurktschiev T, Hanefeld M. The lipid triad in type 2 diabetes - prevalence and relevance of hypertriglyceridaemia/low high-density lipoprotein syndrome in type 2 diabetes. Exp Clin Endocrinol Diabetes 2004; 112:75-9.
5. Clark JM. The epidemiology of nonalcoholic fatty liver disease in adults. J Clin Gastroenterol 2006; 40 Suppl 1:S5-10.
6. Foster GD, Wyatt HR, Hill JO, et al. A randomized trial of a low-carbohydrate diet for obesity. N Engl J Med 2003; 348: 2082-90.
7. Dansinger ML, Gleason JA, Griffith JL, Selker HP, Schaefer EJ. Comparison of the Atkins, Ornish, Weight Watchers, and Zone diets for weight loss and heart disease risk reduction: a randomized trial. Jama 2005; 293:43-53.

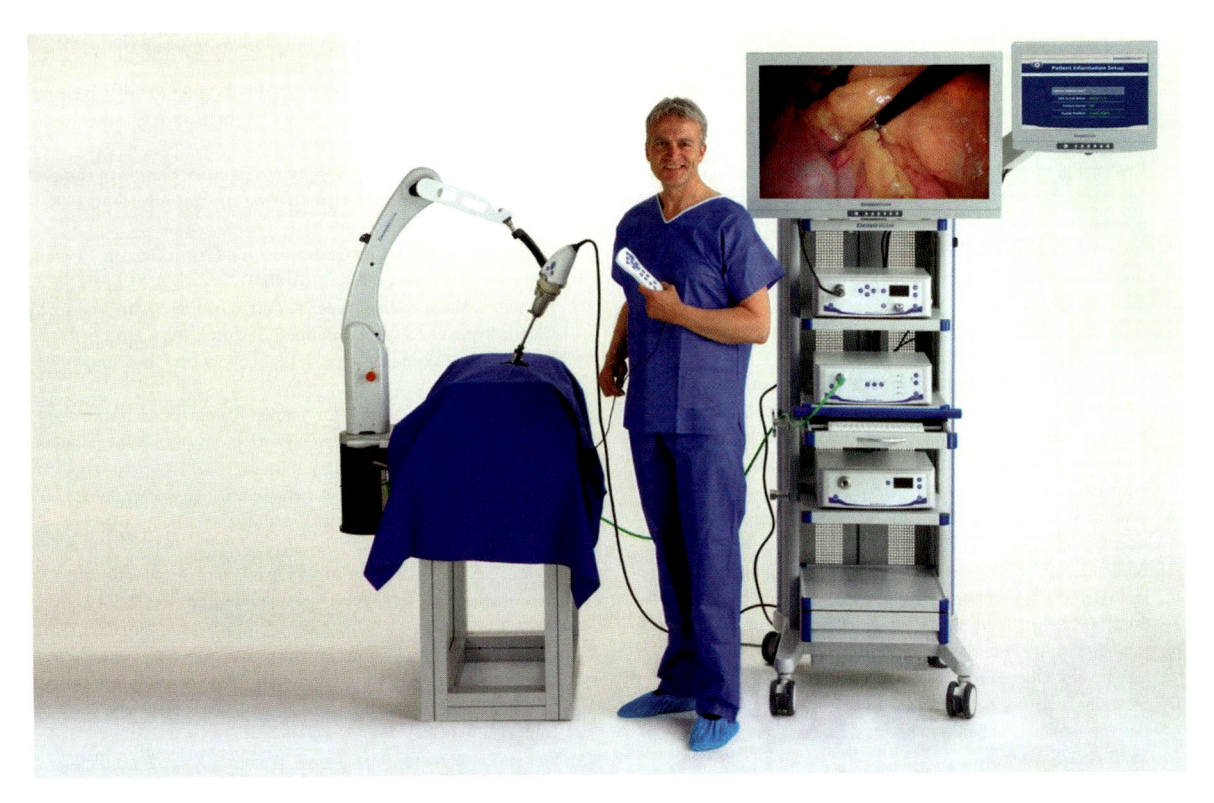

◘ **Fig. 33.1.** View of High-Tec 3D Einstein-Vision Equipment

8. Stern L, Iqbal N, Seshadri P, et al. The effects of low-carbohydrate versus conventional weight loss diets in severely obese adults: one-year follow-up of a randomized trial. Ann Intern Med 2004; 140:778-85.

9. Church TS, Earnest CP, Skinner JS, Blair SN. Effects of different doses of physical activity on cardiorespiratory fitness among sedentary, overweight or obese postmenopausal women with elevated blood pressure: a randomized controlled trial. Jama 2007; 297:2081-91.

10. Christensen R, Kristensen PK, Bartels EM, Bliddal H, Astrup AV. [A meta-analysis of the efficacy and safety of the anti-obesity agent Rimonabant]. Ugeskr Laeger 2007; 169:4360-3.

11. Erondu N, Addy C, Lu K, et al. NPY5R antagonism does not augment the weight loss efficacy of orlistat or sibutramine. Obesity (Silver Spring) 2007; 15:2027-42.

12. Gantz I, Erondu N, Mallick M, et al. Efficacy and safety of intranasal peptide YY3-36 for weight reduction in obese adults. J Clin Endocrinol Metab 2007; 92:1754-7.

13. Sloth B, Holst JJ, Flint A, Gregersen NT, Astrup A. Effects of PYY1-36 and PYY3-36 on appetite, energy intake, energy expenditure, glucose and fat metabolism in obese and lean subjects. Am J Physiol Endocrinol Metab 2007; 292:E1062-8.

14. Sloth B, Davidsen L, Holst JJ, Flint A, Astrup A. Effect of subcutaneous injections of PYY1-36 and PYY3-36 on appetite, ad libitum energy intake, and plasma free fatty acid concentration in obese males. Am J Physiol Endocrinol Metab 2007; 293:E604-9.

15. Moy J, Pomp A, Dakin G, Parikh M, Gagner M. Laparoscopic sleeve gastrectomy for morbid obesity. Am J Surg 2008; 196:e56-9.

16. Suter M, Jayet C, Jayet A. Vertical banded gastroplasty: long-term results comparing three different techniques. Obes Surg 2000; 10:41-6; discussion 47.

17. Baltasar A, Serra C, Perez N, Bou R, Bengochea M, Ferri L. Laparoscopic sleeve gastrectomy: a multi-purpose bariatric operation. Obes Surg 2005; 15:1124-8.

18. del Amo DA, Diez MM, Guedea ME, Diago VA. Vertical banded gastroplasty: is it a durable operation for morbid obesity? Obes Surg 2004; 14:536-8.

19. Favretti F, Cadiere GB, Segato G, et al. Laparoscopic Adjustable Silicone Gastric Banding: Technique and Results. Obes Surg 1995; 5:364-371.

20. Favretti F, Cadiere GB, Segato G, et al. Laparoscopic Placement of Adjustable Silicone Gastric Banding: Early Experience. Obes Surg 1995; 5:71-73.

21. Hess DS, Hess DW. Biliopancreatic diversion with a duodenal switch. Obes Surg 1998; 8:267-82.

22. Marceau P, Hould FS, Simard S, et al. Biliopancreatic diversion with duodenal switch. World J Surg 1998; 22:947-54.

23. Marceau P, Biron S, Bourque RA, Potvin M, Hould FS, Simard S. Biliopancreatic Diversion with a New Type of Gastrectomy. Obes Surg 1993; 3:29-35.

24. Scopinaro N, Adami GF, Marinari GM, et al. Biliopancreatic diversion. World J Surg 1998; 22:936-46.

25. Brolin RE, Kenler HA, Gorman JH, Cody RP. Long-limb gastric bypass in the superobese. A prospective randomized study. Ann Surg 1992; 215:387-95.

26. Rutledge R. The mini-gastric bypass: experience with the first 1,274 cases. Obes Surg 2001; 11:276-80.

27. Sjostrom L, Narbro K, Sjostrom CD, et al. Effects of bariatric surgery on mortality in Swedish obese subjects. N Engl J Med 2007; 357:741-52.

28. Adams TD, Gress RE, Smith SC, et al. Long-term mortality after gastric bypass surgery. N Engl J Med 2007; 357:753-61.

29. Sundbom M, Karlson BM. Low Mortality in Bariatric Surgery 1995 Through 2005 in Sweden, in Spite of a Shift to More Complex Procedures. Obes Surg 2008.

30. Pories WJ, Swanson MS, MacDonald KG, et al. Who would have thought it? An operation proves to be the most effective therapy for adult-onset diabetes mellitus. Ann Surg 1995; 222:339-50; discussion 350-2.

31. Hickey MS, Pories WJ, MacDonald KG, Jr., et al. A new paradigm for type 2 diabetes mellitus: could it be a disease of the foregut? Ann Surg 1998; 227:637-43; discussion 643-4.

32. Rubino F, Gagner M. Potential of surgery for curing type 2 diabetes mellitus. Ann Surg 2002; 236:554-9.

33. Rubino F, Forgione A, Cummings DE, et al. The mechanism of diabetes control after gastrointestinal bypass surgery reveals a role of the proximal small intestine in the pathophysiology of type 2 diabetes. Ann Surg 2006; 244:741-9.

34. Lamounier RN, Pareja JC, Tambascia MA, Geloneze B. Incretins: clinical physiology and bariatric surgery--correlating the entero-endocrine system and a potentially anti-dysmetabolic procedure. Obes Surg 2007; 17:569-76.

35. Katergari SA, Milousis A, Pagonopoulou O, Asimakopoulos B, Nikolettos NK. Ghrelin in pathological conditions. Endocr J 2008; 55:439-53.

36. Mognol P, Chosidow D, Marmuse JP. Laparoscopic sleeve gastrectomy as an initial bariatric operation for high-risk patients: initial results in 10 patients. Obes Surg 2005; 15:1030-3.

37. Weiner RA, Weiner S, Pomhoff I, Jacobi C, Makarewicz W, Weigand G. Laparoscopic sleeve gastrectomy--influence of sleeve size and resected gastric volume. Obes Surg 2007; 17:1297-305.

38. Fobi MA. Placement of the GaBP ring system in the banded gastric bypass operation. Obes Surg 2005; 15:1196-201.

39. Mason EE, Ito C. Gastric bypass in obesity. Surg Clin North Am 1967; 47:1345-51.

40. Mason EE, Doherty C, Cullen JJ, Scott D, Rodriguez EM, Maher JW. Vertical gastroplasty: evolution of vertical banded gastroplasty. World J Surg 1998; 22:919-24.

41. Capella JF, Capella RF. The weight reduction operation of choice: vertical banded gastroplasty or gastric bypass? Am J Surg 1996; 171:74-9.

42. Fobi MA. Vertical Banded Gastroplasty vs Gastric Bypass: 10 years follow-up. Obes Surg 1993; 3:161-164.

43. Howard L, Malone M, Michalek A, Carter J, Alger S, Van Woert J. Gastric Bypass and Vertical Banded Gastroplasty- a Prospective Randomized Comparison and 5-Year Follow-up. Obes Surg 1995; 5:55-60.

44. Langer FB, Bohdjalian A, Felberbauer FX, et al. Does gastric dilatation limit the success of sleeve gastrectomy as a sole operation for morbid obesity? Obes Surg 2006; 16:166-71.

45. Fobi M, Lee H, Igwe D, et al. Band erosion: incidence, etiology, management and outcome after banded vertical gastric bypass. Obes Surg 2001; 11:699-707.

46. Meir E, Van Baden M. Adjustable silicone gastric banding and band erosion: personal experience and hypotheses. Obes Surg 1999; 9:191-3.

47. Ueda K, Gagner M, Milone L, Bardaro SJ, Gong K. Sleeve gastrectomy with wrapping using polytetrafluoroethylene to prevent gastric enlargement in a porcine model. Surg Obes Relat Dis 2008; 4:84-90.

48. Weiner RA, Korenkov M, Matzig E, Weiner S, Karcz WK, Junginger T. Early results with a new telemetrically adjustable gastric banding. Obes Surg 2007; 17:717-21.

33

49. Dumonceau JM. Evidence-based review of the Bioenterics intragastric balloon for weight loss. Obes Surg 2008; 18:1611-7.

50. Fobi M. Banded gastric bypass: combining two principles. Surg Obes Relat Dis 2005; 1:304-9.

51. Schrag HJ, Ruthmann O, Doll A, Goldschmidtboing F, Woias P, Hopt UT. Development of a novel, remote-controlled artificial bowel sphincter through microsystems technology. Artif Organs 2006; 30:855-62.

52. Xu J, McNearney TA, Chen JD. Gastric/intestinal electrical stimulation modulates appetite regulatory peptide hormones in the stomach and duodenum in rats. Obes Surg 2007; 17:406-13.

53. Wang GJ, Yang J, Volkow ND, et al. Gastric stimulation in obese subjects activates the hippocampus and other regions involved in brain reward circuitry. Proc Natl Acad Sci U S A 2006; 103:15641-5.

54. Xu L, Sun X, Tang M, Chen JD. Involvement of the hippocampus and neuronal nitric oxide synapse in the gastric electrical stimulation therapy for obesity. Obes Surg 2009; 19:475-83.

55. Xu L, Sun X, Tang M, Chen JD. Involvement of the Hippocampus and Neuronal Nitric Oxide Synapse in the Gastric Electrical Stimulation Therapy for Obesity. Obes Surg 2008.

56. Bohdjalian A, Prager G, Aviv R, et al. One-year experience with Tantalus: a new surgical approach to treat morbid obesity. Obes Surg 2006; 16:627-34.

57. Champion JK, Williams M, Champion S, Gianos J, Carrasquilla C. Implantable gastric stimulation to achieve weight loss in patients with a low body mass index: early clinical trial results. Surg Endosc 2006; 20:444-7.

58. Cigaina V. Gastric pacing as therapy for morbid obesity: preliminary results. Obes Surg 2002; 12 Suppl 1:12S-16S.

59. Cigaina V, Hirschberg AL. Gastric pacing for morbid obesity: plasma levels of gastrointestinal peptides and leptin. Obes Res 2003; 11:1456-62.

60. Cigaina V. Long-term follow-up of gastric stimulation for obesity: the Mestre 8-year experience. Obes Surg 2004; 14 Suppl 1:S14-22.

61. D'Argent J. Gastric electrical stimulation as therapy of morbid obesity: preliminary results from the French study. Obes Surg 2002; 12 Suppl 1:21S-25S.

62. De Luca M, Segato G, Busetto L, et al. Progress in implantable gastric stimulation: summary of results of the European multicenter study. Obes Surg 2004; 14 Suppl 1:S33-9.

63. Favretti F, De Luca M, Segato G, et al. Treatment of morbid obesity with the Transcend Implantable Gastric Stimulator (IGS): a prospective survey. Obes Surg 2004; 14:666-70.

64. Hoeller E, Aigner F, Margreiter R, Weiss H. Intragastric stimulation is ineffective after failed adjustable gastric banding. Obes Surg 2006; 16:1160-5.

65. Shikora SA. „What are the yanks doing?" the U.S. experience with implantable gastric stimulation (IGS) for the treatment of obesity - update on the ongoing clinical trials. Obes Surg 2004; 14 Suppl 1:S40-8.

66. Shikora SA. Implantable Gastric Stimulation - the surgical procedure: combining safety with simplicity. Obes Surg 2004; 14 Suppl 1:S9-13.

67. Shikora SA, Bergenstal R, Bessler M, et al. Implantable gastric stimulation for the treatment of clinically severe obesity: results of the SHAPE trial. Surg Obes Relat Dis 2009; 5:31-7.

68. Bugajski AJ, Gil K, Ziomber A, Zurowski D, Zaraska W, Thor PJ. Effect of long-term vagal stimulation on food intake and body weight during diet induced obesity in rats. J Physiol Pharmacol 2007; 58 Suppl 1:5-12.

69. Sobocki J, Fourtanier G, Estany J, Otal P. Does vagal nerve stimulation affect body composition and metabolism? Experimental study of a new potential technique in bariatric surgery. Surgery 2006; 139:209-16.

70. Pardo JV, Sheikh SA, Kuskowski MA, et al. Weight loss during chronic, cervical vagus nerve stimulation in depressed patients with obesity: an observation. Int J Obes (Lond) 2007; 31:1756-9.

71. Sani S, Jobe K, Smith A, Kordower JH, Bakay RA. Deep brain stimulation for treatment of obesity in rats. J Neurosurg 2007; 107:809-13.

72. Halpern CH, Wolf JA, Bale TL, et al. Deep brain stimulation in the treatment of obesity. J Neurosurg 2008; 109:625-34.

73. Tarnoff M, Shikora S, Lembo A, Gersin K. Chronic in-vivo experience with an endoscopically delivered and retrieved duodenal-jejunal bypass sleeve in a porcine model. Surg Endosc 2008; 22:1023-8.

74. Tarnoff M, Shikora S, Lembo A. Acute technical feasibility of an endoscopic duodenal-jejunal bypass sleeve in a porcine model: a potentially novel treatment for obesity and type 2 diabetes. Surg Endosc 2008; 22:772-6.

75. Gersin KS, Keller JE, Stefanidis D, et al. Duodenal- jejunal bypass sleeve: a totally endoscopic device for the treatment of morbid obesity. Surg Innov 2007; 14:275-8.

76. Rodriguez-Grunert L, Galvao Neto MP, Alamo M, Ramos AC, Baez PB, Tarnoff M. First human experience with endoscopically delivered and retrieved duodenal-jejunal bypass sleeve. Surg Obes Relat Dis 2008; 4:55-9.

77. Tarnoff M, Rodriguez L, Escalona A, et al. Open label, prospective, randomized controlled trial of an endoscopic duodenal-jejunal bypass sleeve versus low calorie diet for pre-operative weight loss in bariatric surgery. Surg Endosc 2009; 23:650-6.

78. Santoro S, Malzoni CE, Velhote MC, et al. Digestive Adaptation with Intestinal Reserve: a neuroendocrine-based operation for morbid obesity. Obes Surg 2006; 16:1371-9.

79. Boza C, Gagner M, Devaud N, Escalona A, Munoz R, Gandarillas M. Laparoscopic sleeve gastrectomy with ileal transposition (SGIT): A new surgical procedure as effective as gastric bypass for weight control in a porcine model. Surg Endosc 2008; 22:1029-34.

80. Mason EE. Ileal [correction of ilial] transposition and enteroglucagon/GLP-1 in obesity (and diabetic?) surgery. Obes Surg 1999; 9:223-8.

81. Cohen RV, Schiavon CA, Pinheiro JS, Correa JL, Rubino F. Duodenal-jejunal bypass for the treatment of type 2 diabetes in patients with body mass index of 22-34 kg/m2: a report of 2 cases. Surg Obes Relat Dis 2007; 3:195-7.

82. Mingrone G, DeGaetano A, Greco AV, et al. Reversibility of insulin resistance in obese diabetic patients: role of plasma lipids. Diabetologia 1997; 40:599-605.

83. Noya G, Cossu ML, Coppola M, et al. Biliopancreatic diversion preserving the stomach and pylorus in the treatment of hypercholesterolemia and diabetes type II: results in the first 10 cases. Obes Surg 1998; 8:67-72.

84. Arner P, Pollare T, Lithell H. Different aetiologies of type 2 (non-insulin-dependent) diabetes mellitus in obese and non-obese subjects. Diabetologia 1991; 34:483-7.

85. Bolinder J, Lithell H, Skarfors E, Arner P. Effects of obesity, hyperinsulinemia, and glucose intolerance on insulin action in adipose tissue of sixty-year-old men. Diabetes 1986; 35:282-90.

86. Kolterman OG, Gray RS, Griffin J, et al. Receptor and postreceptor defects contribute to the insulin resistance in noninsulin-dependent diabetes mellitus. J Clin Invest 1981; 68:957-69.

87. Elton CW, Tapscott EB, Pories WJ, Dohm GL. Effect of moderate obesity on glucose transport in human muscle. Horm Metab Res 1994; 26:181-3.
88. Melton LJ, 3rd, Palumbo PJ, Dwyer MS, Chu CP. Impact of recent changes in diagnostic criteria on the apparent natural history of diabetes mellitus. Am J Epidemiol 1983; 117:559-65.

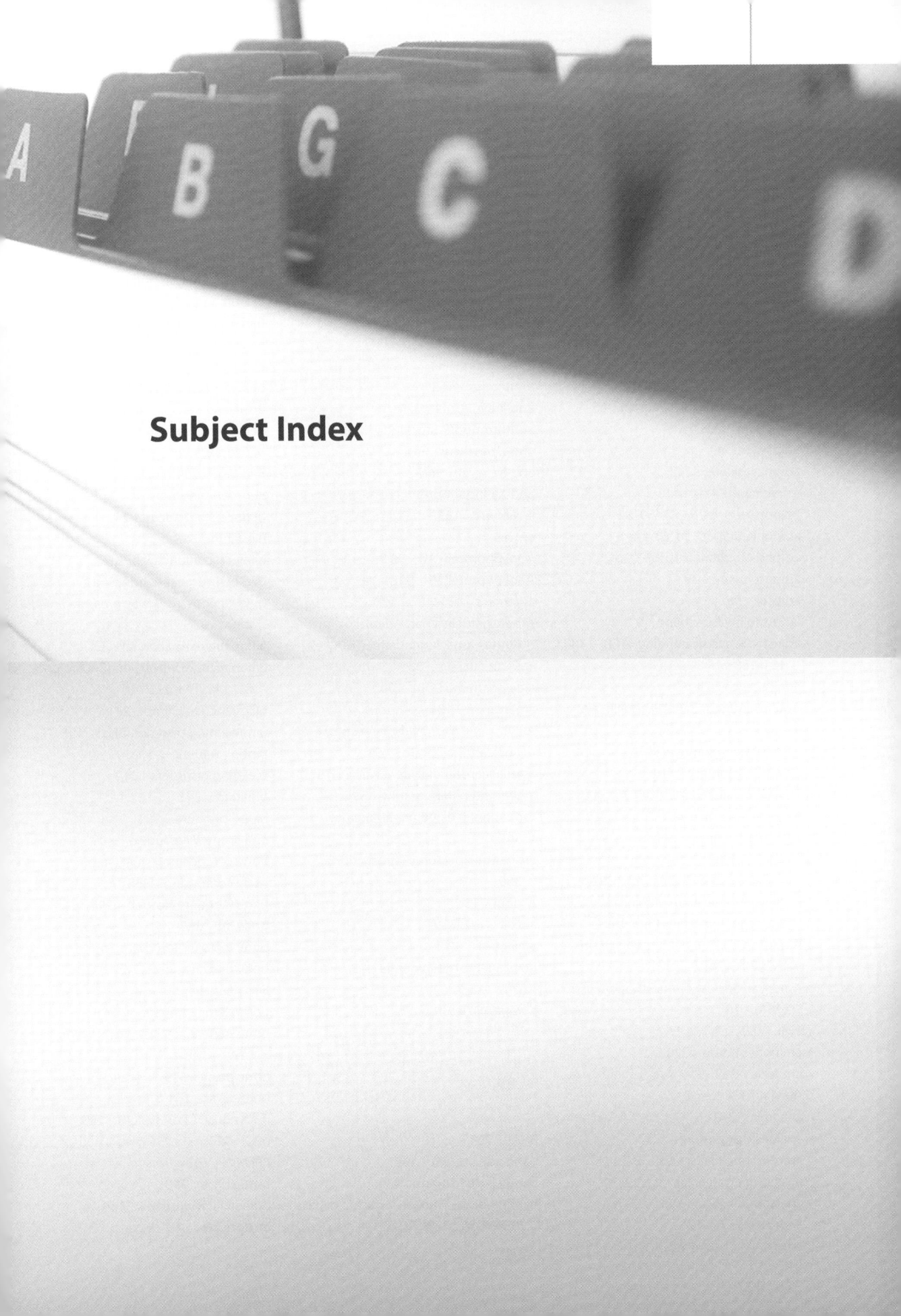

Subject Index

Printing and Binding: Stürtz GmbH, Würzburg